Obstetric
Evidence Based Guidelines

SERIES IN MATERNAL-FETAL MEDICINE

Published in association with the *Journal of Maternal-Fetal and Neonatal Medicine*

Editors in Chief:

Gian Carlo Di Renzo and Dev Maulik

Recent and Forthcoming Titles

Vincenzo Berghella, *Maternal-Fetal Evidence Based Guidelines,* second edition
ISBN 9781841848228

Howard Carp, *Recurrent Pregnancy Loss: Causes, Controversies and Treatment*
ISBN 9780415421300

Fabio Facchinetti, Gustaaf A. Dekker, Dante Baronciani, George Saade, *Stillbirth: Understanding and Management*
ISBN 9780415473903

Moshe Hod, Lois Jovanovic, Gian Carlo Di Renzo, Alberto de Leiva, Oded Langer, *Textbook of Diabetes and Pregnancy,* second edition
ISBN 9780415425606

Michael S. Marsh, Lina A.M. Nashef, Peter A. Brex, *Neurology and Pregnancy: Clinical Management*
ISBN 9781841846521

Simcha Yagel, Norman H. Silverman, Ulrich Gembruch, *Fetal Cardiology: Embryology, Genetics, Physiology, Echocardiographic Evaluation, Diagnosis and Perinatal Management of Cardiac Diseases,* second edition
ISBN 9780415432658

Obstetric
Evidence Based Guidelines

Second Edition

Edited by

Vincenzo Berghella, MD, FACOG

Director, Division of Maternal-Fetal Medicine
Professor, Department of Obstetrics and Gynecology
Jefferson Medical College of Thomas Jefferson University
Philadelphia, Pennsylvania
USA

informa
healthcare

New York London

First published in 2012 by Informa Healthcare, 119 Farringdon Road, London EC1R 3DA, UK
Simultaneously published in the USA by Informa Healthcare, 52 Vanderbilt Avenue, 7th Floor, New York, NY 10017, USA

Informa Healthcare is a trading division of Informa UK Ltd. Registered Office: 37–41 Mortimer Street, London W1T 3JH, UK. Registered in England and Wales number 1072954

A CIP record for this book is available from the British Library

Library of Congress Cataloging-in-Publication Data available on application

ISBN-10: 1841848247
ISBN-13: 9781841848242
eISBN: 9781841848259
Maternal-Fetal and Obstetric Evidence Based Guidelines – Two-Volume Set, Second Edition, ISBN-10: 1841848263; ISBN-13: 978-1841848266

Orders may be sent to: Informa Healthcare, Sheepen Place, Colchester, Essex CO3 3LP, UK
Telephone: +44 (0)20 7017 5540
Email: CSDhealthcarebooks@informa.com
Website: http://informahealthcarebooks.com

For corporate sales please contact: CorporateBooksIHC@informa.com
For foreign rights please contact: RightsIHC@informa.com
For reprint permissions please contact: PermissionsIHC@informa.com

Typeset by MPS Ltd, Delhi

Printed and bound by CPI Group (UK) Ltd, Croydon, CR0 4YY

To Paola, Andrea, Pietro, mamma, and papà,
for giving me the serenity, love, and strength at home now, then, and in the future
to fulfill my dreams and spend my talents as best as possible.

To all those who loved the first edition

To the health of mothers and babies

And, as I often toast: To the next generation!

Introduction

To me, pregnancy has always been the most fascinating and exciting area of interest, as care involves not one but at least two persons—the mother and the fetus—and leads to the miracle of a new life. I was a third-year medical student, when, during a lecture, a resident said: "I went into obstetrics because this is the easiest medical field. Pregnancy is a physiologic process, and there isn't much to know. It's simple." I knew from my "classic" background that "obstetrics" means to "stand by, stay near," and that indeed pregnancy used to receive no medical support at all.

After over 20 years practicing obstetrics, I know now that while physiologic and at times simple, obstetrics and maternal-fetal medicine can be the **most complex of the medical fields**: pregnancy is based on a different physiology than for nonpregnant women, can include any medical disease, requires surgery, etc. It is not so simple. In fact, ignorance can kill, in this case with the health of the woman and her baby both at risk. Too often I have gone to a lecture, journal club, rounds, or other didactic event to hear presented only one or a few articles regarding the subject, without the presenter reviewing the pertinent best literature and data. It is increasingly difficult to read and acquire as knowledge all that is published, certainly in obstetrics, with about 3000 scientific manuscripts published monthly on this subject. Some residents or even authorities would state at times that "there is no evidence" on a topic. We indeed used to be the field with the worst use of randomized trials (1). As the best way to find something is to look for it, my coauthors and I searched for the best evidence. On careful investigation, indeed there are data on almost everything we do in obstetrics, especially on our interventions. Indeed, **our field is now the pioneer for numbers of meta-analysis and extension of work for evidence-based reviews** (2). Obstetricians are now blessed with lots of data, and should make the best use of it.

The **aims** of this book are to **summarize the best evidence available in the obstetrics and maternal-fetal medicine literature**, and make the results of randomized trials and meta-analyses **easily accessible to guide clinical care**. The intent is to bridge the gap between knowledge (the evidence) and its easy application. To reach these goals, we reviewed all trials on effectiveness of interventions in obstetrics. **Millions of pregnant women have participated in thousands of properly conducted randomized controlled trials.** The efforts and sacrifice of mothers and their fetuses for science should be recognized at least by the physicians' awareness and understanding of these studies. Some of the trials have been summarized in over 400 Cochrane reviews, with hundreds of other meta-analyses also published in obstetrical topics (Table 1). All of the Cochrane reviews, other meta-analyses and trials in obstetrics and maternal-fetal medicine were reviewed and referenced. The material presented in single trials or meta-analyses is too detailed to be readily translated to advice for the busy clinician who needs to make dozens of clinical decisions a day. Even the Cochrane Library, the undiscussed leader for evidence-based medicine efforts, has been criticized for its lack of flexibility and relevance in failing to be more easily understandable and clinically readily usable (3). It is the gap between research and clinicians that needed to be filled, making sure that proven **interventions** are clearly highlighted and are included in today's care. Like all pilots fly planes under similar rules to maximize safety, all obstetricians should manage all aspects of pregnancy with similar, evidence-based rules. Indeed **only interventions that have been proven to provide benefit should be used routinely**. However, **primum non nocere**: interventions that have clearly been shown to be not helpful or indeed harmful to mother and/or baby should be avoided. Another aim of the book is to make sure the pregnant woman and her unborn child are not penalized by the medical community. In most circumstances, medical disorders of pregnant women can be treated as in nonpregnant adults. Moreover, there are several effective interventions for preventing or treating specific pregnancy disorders.

Table 1   Obstetrical Evidence

Over 400 current Cochrane reviews
Hundreds of other current meta-analyses
More than 1000 RCTs
Millions of pregnant women randomized

Abbreviation: RCTs, randomized controlled trials.

Evidence-based medicine is the concept of treating patients according to the best available evidence. While George Bernard Shaw said: "I have my own opinion, do not confuse me with the facts," this can be a deadly approach, especially in medicine, and compromise two or more lives at the same time in obstetrics and maternal-fetal medicine. What should be the basis for our interventions in medicine? Meta-analyses provide a comprehensive summary of the best research data available. As such, they provide the best guidance for "effective" clinical care (4). It is unscientific and unethical to practice medicine or to teach or conduct research without first knowing all that has already been proven (4). In the absence of trials or meta-analyses, lower level evidence is reviewed. This book aims at providing a current systematic review of the evidence, **so that current practice and education, as well as future research, can be based on the full story from the best-conducted research, not just the latest data or someone's opinion** (Table 2). These evidence-based guidelines cannot be used as a "cookbook," or a document dictating the best care. The knowledge from the best evidence presented in the guidelines needs to be integrated with other knowledge gained from clinical judgment, individual patient circumstances, and patient preferences, to lead to best medical practice. These are guidelines, not rules. Even the best scientific studies are not always perfectly related to any given individual, and clinical judgment must still be applied to allow the best "particularization" of the best knowledge for the individual, unique patient. Evidence-based medicine informs clinical judgment but does not substitute it. It is important to understand though that greater clinical experience by the physician actually correlates with inferior quality of care, if not integrated with knowledge of the best evidence (5). The appropriate treatment is given in only 50% of visits to general physicians (5). At times, limitations in resources may also limit the applicability of the guidelines, but should not limit the physicians' knowledge. Guidelines and clinical pathways based on evidence not only point to the right management but can also decrease medicolegal risk (6).

We aimed for brevity and clarity. Suggested management of the healthy or sick mother and child is stated as straightforwardly as possible, **for everyone to easily understand and implement** (Table 3). If you find the Cochrane reviews, scientific

Table 2   Aims of This Book

- Improve the health of women and their children
- "Make it easy to do it right"
- Implement the best clinical care based on science (evidence), not opinion
- Research ideas
- Education
- Develop lectures
- Decrease disease, use of detrimental interventions, and therefore costs
- Reduce medicolegal risks

Table 3   This Book Is For

- Obstetricians
- Midwives
- Family medicine and others (practicing obstetrics)
- Residents
- Nurses
- Medical students
- MFM attendings
- MFM fellows
- Other consultants on pregnancy
- Lay public who wants to know "the evidence"
- Politicians responsible for health care

Abbreviation: MFM, maternal-fetal medicine.

manuscripts, and books difficult to "translate" into care of your patients, this book is for you. We wanted to prevent information overload. However, "everything should be made as simple as possible, but not simpler" (A. Einstein). Key management points are highlighted at the beginning of each guideline, and in bold in the text. The chapters are divided into two volumes, one on obstetrics and one on maternal-fetal medicine; cross-references to chapters in *Maternal-Fetal Evidence Based Guidelines* have been noted in the text where applicable. Please contact us (vincenzo.berghella@jefferson.edu) for any comments, criticisms, corrections, missing evidence, etc.

I have the most fun discovering the best ways to alleviate discomfort and disease. The search for the best evidence for these guidelines has been a wonderful, stimulating journey. Keeping up with evidence-based medicine is exciting. The most rewarding part, as a teacher, is the dissemination of knowledge. I hope, truly, that this effort will be helpful to you, too.

REFERENCES

1. Cochrane AL. 1931–1971: a critical review, with particular reference to the medical profession. In: Medicines for the Year 2000. London: Office of Health Economics, 1979:1–11. [Review]
2. Dickersin K, Manheimer E. The Cochrane Collaboration: evaluation of health care and services using systematic reviews of the results of randomized controlled trials. Clinic Obstet Gynecol 1998; 41:315–331. [Review]
3. Summerskill W. Cochrane Collaboration and the evolution of evidence. Lancet 2005; 366:1760. [Review]
4. Chalmers I. Academia's failure to support systematic reviews. Lancet 2005; 365:469. [III]
5. Arky RA. The family business—to educate. N Engl J Med 2006; 354:1922–1926. [Review]
6. Ransom SB, Studdert DM, Dombrowski MP, et al. Reduced medico-legal risk by compliance with obstetric clinical pathways: a case-control study. Obstet Gynecol 2003; 101:751–755. [II-2]

How to "Read" This Book

The knowledge from randomized controlled trials (RCTs) and meta-analyses is summarized and easily available for clinical implementation. Key management points are highlighted at the beginning of each guideline, and in bold in the text. Relative risks and 95% confidence intervals from studies are generally not quoted, unless trends were evident. Instead, the straight recommendation for care is made if one intervention is superior to the other, with the percent improvement often quoted to assess degree of benefit. If there is insufficient evidence to compare to interventions or managements, this is clearly stated.

References: Cochrane reviews with 0 RCT are not referenced, and, instead of referencing a meta-analysis with only one RCT, the actual RCT is usually referenced. RCTs that are already included in meta-analyses are not referenced, for brevity and because they can be easily accessed by reviewing the meta-analysis. If new RCTs are not included in meta-analysis, they are obviously referenced. Each reference was reviewed and evaluated for quality according to a modified method as outlined by the U.S. Preventive Services Task Force (http://www.ahrq.gov):

I	Evidence obtained from at least one properly designed randomized controlled trial.
II-1	Evidence obtained from well-designed controlled trials without randomization.
II-2	Evidence obtained from well-designed cohort or case-control analytic studies, preferably from more than one center or research group.
II-3	Evidence obtained from multiple time series with or without the intervention. Dramatic results in uncontrolled experiments could also be regarded as this type of evidence.
III (review)	Opinions of respected authorities, based on clinical experience, descriptive studies, or reports of expert committees.

These levels are quoted after each reference. For RCTs and meta-analyses, the number of subjects studied is stated, and, sometimes, more details are provided to aid the reader to understand the study better.

Contents

Contributors

Alfred Abuhamad Division of Maternal-Fetal Medicine, Eastern Virginia Medical School, Norfolk, Virginia, U.S.A.

Alexi E. Achenbach Department of Obstetrics and Gynecology, Good Samaritan Hospital, Lebanon, Pennsylvania, U.S.A.

Brittany L. Anderson Department of Psychology, Old Dominion University, Norfolk, Virginia, U.S.A.

Marianna Andreani Department of Obstetrics and Gynecology, University of Milano-Bicocca, Monza, Italy

Valerie A. Arkoosh Departments of Anesthesia and Critical Care and of Obstetrics and Gynecology, University of Pennsylvania School of Medicine, Philadelphia, Pennsylvania, U.S.A.

Michele Berghella Department of Obstetrics and Gynecology, Ospedale Civile Santo Spirito, Pescara, Italy

Vincenzo Berghella Division of Maternal-Fetal Medicine, Department of Obstetric and Gynecology, Jefferson Medical College of Thomas Jefferson University, Philadelphia, Pennsylvania, U.S.A.

Sean C. Blackwell Division of Maternal-Fetal Medicine, Department of Obstetrics and Gynecology, University of Texas Health Science Center, Houston, Texas, U.S.A.

Geoffrey Bowers Department of Obstetrics and Gynecology, Jefferson Medical College of Thomas Jefferson University, Philadelphia, Pennsylvania, U.S.A.

Elizabeth Brass Division of Maternal-Fetal Medicine, Department of Obstetrics and Gynecology, Oregon Health and Science University, Portland, Oregon, U.S.A.

Suneet P. Chauhan Division of Maternal-Fetal Medicine, Eastern Virginia Medical School, Norfolk, Virginia, U.S.A.

Beatrice A. Chen Department of Obstetrics, Gynecology and Reproductive Sciences, University of Pittsburgh, Pennsylvania, U.S.A.

Sandra D. Dayaratna Department of Obstetrics and Gynecology, Jefferson Medical College of Thomas Jefferson University, Philadelphia, Pennsylvania, U.S.A.

Gary Emmett Department of General Pediatrics, Thomas Jefferson University and A I DuPont Hospital for Children, Philadelphia, Pennsylvania, U.S.A.

Aileen M. Gariepy Department of Obstetrics and Gynecology and Reproductive Sciences, Yale School of Medicine, New Haven, Connecticut, U.S.A.

Alessandro Ghidini The Brock Perinatal Diagnostic Center, Inova Alexandria Hospital, Alexandria, Virginia, and Division of Maternal-Fetal Medicine, Georgetown University, Washington, D.C., U.S.A.

Ariella B. Glazer Department of Obstetrics and Gynecology, Hospital of the University of Pennsylvania, Philadelphia, Pennsylvania, U.S.A.

Jay Goldberg Division of General Obstetrics and Gynecology, Jefferson Medical College of Thomas Jefferson University, Philadelphia, Pennsylvania, U.S.A.

William Grobman Division of Maternal-Fetal Medicine, Department of Obstetrics and Gynecology, Feinberg School of Medicine, Northwestern University, Chicago, Illinois, U.S.A.

Nancy W. Hendrix Division of Genetics, Department of Obstetrics and Gynecology, Magee Women's Hospital, University of Pittsburgh Medical Center, Pittsburgh, Pennsylvania, U.S.A.

Colleen Horan Department of Obstetrics and Gynecology, Jefferson Medical College of Thomas Jefferson University, Philadelphia, Pennsylvania, U.S.A.

Thomas M. Jenkins Prenatal Diagnosis, Legacy Center for Maternal-Fetal Medicine, Portland, Oregon, U.S.A.

Cheung K. Kim Department of Obstetrics and Gynecology, Jefferson Medical College of Thomas Jefferson University, Philadelphia, Pennsylvania, U.S.A.

Dawnette Lewis Division of Maternal-Fetal Medicine, Department of Obstetrics and Gynecology, North Shore University Hospital, New York University School of Medicine, Manhasset, New York, U.S.A.

Anna Locatelli Department of Obstetrics and Gynecology, University of Milano-Bicocca, Monza, Italy

Melissa I. March Department of Maternal-Fetal Medicine, Beth Israel Deaconess Medical Center, Boston, Massachusetts, U.S.A.

Amen Ness Division of Maternal-Fetal Medicine, Department of Obstetrics and Gynecology, Stanford University Medical Center, Stanford, California, U.S.A.

George Patounakis Department of Obstetrics and Gynecology, Jefferson Medical College of Thomas Jefferson University, Philadelphia, Pennsylvania, U.S.A.

Sarah Poggi The Brock Perinatal Diagnostic Center, Inova Alexandria Hospital, Alexandria, Virginia, and Division of Maternal-Fetal Medicine, Georgetown University, Washington, D.C., U.S.A.

Norman G. Rosenblum Division of Gynecologic Oncology, Department of Obstetrics and Gynecology, Jefferson Medical College of Thomas Jefferson University, Philadelphia, Pennsylvania, U.S.A.

Kelly E. Ruhstaller Division of Maternal-Fetal Medicine, Department of Obstetrics and Gynecology, Christiana Care Health System, Newark, Delaware, U.S.A.

Rolf Alexander Schlichter Department of Anesthesia and Critical Care, University of Pennsylvania School of Medicine, Philadelphia, Pennsylvania, U.S.A.

Adele Schneider Division of Genetics, Department of Pediatrics, Albert Einstein Medical Center, Philadelphia, Pennsylvania, U.S.A.

Anthony C. Sciscione Division of Maternal-Fetal Medicine, Department of Obstetrics and Gynecology, Christiana Care Health System, Newark, Delaware, U.S.A.

Sally Segel Department of Maternal-Fetal Medicine, The Vancouver Clinic, Portland, Oregon, U.S.A.

Melissa Skibo Department of General Pediatrics, Thomas Jefferson University Hospital, Philadelphia, Pennsylvania, U.S.A.

Allison M. Stuebe Division of Maternal-Fetal Medicine, Department of Obstetrics and Gynecology and Department of Maternal and Child Health, Gillings Global School of Public Health, University of North Carolina, Chapel Hill, North Carolina, U.S.A.

Carol Sudtelgte Division of Maternal-Fetal Medicine, Department of Obstetrics and Gynecology, Jefferson Medical College of Thomas Jefferson University, Philadelphia, Pennsylvania, U.S.A.

Jorge E. Tolosa Division of Maternal-Fetal Medicine, Department of Obstetrics and Gynecology, Oregon Health and Science University, Portland, Oregon, U.S.A.

Candice T. Tong Department of Obstetrics and Gynecology, Golden Valley Health Center, Modesto, California, U.S.A.

Patrizia Vergani Department of Obstetrics and Gynecology, University of Milano-Bicocca, Monza, Italy

John F. Visintine Division of Maternal-Fetal Medicine, Driscoll Children's Hospital, Corpus Christi, Texas, U.S.A.

List of Abbreviations

Ab	antibody
AC	abdominal circumference
ACA	anticardiolipin antibody
ACOG	American College of Obstetricians and Gynecologists
ACS	acute chest syndrome
ADR	autosomic dysreflexia
AF	amniotic fluid
AFI	amniotic fluid index
AFP	alpha-fetoprotein
AFV	amniotic fluid volume
Ag	antigen
AIDS	acquired immune deficiency syndrome
ALT	alanine aminotransferase
ANA	antinuclear antibodies
aPT	activated prothrombin time
APS	antiphospholipid syndrome
aPTT	activated partial thromboplastin time
AROM	artificial rupture of membranes
ART	assisted reproductive technologies
ARV	antiretroviral therapy
ASA	aspirin
ASD	atrial septal defect
AST	aspartate aminotransferase
AT III	antithrombin III
AZT	ziduvudine
bid	"bis in die," i.e., twice per day
BPD	biparietal diameter
BPD	bronchopulmonary dysplasia
BPP	biophysical profile
BMI	body mass index
BP	blood pressure
CAP	community-acquired pneumonia
CBC	complete blood count
CDC	Center for Disease Control
CF	cystic fibrosis
CHD	congenital heart defect
CL	cervical length
CMV	cytomegalovirus
CNS	central nervous system
CRL	crown-rump length
CSE	combined spinal epidural
CSF	cerebrospinal fluid
CT	computerized tomography
CVS	chorionic villus sampling
D&C	dilation and curettage
DES	diethylstilbestrol
DIC	disseminated intravascular coagulation
DM	diabetes mellitus
DNA	deoxyribonucleic acid
DRVVT	dilute Russell's viper venom time
DV	ductus venosus
DVP	deepest vertical pocket
DVT	deep vein thrombosis

ECV	external cephalic version
EDC	estimated date of confinement
EDD	estimated date of delivery (synonym of EDC)
EKG	electrocardiogram
EPF	early pregnancy failure
EVA	electric vacuum aspiration
FBS	fetal blood sampling
FDA	Federal Drug Administration
FFN	fetal fibronectin
FGR	fetal growth restriction
FHR	fetal heart rate
FISH	fluorescent in situ hybridization
FLM	fetal lung maturity
FOB	father of baby
FPR	false positive rate
FTS	first-trimester screening
FVL	factor V Leiden
g	grams
GA	gestational age
GBS	group B streptococcus
GDM	gestational diabetes
GI	gastrointestinal
HAART	highly active antiretroviral therapy
HAV	hepatitis A virus
HBV	hepatitis B virus
HBsAg	hepatitis B surface antigen
HCG	human chorionic gonadotroponin
Hct	hematocrit
HCV	hepatitis C virus
HG	hyperemesis gravidarum
Hgb	hemoglobin
HIE	hypoxic-ischemic encephalopathy
HIV	human immunodeficiency virus
HR	heart rate
HSV	herpes simplex virus
HTN	hypertension
ICU	intensive care unit
IUGR	intrauterine growth restriction (synonym of FGR)
IV	intravenous
IVH	intraventricular hemorrhage
L&D	labor and delivery floor
LA	lupus anticoagulant
Lab	laboratory
LFT	liver function tests
LMP	last menstrual period
LBW	low birth weight (infants)
LMW	low molecular weight
LMWH	low-molecular-weight heparin
LR	likelihood ratio
MAS	meconium aspiration syndrome
MCA	middle cerebral artery
MCV	mean corpuscular volume
MOM	multiple of the median
MRI	magnetic resonance imaging
MSD	mean sac diameter
MTHFR	methylenetetrahydrofolate reductase
MVA	manual vacuum aspiration
MVP	maximum vertical pocket
NA	not available
NAIT	neonatal alloimmune thrombocytopenia
NEC	necrotizing enterocolitis
NIH	National Institute of Health

NIH	nonimmune hydrops
NRFS	nonreassuring fetal status
NRFHR	nonreassuring fetal heart rate
NRFHT	nonreassuring fetal heart testing
NSAIDS	nonsteroidal anti-inflammatory drugs
NT	nuchal translucency
NTD	neural tube defects
NST	nonstress test
n/v	nausea and/or vomiting
OR	operating room
PC	protein C
PCR	polymerase chain reaction
PE	pulmonary embolus
PF	pregnancy failure
PFT	pulmonary function tests
PGM	prothrombin gene mutation
PID	pelvic inflammatory disease
PL	pregnancy loss
PNC	prenatal care
po	"per os," i.e., by mouth
PPH	postpartum hemorrhage
PRCD	Planned repeat cesarean delivery
PS	protein S
PT	prothrombin time
PTB	preterm birth
PTT	partial thromboplastin time
PPROM	premature preterm rupture of membranes
pRBC	packed red blood cells
PROM	preterm rupture of membranes
PSV	peak systolic velocity
PTL	preterm labor
PTU	propylthiouracil
PUBS	percutaneous umbilical blood sampling
qd	once a day
qid	four times per day
qhs	before bedtime
QS	quadruple screen
RBC	red blood cell
RCT	randomized controlled trial
RDS	respiratory distress syndrome
RNA	ribonucleic acid
ROM	rupture of membranes
RPR	rapid plasma reagin
RR	respiratory rate
Rx	treatment
SAB	spontaneous abortion
SC	subcutaneous
SCI	spinal cord injury
SDP	single deepest pocket
SIDS	sudden infant death syndrome
SLE	systemic lupus erythematosus
SPTB	spontaneous preterm birth
STD	sexually transmitted diseases (synonym of STI)
STI	sexually transmitted infections
STS	second-trimester screening
TB	tuberculosis
TG	*Toxoplasma gondii*
tid	three times per day
TOL	trial of labor
TRAP	twin reversal arterial perfusion
TSH	thyroid-stimulating hormone
TSI	thyroid-stimulating immune globulins

TTTS	twin-twin transfusion syndrome
TVU	transvaginal ultrasound
UA	umbilical artery
UFH	unfractionated heparin
U/S (or u/s)	ultrasound
VBAC	vaginal birth after cesarean
VDRL	venereal disease research laboratory
VSD	ventricular septal defect
VTE	venous thromboembolism
WHO	World Health Organization

Preconception care[a]

Vincenzo Berghella

KEY POINTS

- Preconception care is a **set of interventions that aim to identify and modify biomedical, behavioral, and social risks to a woman's health or pregnancy outcome through prevention and management. The foundation of preconception care is prevention.**
- **Preconception care should occur any time any health care provider sees a reproductive-age woman** (e.g., 15–44 years old).
- **Personal and family history, physical exam, laboratory screening, reproductive plan, nutrition, supplements, weight, exercise, vaccinations, and injury prevention** should be reviewed in all reproductive-age women.
- **Folic acid 400 μg/day**, as well as proper diet and exercise, should be encouraged.
- Regarding **vaccinations**, women should receive the **influenza** vaccine if planning pregnancy during flu season; the **rubella** and **varicella** vaccines if there is no evidence of immunity to these viruses; and **tetanus/diphtheria/pertussis** if lacking adult vaccination.
- **Specific interventions** to reduce morbidity and mortality for both the woman and her baby should be offered to those identified with chronic diseases or exposed to teratogens or illicit substances.

HISTORY

Preconception care has ancient origins. Plutarch (46–120 C.E.) wrote that the ancient Spartans "[...] ordered the maidens to exercise [...], to the end that the fruit they conceived might [...] take firmer root and find better growth" (1).

DEFINITION

Preconception care is a **set of interventions that aim to identify and modify biomedical, behavioral, and social risks to a woman's health or pregnancy outcome through prevention and management** (2,3). This care has also been called prepregnancy, interpregnancy care, or periconceptional medicine (4).

AIM AND EFFECTIVENESS

The foundation of preconception care is prevention. Prevention of disease is the most effective form of medicine, and health care should shift from the delivery of procedure-based acute care to the provision of counseling-based preventive care (5,6). For example, the two leading causes of death in the first year of life—birth defects and disorders caused by preterm

birth (PTB)—can both be significantly reduced by preconception care. General practitioner–initiated preconception counseling not only can decrease adverse pregnancy outcomes but also reduces anxiety in reproductive-age women (7).

TIMING AND TARGET POPULATION

The time that people should start caring for a pregnancy is not after, but before, conception. **Preconception care should occur any time any health care provider sees a reproductive-age woman**. A reproductive-age woman is usually defined as one between **15 and 44 years** of age, but occasionally even younger or older women contemplate, or at least are at risk of, pregnancy. The first prenatal visit is "months too late!" (8). It often happens after first-trimester exposure to a potential teratogen has already occurred. There are about 1 billion reproductive-age women worldwide. In the United States, as an example, only about half of pregnancies are planned. As women get pregnant later in life, disease prevalence and medication exposures increase. Approximately 80% of reproductive-age U.S. women have dental disease, 66% are obese or overweight, 55% drink alcohol, 11% smoke, 9% have diabetes, 6% asthma, 3% hypertension, and 3% cardiac disease (2). The incidences of many of these conditions, even among pregnant women, are on the rise.

While some beneficial interventions could be started as soon as a pregnancy is diagnosed, this is unrealistic. Many of the preventive measures take time, often months, such as quitting smoking, losing weight, folic acid supplementation, and stabilization of medical conditions with effective and safe medications.

OPPORTUNITIES FOR PRECONCEPTION CARE

By age 25, about 50% of U.S. women have had at least one birth. The highest fertility rate occurs in 25- to 30-year-old women. By age 44, >85% have given birth at least once. About 84% of reproductive-age women, when asked, answer that they had a health care visit within the prior year (6). Therefore, **universal preconception care can be achieved if health care providers make it a priority and plan for it at every opportunity** (Table 1.1). The approach should be "**every reproductive-age woman, every time**" (6). **Every reproductive-age woman should be asked at every health care encounter: "Are you considering pregnancy?" and "Could you possibly become pregnant?"** Increased awareness of preconception care can be accomplished through improving health resources, public outreach, and advertising. Despite its great effectiveness, not all health care plans cover preconception care. **A preconception visit (or often more than one) should be standard primary care**, as stated by the Center for Disease Control in 2006 (2). It should be as routine, if not more so, as prenatal care, as should the screening and interventions associated with

---

[a]This chapter has been modified from Berghella V, Buchanan E, Pereira L, et al. Preconception care. Obstet Gynecol Surv 2010; 65(2):119–131. [Review].

it. A clear political will to drive the funding and insurance coverage for preconception care is required.

Therefore, providers of all specialties should be aware of the evidence-based recommendations (Tables 1.1–1.8).

Table 1.1 Visits That Are Opportunities for Preconception Care

- Adolescent (first gynecological exam)
- Any to a doctor during reproductive years (15–44 years old)
- College—Graduate school health
- Family planning, contraception prescribing, and counseling
- Annual ob-gyn
- Postpartum
- Pregnancy test (especially if negative)
- Health maintenance
- Medical work
- Emergency visit
- Fertility
- (Pre-)marriage

Table 1.2 Topics to be Reviewed in Preconception Care

Screening for risk assessment
- Personal and family history, physical exam, and laboratory screening

Preventive health
- Reproductive plan
- Nutrition, supplements, weight, and exercise
- Vaccinations
- Injury prevention

Specific individual issues/"exposures"
- Chronic diseases
- Medications (teratogens)
- Substance abuse/environmental hazards and toxins

Source: Modified from Refs. 2, 11.

Table 1.3 Preconception Screening Assessment for all Reproductive-Age Women (15–44 Years Old)

History
  Reason for visit
  Health status: obstetrical, gynecological, medical, surgical, and family history
  Use of prescription, over-the-counter, complementary, and alternative medicines
  Allergies (to medications or other)
  Tobacco, alcohol, other drug use
  Work-related exposures
  Dietary/Nutrition assessment
  Physical activity
  Urinary and fecal incontinence
Physical examination
  Height, weight, body mass index (BMI)
  Blood pressure
  Head
  Neck: adenopathy and thyroid
  Breasts
  Heart, lungs
  Abdomen
  Pelvic examination
  Skin
Laboratory testing
  Rubella titer[a]
  Varicella titer[a]
  Human immunodeficiency virus (HIV) testing[b]
  Cervical cytology[c]
  Chlamydia testing (if aged 25 years or younger and sexually active)

(Continued)

Table 1.3 Preconception Screening Assessment for all Reproductive-Age Women (15–44 Years Old) *(Continued)*

Evaluation and counseling
  Sexuality and reproductive planning
    High-risk behaviors
    Discussion of a reproductive health plan
    Contraceptive options for prevention of unwanted pregnancy, including emergency contraception
    Genetic counseling
  Sexually transmitted diseases
    - Partner selection
    - Barrier protection
  Sexual function
Fitness and nutrition
  Dietary/Nutrition assessment
  Exercise program
  Folic acid supplementation (0.4 mg/day)
  Calcium intake
Psychosocial evaluation
  Abuse/neglect/violence (physical, sexual, and emotional)
  Sexual practices
  Lifestyle/stress
  Sleep disorders
  Home and work (including satisfaction, and environmental hazards)
  Interpersonal/family relationships; social support
  Depression (suicide)
  Criminality
  Education
  Language and culture
  Health insurance status; coverage; access; public programs
Cardiovascular risk factors
  Family history
  Hypertension
  Dyslipidemia
  Obesity
  Diabetes mellitus
Health/Risk behaviors
  Hygiene (including dental)
  Injury prevention
    - Safety belts and helmets
    - Occupational hazards
    - Recreational hazards
    - Firearms
    - Hearing
    - Exercise and sports involvement
  Breast self-examination
Vaccinations
  See Table 1.5

[a]Unless documented immunity.
[b]HIV screening should be offered as routine to all women of reproductive age, under an "opt-out" policy. Physicians should be aware of and follow their states'/countries' HIV screening requirements.
[c]Annually beginning no later than age 21 years; every 2 to 3 years after three consecutive negative test results if age 30 years or older with no history of cervical intraepithelial neoplasia 2 or 3, immunosuppression, HIV infection, or diethylstilbestrol exposure in utero.
Source: Modified from Refs. 1, 11, 14.

Organizations representing family and internal medicine, obstetrics and gynecology, nurse midwifery, nursing, public health, diabetes, neurology, cardiology, and many other associations have supported recommendations for preconception care. Unfortunately, practitioners seldom implement them (9), even though it is an opportunity to optimize the health of the woman independent of whether she is planning pregnancy (6). Only one out of six obstetrician-gynecologists (ob-gyns) or family physicians provides preconception care to the majority of women for whom they provide prenatal care (10).

Preconception care may often need to be **multidisciplinary care**. Prior to pregnancy, a woman can have numerous different medical problems affecting different specialties, and her care should occur in close collaboration between the different fields involved. **Maternal physiology is different than nonpregnant adult physiology.** An entire field, **maternal-fetal medicine**, is dedicated to the care of pregnancies with maternal or fetal problems, and these specialists are particularly adept at directing best practices for preconception counseling. Preconception care occurs best if all practitioners, including primary and specialty care, either directly implement or appropriately refer for implementation of effective preconception screening and intervention. The worse scenario is the belief that a positive pregnancy test is a good reason to "stop all medicines" thereby stopping disease treatment. Prevent panic: get women ready for a healthy pregnancy before contraception is stopped.

CONTENT OF PRECONCEPTION CARE

Topics pertinent to optimizing preconception health and therefore future maternal and perinatal outcome should be discussed. Topics to be discussed in preconception care are listed in Table 1.2 (2,11). Further research is needed to determine the best content of preconception care and the most effective way to implement it (12,13).

UNIVERSAL SCREENING AND RELATED INTERVENTIONS
History, Exam, and Laboratory Screen

Suggested preconception screening assessment is shown in Table 1.3 (11,14). A **questionnaire should be completed ahead of time**, either on paper or online, to review this extensive list. A standardized form improves the completeness of preconception screening, which necessitates time and commitment (15). This standardized preconception form should be integrated into the permanent record of all reproductive-age woman. In a randomized trial, women assigned to be screened with a preconception risk survey were found to have an average of nine risk factors, supporting the facts that even low-risk women may benefit from preconception screening (12).

History should be detailed, especially when pertinent positives are detected. **Prior inpatient and outpatient medical records should be reviewed.** Women should be empowered with easy access to their records (best if electronic), to facilitate multispecialty care coordination. Personal prenatal medical record access has been associated with increased maternal control, satisfaction during pregnancy, and increased availability of antenatal records during hospital attendance (16).

Prior **obstetrical and gynecological history**, including prior pregnancy complications, should be reviewed. Other reproductive issues should also be assessed: fertility, including the possibility of assisted reproductive technology needs, sexuality (in particular high-risk behaviors), contraception, partner selection, and sexual function. Several social issues need to be reviewed as well (Table 1.3).

All couples should have a basic screen for family history of **heritable genetic disorders**, with a pedigree to at least the second prior generation. Women belonging to an ethnic group at increased risk for a recessive condition (Table 1.4) should be offered appropriate screening. All couples should be made aware of the option for **cystic fibrosis** (CF) screening, especially those who have a family history of CF, are in a high-risk

group, or are reproductive partners of individuals with CF (17). Women with a specific indication for genetic testing should be referred for formal genetic counseling (see chap. 6).

Physical exam details are shown in Table 1.3. Pelvic exam may include cytologic and sexually transmitted infection screening for women with certain risk factors. **Laboratory tests** are done routinely (Table 1.3), and depending on risk factors (Table 1.4) (11,18).

Reproductive Health Plan

Asking a reproductive-age woman, and therefore inducing her to think about, her reproductive health plan should be a priority of any medical visit (19). Such a plan should address the desire (or not) for children; the optimal number, spacing, and timing of pregnancies; contraception to achieve this plan; opportunities to improve her health and therefore a successful reproductive life; and age-related changes in fertility (19). Having a reproductive health plan reduces unintended pregnancies, age-related infertility, and fetal exposure to teratogens (2). Very few women know that a **short interpregnancy interval (i.e., <6 months from the end of last pregnancy to the next conception)** is associated with increased incidence of both small-for-gestational-age and low–birth weight neonates (20). Folic acid depletion may be the etiology for these increased risks (21). Education and **contraception advice** are necessary to aim for the wished reproductive plan, avoid unplanned pregnancies, and optimize the 18- to 24-month interpregnancy interval goal. In a nonrandomized study, preconception care decreased the number of unintended pregnancies (22).

All women should be counseled that 2% to 3% of babies are born with minor (usually) or major anomalies. Screening and diagnostic options to detect aneuploidy and birth defects should be reviewed so that women may consider their options in relation to their personal values.

Nutrition, Weight, and Exercise

Lifelong habits of healthy diet and regular exercise should be established preconceptionally (23). Proper diet and exercise can prevent several complications of pregnancy, including gestational diabetes and hypertensive complications (24). Some studies suggest a correlation between a diet high in fruits, vegetables, nuts, and legumes, less than two servings of meat weekly and at least two servings of fish weekly (the "Mediterranean Diet") with decreased rates of infertility and PTB (25–27).

In addition to following a healthy diet, issues of food safety are important to review. All meat, seafood, and shellfish should be **thoroughly cooked**. Eating at least 12 oz of **fish** weekly is associated with several benefits, including a lower rate of PTB (see chap. 16), but women must avoid >2 serving/wk of shark, swordfish, king mackerel, some tuna, or tilefish, all of which may contain high concentrations of methyl mercury. Albacore (white) tuna has more mercury than canned, light tuna (28). Other recommendations include **eating only pasteurized eggs and dairy products and washing raw fruits and vegetables** before eating. Women should try to obtain a minimum daily iodine intake of 150 μg/day. Education about proper hand, food, and cooking utensil hygiene is important, especially in developing countries.

Body mass index (BMI) should be calculated at least annually for reproductive-age women (29). For women whose BMI falls outside the normal range (28–34), preconception counseling is extremely important. **Formal nutritional counseling should be offered and goals set to avoid pregnancy**

Table 1.4 Preconception Laboratory Screening Depending on Risk Factors

Personal history:

    Age:
- >35: fasting glucose

    Race:
- African-American: fasting glucose; hemoglobin electrophoresis (for sickle cell disease)
- Hispanic: fasting glucose
- Native American: fasting glucose
- Pacific Islander: fasting glucose
- Mediterranean: mean corpuscular volume (MCV) screening (for thalassemia)
- Ethnic testing: Ashkenazi—familial dysautonomia; Tay–Sachs; Canavan; Fanconi anemia type C; Niemann–Pick disease type A; Bloom's syndrome; Gaucher disease; glycogen storage 1a; maple syrup urine disease; mucolipidosis type IV

    Prior obstetrical history:
- Prior birth of a newborn weighting more than 9 lb or >4500 g (macrosomia): fasting glucose
- History of gestational diabetes mellitus: fasting glucose
- Prior unexplained fetal death: check autopsy and karyotype of fetal death; antiphospholipid antibody testing; fasting glucose
- Prior infant with congenital anomaly (if not screened in that pregnancy): fasting glucose
- Prior recurrent unexplained early pregnancy loss: antiphospholipid antibody testing; study of uterine anatomy; parental karyotype

    Prior medical history:
- Metabolic syndrome/obesity; family history of lipid or coronary disorders: cholesterol/lipid profile
- Diabetes: lipid profile; hemoglobin A1c; cardiac and renal baseline function assessment; ophthalmologic exam
- Hypertension: fasting glucose; baseline cardiac, renal, and liver functions
- Multiple coronary heart disease risk factors (e.g., tobacco use, hypertension): lipid profile
- High-density lipoprotein cholesterol level ≤35 mL/dL: fasting glucose
- Triglyceride level ≥250 mg/dL: fasting glucose
- History of impaired glucose tolerance or impaired fasting glucose: fasting glucose
- Chronic use of steroids: fasting glucose
- Polycystic ovary syndrome: fasting glucose
- History of vascular disease: fasting glucose
- Marfan syndrome: echocardiogram for assessment of aortic root; eye exam for lens
- History of STD, drug abuse, etc.: HIV, Hep C
- Recipients of blood from donors who later tested positive for HCV infection: Hep C
- Recipients of blood or blood-component transfusion or organ transplant before July 1992: Hep C
- Recipients of clotting factor concentrates before 1987: Hep C
- Chronic (long-term) hemodialysis: Hep C
- History of transfusion from 1978 to 1985: HIV
- Invasive cervical cancer: HIV
- HIV infection: STD screening; PPD
- Medical risk factors known to increase risk of TB if infected: PPD
- Not sure if had varicella infection in past: varicella titer

Social history:
- HIV or TB contact, IV drug use, etc.: TB testing
- History of injecting illegal drugs: Hep C; HIV; STD screening (chlamydia, gonorrhea, syphilis, etc.); PPD
- Occupational percutaneous or mucosal exposure to HCV-positive blood: Hep C
- More than one sexual partner since most recent HIV test or a sex partner with more than one sexual partner since most recent HIV test: HIV
- Seeking treatment for STDs: HIV
- History of prostitution: STD screening; HIV
- Past or present sexual partner who is HIV positive or bisexual or injects drugs: HIV
- Long-term residence or birth in an area with high prevalence of HIV infection: HIV
- Adolescents who are or ever have been sexually active: HIV
- Adolescents entering detention facilities: HIV; STD screening
- Offer to women seeking preconception evaluation: HIV (all women should be screened)
- History of multiple sexual partners or a sexual partner with multiple contacts: STD screening
- Sexual contact with individuals with culture-proven STD: STD screening
- History of repeated episodes of STDs: STD screening
- Attendance at clinics for STDs: STD screening
- All sexually active women aged 25 years or younger: chlamydia
- All sexually active adolescents: gonorrhea
- Close contact with individuals known or suspected to have TB: PPD
- Born in country with high TB prevalence: PPD
- Medically underserved: PPD
- Low income: PPD
- Alcoholism: PPD
- Resident of long-term care facility (e.g., correctional institutions, mental institutions, and nursing homes and facilities): PPD
- Health professional working in high-risk health care facilities: PPD

Family history:
- Family history of diabetes mellitus: fasting glucose
- Family history of diabetes; history of gestational diabetes, overweight/obese, hypertension, high-risk ethnic group (African-American, Hispanic, Native American): fasting glucose every 3 years

(Continued)

Table 1.4 Preconception Laboratory Screening Depending on Risk Factors (*Continued*)

- Family history suggestive of familial hyperlipidemia: lipid profile
- Family history of premature (age < 50 years for men, age < 60 years for women) cardiovascular disease: lipid profile
- Colorectal cancer or adenomatous polyps in first-degree relative younger than 60 years or in two or more first-degree relatives of any ages; family history of familial adenomatous polyposis or hereditary nonpolyposis colon cancer: colonoscopy
- First-degree relative (i.e., mother, sister, or daughter) or multiple other relatives who have a history of premenopausal breast or breast or ovarian cancer: mammography
- Family history of Marfan syndrome: echocardiogram for assessment of aortic root; eye exam for lens
- Family history of breast cancer: mammography
- Family history of thyroid disease: TSH

Physical examination:
- Overweight (BMI ≥ 25): fasting glucose
- Hypertension: fasting glucose

Laboratory screening:
- Persistently abnormal alanine aminotransferase levels: Hep C
- Glycosuria: fasting glucose

Abbreviations: STDs, sexually transmitted diseases; HIV, human immunodeficiency virus; Hep C, hepatitis C; HCV, hepatitis C virus; PPD, purified protein derivative; TB, tuberculosis; IV, intravenous; TSH, thyroid-stimulating hormone; BMI, body mass index.
Source: Modified from Ref. 11.

until optimal weight is achieved. Women with low BMI should be screened for eating disorders. In overweight and obese women, **calorie and portion-size control** may be the most effective methods of sustained preconception weight loss. Postpartum individual counseling on diet and physical activity increased the proportion of women returning to prepregnancy weight from 30% to 50% in one randomized trial (30).

An exercise routine that can be started preconceptionally and safely continued in pregnancy may include yoga; brisk walking (including hiking and backpacking); jogging; swimming; biking; cross-country skiing; and using fitness equipment such as an elliptical trainer, treadmill, or stationary bike. Women should be given standard advice for engaging in regular physical activity for 30 to 60 min/day for five or more days per week.

Supplements

The preconception intervention with the most evidence-based data to support its efficacy is **folic acid supplementation**. Folic acid supplementation is recommended, with a **minimum of 400 μg/day** for all women [93% decrease in neural tube defects (NTDs)], and **4 mg/day for women with prior children with NTDs** (69% decrease in recurrent NTDs) (31).

Supplementation should start at least 1 month before conception and continue until at least 28 days after conception (time of neural tube closure). Given the unpredictability of planned conception, all reproductive-age women should be on folic acid supplementation from menarche to menopause. Women taking antiseizure medications, other drugs that might interfere with folic acid metabolism, those with homozygous methylenetetrahydrofolate reductase (MTHFR) enzyme mutations, or those who are obese may need higher doses of folic acid supplementation. As increases in baseline serum folate level are directly proportional with a decrease in the incidence of NTD, some experts have advocated 5 mg of folic acid per day as optimal universal supplementation (32). Folic acid supplementation has also been associated with a decrease in the risk of congenital anomalies other than NTDs (e.g., cardiac, facial clefts) (33).

The overall benefits or risks of fortifying basic foods such as grains with added folate have been associated with a 140 to 200 μg/day increase in supplementation and a 20% to 50% decrease in incidence of NTD (34). Education with provision of printed material (31,35), computerized counseling (36), and learner-centered nutrition education (37) all increase the awareness of the folate/NTDs association and the use of the folate supplements. These interventions may be effective in increasing the prophylactic use of additional preconception care activities.

There is insufficient evidence to justify the routine use of other supplements in reproductive-age women, especially in the developed world, unless a nutritional deficiency has been identified. It is important to obtain a **minimum daily iodine intake of 150 μg/day** and 10,000 IU daily of vitamin A (as beta-carotene) if deficiencies in these nutrients are identified. The use of certain supplements may be detrimental, especially if excessive amounts of lipid-soluble vitamins such as vitamin A (>10,000 IU/day) are taken, since they can be teratogenic. All supplements, including alternative and complementary medicines, should be reviewed (see also chap. 2) (38,39).

Vaccines

Preconception vaccination for the prevention of fetal and maternal disease is an important preconception intervention (Table 1.5) (see also chap. 38 in *Maternal-Fetal Evidence Based Guidelines*). **Maternal immunity to infections such as rubella and varicella** should be assessed for potential vaccination of nonimmune women, thus eliminating their risk for congenital syndromes associated with these viruses. Vaccination with live attenuated viruses should occur at least 4 weeks prior to conception due to theoretical risk of live virus affecting the fetus.

Annual influenza vaccination for women and their partners contemplating pregnancy will reduce the chance of maternal prenatal infection, a time during which higher morbidity has been documented. Influenza vaccination for new mothers and other close contacts of the newborn will reduce risk of infection for the child who is unable to receive vaccination until 6 months of age. Through this process of "cocooning," the newborn is protected from the high morbidity and mortality rates associated with influenza in the first year of life (40).

Hepatitis B vaccination should be offered to all susceptible women of reproductive age in regions with intermediate and high rates of endemicity [where ≥2% of the population is hepatitis B surface antigen (HBsAg) positive]. Perinatal transmission of hepatitis B results in 90% chance of chronic

Table 1.5 Recommended Preconception Vaccinations

All reproductive-age women
During flu season: **Influenza**
No evidence of immunity to rubella: **MMR**
No evidence of immunity to varicella: **Varicella**
No adult Td vaccination in last 2 years: **Tetanus/Diphtheria/Pertussis (Tdap)**
Hepatitis B nonimmune: **Hepatitis B vaccine**
Age
All girls and women 9 to 26 years old: HPV
All persons 18 years old and younger without immunity to hepatitis B infection: Hepatitis B
Occupational
Health care workers: Hepatitis B, Influenza, MMR, Varicella
Public safety workers who have exposure to blood in the workplace: Hepatitis B
Students in schools of medicine, dentistry, nursing, laboratory technology, and other allied health professions: Hepatitis B
Staff of institutions for the developmentally disabled: Hepatitis B
Individuals who work with HAV-infected nonhuman primates or with HAV in a research laboratory setting: Hepatitis A
Military recruits: Meningococcus
Microbiologists routinely exposed to *Neisseria meningitidis* isolates: Meningococcus
Social history/Living situation
Individuals with more than one sexual partner in the previous 6 months: Hepatitis B
Household contacts and sexual partners of individuals with chronic hepatitis B infection: Hepatitis B
Inmates of correctional facilities: Hepatitis B
Clients of institutions for the developmentally disabled: Hepatitis B
Illegal injected drug users: Hepatitis B
Illegal drug users (injected and noninjected): Hepatitis A
Exposure to environment where pneumococcal outbreaks have occurred: Pneumococcus
Native Alaskan/Native American: Pneumococcus
Alcohol abuse: Pneumococcus
Tobacco smoking: Pneumococcus
Residents of long-term care facilities: Influenza, Pneumococcus
First-year college students living in dormitories: Meningococcus
Travel/Immigration
Individuals traveling to or working in countries that have high or intermediate endemicity of hepatitis A: Hepatitis A
International travelers who will be in countries with high or intermediate prevalence of chronic hepatitis B infection for more than 6 months: Hepatitis B
Travel to areas hyperendemic or epidemic for *Neisseria meningitides*: Meningococcus
Pulmonary conditions
Chronic pulmonary disorders, including asthma: Pneumococcus
Cardiac conditions
Chronic cardiovascular disorders (e.g., CHF, cardiomyopathies): Influenza, Pneumococcus
Renal conditions
Chronic metabolic diseases, including renal dysfunction: Influenza, Pneumococcus
Nephrotic syndrome: Pneumococcus
End-stage renal disease including those on dialysis: Hepatitis B
Endocrine conditions
Diabetes mellitus: Influenza, Pneumococcus
Hematologic/Immunologic conditions
Prior transfusions: Hepatitis A, Hepatitis B
Patients with clotting factor disorders (those who receive clotting factor concentrates): Hepatitis A
Chronic illness, such as functional asplenia (e.g., sickle cell disease) or splenectomy: Pneumococcus
Immunocompromised patients (e.g., HIV infection, hematologic or solid malignancies, chemotherapy, steroid therapy): Pneumococcus
Adults with anatomic or functional asplenia: Pneumococcus, Meningococcus
Terminal complement component deficiencies: Meningococcus
Infectious conditions
Individuals with a recently acquired or recent evaluation for STI: Hepatitis B
All clients in STD clinics: Hepatitis B
HIV: Hepatitis B, Influenza, Pneumococcus, consider Meningococcus
GI/Hepatic conditions
Chronic liver disease: Hepatitis A, Hepatitis B, Pneumococcus
Neurologic conditions
Cerebrospinal fluid leaks: Pneumococcus

Abbreviations: MMR, measles, mumps, and rubella; HPV, human papillomavirus; HAV, hepatitis A virus; CHV, congestive heart failure; HIV, human immunodeficiency virus; STI, sexually transmitted infection; STD, sexually transmitted disease.
Source: Modified from Ref. 11 (see also chap. 38 in *Maternal-Fetal Evidence Based Guidelines*).

Table 1.6 Preconception Interventions for All Women

Intervention	Prevention of
Folic acid 400 μg/day[a]	NTDs, and also probably cardiac defects, facial clefts
Vaccinations	Maternal/Perinatal infection[b] (Table 1.5)
Proper diet and exercise	Obesity, diabetes, hypertensive diseases, and their consequences
Injury prevention (e.g., seat belts, helmets)	Physical trauma
Screen for specific risk factors	Table 1.7

[a]Consider higher dose, especially for women taking antiseizure medications, other drugs that might interfere with folic acid metabolism, those with homozygous MTHFR enzyme mutations, or those who are obese.
[b]By decreasing perinatal transmission, also decrease congenital defects caused by infection.
Abbreviations: NTDs, neural tube defects; STD, sexually transmitted disease; MTHFR, methylenetetrahydrofolate reductase.

infection in the newborn, which places the child at risk for future cirrhosis and hepatocellular carcinoma. In regions of low prevalence, vaccination should be targeted to high-risk groups (Table 1.5).

Tetanus vaccination should remain up-to-date in reproductive-age women, particularly in regions of the world where maternal and neonatal tetanus is prevalent (41). This has been shown to markedly reduce the incidence of tetanus related to parturition. Due to increasing prevalence and the high morbidity and mortality rates of neonatal pertussis, vaccination (in combination with tetanus and diphtheria) is recommended for all women and their partners of reproductive age who have not been immunized in their adult lives (since age 11 years) (42). It is well documented that 75% of cases of neonatal pertussis have a family member as the index case (43). Again, through the concept of cocooning, the incidence of neonatal pertussis can be reduced.

Other vaccination recommendations based on medical, occupational, or social risks are described in Table 1.5.

Injury Prevention
The second leading cause of death in reproductive-age women is accidents. Use of **seat belts** and **helmets** should be reviewed and strongly encouraged where appropriate. Inquiry should be made regarding occupational and recreational hazards. Possession and use of firearms should be evaluated.

Universal Recommendations
Preconception recommendations for all women are listed in Table 1.6. Reproductive-age women should be aware of these evidence-based recommendations, both through their doctors and through public awareness campaigns. Several online resources are available (44–47). Women and their partners should take more responsibility for their care and the future health of their offspring, and implement the health and lifestyle changes recommended.

SPECIFIC INDIVIDUAL ISSUES
Chronic Diseases
The incidences of several medical disorders such as obesity, diabetes mellitus, and hypertension are high and on the rise in reproductive-age women. There is literature for evidence-based recommendations on each disease or condition that can involve the reproductive-age woman and affect her reproductive health (4,14,48). Full review of each is behind the scope of this chapter (see individual chapters in *Maternal-Fetal Evidence Based Guidelines*). Some common conditions are discussed for brief preconception management review (Table 1.7).

Diabetes
Diabetes (see chaps. 4 and 5 in *Maternal-Fetal Evidence Based Guidelines*) is associated with an increased risk of congenital anomalies, in particular cardiac defects and NTDs, if poorly controlled in the first weeks of pregnancy. The risk of congenital anomalies is related to long-term diabetic control, reflected in the level of glycosylated hemoglobin (**HgB A1c): <7% = no increased risk** (2–3% baseline); 7% to 9% = 15%; 9% to 11% = 23%; >11% = 25% (33). **It has been estimated that euglycemia (with normal HgB A1c) during the first trimester, which can only be achieved through attentive preconception counseling, could prevent >100,000 U.S. pregnancy losses or birth defects per year** (2). The benefits of preconception diabetes care have been previously demonstrated (49,50), even in teenagers (51). Preconception care is also essential for counseling of the woman with conditions severe enough to make a successful pregnancy extremely unlikely. The diabetic woman with either ischemic heart disease, untreated proliferative retinopathy, creatinine clearance <50 mL/min, proteinuria >2 g/24 hr, creatinine >2 mg/dL, uncontrolled hypertension, or gastropathy should be told not to get pregnant before the above conditions can be improved, and counseled regarding adoption if the conditions cannot be improved (52). The frequency of fetal/infant and maternal morbidity and mortality are reduced in diabetic women seeking consultation in preparation for pregnancy, but unfortunately only about one-third of these women receive such consultation (53). The preconception consultation affords the opportunity to screen for vascular consequences of the diabetes, with **ophthalmologic, electrocardiogram (EKG), and renal evaluation via a 24-hour urine collection for total protein and creatinine clearance**, and determine ancillary pregnancy risks. A **thyroid-stimulating hormone (TSH)** should be checked, as 40% of young women with type 1 diabetes have hypothyroidism. Proliferative retinopathy should be treated with laser before pregnancy.

Diabetes evaluation should emphasize the importance of tight glycemic control, with normalization of the HgB A1c to at least <7%. To achieve euglycemia, **diet, glucose monitoring, and exercise** are always stressed. **If euglycemia is not achieved with these means, oral hypoglycemic agents or insulins are utilized**, and their regimens should be optimized preconceptionally. Of the oral hypoglycemic agents, **glyburide and glucophage can be used**, and probably continued during pregnancy. The original safety data available for glyburide showed that it did not cross the placenta in appreciable amounts (54), but recent data have shown a 70% level in umbilical blood compared to maternal blood (55). The other oral hypoglycemic agents should not be used for preconception glycemic control, as there is no sufficient evidence for their safety and efficacy in pregnancy. **A common insulin regimen currently used by diabetologists is long-acting (e.g., glargine)**

Table 1.7 Preconception Interventions for Women with Selected Specific Risk Factors

Risk factor/Population	Intervention	Prevention of
Smoking	Smoking cessation	PTB, LBW, etc.
Alcohol	Avoid all alcohol intake	Congenital anomalies, mental retardation
Other drugs of abuse	Avoid all drugs of abuse	PTB, IUGR, neonatal withdrawal, etc. (Effect depends on drug of abuse)
Teratogenic drugs	Avoid teratogenic drugs (Table 1.8)	Congenital anomalies
Supplements and over-the-counter medications	Review and counsel: Avoid excess of recommended daily allowance (RDA)	Congenital anomalies
Diabetes	Hemoglobin A1c <7%; screening for asymptomatic bacteriuria	Congenital anomalies, length of NICU admission, perinatal mortality and long-term health consequences in infant; miscarriage; maternal hospitalizations, maternal renal disease
Obesity	Diet and exercise to achieve normal BMI; screening for diabetes	Infertility, fetal NTDs, PTB, CD, HTN disorders, diabetes, VTE
Hypertension	Avoid angiotensin-converting enzyme inhibitors and angiotensin-receptor blockers. If long-standing HTN, assess for renal disease, ventricular hypertrophy, and retinopathy	Congenital anomalies, HTN complications, CD, IUGR, placental abruption, PTB, perinatal death
Hypothyroidism	Thyroxine supplementation to maintain normal TSH (0.5–2.0 μU/mL)	Infertility, maternal HTN, preeclampsia, abruption, anemia, PTB, LBW, fetal death, possibly neurological problems in infant
Hyperthyroidism	Propylthiouracil (PTU) supplementation to maintain FT4 in high normal range, and TSH in low normal range	Spontaneous pregnancy loss, PTB, preeclampsia, fetal death, FGR, maternal congestive heart failure, and thyroid storm; neonatal Graves' disease
Seizure disorders	Lowest dose of safest effective anticonvulsant monotherapy; folic acid 4 mg/day	Congenital anomalies
Asthma	Management following National Asthma Education and Prevention Program (NAEPP)	PTB, LBW, preeclampsia, perinatal mortality
Systemic lupus erythematosus	≥6 months of quiescence on stable therapy	HTN, preeclampsia, PTB, fetal death, IUGR, neonatal lupus
HIV	Initiate or modify antiviral agents with goals of the following: (*i*) HIV-1 RNA viral load level <1000 copies/mL or below the limit of detection of the assay; (*ii*) avoid teratogenic agents	Perinatal HIV infection
PKU	Low-phenylalanine diet	PKU-related mental retardation
Sexually transmitted disease (e.g., chlamydia)	Screen at risk populations (Tables 1.3 and 1.4)	Ectopic pregnancy
Social issues (e.g., abuse)	Counseling; Referral to appropriate agency	Physical and emotional trauma and their consequences

Abbreviations: PTB, preterm birth; LBW, low birth weight; IUGR, intrauterine growth restriction; NICU, neonatal intensive care unit; BMI, body mass index; NTD, neural tube defects; CD, cesarean delivery; HTN, hypertension; VTE, venous thromboembolism; TSH, thyroid-stimulating hormone; FT4, free thyroxine; FGR, fetal growth restriction; HIV, human immunodeficiency virus; RNA, ribonucleic acid; PKU, phenylketonuria.

and short-acting (e.g., lispro). This is a safe and effective regimen in pregnancy, too. Women compliant with insulin pumps should continue this regimen.

Hypertension

Hypertension (see chap. 1 in *Maternal-Fetal Evidence Based Guidelines*) is associated with several maternal [worsening hypertension; superimposed preeclampsia; severe preeclampsia; eclampsia; hemolysis, elevated liver enzyme levels, and a low platelet count (HELLP) syndrome; cesarean delivery] and fetal (growth restriction; oligohydramnios; placental abruption; PTB; perinatal death) risks in pregnancy. **Serum creatinine, 24-hour urine for total protein and creatinine clearance, EKG, and ophthalmologic exam** are suggested, especially in women with long-standing or severe hypertension. It is important to identify cardiovascular risk factors, any reversible cause of hypertension, and assess for target organ damage or cardiovascular disease. If hypertension is newly diagnosed and has not been evaluated previously, a medical consult may be indicated to assess for any of these factors. Secondary hypertension, target organ damage (left ventricular dysfunction,

retinopathy, dyslipidemia, microvascular disease, and prior stroke), maternal age >40, previous pregnancy loss, systolic blood pressure ≥180 mmHg, or diastolic blood pressure ≥110 mmHg are associated with higher risks in pregnancy. Abnormalities should be addressed and managed appropriately. If, for example, serum creatinine is >1.4 mg/dL, the woman should be aware of increased risks in pregnancy (pregnancy loss, reduced birth weight, PTB, and accelerated deterioration of maternal renal disease). Even mild renal disease (creatinine 1.1–1.4 mg/dL) with uncontrolled hypertension is associated with 10-fold higher risk of fetal loss. Preconception prevention can be enormously effective. **Thirty minutes of exercise three times per week in all women with hypertension and weight reduction if overweight are recommended**. Restriction of sodium intake to the same <2.4 g sodium daily intake recommended for essential hypertension is beneficial in nonpregnant adults. If antihypertensive medical therapy is necessary, **angiotensin-converting enzyme (ACE) inhibitors and angiotensin II (AII) receptor antagonists should be discontinued** as they are associated with birth defects, fetal growth restriction, oligohydramnios, neonatal

Table 1.8 Teratogens

Prescribed drugs
- Androgens and testosterone derivatives (e.g., danazol)
- Angiotensin-converting enzyme (ACE) inhibitors (e.g., enalapril, captopril) and angiotensin II receptor blockers
- Coumadin derivatives (e.g., warfarin)
- Carbamazepine
- Diethylstilbestrol
- Folic acid antagonists (methotrexate and aminopterin)
- HMG-CoA reductase inhibitors (statins)
- Lithium
- Phenytoin
- Primidone
- Streptomycin and kanamycin
- Tetracycline
- Thalidomide and leflunomide
- Trimethadione and paramethadione
- Valproic acid
- Vitamin A above RDA, and its derivatives (e.g., isotretinoin, etretinate, and retinoids)

Chemicals
- Lead
- Mercury

Drugs of abuse
- Alcohol
- Cocaine

Infections
- Cytomegalovirus
- Rubella
- Syphilis
- Toxoplasmosis
- Varicella

Radiation

Abbreviations: HMG-CoA, 3-hydroxy-3-methyl-glutaryl-CoA reductase; RDA, recommended daily allowance.
Source: Modified from Refs. 56, 57.

renal failure, and neonatal death in pregnancy. All other antihypertensive agents should be used at the lowest effective dose, and are probably safe if started preconceptionally and continued in pregnancy.

Seizure Disorders
Conception should be deferred until seizures are well controlled on the minimum effective dose of medication (see chap. 19 in *Maternal-Fetal Evidence Based Guidelines*). **Monotherapy is preferable.** Lamotrigine has been reported to be first-line therapy for nonpregnant adults for partial seizures (56,57), and associated with a low incidence of major malformations (58), but not in all studies (59). The best choice is the antiepileptic drug (AED) that best controls the seizures. The AEDs are usually FDA category C (human risk unknown, but none proven yet) except for the following AEDs that are known potential teratogens: carbamazepine, primidone, phenytoin, and valproate (Table 1.8). These four AEDs should therefore be avoided if possible, by using a different therapy beginning in the preconception period. **Women who have been seizure-free for ≥2 years with a normal electroencephalogram (EEG) may be eligible to stop anticonvulsant therapy after consulting with a neurologist** (60).

Medications/Teratogens

Detailed discussion regarding prescribed and over-the-counter medications should occur at the preconception visit. The indication, safety, effectiveness, and necessity of each drug need to be reviewed. Often, women and their doctors stop efficacious and necessary medications as soon as the woman finds out she is pregnant, compromising the health of both the woman and her baby. **The vast majority of prescribed medications are safe in pregnancy, even in the first trimester. Only a few drugs, chemicals, infections, or radiation are proven teratogens** (Table 1.8) (61,62). These should be avoided, except in rare circumstances (e.g., the woman with mechanical cardiac valves who accepts the teratogenic risk of warfarin). This medication counseling is often a crucial part of preconception care and can save and ameliorate significantly the health of a future offspring. Great resources exist on the Web for up-to-date teratologic information (63–65).

Substance abuse/Environmental hazards/Toxins

Tobacco smoking during pregnancy is associated with increased risks of several complications (see chap. 22 in *Maternal-Fetal Evidence Based Guidelines*). The benefits of smoking cessation are tremendous: prevention of 10% of perinatal deaths, 35% of low–birth weight births, and 15% of preterm deliveries (66). Smoking only 1 to 5 cigarettes/day is associated with a 55% higher incidence of low birth weight compared to nonsmokers. Reproductive-age women should be informed of other smoking-related diseases, such as ischemic heart disease, cancer, lung diseases, pneumonia, stroke, and congestive heart failure. Women at greatest risk for smoking are those <25 years old with less than a high school education. Smoking makes a major contribution to disparities in mortality (67). Smoking cessation programs are associated with a 6% increase in smoking cessation, and decreases in incidences of low birth weight (by 19%) and PTB (by 16%) (68). **Support and reward techniques** to help quit smoking are one of the best form of evidence-based medicine, supported by over 20 high-quality randomized trials. The "5 As" for screening and interventions to prevent smoking in pregnancy are **Ask, Advise, Assess, Assist, and Arrange** (69). **Counseling with behavioral and educational interventions is associated with highest cessation rates. If necessary, most pharmacotherapies are effective preconception**, but contraindicated or with uncertain safety and efficacy during pregnancy. Nicotine replacement therapy (e.g., patch, gum, and bupropion) is safe and effective in reproductive-age women, but there is insufficient evidence for recommending them in pregnant smokers. Nicotine replacement therapy is associated with known adverse fetal effects, and nicotine is detected in breast milk. Possibly the best prevention of the adverse effects of smoking on pregnancy is achieved by avoiding sale of tobacco to young people, prohibition of smoking in public places, increase in tobacco taxation, workplace smoking cessation programs, and banning of tobacco sponsorship of sporting and cultural events.

Numerous recreational drug exposures have adverse pregnancy effects (see chap. 23 in *Maternal-Fetal Evidence Based Guidelines*). This list is extensive and includes, but not limited to, common recreational drugs such as alcohol, cannabinoids, cocaine, heroin, and methamphetamines. Working to ensure that women with substance abuse issues engage in safe sex practices and family planning is a constant challenge, and these women are disproportionately overrepresented among women with unplanned pregnancies.

REFERENCES
1. Plutarch: Lycurgus 14 (trans. John Dryden). New York, USA: Random House, 1932:59–60. [Historical reference]
2. Johnson K, Posner SF, Biermann J, et al. Recommendations to improve preconception health and health care—United States. A report of the CDC/ATSDR Preconception Care Work Group and

the Select Panel on Preconception Care. MMWR Morb Mortal Wkly Rep 2006; 55(RR-6):1–23. Available at: http://www.cdc.gov/mmwR/preview/mmwrhtml/rr5506a1.htm. Accessed January 19, 2009. [Review]

3. Berghella V, Buchanan E, Pereira L, et al. Preconception care. Obstet Gynecol Surv 2010; 65(2):119–131. [Review].

4. Greer I, Steegers E. Periconceptional medicine. London, UK and New York, USA: Informa Healthcare, 2008. [Review]

5. The U.S. Preventative Services Task Forces' Guide to Clinical Preventive Services, 2006. Available at: http://www.ahrq.gov/clinic/uspstfix.htm. Accessed January 18, 2009. [Guideline]

6. Atrash H, Jack BW, Johnson K, et al. Where is the "W"oman in MCH? Am J Obstet Gynecol 2008; 199(6B):S259–S265. [Review]

7. de Jong-Potjer LC, Elsinga J, le Cessie S, et al. GP-initiated preconception counselling in a randomised controlled trial does not induce anxiety. BMC Fam Pract 2006; 7:66. [RCT]

8. Rabin R. That prenatal visit may be months too late. The New York Times, November 28, 2006. Available at: http://www.nytimes.com/2006/11/28/health/28natal.html. Accessed March 13, 2009. [Magazine article]

9. Williams J, Abelman S, Fassett E, et al. Health care provider knowledge and practices regarding folic acid, United States 2002-03. Matern Child Health J 2006; 10(5 suppl):s67–s72. [II-3]

10. Henderson JT, Weisman CS, Grason H. Are two doctors better than one? Women's physician use and appropriate care. Women Health Iss 2002; 12:138–149. [III]

11. American College of Obstetricians and Gynecologists. Primary and preventive care: periodic assessments. ACOG Committee Opinion No. 357. Obstet Gynecol 2006; 108:1615–1622. [Review]

12. Jack BW, Culpepper L, Babcock J, et al. Addressing preconception risks identified at the time of a negative pregnancy test: a randomized trial. J Fam Pract 1998; 47:33–38. [II-3]

13. Lumley J, Donohue L. Aiming to increase birth weight: a randomized trial of pre-pregnancy information, advice and counseling in inner-urban Melbourne. BMC Public Health 2006; 6:299–310. [RCT]

14. Jack BW, Atrash H, Coonrod DV, et al. The clinical content of preconception care: an overview and preparation of this supplement. Am J Obstet Gynecol 2008; 199(6B):S266–S279. [Review]

15. Bernstein PS, Sanghvi T, Merkatz IR. Improving preconception care. J Repro Med 2000; 45:546–552. [Review]

16. Brown HC, Smith HJ. Giving women their own case notes to carry during pregnancy. Cochrane Database Syst Rev 1, 2009. [Meta-analysis]

17. American College of Obstetricians and Gynecologists and American College of Medical Genetics. Preconception and prenatal carrier screen for cystic fibrosis: clinical and laboratory guidelines. Washington, DC: ACOG/ACMG, 2001. [Guideline]

18. American College of Obstetricians and Gynecologists. Primary and preventive care: periodic assessments. ACOG Committee Opinion No. 357. Obstet Gynecol 2006; 108(6):1615–1622. [Review]

19. American College of Obstetricians and Gynecologists. The importance of preconception care in the continuum of women's health care. ACOG Committee Opinion No. 313. Obstet Gynecol 2005; 106:665–666. [Review]

20. Zhu B-P, Rolfs RT, Nangle BE, et al. Effect of interval between pregnancies on perinatal outcomes. N Engl J Med 1999; 340:589–594. [II-2]

21. Smits LJ, Essed GGM. Short interpregnancy intervals and unfavourable pregnancy outcome: role of folate depletion. Lancet 2001; 358:2074–2077. [Review]

22. Moos MK, Bangdiwala SI, Meibohm AR, et al. The impact of a preconceptional health promotion program on intendedness of pregnancy. Am J Perinatol 1996; 13:103–108. [II-3]

23. United States Department of Agriculture. MyPyramid.gov. Available at: http://www.mypyramid.gov/. Accessed March 13, 2009. [Guideline]

24. Tieu J, Crowther CA, Middleton P. Dietary advice in pregnancy for preventing gestational diabetes mellitus. Cochrane Database Syst Rev 2008; 2:CD006674. [Meta-analysis]

25. Mikkelsen TB, Osterdal ML, Knudsen VK, et al. Association between a Mediterranean-type diet and risk of preterm birth among Danish women: a prospective cohort study. Acta Obstet Gynecol Scand 2008; 87(3):325–330. [II-1]

26. Vujkovic M, Steegers EA, Looman CW, et al. The maternal Mediterranean dietary pattern is associated with a reduced risk of spina bifida in the offspring. BJOG 2009; 116(3):408–415. [II-1]

27. Vujkovic M, de Vries JH, Lindemans J, et al. The preconception Mediterranean dietary pattern in couples undergoing in vitro fertilization/intracytoplasmic sperm injection treatment increases the chance of pregnancy. Fertil Steril 2010; 94(6):2096–2101 [Epub March 1, 2010]. [II-2].

28. U.S. Department of Health and Human Services and U.S. Environmental Protection Agency. What you need to know about mercury in fish and shellfish. 2004 EPA and FDA advice for women who might become pregnant, women who are pregnant, nursing mothers, young children. Washington, DC: U.S. Environmental Protection Agency, 2004. Available at: http://www.cfsan.fda.gov/~dms/admehg3.html. Accessed February 23, 2009). [Review]

29. National Institute of Health Publication No. 98-4083. Clinical Guidelines on the Identification, Evaluation, and Treatment of Overweight and Obesity in Adults: The Evidence Report. NHLBI (National Heart, Lung, and Blood Institute), 1998. [Guideline]

30. Kinnunen TI, Pasanen M, Aittasalo M, et al. Reducing postpartum weight retention - a pilot trial in primary health care. Nutr J 2007; 6:21–30. [II-2]

31. De-Regil LM, Fernández-Gaxiola AC, Dowswell T, et al. Effects and safety of periconceptional folate supplementation for preventing birth defects. Cochrane Database Syst Rev 2010; (10): CD007950 [review]. [Meta-analysis]

32. Wald NJ. Folic acid and the prevention of neural-tube defects. N Engl J Med 2004; 350:101–103. [Review]

33. Wilcox AJ, Lie RT, Solvoll K, et al. Folic acid supplements and risk of facial clefts: national population based case-control study. Br Med J 2007; 334(7591):464. [II-3]

34. Honein MA, Paulozzi LJ, Mathews TJ, et al. Impact of folic acid fortification of the U.S. food supply on the occurrence of neural tube defects. JAMA 2001; 285:2981–2986. [II-1]

35. Watson MJ, Watson LF, Bell RJ, et al. A randomized community intervention trial to increase awareness and knowledge of the role of periconceptional folate in women of child-bearing age. Health Expect 1999; 2:255–265. [RCT]

36. Scwartz EB, Sobota M, Gonzales R, et al. Computerized counseling for folate and use: a randomized controlled trial. Am J Prev Med 2008; 35:606–607. [RCT]

37. Cena ER, Heneman K, Espinosa-Hall G, et al. Learner-centered nutrition education improves folate intake and food-related behaviors in non-pregnant, low-income women of childbearing age. J Am Diet Assoc 2008; 108:1627–1635. [RCT]

38. Mahomed K, Gulmezoglu AM. Maternal iodine supplements in areas of deficiency. Cochrane Database Syst Rev 1, 2009. [Systematic review].

39. van den Broek N, Dou L, Othman M, et al. Vitamin A supplementation during pregnancy for maternal and newborn outcomes. Cochrane Database Syst Rev 2010; (11):CD001996. [Meta-analysis].

40. Fiore AE, Shay DK, Broder K, et al. Prevention and control of influenza. MMWR 2008; 57(RR-7):1–60. [Guideline]

41. Tetanus vaccine: WHO position paper. Wkly Epidemiol Rec 2006; 81:198–208. [Review]

42. Kretsinger K, Broder KR, Cortese MM, et al. Preventing tetanus, diphtheria, and pertussis among adults: use of tetanus toxoid, reduced diphtheria toxoid and acellular pertussis vaccine. MMWR Recomm Rep 2006; 55(RR-17):1–37. [Guideline]

43. Bisgard KM, Pascual FB, Ehresmann KR, et al. Infant pertussis: who was the source? Ped Inf Dis J 2004; 23(11):985–989. [Review]

44. Department of Health and Human Services Centers for Disease Control and Prevention (CDC). Available at: http://www.cdc.gov/ncbddd/preconception/default.htm. Accessed March 13, 2009. [Guideline]

45. U.S. National Library of Medicine and the National Institutes of Health, Medline Plus. Available at: http://www.nlm.nih.gov/medlineplus/preconceptioncare.html. Accessed March 13, 2009. [Guideline]

46. March of Dimes. Available at: http://www.marchofdimes.com. Accessed March 13, 2009. [Guideline]

47. The American College of Obstetricians and Gynecologists (ACOG). Available at: http://www.acog.org. Accessed March 13, 2009. [Review]

48. Berghella V. Maternal-fetal evidence based guidelines. London, UK and New York, USA: Informa Healthcare, 2007. [Review]

49. Moos MK. Preconception Health Promotion: A Focus for Women Wellness. 2nd ed. White Plaines, NY: March of Dimes, 2003. [Review]

50. Pearson DWM, Kernahhan D, Lee R, et al. The relationship between pre-pregnancy care and early pregnancy loss, major congenital anamoly or perinatal death in type I diabetes mellitus. Br J Obstet Gynecol 2007; 114:104–107. [II-2]

51. Charron-Prochownik D, Ferons-Hannan M, Sereika S, et al. Randomized efficacy trial of early preconception counseling for diabetic teens. Diabetes Care 2008; 31:1327–1330. [RCT]

52. American Diabetes Association. Preconception care of women with diabetes. Diabetes Care 2004; 27(suppl 1):S76–S78. [Review]

53. Korenbrot CC, Steinberg A, Bender C, et al. Preconception care: a systematic review. Matern Child Health J 2002; 6(2):75–88. [Review]

54. Langer O, Conway DL, Berkus MD, et al. A comparison of glyburide and insulin in women with gestational diabetes. N Engl J Med 2000; 343:1134–1138. [RCT]

55. Hebert MF, Ma X, Naraharisetti SB, et al. for the Obstetric-Fetal Pharmacology Research Unit Network. Are we optimizing gestational diabetes treatment with glyburide? The pharmacologic basis for better clinical practice. Clin Pharmacol Ther 2009; 85:607–614. [Review]

56. Marson AG, Al-Kharusi AM, Appleton R, et al. The SANAD study of effectiveness of carbamazepine, gabapentin, lamotrigine, oxcarbazepine, or topiramate for treatment of partial epilepsy: an unblended randomized controlled trial. Lancet 2007; 369:1000–1015. [RCT]

57. French JA. First-choice drug for newly diagnosed epilepsy. Lancet 2007; 369:970–971. [Review]

58. Meador KJ, Penovich P. What is the risk of orofacial clefts from lamotrigine exposure during pregnancy? Neurology 2008; 71:706–707. [II-1]

59. Holmes LB, Baldwin EJ, Smith CR, et al. Increased frequency of isolated cleft palate in infants exposed to lamotrigine during pregnancy. Neurology 2008; 70:2152–2158. [II-2]

60. Report of the Quality Standards Subcommittee of the American Academy of Neurology. Practice parameter: management issues for women with epilepsy (summary statement). Neurology 1998; 51(4):944–948. [Guideline]

61. American College of Obstetricians and Gynecologists. Teratology. ACOG Educational Bulletin No. 236. Washington, DC: ACOG, 1997. [Review]

62. Dunlop AL, Gardiner PM, Shellhaas CS, et al. The clinical content of preconception care: the use of medications and supplements among women of reproductive age. Am J Obstet Gynecol 2008; 12:s367–s372. [Review]

63. Thomson Reuters Healthcare. Available at: http://www.micromedex.com. Accessed March 13, 2009. [Review]

64. Reprotox. An Information System on Environmental Hazards to Human reproduction and Development. Available at: http://www.reprotox.org. Accessed March 13, 2009. [Review]

65. OTIS. Organization of Teratology Information Specialists. Available at: http://www.otispregnancy.org. Accessed March 13, 2009. [Review]

66. U.S. Department of Health and Human Services. The Health Benefits of Smoking Cessations: U.S. Department of Health and Human Services, Public Health Service, Centers for Disease Control, Center for Chronic Disease Prevention and Health Promotion, Office on Smoking and Health, 1990. [Review]

67. Wong MD, Shapiro MF, Boscardin WJ, et al. Contribution of major diseases to disparities in mortality. N Engl J Med 2002; 347 (20):1585–1592. [Review]

68. Lumley J, Oliver SS, Chamberlain C, et al. Interventions for promoting smoking cessation during pregnancy. Cochrane Database Syst Rev 2008; 4:CD001055. [Meta-analysis]

69. Fiore MC, Bailey WC, Cohen SJ, et al. Treating tobacco use and dependence. Quick reference guide for clinicians. Rockville, MD: U.S. Department of Health and Human Services. Public Health Service, 2000. [Guideline]

2

Prenatal care

Carol Sudtelgte

KEY POINTS

- **Prenatal care is of benefit to pregnant women, especially those with modifiable risk factors.**
- **Most women can be offered midwife-led models of care,** and women should be encouraged to ask for this option. Continuity of care by midwives has been associated with improved patient satisfaction. Caution should be exercised in applying this advice to women with substantial medical or obstetric complications.
- **Group prenatal care should be promoted,** as it has been associated reduction in preterm birth (PTB), greater satisfaction with care, and higher breastfeeding initiation. **In the developing world, participatory intervention with women's groups** is associated with **decreased maternal and neonatal mortality.**
- **Women should be allowed to carry their record.**
- Prenatal care usually consists of 7 to 12 visits per pregnancy, with a prenatal visit ideally at 11 to 14 weeks for aneuploidy screening, followed by visits about every 4 weeks approximately at 16, 20, 24, and 28 weeks; about every 3 weeks to 34 to 36 weeks, then weekly until delivery. **In settings with limited resources** where the number of visits is already low, **reduced visits programs of antenatal care (<5) are associated with an increase in perinatal mortality** compared to standard care.
- See Table 2.1 for screening and interventions at different times in pregnancy.
- **Early ultrasonography** should be used to determine the estimated date of confinement (EDC) if there is any uncertainty regarding last menstrual period (LMP).
- Content issues that should be included in prenatal care are drugs and environment, lifestyle, nutrition, supplements, vaccinations, prenatal education, and others.
- **Regular exercise is beneficial to overall maternal fitness and sense of well-being,** as well as associated with prevention of excessive weight gain.
- Most studies report that **sexual activity** is associated with **better pregnancy outcomes,** probably because women who are sexually active are healthier to begin with compared to women with less sexual activity.
- **Balanced energy/protein supplementation** is associated with modest increases in maternal weight gain and in mean birth weight, and **reduction in risk of small-for-gestational-age (SGA), stillbirth, and neonatal death.** High-protein and isocaloric protein supplementations should be avoided, as they are associated with increased risk of SGA.
- **Suggested weight gain in pregnancy is shown in** Table 2.4. **Women who are underweight are at increased risk for low birth weight (LBW) and PTB and have better outcomes with a higher total weight gain. Excessive weight gain in women with normal body mass index (BMI) can be prevented with dietary and lifestyle counseling.**
- **Folic acid supplementation is recommended for neural tube defect (NTD) prevention,** with 400 μg/day for all women, and 4 mg/day for women with prior children with NTD. All reproductive-age women should be on folic acid supplementation.
- Immunity to **rubella, varicella, hepatitis B, influenza, tetanus, and pertussis should be assessed at the first prenatal visit. Ideally needed vaccinations would be provided preconception.**
- **Prenatal education directed at specific objectives has been demonstrated to be effective.**
- **Implementation of community-based interventional care packages is associated with a trend for reduction in maternal mortality, and with significant reductions in maternal morbidity, neonatal mortality, stillbirths, and perinatal mortality.**
- **Perineal massage with sweet almond oil for 5 to 10 minutes daily from 34 weeks until delivery is associated with a significantly higher chance of intact perineum.**
- **Antenatal classes with training to prepare for labor and delivery** are associated with **arriving to L&D ward more often in active labor,** and **using less epidural analgesia.**
- **Identifying mothers "at-risk" assists the prevention of postpartum depression compared to intervening on the general population.**
- **Breastfeeding is the best feeding method for most infants** and should be **strongly encouraged. Counseling and education** facilitate breastfeeding success.
- **Unsensitized RhD-negative women should be offered anti-D immunoglobulin prophylaxis.**
- **Sweeping or "stripping" of membranes** during cervical exam at ≥38 weeks **reduces the rate of postterm delivery.**
- **Massage with Trofolastin cream** (*Centella asiatica* extract, α-tocopherol, and collagen elastin hydrolases) applied daily **decreases the development of stretch marks. Massage with Verum ointment** (tocopherol, panthenol, hyaluronic acid, elastin, and menthol) also **decreases the development of stretch marks.**
- **Magnesium lactate or citrate chewable tablets** 5 mmol in the morning and 10 mmol in the evening for 3 weeks for women with leg cramps are associated with **significant improvement in persistent leg cramps.**
- **Water gymnastics** for 1 hour weekly starting at <19 weeks **reduces back pain** in pregnancy and allows more women to continue to work, with no adverse effects. **Both physiotherapy and acupuncture** starting <32 weeks for 10 sessions **might reduce back and pelvic pain.**
- **Exercise, increase in water intake, dietary counseling, and certain foods (e.g., prunes)** have shown relief in constipation. If these self-help measures are inadequate, the pregnant woman should then try **daily bran or wheat fiber supplements. Docusate sodium** is an effective **stimulant laxative.**

Table 2.1 Suggested Prenatal Care Counseling, Screening, and Intervention

Initial visit ≤14 wk	Visits at: 14–24 wk	24–28 wk	28–34 wk	34–41 wk
Assessments/Procedures				
• Complete history and risk identification • Assessment of EDB by LMP and sizing; ultrasound if indicated • Baseline BP screening • Weight and BMI • Screening for domestic abuse • Vaccines according to risk status and season • Referral for specialist care according to history • Offer 11–13 6/7 wk aneuploidy screening ultrasound	• Fetal heart tones • Fundal height • Fetal movement • BP • Weight • Screening ultrasound for anatomy	• Fetal heart tones • Fundal height • Fetal movement • BP • Weight • Rh immunoglobulin if indicated • Screening for domestic abuse	• Fetal heart tones • Fundal height • Fetal movement • BP • Weight	• Fetal heart tones • Fundal height/EFW • Fetal movement • Fetal presentation • BP • Weight • Sweeping of membranes starting at ≥38 wk
Laboratory tests				
• Multiple-marker aneuploidy screen • CBC; Blood type, Rh, antibody screen; Rubella IgG; RPR; HBsAg; HIV • Urine dipstick for protein and glucose • Urinalysis and urine culture • Gonorrhea/Chlamydia[a] • Pap[a] • Additional testing as directed by history and PE[a]	• Multiple-marker aneuploidy screen • Urine dipstick for protein if indicated	• Gestational diabetes screen; repeat CBC and antibody screen • Antibody screen if indicated • Urine dipstick for protein	• Urine dipstick for protein	• Group B Strep • Urine dipstick for protein • HIV
Education/Counseling				
• Cessation of harmful substances • Exercise/Activity • Nutrition • Nutrition • Weight gain • Supplements • Food safety • Breastfeeding	• Review and discuss results of testing	• Preterm labor s/sx	• Preterm labor s/sx • Preeclampsia s/sx	• Labor symptoms/when to call • Preeclampsia s/sx • Post-dates management • Breastfeeding
Education/Counseling not limited to specific weeks gestation				
• Danger signs • Dental care • Family planning		• Labor preparation, options, s/sx to report • Travel • TOLAC		

[a]See text, only in certain circumstances.
Abbreviations: EDB, expected date of birth; LMP, last menstrual period; BP, blood pressure; BMI, body mass index; EFW, estimation of fetal weight; RPR, rapid plasma regain; HIV, human immunodeficiency virus; CBC, complete blood count; PE, physical exam; TOLAC, trial of labor after cesarean; s/sx, signs and symptoms.
Source: Adapted from a review of current prenatal care guidelines from four major groups: U.S. Veterans Health Administration, Department of Veteran Affairs, and Health Affairs, Department of Defense; Institute for Clinical Systems Improvement; the American Academy of Pediatrics and the American College of Obstetricians and Gynecologists; and the American Academy of Family Physicians (105).

DEFINITION

Prenatal care is the care provided to pregnant women with the aim to prevent complications and decrease the incidence of perinatal and maternal morbidity/mortality (1). This care consists of health promotion, risk assessment, and intervention linked to the risks and conditions uncovered. These activities require the cooperative and coordinated efforts of the woman, her family, her prenatal care providers, and other specialized providers. Prenatal care begins when conception is first considered and continues until labor begins. The objectives of prenatal care for the mother, infant, and family relate to outcomes through the first year following birth (1).

PURPOSE

Prenatal care developed, historically, to reduce the incidence of LBW and preterm infants (2). It has evolved to encompass a broader purpose; to identify pregnancies with maternal or fetal conditions associated with morbidity/mortality, to provide interventions to prevent or treat such complications, and to provide education support and health promotion that can have lasting effects on the health of an entire family (3). Care should be systematic, evidence based, and should result in informed shared decision-making between the patient and the provider.

EFFECTIVENESS

Prenatal care is of benefit to pregnant women. Nonetheless, the value of prenatal care is controversial, as there is no definite evidence that prenatal care improves birth outcomes. **There are no randomized control trials (RCTs) of prenatal care versus no prenatal care.** Most studies are observational, comparing outcomes in women who have had prenatal care to those without prenatal care. While some results show benefit, others do not. Selection bias (women who self-select to prenatal care usually are more inclined to have better outcomes) leads to confounding bias (e.g., risk factors associated with LBW and neonatal death are also risk factors for inadequate prenatal care).

There are other sources that indirectly demonstrate the beneficial effects of prenatal care. There are worse outcomes in programs with significantly less (<5) numbers of prenatal visits (4). Also, studies demonstrate a reduction in poor outcomes in high-risk pregnancies with enhanced prenatal care (5) (see subsection "Number and Timing of Visits"). In addition, women indicate dissatisfaction with a reduced schedule of prenatal visits indicating a perceived benefit by women (4). Specific interventions for specific risks may reduce morbidity and mortality. Prenatal care is probably of most benefit to medically high-risk women (2).

ORGANIZATIONAL ISSUES
Health Care Provider
There is no evidence that physicians need to be involved in the prenatal care of every woman experiencing an uncomplicated pregnancy. The effect of midwife-led care compared to physician-led care or to other provider-led care has been evaluated mostly for the whole pregnancy, including together both antepartum care and care during labor and delivery (see also chap. 7). Therefore it is difficult to assess the effect of midwife-led care just on antepartum care. From the evidence from both antepartum and L&D care, **most women can be offered midwife-led models of care and women should be encouraged to ask for this option. Caution should be exercised in applying this advice to women with substantial medical or obstetric complications.** In a meta-analysis, women, the vast majority low risk, who had midwife-led models of care, were **less likely to experience antenatal hospitalization**, and **less likely to experience fetal loss before 24 weeks' gestation** [relative risk (RR) 0.79, 95% confidence interval (CI) 0.65–0.97], although there were no statistically significant differences in fetal loss/neonatal death of at least 24 weeks (RR 1.01, 95% CI 0.67–1.53) or in fetal/neonatal death overall (RR 0.83, 95% CI 0.70–1.00) (6) (see also chap. 7). It is not clear whether these associations are due to greater continuity of care or to midwifery care (6).

Group Prenatal Care
In a meta-analysis, educational interventions were the focus of group prenatal care, and no consistent results were found. Sample sizes were very small to moderate. No data were reported concerning anxiety, breastfeeding success, or general social support. Knowledge acquisition, sense of control, factors related to infant-care competencies, and some labor and birth outcomes were measured. The largest of the included studies (n = 1275) examined an educational and social support intervention to increase vaginal birth after cesarean section. This high-quality study showed similar rates of vaginal birth after cesarean section in "verbal" and "document" groups (RR 1.08, 95% CI 0.97–1.21) (7). One large, more recent RCT demonstrated significant **reduction in PTB, greater satisfaction with care, and higher breastfeeding initiation** at no added cost for group prenatal care over standard care in a group of medically low-risk (but socially at-risk) women in an urban clinic (5). In this study, group care included, among other interventions, continuity of care from a single provider, patient keeping

copies of their records, no waiting time at visits, about 20 hours of provider/patient time, with 8 to 10 women in each group session. **In the developing world, participatory intervention with women's groups** is associated with **decreased maternal and neonatal mortality** in several large cluster-randomized trials (8–10). In one of these studies, participatory care involved a female facilitator convening nine women's group meetings every month. The facilitator supported groups through an action-learning cycle in which they identified local perinatal problems and formulated strategies to address them (8). This strategy holds great promise in decreasing maternal and perinatal deaths among the most vulnerable in our world. **Group prenatal care should be promoted** and further studied among more diverse populations.

Prenatal Record
A formal, structured record should be used for documenting care during the pregnancy. Structured records with reminder aids help ensure that providers incorporate evidence-based guidelines into clinical practice. There is no trial comparing different records. **Women should be allowed to carry their record.** Carrying the record is **associated with increased maternal control and satisfaction during pregnancy, increased availability of antenatal records during hospital attendance, but also with more operative deliveries** (11). More women in the case-notes-carrying group would prefer to hold their antenatal records in another pregnancy (11).

Number and Timing of Visits
There is insufficient evidence to recommend an ideal schedule of prenatal visits for all pregnant women. The most important visit to optimize pregnancy outcomes is the **preconception visit** (see chap. 1). A visit early, soon after the pregnancy test is positive, and in time to establish location and number of embryo(s), usually at around 6 to 8 weeks, is also desirable.

At this early visit, each woman should be assessed for risk factors (see Tables 1.3 and 1.4 in chap. 1). The frequency of subsequent visits can be determined based on risk factors.

In developed countries, **prenatal care usually consists of 7 to 12 visits per pregnancy, with a prenatal visit ideally at 11 to 14 weeks for aneuploidy screening** (see chaps. 5 and 6), **followed by visits about every 4 weeks approximately at 16, 20, 24, and 28 weeks; about every 3 weeks to 34 to 36 weeks, then weekly until delivery** (Table 2.1). Uncomplicated multiparous women may need fewer visits than uncomplicated nulliparous ones. Individual patient needs and risk factors should be assessed at the first prenatal visit and reassessed at each appointment thereafter.

A small reduction in the traditional number of prenatal visits in both developed and developing countries has *not* been associated with adverse biological maternal or perinatal outcomes, but women may feel less satisfied with fewer visits (4). But, **in settings with limited resources where the number of visits is already low, reduced antenatal visits (<5) are associated with an increase in perinatal mortality compared to standard care** (4). **In addition, women in high-resource settings were more often dissatisfied with a reduced schedule of visits (defined as eight). The schedule of visits should be determined by the purpose of the appointment. A minimum of four prenatal care visits is recommended even for low-risk women** (4).

STRUCTURE
Initial Visit

Ideally, this visit should occur prior to 12 weeks of gestation. Women should receive *written* information regarding their pregnancy care services, the proposed schedule of visits, screening tests that will be offered, and lifestyle issues, such as nutrition and exercise. Major parts of the visit include history, risk identification, physical exam, laboratory testing, education for health promotion, and a detailed plan of care for any risks identified (see Table 2.1) (see also chap. 1, Tables 1.2–1.5).

History

A comprehensive history should be performed, preferably using standardized record forms (e.g., www.acog.org). Risk assessment should be performed with detailed review of systems. In particular, the woman who may require additional care or referral should be identified. **Early ultrasonography should be used to determine the EDC if there is any uncertainty regarding LMP.** Accuracy of EDC is critical for timing of screening tests and appropriate interventions, managing complications, and consideration of post-dates induction. It also provides early identification of multiple pregnancies (see "Ultrasonography" below and chap. 4). Content issues such as drugs, environment, lifestyle, nutrition, supplements, vaccinations, prenatal education, and others should be discussed (see "Content of Prenatal Care"). Prenatal diagnosis and screening for aneuploidy (chap. 5) and genetic screening (chap. 6) should be reviewed.

Physical Exam

The physical exam should be both general (Table 2.1) and directed by any risks identified in the history (see chap. 1).

Weight and height should be determined at the initial prenatal visit, in order to determine BMI [**BMI** = weight (kg)/ height squared (m^2)]. BMI should be based on weight at time of conception or the earliest known weight in pregnancy. Categories of BMI are in Table 2.2. Women with **obesity** are at increased risk for diabetes, shoulder dystocia, cesarean section, and other complications, and have better outcomes with a lower (or no) total weight gain. Women who are underweight (<50 kg or <120 lb) also are at increased risk for LBW and PTB, and have better outcomes with a higher total weight gain (see subsection "Nutrition").

Blood Pressure is recommended at each prenatal visit. Initial blood pressure evaluation may help to identify women with chronic hypertension, while subsequent blood pressure readings aid in preeclampsia screening. A diastolic blood pressure of ≥80 at booking is associated with later risks of preeclampsia (12). There are significant risks associated with hypertension and preeclampsia in pregnancy. This simple, inexpensive, and widely accepted screening tool may help to identify abnormal trends in blood pressure over time. Blood pressure should be taken in the sitting position using an appropriately sized cuff and correct technique (see chap. 1 in *Maternal-Fetal Evidence Based Guidelines*).

Table 2.2 Body Mass Index (BMI) Categories

Weight category	BMI
Underweight	<18.5
Normal weight	18.5–24.9
Overweight	25–29.9
Obesity (class I)	30–34.9
Obesity (class II)	35–39.9
Extreme obesity (class III)	≥40

Pelvic Exam

Routine pelvic exam early in pregnancy is not as accurate for assessment of gestational age as ultrasound (see chap. 4) and not a reliable predictive test of PTB or cephalopelvic disproportion later in pregnancy (see also chaps. 7 and 16). It is not recommended for these assessments. Abdominal and pelvic examination to detect gynecologic pathology can be included in the initial examination.

Laboratory Screening

Recommended initial universal laboratory screening is listed in Table 2.1. Other lab testing may be ordered if other risks/conditions are present.

ABO/Rh (D) type and antibody screen. Testing for blood group, Rh status, and atypical red cell antibodies at the initial visit is recommended. Unsensitized RhD-negative women should be offered anti-D immunoglobulin at 28 weeks (see chap. 52 in *Maternal-Fetal Evidence Based Guidelines*). Anti-D immunoglobulin should also be offered for any invasive procedure [e.g., amniocentesis, chorionic villus sampling (CVS), percutaneous umbilical blood sampling (PUBS)], for second- or third-trimester bleeding, for partial molar pregnancies, spontaneous abortion, and elective termination, and for any condition that might be associated with fetal-maternal hemorrhage, such as abdominal trauma, external cephalic version, or placental abruption. It may also be offered for any first-trimester threatened abortion, and for ectopic pregnancy, although the evidence is not as strong, and it is probably not cost-effective or necessary unless the bleeding is significant. For the RhD-negative woman with a known RhD-negative father of the pregnancy, anti-D immunoglobulin can be deferred. Du-positive women do not need anti-D immunoglobulin (see chap. 52 in *Maternal-Fetal Evidence Based Guidelines*).

Complete blood count. Recommended at the first prenatal visit to identify anemia [hemoglobin and hematocrit], and to screen for thalassemia [mean corpuscular volume (MCV)]. Pregnant women identified with anemia (Hgb < 11.0 g/dL in first trimester) should be treated as per chapter 14 in *Maternal-Fetal Evidence Based Guidelines*. Initial determination of platelet count (optimally also before pregnancy) may help with later diagnosis of hemolysis, elevated liver enzyme levels, and a low platelet count (HELLP) syndrome, gestational thrombocytopenia, or neonatal alloimmune thrombocytopenia, and with screening for idiopathic thrombocytopenia purpura (ITP).

Rubella antibody. Screen all women at first encounter. Nonimmune pregnant women should be counseled to avoid exposure and seek immunization postpartum (see chap. 38 in *Maternal-Fetal Evidence Based Guidelines*).

Syphilis screening. All pregnant women should be screened with a serologic test for syphilis at the first prenatal visit. Women who are at high risk, live in areas of high syphilis morbidity, or are previously untested should be screened at 28 weeks and again at delivery (see chap. 35 in *Maternal-Fetal Evidence Based Guidelines*).

HBsAg. Screen at initial encounter, and rescreen high-risk populations in third trimester. Postnatal intervention is recommended in all HBsAg-positive women to reduce the risk of viral transmission to the neonate. Pregnancy and breastfeeding are not contraindications to immunization in women who are at risk for acquisition of the hepatitis B virus (see chap. 30 in *Maternal-Fetal Evidence Based Guidelines*).

HIV serology. Screening is recommended for all pregnant women. The "opt-out" approach is recommended. It should be emphasized that testing not only provides the opportunity to maintain maternal health, but interventions can be offered to dramatically reduce the risk of viral transmission to the fetus (see chap. 32 in *Maternal-Fetal Evidence Based Guidelines*).

Urine dipstick for protein. Screening for proteinuria should occur at the initial visit and routinely after 20 weeks in women at risk for preeclampsia. Urine dipsticks for protein do not reliably detect the variable elevations in albumin that may occur in preeclampsia and may not be indicated at each visit in low-risk women (13). In women at high risk for preeclampsia, the 24-hour collection is a reasonable screen for proteinuria as a baseline at the first prenatal visit, and when other signs/symptoms of preeclampsia are present (see chap. 1 in *Maternal-Fetal Evidence Based Guidelines*).

Urine dipstick for glucose. Glycosuria ≥ 250 mg/dL on urine dipstick in the first or second trimester is associated with abnormal gestational diabetes (GDM) screening later in pregnancy. Presence of significant glycosuria before 24 to 28 weeks is an indicator for earlier gestational glucose screening (see chaps. 4 and 5 in *Maternal-Fetal Evidence Based Guidelines*).

Urine culture for asymptomatic bacteriuria. Screening for bacteriuria is recommended at the first prenatal visit for all women. Pregnant women with asymptomatic bacteriuria are at increased risk for symptomatic infection and pyelonephritis. There is also as a positive relationship between untreated bacteriuria and LBW/PTB. Treatment of asymptomatic bacteriuria prevents these complications (see chap. 16 in *Maternal-Fetal Evidence Based Guidelines*).

Cervical cancer screening. Cervical cancer screening should be obtained if not current according to guidelines. Pap smear screening should be initiated at age 21, regardless of onset of sexual activity. Routine screening intervals can be extended to every 2 years for women in their 20s, and every 3 years in women over 30 who have had three consecutive normal Pap smears (see chap. 31).

Selective (Only Women with Risk Factors) Laboratory Screening
Hepatitis C serology. A test for hepatitis C antibodies should be performed in pregnant women at increased risk for exposure, such as those with a history of IV drug abuse, exposure to blood products or transfusion, organ transplants, kidney dialysis, etc. (see chap. 31 in *Maternal-Fetal Evidence Based Guidelines*).

Chlamydia screening. All women of age <25 years (strongest risk factor), multiple sex partners, new partner within past 3 months, single marital status, inconsistent use of barrier contraception, previous or concurrent sexually transmitted infection (STI), vaginal discharge, mucopurulent cervicitis, friable cervix, or signs of cervicitis on physical examination should be screened. Some agencies advocate universal chlamydia screening. Rescreen in the third trimester if at increased risk for infection. Screening using polymerase chain reaction (PCR) technology is most accurate (see chap. 34 in *Maternal-Fetal Evidence Based Guidelines*).

Gonorrhea screening. All women of age <25 years, prior STI, multiple sexual partners, having a partner with a past history of any sexually transmitted disease (STD), sex work, drug use, and inconsistent condom use should be screened for gonorrhea. Some agencies advocate universal gonorrhea screening. Rescreen in the third trimester if at increased risk for infection. Screening using PCR technology is most accurate (see chap. 33 in *Maternal-Fetal Evidence Based Guidelines*).

Bacterial vaginosis. There is **no benefit** to routine screening and treatment for asymptomatic bacterial vaginosis. Consideration can be given to screening and treating women with a prior PTB. Those women who are symptomatic should be

Table 2.3 Prevention of Food-Borne Illnesses

Food-borne illness to avoid	Preventive strategy
Listeriosis	Cook meat thoroughly including luncheon meats; avoid raw or smoked meats or fish, pates, unpasteurized cheese, and raw milk.
Toxoplasmosis	Cook meat and wash fruits and vegetables thoroughly; avoid cat litter; wear gloves when gardening outdoors.
Escherichia coli and Salmonella	Follow food-handling guidelines above.
Methylmercury	Avoid consumption of large, mercury-containing fish.

screened (see chap.16 in *Maternal-Fetal Evidence Based Guidelines*).

Genital herpes. Routine serologic or other screening for herpes simplex virus (HSV) in asymptomatic pregnant women is not recommended. In the absence of lesions during the third trimester, routine serial cultures are not indicated for women with a history of recurrent genital herpes (see chap. 49 in *Maternal-Fetal Evidence Based Guidelines*).

Varicella. Screening is indicated if a woman has had neither past infection nor vaccination. Varicella vaccine (live attenuated) is not recommended during pregnancy, but seronegative women should be advised to take appropriate precautions (see chaps. 38 and 50 in *Maternal-Fetal Evidence Based Guidelines*).

Tuberculosis. Postpartum depression screening can be offered to high-risk women at any gestational age in pregnancy, and follow-up chest X ray is recommended for recent converters. High-risk factors include human immunodeficiency virus (HIV) disease, homeless or impoverished women, prisoners, recent immigrants from areas where tuberculosis is prevalent, and others (see chap. 24 in *Maternal-Fetal Evidence Based Guidelines*).

CMV. Routine testing is not recommended. Good hand washing and practicing universal precautions are recommended to prevent transmission (14) (see chap. 46 in *Maternal-Fetal Evidence Based Guidelines*).

Parvovirus. Routine screening is not recommended, but can be considered for high-risk groups (see chap. 48 in *Maternal-Fetal Evidence Based Guidelines*).

Toxoplasmosis. Universal screening is not recommended. Education regarding prevention of disease should be addressed (Table 2.3) (see chap. 47 in *Maternal-Fetal Evidence Based Guidelines*).

Follow-up Visits
Follow-up visits should provide for the following:

- Follow-up physical exam, laboratory screening, and testing as indicated
- Ongoing assessment of risk factors and plan for intervention as indicated
- Education and health promotion directed to individual plan of care
- Opportunity for discussion and questions

Follow-up Physical Exam

- **Weight:** Usually done at each visit, as optimal weight gain (Table 2.4) is associated with better outcomes. Excessive fast weight gain can be a sign of preeclampsia.

Table 2.4 Institute of Medicine Recommended Total Weight Gain in Pregnancy by Prepregnancy BMI [kg (lb)]

BMI	Singleton	Twin
<18.5	12.5–18 (27–40)	Insufficient information
18.5–24.9	11.5–16 (25–35)	17–25 (37–55)
25.0–29.9	7–11.5 (15–25)	14–23 (31–51)
≥30[a]	5–9 (11–20)	11–19 (24–41)

[a]See Table 2.6 for our recommendations.
Source: From Ref. 38.

- **Blood pressure:** Should be performed and recorded at each visit.
- **Fetal heart tones:** Should be performed and recorded at each visit after the first trimester.
- **Symphyseal-fundal height measurement:** Can be performed at each visit from the 24th through 41st weeks. Fundal height measurement may help to detect fetal growth restriction (FGR) and macrosomia, but there is poor intra- and inter-user reliability. There is probably some value in evaluating trends and although it will not impact on the underlying condition, it may affect decision-making on fetal surveillance. **There is insufficient evidence to show whether this measurement has any impact, beneficial or not, on pregnancy outcomes, with no effect in the only one trial** (15) (see also chap. 44 in *Maternal-Fetal Evidence Based Guidelines*).
- **Cervical examination:** Routine digital examination of the cervix is not recommended as a screening measure for prevention of PTB (see chap. 16 in *Maternal-Fetal Evidence Based Guidelines*).

    Sweeping or "stripping" of membranes during cervical exam at ≥38 weeks reduces the rate of postterm delivery (see chap. 24). Cervical examination may assist in the identification of abnormal presentation, and therefore the opportunity to offer appropriate intervention (i.e., version).
- **Fetal movement:** There is no evidence that formalized kick counts reduce the incidence of fetal death in the healthy singleton (16) (see chap. 55 in *Maternal-Fetal Evidence Based Guidelines*). Nonetheless, women may be instructed to be aware of daily fetal movements from at or around 28 weeks.
- **Leopold's maneuvers:** Perform at each visit from 34 weeks to estimate fetal weight and determine presentation. Ultrasound can be used to confirm findings, and interventions may be offered (17,18).
- **Clinical pelvimetry:** Measurement of the bony birth canal is of limited, unproven value in predicting dystocia during delivery (see chaps. 7 and 8).
- **Routine evaluation for edema:** Edema has traditionally been a part of the evaluation for preeclampsia, but by itself, it is neither specific nor sensitive.

Follow-up Laboratory Screening

- **11 to 13 6/7 weeks: Serum aneuploidy screening, with nuchal translucency screening by ultrasound** (see below), should be offered to every pregnant woman (see chap. 5) (Table 2.1).
- **14 to 21 weeks:** The second part of serum aneuploidy screening (best at 16–18 weeks) should be offered to all pregnant women interested in prenatal diagnosis of aneuploidy (see chap. 5). Counseling regarding the variety of screening options and the limitations of testing should be made available to all pregnant women.

- **24 to 28 weeks:** Women with risk factors for GDM should be screened with either one-step or two-step tests, since intervention (diet, exercise, glucose monitoring, and, as necessary, medical therapy) prevents maternal and perinatal morbidities (see chap. 5 in *Maternal-Fetal Evidence Based Guidelines*). Universal **glucose challenge screening for GDM** is the most sensitive approach, but the following women are at low risk and less likely to benefit from testing (must meet all of the following criteria): age <25 years; ethnic origin of low-risk (not Hispanic, African, Native American, South or East Asian, or Pacific Islander); BMI <25; no previous personal or family history of impaired glucose tolerance; and no previous history of adverse obstetric outcomes associated with GDM. Antibody screening and hemoglobin and hematocrit are also repeated. Repeat screening of rapid plasma reagin (RPR) [or venereal disease research laboratory (VDRL)] and HIV in the early third trimester and at delivery can be considered for high-risk populations (see chaps. 32 and 35 in *Maternal-Fetal Evidence Based Guidelines*).
- **35 to 37 weeks: Group B Streptococcus (GBS)** is a significant cause of morbidity and mortality in neonates. Approximately 10% to 30% of pregnant women are asymptomatically colonized with GBS in the vagina or rectum. Vertical transmission of this organism from mother to fetus occurs most commonly after onset of labor or rupture of membranes. All women should be screened for GBS colonization by rectovaginal culture at 35 to 37 weeks of gestation. Colonized women should be treated with IV antibiotics (penicillin is first choice if not allergic) in labor or with rupture of membranes (see chap. 37 in *Maternal-Fetal Evidence Based Guidelines*).

Ultrasonography (see chap. 4)

Ultrasound has not been proven harmful to mother or fetus.

- **First-trimester "fetal dating" ultrasonography (before 14 weeks' gestation):** First-trimester ultrasound is more accurate than LMP to determine gestational age. First-trimester ultrasound also allows earlier detection of multiple pregnancies, aneuploidy screening with nuchal translucency, and diagnosis of nonviable pregnancies.
- **Second-trimester "fetal anatomy" ultrasound:** Generally, women are offered an ultrasound at 18 to 22 weeks' gestation to screen for structural anomalies. Routine use of ultrasound reduces the incidence of postterm pregnancies and rates of induction of labor for postterm pregnancy, increases early detection of multiple pregnancies, increases earlier detection of major fetal anomalies when termination of pregnancy is possible, increases detection rates of fetal malformations, and decreases admission to special care nursery (19,20). Given the benefits mentioned, all pregnant women should be offered a second-trimester ultrasound. No significant differences are detected for substantive clinical outcomes such as perinatal mortality, possibly because of insufficient data.
- **Third-trimester "fetal growth" ultrasound:** In low-risk or unselected populations, routine third-trimester ultrasound has not been associated with improvements in perinatal mortality (21). Selective ultrasound in later pregnancy is of benefit in specific situations, such as calculation of interval growth for suspected FGR, assessment of amniotic fluid index for suspect oligo- or hydramnios, and assessment of malpresentation (see chap. 4).

- Routine umbilical artery or other Doppler ultrasound in low-risk or unselected patients has not been shown to be of benefit.

CONTENT OF PRENATAL CARE

The content of prenatal care is extensive and reviewed in detail not only in this chapter but also in most other chapters in this book, as well as its companion, *Maternal-Fetal Evidence Based Guidelines*. In chapter 1, "Preconception Care," see Table 1.2 for topics to be reviewed, Table 1.3 for screening, Table 1.4 for laboratory tests, Table 1.5 for vaccinations, Table 1.6 for interventions for all women, and Table 1.7 for interventions for women with risk factors. Prenatal care usually incorporates, among other things, the following:

- **Prenatal education and reassurance** (regarding drugs, environment, lifestyle, nutrition, supplements, vaccinations, preventive measures, preparation for labor and delivery, depression, breastfeeding, etc.)
- Provision of evidence-based screening tests at appropriate intervals (Table 2.1)
- Risk assessment
- Problem-oriented visits as needed
- Condition-specific care for high-risk patients

Content issues that should be included in prenatal care such as drugs and environment, lifestyle, nutrition, supplements, vaccinations, prenatal education, and others are described below.

Drugs and Environment
Substance Abuse
Screening for use and counseling for cessation of tobacco, alcohol, and recreational or illicit drug use is recommended (see chaps. 22 and 23 in *Maternal-Fetal Evidence Based Guidelines*). Maternal smoking as well as exposure to secondhand smoke is hazardous to both the woman and her fetus. Offers of personal advice and educational material tailored to pregnancy are shown to increase smoking cessation by 70% and reduce LBW and PTB (22–24).

Alcohol use at any level in pregnancy cannot be supported although deleterious effects at low-moderate levels are difficult to quantify (25). The evidence from the limited number of studies suggests that **psychological and educational interventions may result in increased abstinence from alcohol, and a reduction in alcohol consumption among pregnant women.** However, results were not consistent, and the paucity of studies, the number of total participants, the high risk of bias of some of the studies, and the complexity of interventions limit our ability to determine the type of intervention that would be most effective in increasing abstinence from, or reducing the consumption of, alcohol among pregnant women (26). Counseling may be effective in reducing substance abuse in pregnancy, although women with addictions will need specialized interventions. There is insufficient evidence to recommend the routine use of home visits for women with a drug or alcohol problem (27).

Over-the-Counter, Alternative/Complementary, and Prescription Medications
Because of the possibility of adverse fetal effects, medication use, including alternative remedies, should be limited to circumstances where benefit outweighs risk. Beneficial medications should be continued in pregnancy when safe for both mother and fetus (see specific disease guidelines in *Maternal-Fetal Evidence Based Guidelines*).

Environmental/Occupational Risks and Exposures
In general, working is not associated with poor pregnancy outcome. Some workplace exposures, such as toxic chemicals, radiation (>5 rad), heavy repeated lifting, prolonged (>8 hours) standing, excessive (>80/wk) work hours, and high fatigue score may be associated with pregnancy complications, but there is insufficient evidence on the effect of avoidance of these risks (see also chap. 16). There is insufficient safety data for paint, solvents, hair dyes, fumes, anesthetic drugs, etc., with no absolute evidence of harm. Hot tubs, saunas, etc. should avoid temperatures >102°F to avoid risk of dehydration, especially in first trimester. After 14 weeks, all these exposures are probably not harmful.

Domestic Violence
Domestic violence against pregnant women is associated with increased risk of PTB, LBW, second- and third-trimester bleeding, and fetal injury. Domestic violence may escalate during pregnancy. As such, providers need to be alert to signs and symptoms of abuse and provide opportunities for private disclosure.

Lifestyle
Exercise
Regular exercise during low-risk pregnancies is beneficial as it increases overall maternal fitness and sense of well-being, with insufficient data to assess impact on maternal or fetal outcomes or assess effect in high-risk pregnancies (28). There is no reported effect on PTB, LBW, or other maternal or perinatal outcome (28). In a meta-analysis, **exercise was associated with a lower (by 600 g) gestational weight gain** (29). Possible maternal benefits include improved cardiovascular function, limited pregnancy weight gain, decreased musculoskeletal discomfort, reduced incidence of muscle cramps and lower limb edema, mood stability, and attenuation of GDM and gestational hypertension. Fetal benefits include decreased fat mass, improved stress tolerance, and advanced neurobehavioral maturation (30). **Twenty minutes of light exercise five times a week** has not been associated with detrimental effects. Exercise in pregnancy should still increase heart rate (up to 140 is safe with normal cardiac function, and this may vary by age and exercise tolerance). **Walking, swimming, and other sports with low chance of loss of balance are recommended.** Avoid contact sports and sports with high chance of loss of balance. Avoid hypoglycemia and dehydration.

Travel
Counseling should include the proper use of passenger restraint systems in automobiles, reduction of risk of venous thromboembolism during long-distance air travel by walking and exercise, and provision of care and prevention of illness during travel abroad.

Sex and Sexuality
Intercourse has not been associated with adverse outcomes in pregnancy. Women have a progressive decrease in sexual desire during the pregnancy, most markedly in the third trimester. Couples are often concerned that intercourse may harm the pregnancy. This is associated with progressively decreasing frequency of sexual intercourse in pregnancy (31). Most women desire more communication regarding sex in pregnancy by their care providers. Health care provider counseling should be reassuring, in the absence of pregnancy complications. Semen is a source of prostaglandin, pyospermia

is associated with preterm premature rupture of membranes (PPROM), and orgasms and nipple stimulation do increase contractions (32). Therefore, sexual intercourse may be detrimental in women with cervical dilatation and/or shortening but this is not well studied. PTB and other complications of pregnancy do not seem increased in most studies of sex in pregnancy. **Most studies report that sexual activity is associated with better pregnancy outcomes**, probably because women who are sexually active are healthier to begin with compared to women with less sexual activity (33).

Nutrition

Energy/Protein Supplementation
In five trials (1135 women), nutritional advice to increase energy and protein intakes was successful in achieving those goals, but no consistent benefit was observed on pregnancy outcomes.

In 13 trials (4665 women), **balanced energy/protein supplementation** was associated with modest increases in maternal weight gain and in mean birth weight, and a substantial **reduction in risk of SGA birth**. These effects did not appear greater in undernourished women. No significant effects were detected on PTB, but **significantly reduced risks were observed for stillbirth and neonatal death**.

In two trials (529 women), **high-protein supplementation was associated with** a small, nonsignificant increase in maternal weight gain but a nonsignificant reduction in mean birth weight, a **significantly increased risk of SGA birth**, and a nonsignificantly increased risk of neonatal death. In three trials, involving 966 women, **isocaloric protein supplementation was also associated with an increased risk of SGA birth**.

In four trials (457 women), energy/protein restriction of pregnant women who were overweight, or exhibited high weight gain, significantly reduced weekly maternal weight gain and mean birth weight but had no effect on pregnancy-induced hypertension or preeclampsia (34) (see also chap. 3 in *Maternal-Fetal Evidence Based Guidelines*).

Cholesterol-Lowering Diet
A cholesterol-lowering diet with omega-3 fatty acids and dietary counseling does not affect cord or neonatal lipids but is associated with a 90% reduction in preterm delivery <37 weeks in one trial (35) (see also chap. 16).

Low–Glycemic Index Diet
A low–glycemic index diet appears to be beneficial to both mother and child in reducing the incidence of abnormal glucose tolerance tests, large-for-gestational-age (LGA) infants, and ponderal indices. The numbers of studies and subjects are small, however, and therefore considered inconclusive (36).

Antigen Avoidance Diet
In high-risk women, an antigen avoidance diet (e.g., avoiding chocolate and nuts) in pregnancy is not associated with a reduction in the incidence of a child's development of atopic

Table 2.5 Food Safety in Pregnancy

Clean: Wash hands thoroughly with soap and water, before and after handling food, using the bathroom, changing diapers, or handling pets. Wash cutting boards, dishes, utensils, and countertops with soap and water. Rinse raw fruits and vegetables well, under running water.
Separate: Separate raw meats and seafood from fresh or prepared foods. Use a separate cutting board for raw meats and seafood. Place prepared food on a clean plate.
Cook: Cook foods thoroughly. Avoid allowing foods to sit at temperatures between 40°F and 140°F (4°C and 60°C). Discard foods left out at room temperature for more than 2 hours. Avoid foods made with raw eggs.
Chill: Maintain refrigerator temperature at 40°F (4°C) or below and the freezer at 0°F (−18°C).

diseases; and such diet may be detrimental, as it is associated with a decrease in BW (37).

Food Safety
Food safety and prevention of food-borne illness and infection are suggested in Tables 2.3 and 2.5.

BMI and Weight Gain
BMI is utilized in counseling a woman on optimal weight gain in pregnancy (Table 2.2).

Suggested weight gain in pregnancy is shown in Table 2.4 (38). Women who are underweight are at increased risk for LBW and PTB and have better outcomes with a higher total weight gain (39–41). Excessive weight gain in women with normal BMI can be prevented with dietary and lifestyle counseling (42,43). Obesity is associated with cardiovascular disease; diabetes; hypertension; stroke; osteoarthritis; gallstones; increased incidence of endometrial, breast, and colon cancer; cardiomyopathy; fatty liver; obstructive sleep apnea; urinary tract infections; other complications; and, most importantly, mortality. Prepregnancy obesity and excessive gestational weight gain are associated with increased risk of childhood obesity. Obese pregnant women are specifically at increased risk for miscarriage, congenital malformations, GDM, hypertension, preeclampsia, stillbirth, cesarean birth, labor abnormalities, macrosomia, anesthesia complications, wound infection, and thromboembolism. These women have better outcomes with lower (or no) total weight gain (39,44–50) (Table 2.6) (see also chap. 3 in *Maternal-Fetal Evidence Based Guidelines*).

Caffeine
The evidence is insufficient to make recommendations regarding caffeine intake. Based on non-RCT data, a maximum of three servings of caffeine a day has been suggested. Reducing the caffeine intake of regular coffee drinkers (3+ cups/day) during the second and third trimester by an average of 182 mg/day did not affect birth weight or length of gestation in one RCT (51).

Table 2.6 Weight Gain Suggestions for Overweight and Obese Women

Prepregnancy weight category	Our suggested total weight gain range (lb)	IOM recommendations (lb)
Overweight (BMI 25–29.9 kg/m^2)	6–20 (2.7–9.0 kg)	15–25 (6.8–11.4 kg)
Class I obesity (BMI 30–34.9 kg/m^2)	5–15 (2.3–6.8 kg)	11–20 (5–9.1 kg)
Class II obesity (BMI 35–39.9 kg/m^2)	−9–9 (−4.0–4.0 kg)	11–20 (5–9.1 kg)
Class III obesity (BMI >40 kg/m^2)	−15–0 (−6.8–0 kg)	11–20 (5–9.1 kg)

Abbreviation: IOM, Institute of Medicine.

Supplements

Multivitamin

There is **insufficient evidence** to suggest replacement of iron and folate supplementation with a multiple-micronutrient supplement. A reduction in the number of LBW and SGA babies and maternal anemia has been found with a multiple-micronutrient supplement compared to supplementation with two or less micronutrients or none or a placebo, but analyses revealed no added benefit of multiple-micronutrient supplements compared with iron and folic acid supplementation (52,53). These results are limited by the small number of studies available. There is also insufficient evidence to identify which micronutrients are more effective, to assess adverse effects, and to say that excess multiple-micronutrient supplementation during pregnancy is harmful to the mother or the fetus (52,53). Therefore, there is **insufficient evidence** to recommend routine multivitamin supplementation for all women, or even only for women who are underweight, have poor diets, smokers, substance abusers, vegetarians, multiple gestations, or others. **Excess (>1) prenatal vitamin intake per day should be avoided. No prenatal multivitamin supplement has been shown to be superior to another.** Use of multivitamin supplement not specific for pregnancy should be discouraged, as often excess doses can pose risks to the pregnancy. Each supplement, including each vitamin supplement, should be studied for safety and efficacy individually.

Folic Acid

Folic acid supplementation is recommended, with minimum 400 μg/day for all women (93% decrease in NTDs), and 5 mg/day for women with prior children with NTD (69% decrease in NTD) (54,55). Supplementation should start at least 1 month before conception and continue until at least 28 days after conception (time of neural tube closure). Given the unpredictability of conception and that 50% of pregnancies are unplanned, all reproductive-age women should be on folic acid supplementation. Because in several countries the baseline serum folate level is only 5 ng/mL, and increases in this level are directly proportional with a decrease in the incidence of NTD, some experts have advocated 5 mg of folic acid per day as optimal supplementation (56). No increase in ectopic pregnancy, miscarriage, or stillbirth has been associated with folate supplementation, but it might increase (nonsignificant trend) the incidence of multiple gestations by 40% (56,57). Folic acid supplementation has been associated (one non-RCT study) with decrease in severe language delay at 3 years of age (58). Fortifying basic foods such as grains with added folate is associated with an increase in supplementation of only 140 to 200 μg/day, and with only a 20% to 50% decrease in incidence of NTD, with the potential for large-scale prevention (57). Women taking antiseizure medications, other drugs that might interfere with folic acid metabolism, those with homozygous methylenetetrahydrofolate reductase (MTHFR) enzyme mutations, or those who are obese may need higher doses of folate supplementation. Women with first-trimester diabetes mellitus or exposure to valproic acid or high temperatures might not experience decrease in NTD risk with folate supplementation due to these risks (see also chap. 1).

Vitamin A

In pregnancy, some extra vitamin A is required for growth and tissue maintenance in the fetus, for providing fetal reserves, and for maternal metabolism (59). However, vitamin A in its synthetic form as well as in large doses as retinol (preformed vitamin A found in cod liver oil and chicken or beef liver) is teratogenic. It is recommended that pregnant women ingest vitamin A as β-carotene and limit the ingestion of retinol during pregnancy (60). In vitamin A–deficient populations (where night blindness is present), and in HIV-positive women, vitamin A supplementation reduces maternal night blindness and anemia (59).**Excess vitamin A intake can cause birth defects and miscarriages at doses >25,000 IU/day.** Vitamin A supplements should be avoided, with maximum daily intake prior to and during pregnancy probably 5000 IU and certainly ≤10,000 IU, respectively. **Vitamin A supplementation may be beneficial in women with vitamin A deficiency, especially in prevention of night blindness, in developing countries** (59,60). Optimal duration of supplement use cannot be evaluated. One large population-based trial in Nepal shows a possible beneficial effect on maternal mortality after weekly vitamin A supplements. Night blindness, associated with vitamin A deficiency, was assessed in a nested case-control study within this trial and found to be reduced but not eliminated. There is insufficient evidence to support vitamin A supplementation as an intervention for anemia (59,60).

Vitamin B6 (Pyridoxine)

There is **insufficient evidence** to evaluate pyridoxine supplementation during pregnancy. There are few trials, reporting few clinical outcomes and mostly with unclear trial methodology and inadequate follow-up. There is not enough evidence to detect clinical benefits of vitamin B6 supplementation in pregnancy and/or labor other than one trial suggesting protection against dental decay (61). For the aim of decreasing dental decay or missing/filled teeth, pyridoxine supplementation 20 mg/day (lozenges or capsules) is associated with decreased incidence of these outcomes in pregnant women (62).

Vitamin C

The **data are insufficient** to assess if vitamin C supplementation either alone or in combination with other supplements is beneficial during pregnancy for either low- or high-risk women. There may be an associated increased risk of PTB with vitamin C supplementation (RR 1.38, 95% CI 1.04–1.82, 3 trials, 583 women) (63). Except for this difference, no other difference in outcome is noted between vitamin C supplementation versus no treatment or placebo. There are very limited trials available to assess whether vitamin C supplementation may be useful for all pregnant women. Usually the women involved in the trials were either at high risk of preeclampsia or PTB or the women had established severe early-onset preeclampsia (see also chap. 1 in *Maternal-Fetal Evidence Based Guidelines*). No difference is seen between women supplemented with vitamin C alone or in combination with other supplements compared with placebo for the risk of stillbirth, neonatal death, LBW, or intrauterine growth restriction (63).

Vitamin D

There is insufficient evidence to evaluate the effects of vitamin D supplementation during pregnancy (64). Vitamin D 1000 IU/day in the third trimester is associated with no consistent effect on incidence of LBW (64). **Neonatal hypocalcemia is less common** with vitamin D supplementation compared to placebo (64). There are limited data to assess any benefit of vitamin D supplements for complete vegetarians and women with extremely limited exposure to sunlight.

Vitamin E

There is **insufficient evidence** to assess if vitamin E supplementation either alone or in combination with other supplements is beneficial during pregnancy (65). There are no trials available to assess whether vitamin E supplementation may be useful for all pregnant women, or if vitamin E may be beneficial when used alone. All evidence tested women at high risk of preeclampsia or with established preeclampsia and assessed vitamin E in combination with other supplements (usually vitamin C) (see chap. 1 in *Maternal-Fetal Evidence Based Guidelines*). Compared to placebo, vitamin E in combination with other supplements during pregnancy is associated with similar risk of stillbirth, neonatal death, perinatal death, PTB, preeclampsia, intrauterine growth restriction, and LBW (65).

Magnesium

Numerous studies demonstrate an association between magnesium supplementation and decreased incidences of LBW, SGA, antenatal hospitalization, and antenatal hemorrhage. The majority of RCTs are of poor quality and the one judged to be of high quality did not support these associations. There is **insufficient high-quality evidence** to show that dietary magnesium supplementation during pregnancy is beneficial (66). Including high- and low-quality trials, oral magnesium treatment from before the 25th week of gestation is associated with a lower frequency of PTB, a lower frequency of LBW, and fewer SGA infants compared with placebo (67). In addition, magnesium-treated women have less hospitalization during pregnancy and fewer cases of antepartum hemorrhage than placebo-treated women. Incidences of preeclampsia and all other outcomes are similar. In the analysis of one high-quality trial, no differences between magnesium and placebo groups are seen. Poor-quality trials are likely to have resulted in a bias favoring magnesium supplementation (67).

Calcium

Calcium supplementation is associated with a **reduction of the incidence of preeclampsia in pregnancy in all women, particularly for women at high risk of hypertension and in women with low dietary calcium intake** (e.g., <600 mg/day) (67). The minimum dose in the Cochrane review was 1 g/day. Further research is needed to determine whether dietary sources of calcium confer the same benefit and at what amount. There is insufficient evidence to determine optimum dosage and the effect on other important maternal and fetal outcomes. There is no overall reduction in preterm delivery, although there is **reduction in PTB among women at high risk of developing hypertension**. There is no evidence of any effect of calcium supplementation on stillbirth or death before discharge from hospital. In women at high risk of hypertension, calcium supplementation is associated with fewer babies with birth weight <2500 g. In one study, childhood systolic blood pressure >95th percentile was reduced (67) (see also chap. 1 in *Maternal-Fetal Evidence Based Guidelines*).

Iron

There is no evidence to advise against a policy of routine iron and folate supplementation in pregnancy. Iron supplementation is associated with **prevention of low hemoglobin at birth or at 6 weeks postpartum** (68). Iron supplementation, however, has no detectable effect on any substantive measures of either maternal or fetal outcome. One trial, with the largest number of participants of selective versus routine supplementation, shows an increased likelihood of cesarean section and postpartum blood transfusion, but a lower perinatal mortality

rate (up to 7 days after birth). There are few data derived from communities where iron deficiency is common and anemia is a serious health problem (68). There is limited evidence for daily versus intermittent supplementation. High-dose supplementation (80 mg daily) has no clinical advantage over low-dose supplementation (20 mg daily) and is associated with more gastrointestinal (GI) side effects. One RCT suggests adverse effects of hemoconcentration from iron supplementation in nonanemic women (68). For iron supplementation for women with anemia, see chapter 14 in *Maternal-Fetal Evidence Based Guidelines*.

Zinc

There is insufficient evidence to evaluate fully the effect of zinc supplementation during pregnancy. Zinc supplementation is associated with **significant reduction in PTB** (RR 0.86, 95% CI 0.76–0.98; 13 RCTs; 6854 women). These studies were primarily from a low social-economic population and **may reflect overall poor nutrition**. The reductions in induction of labor and cesarean delivery are from small studies, with no other differences detected between groups of women who had zinc supplementation and those who had either placebo or no zinc during pregnancy. There is insufficient evidence to assess the best dose, gestational age and duration, and population for zinc supplementation in pregnancy (69).

Iodine

Iodine is essential for normal fetal thyroid and brain development. Iodine supplementation **in populations with low iodine intake and high levels of endemic cretinism** results in an important reduction in the incidence of the condition with no apparent adverse effects. Iodine supplementation is associated with **a reduction in deaths during infancy and early childhood, with decreased endemic cretinism at the age of 4 years and better psychomotor development scores between 4 to 25 months of age** (28). There is little data, however, on the safety of routine iodine supplementation in populations with normal or low normal iodine levels. Some data suggest an increased risk of fetal and maternal hypothyroidism from iodine supplementation. The upper levels of safety have not been established (70,71).

Vaccinations

Immunity to **rubella, varicella, hepatitis B, influenza, tetanus, and pertussis should be assessed at the first prenatal visit. Ideally, needed vaccinations would be provided preconception.** There is no vaccine that is more dangerous to a pregnant woman or her fetus than the disease it is designed to prevent. Recombinant, inactivated, and subunit vaccines, as well as toxoids, and immunoglobulins pose no threat to a developing fetus. Inactivated influenza vaccine should be given (by injection, as killed virus) to all pregnant women during the influenza season. The live attenuated form of the vaccine (intranasal spray) should not be given during pregnancy. Hepatitis B vaccine can be safely given in pregnancy. Tdap vaccination is given before postpartum discharge from the hospital. For pregnancies at high risk for neonatal tetanus or pertussis, Tdap may be used during pregnancy (see Table 1.5 in chap. 1, and chap. 38 in *Maternal-Fetal Evidence Based Guidelines*).

Abdominal Decompression

Abdominal decompression consists of a rigid dome placed about the abdomen and covered with an airtight suit, with the space around the abdomen decompressed to −50 to −100 mmHg for 15 to 30 seconds out of each minute for 30 minutes once to thrice daily, or with uterine contractions during labor. This is thought to "pump" blood through the intervillous space. There is no evidence to support the use of abdominal decompression in normal pregnancies. There is no difference between the abdominal decompression groups and the control groups for LBW, admission for preeclampsia, low Apgar score, perinatal mortality, and childhood development (72).

Prevention of Complications

Please see specific diseases in each chapter of this book, and its companion, *Maternal-Fetal Evidence Based Guidelines*. Here are reported only some general, nonspecific interventions.

Antibiotic prophylaxis of pregnant women with no specific risk factor or infection is associated with similar incidence of PPROM, PTB, and postpartum endometritis (73,74) (see also chap. 16).

Programs offering **additional social support** (caring family members, friends, and health professionals) for at-risk (e.g., for PTB and LBW) pregnant women are not associated with improvements in any perinatal outcomes, but there is a **reduction in the likelihood of antenatal hospital admission** (RR 0.79, 95% CI 0.68–0.92) and **cesarean birth** (RR 0.87, 95% CI 0.78–0.97) (75).

For issues such as mild hypertension or preeclampsia, small studies suggest that there are no major differences in clinical outcomes for mothers or babies between antenatal day units or hospital admission, but women may prefer day care (76) (see also chap. 1 in *Maternal-Fetal Evidence Based Guidelines*).

Prenatal Education

There is insufficient evidence to assess the effectiveness of formal prenatal education programs. **Prenatal education directed at specific objectives (e.g., promoting breastfeeding and avoiding planned induction of labor) has been demonstrated to be effective** (77,78). Individualized prenatal education directed toward avoidance of a cesarean delivery does not increase the rate of vaginal birth after cesarean section (79). As a part of prenatal care, women should be provided with information and instruction regarding their health, including risk avoidance, breastfeeding, what to expect during labor and birth (see subsection "Preparation for Labor and Delivery"), how to obtain care when labor begins, and the value of a support person during the labor process (see chaps. 7 and 8).

Community Interventions

There is encouraging evidence of the value of integrating maternal and newborn care in community settings through a range of interventions that can be packaged effectively for delivery through a range of community health workers and health promotion groups. Such evidence-based available interventions as immunization to mothers, clean and skilled care at delivery, newborn resuscitation, exclusive breastfeeding, clean umbilical cord care, and management of infections in newborns require facility-based and outreach services. **Implementation of community-based interventional care packages is associated with a trend for reduction in maternal mortality** (RR 0.77, 95% CI 0.59–1.02) **and with significant reductions in maternal morbidity** (RR 0.75, 95% CI 0.61–0.92), **neonatal mortality** (RR 0.76; 95% CI 0.68–0.84), **stillbirths** (RR 0.84, 95% CI 0.74–0.97), **and perinatal mortality** (RR 0.80; 95% CI

0.71–0.91). It also increases the referrals to health facility for pregnancy-related complication by 40% and improves the rates of early breastfeeding by 94% (80).

Preparation for Labor and Delivery

Perineal massage with sweet almond oil for 5 to 10 minutes daily from 34 weeks until delivery is associated with a significantly higher chance of intact perineum compared to no massage in nulliparous, but probably not multiparous women (81–83). For perineal massage in labor, see chapter 8, "Second Stage of Labor."

Women should be provided with written information and instruction regarding what to expect during labor and delivery, how to obtain care when labor begins, and the value of a support person during the labor process (see chaps. 7 and 8).

Compared to no such training, 9 hours of **antenatal classes with training to prepare for labor and delivery** are associated with **arriving to L&D ward more often in active labor** (RR 1.45, 95% CI 1.26–1.65) and **using less epidural analgesia** (RR 0.84, 95% CI 0.73–0.97) (84).

Compared to standard antenatal education, antenatal education focusing on natural childbirth preparation with training in breathing and relaxation techniques is not associated with any effects on maternal or perinatal outcomes, including similar incidences of epidural analgesia, childbirth, or parental stress, in nulliparous women and their partners (85).

Compared to conventional therapy, intensive counseling therapy for fear of childbirth does not affect the incidence of cesarean but is associated with reduced pregnancy- and birth-related anxiety and concerns, and shorter labors in one RCT (86).

In a small RCT, **a specific antenatal education program is associated with a reduction in the mean number of visits to the labor suite before the onset of labor** (4). It is unclear whether this results in fewer women being sent home because they are not in labor (87) (see also chap. 7).

Depression in Pregnancy and the Postpartum Period

Between 14% and 23% of pregnant women will experience a depressive mood disorder while pregnant (88). Maternal anxiety, life stress, history of depression, lack of social support, unintended pregnancy, Medicaid insurance, domestic violence, lower income, lower education, smoking, single status, and poor relationship quality were associated with a greater likelihood of antepartum depressive symptoms in bivariate analyses. Life stress, lack of social support, and domestic violence continued to demonstrate a significant association in multivariate analyses (89). Identification of risk factors and screening for depression will facilitate referral for treatment (see chap. 21 in *Maternal-Fetal Evidence Based Guidelines*).

Between 5% and 7% of women will experience postpartum depression. Risk factors include antenatal depressive symptoms, a history of major depressive disorder, or previous postpartum major depression. If left untreated, postpartum major depression can lead to poor mother-infant bonding, delays in infant growth and development, and an increased risk of anxiety or depressive symptoms in the infant later in life (90). **Identifying mothers at-risk assists the prevention of postpartum depression compared to intervening on the general population.** The provision of **intensive postpartum support provided by public health nurses or midwives** is associated with 32% less postpartum depression. Interventions with **only a postnatal component** appeared to be more beneficial than interventions that also incorporated an antenatal component. **Individual-based interventions** may be more effective than those that are group-based. Women who received multiple-contact intervention are just as likely to experience postpartum depression as those who received a single-contact intervention (91). **There is insufficient evidence to assess the effectiveness of antidepressants given immediately postpartum in preventing postnatal depression in all women or just in high-risk women** (92). Norethisterone enanthate, a synthetic progestogen, 200 mg IM administered once within 48 hours of delivery to unselected women is associated with a significantly higher risk of developing postpartum depression at 6 weeks (93) (see chap. 21 in *Maternal-Fetal Evidence Based Guidelines*).

Breastfeeding
Breastfeeding is the best feeding method for most infants and should be strongly encouraged (see chap. 27). **Counseling and education during pregnancy have been shown to facilitate breastfeeding success** (77). Attitudes of the health care provider are highly associated with breastfeeding success. Antigen avoidance diet during lactation by high-risk women may reduce the child's risk of developing atopic eczema, and may reduce atopic eczema in children already with atopic eczema during the first 12 to 18 months, although more trials are needed (37).

INTERVENTIONS FOR COMMON PREGNANCY COMPLAINTS
Itching
The differential diagnosis of itching in late pregnancy (>32 weeks) is presented in chapter 10 in *Maternal-Fetal Evidence Based Guidelines*. If the itching is not due to liver disease, and if there is no rash, aspirin (600 mg qid) has been reported to decrease itching (94), but because of potential detrimental fetal effects (closure of ductus arteriosus and oligohydramnios) should not be used. If there are both itching and a rash, chlorpheniramine 4 mg tid decreased itching in a small trial (94).

Stretch Marks
Some stretch marks (striae gravidarum) develop in about 50% of women by the end of pregnancy. **Massage with Trofolastin cream (*C. asiatica* extract, α-tocopherol, and collagen elastin hydrolases) applied daily decreases the development of stretch marks by 59% compared to massage with placebo. Massage with Verum ointment (tocopherol, panthenol, hyaluronic acid, elastin, and menthol) decreases the development of stretch marks by 74% compared to no treatment. It is unclear in the study if the massage or the Verum ointment was beneficial.** In women with stretch marks from a previous pregnancy there is no benefit (95). It is unclear which one of the ingredients (or combination) is beneficial, and if massage itself has any effect. There is no proven treatment for stretch marks once they have developed (95).

Leg Cramps
Leg cramps are reported to occur in a reported 34% of pregnant women in the midtrimester (16). **Magnesium lactate or citrate chewable tablets 5 mmol in the morning and 10 mmol in the evening for 3 weeks are associated with one-third of women not having persistent leg cramps** compared to 94% of placebo controls having persistent cramps (96). Multivitamin with mineral supplement might decrease leg cramps, but it is unclear which one of the 12 ingredients (or combination) is beneficial. Sodium chloride is associated with a slight reduction although consideration must be given to potential effect on blood pressure. **Calcium supplements do not decrease leg cramps compared to placebo** (96). Calf stretching prior to bedtime does not decrease nocturnal leg cramps in nonpregnant patients (97).

Back and Pelvic Pain
Back pain is common in pregnancy, given weight gain and its uneven distribution as well as the softening effects of pregnancy hormones on the musculature. **Water gymnastics for 1 hour weekly starting at <19 weeks reduces back pain in pregnancy and allows more women to continue to work, with no adverse effects** (98). A special-shaped pillow (Ozzlo) used for 1 week when laying in a lateral position reduces back pain in late pregnancy and improves sleep compared to a regular pillow, but this pillow is no longer commercially available (99). **Pregnancy-specific exercises, physiotherapy, and acupuncture starting <32 weeks for 10 sessions appear to reduce back and pelvic pain** (98); individual acupuncture sessions are more beneficial than group physiotherapy sessions (98). Education, other exercises, massage, heat therapy, support belts, analgesic therapy, etc. have not been studied in a trial in pregnancy for back pain relief.

Constipation
Constipation is common in pregnancy, probably because of decreased bowel peristalsis (possibly related to increased progesterone). It is reported by nearly 70% of women in the midtrimester (99).

In nonpregnant adults, **exercise, increase in water intake, dietary counseling, and certain foods (e.g., prunes)** have been shown to relieve constipation. If these self-help measures are inadequate, the pregnant woman should then try daily bran or wheat fiber supplements.

Dietary fiber supplements (e.g., 10 mg/day of either corn-based biscuits—"Fibermed"—or 23 g wheat bran) increase the frequency of defecation and are associated with softer stools (99). Women who do not have sufficient benefit from fiber should be offered either stimulant laxatives or bulk-forming laxatives that may be less effective.

Stimulant laxatives (e.g., Senna 14 mg, or dioctyl sodium succinate 120 mg and dihydroxyanthroquinone 100 mg—Normax) are more effective at resolving constipation compared to bulk-forming laxatives (e.g., 10 mL of 60% sterculia and 40% frangula—Normacol standard, or 10 mL of 60% sterculia—Normacol special), but these stimulant laxatives are more likely to be associated with diarrhea and abdominal pain (99). Acceptability was similar between these two types of laxatives (99). **Docusate sodium** is a similar **stimulant laxative**, and it is widely available. These findings in pregnant women are consistent with nonpregnant evidence.

Varicosities and Leg Edema
A small RCT ($n = 69$) shows that rutoside capsules improve leg edema symptoms; however, there are insufficient data to confirm rutoside safety in pregnancy. Another small RCT ($n = 43$) demonstrates a reduction in leg edema with **reflexology**. Compression stockings are not effective compared to simple resting, but studies do not compare compression stockings

to no compression stockings. Leg elevation, compression hosiery, and swimming have not been studied for leg edema/varicosities relief in pregnancy (100).

Hemorrhoids

Hemorrhoids are common during pregnancy with 13% of women complaining of them in the midtrimester. **Oral hydroxyethylrutosides decrease symptoms compared to placebo group in women with hemorrhoids and reduce the signs identified by the health care provider** (101). Rutosides are associated with mild side effects such as GI discomfort, and their safety data in pregnancy are still insufficient. Constipation is a predisposing factor for hemorrhoids and should be treated. Sitz baths, ice, or ointments have been insufficiently studied for treatment of hemorrhoids in pregnancy (101).

Heartburn

Heartburn is common during pregnancy with 53% of women complaining of it in the midtrimester (16).

A consensus document has recommended that lifestyle and dietary modifications should remain first-line treatment for heartburn in pregnancy. The measures include reducing and avoiding intake of reflux-inducing foods (e.g., greasy and spicy foods, tomatoes, highly acidic citrus products, and carbonated drinks) and substances such as caffeine. Nonsteroidal anti-inflammatory drugs (NSAIDs) should also be avoided. Other lifestyle changes to reduce the risk of reflux, such as avoiding lying down within 3 hours after eating, are advised. However, if heartburn is severe enough to warrant this action, medication should begin after consultation with a health care professional. **Antacids, H$_2$ blockers, and proton pump inhibitors** all have acceptable safety profiles for the pregnant woman (102–104).

REFERENCES

1. Rosen MG, Merkatz IR, Hill JG. Caring for our future: a report by the expert panel on the content of prenatal care. Obstet Gynecol 1991; 77(5):782–787. [Review]
2. Alexander GR, Kotelchuck M. Assessing the role and effectiveness of prenatal care: history, challenges, and directions for future research. Public Health Rep 2001; 116(4):306–316. [II-3]
3. Novick G. Centering pregnancy and the current state of prenatal care. J Midwifery Women's Health 2004; 49(5):405–411. [Meta-analysis; 7 RCTs, n = >60,000]
4. Dowswell T, Carroli G, Duley L, et al. Alternative versus standard packages of antenatal care for low-risk pregnancy. Cochrane Database Syst Rev 2010; 10:CD000934. [Meta-analysis]
5. Ickovics JR, Kershaw TS, Westdahl C, et al. Group prenatal care and perinatal outcomes: a randomized controlled trial. Obstet Gynecol 2007; 110(2 pt 1):330–339. [RCT, n = 1047].
6. Hatem M, Sandall J, Devane D, et al. Midwife-led versus other models of care for childbearing women. Cochrane Database Syst Rev 2008; 1(4): CD004667. [11 RCTs, n = 12,276]
7. Gagnon AJ, Sandall J. Individual or group antenatal education for childbirth or parenthood, or both. Cochrane Database Syst Rev 2007; (3):CD002869. [Meta-analysis; 9 RCTs, n = 2284]
8. Manandhar DS, Osrin D, Shrestha BP, et al. Effect of participatory intervention with women's groups on birth outcomes in Nepal: cluster-randomized controlled trial. Lancet 2004; 364:970–979. [RCT, n = 6212]
9. Mushi D, Mpembeni R, Jahn A. Effectiveness of community based safe motherhood promoters in improving the utilization of obstetric care. The case of Mtwara Rural District in Tanzania. BMC Pregnancy Childbirth 2010; 10:14. [II-1]
10. Bhutta ZA, Lassi ZS. Empowering communities for maternal and newborn health. Lancet 2010; 375(9721):1142–1144. [Review]
11. Brown HC, Smith HJ. Giving women their own case notes to carry during pregnancy. Cochrane Database Syst Rev 2005; (3). [Meta-analysis; 3 RCTs, n = 675]
12. Duckitt K, Harrington D. Risk factors for pre-eclampsia at antenatal booking: systematic review of controlled studies. BMJ 2005; 330(7491):565. [II-2]
13. Alto WA. No need for glycosuria/proteinuria screen in pregnant women. J Fam Pract 2005; 54(11):978–983. [II-2]
14. Yinon Y, Farine D, Yudin MH, et al. Cytomegalovirus infection in pregnancy. J Obstet Gynaecol Can 2010; 32(4):348–354. [Review]
15. Lindhard A, Nielsen PV, Mouritsen LA, et al. The implications of introducing the symphyseal-fundal height measurement. A prospective randomized controlled trial. BJOG 1990; 97:675–680. [RCT, n = 1639]
16. Kamysheva BA, Wertheim EH, Skouteris H, et al. Frequency, severity, and effect on life of physical symptoms experienced during pregnancy. J Midwifery Women's Health 2009; 54:43–49. [II-2]
17. Nahum GG. Predicting fetal weight. Are Leopold's maneuvers still worth teaching to medical students and house staff? J Reprod Med 2002; 47(4):271–278. [II-3]
18. McFarlin BL, Engstrom JL, Sampson MB, et al. Concurrent validity of Leopold's maneuvers in determining fetal presentation and position. J Nurse Midwifery 1985; 30(5):280–284. [II-3]
19. Whitworth M, Bricker L, Neilson JP, et al. Ultrasound for fetal assessment in early pregnancy. Cochrane Database Syst Rev 2010; (4):CD007058. [11 trials including 37,505 women]
20. Neilson JP. Ultrasound for fetal assessment in early pregnancy. Cochrane Database Syst Rev 2010; (4):CD000182. [Meta-analysis]
21. Bricker L, Neilson JP, Dowswell T. Routine ultrasound in late pregnancy (after 24 weeks' gestation). Cochrane Database Syst Rev 2009; (1). [Meta-analysis]
22. Mullen PD. Maternal smoking during pregnancy and evidence-based intervention to promote cessation. Prim Care 1999; 26 (3):577–589. [Review]
23. Naughton F, Prevost AT, Sutton S. Self-help smoking cessation interventions in pregnancy: a systematic review and meta-analysis. Addiction 2008; 103(4):566–579. [Meta-analysis]
24. Lumley J, Chamberlain C, Dowswell T, et al. Interventions for promoting smoking cessation during pregnancy. Cochrane Database Syst Rev 2009; (3):CD001055. [Meta-analysis]
25. Henderson J, Gray R, Brocklehurst P. Systematic review of effects of low-moderate prenatal alcohol exposure on pregnancy outcome. BJOG 2007; 114(3):243–252. [II-1]
26. Stade BC, Bailey C, Dzendoletas D, et al. Psychological and/or educational interventions for reducing alcohol consumption in pregnant women and women planning pregnancy. Cochrane Database Syst Rev 2009; (2):CD004228. [Meta-analysis; 4 RCTs, n = 715]
27. Doggett C, Burrett SL, Osborn DA. Home visits during pregnancy and after birth for women with an alcohol or drug problem. Cochrane Database Syst Rev 2005; (4):CD004456. [Meta-analysis; 6 RCTs, n = 709]
28. Kramer MS, McDonald SW. Aerobic exercise for women during pregnancy. Cochrane Database Syst Rev 2010; (6). [14 RCTs, n = 1014]
29. Streuling I, Beyerlein A, Rosenfeld E, et al. Physical activity and gestational weight gain: a meta-analysis of intervention trials. BJOG 2010; 118(3):278–284. [Meta-analysis; 12 RCTs]
30. Melzer K, Schutz Y, Boulvain M, et al. Physical activity and pregnancy: cardiovascular adaptations, recommendations and pregnancy outcomes. Sports Med 2010; 40(6):493–507. [Review]
31. Serati M, Salvatore S, Siesto G, et al. Female sexual function during pregnancy and after childbirth. J Sex Med 2010; 7(8):2782–2790. [Review]
32. Kavanagh J, Kelly AJ, Thomas J. Sexual intercourse for cervical ripening and induction of labour. Cochrane Database Syst Rev 2001; (2):CD003093. [Meta-analysis]
33. Berghella V, Klebanoff M, McPherson C, et al. Sexual intercourse association with asymptomatic bacterial vaginosis and

trichomonas vaginalis treatment in relationship to preterm birth. Am J Obstet Gynecol 2002; 187:1277–1282. [II-2]

34. Kramer MS, Kakuma R. Energy and protein intake in pregnancy. Cochrane Database Syst Rev 2003; (4):CD000032. [Meta-analysis]

35. Khoury J, Henriksen T, Christophersen B, et al. Effect of a cholesterol-lowering diet on maternal, cord, and neonatal lipids, and pregnancy outcome: a randomized clinical trial. Am J Obstet Gynecol 2005; 193:1292–1301. [RCT, $n = 290$]

36. Tieu J, Crowther CA, Middleton P. Dietary advice in pregnancy for preventing gestational diabetes mellitus. Cochrane Database Syst Rev 2009; 3:CD006674. [3 trials, $n = 107$]

37. Kramer MS, Kakuma R. Maternal dietary antigen avoidance during pregnancy or lactation, or both, for preventing or treating atopic disease in the child. Cochrane Database Syst Rev 2006; (3):CD000133. [Meta-analysis; 5 RCTs, $n = 952$]

38. Rasmussen KM, Yaktine AL, eds. Committee to reexamine IOM pregnancy weight guidelines. Weight gain during pregnancy: reexamining the guidelines. Institute of Medicine; National Research Council. JAMA 2009; 302:241–242. [Guideline]

39. Kiel DW, Dodson EA, Artal R, et al. Gestational weight gain and pregnancy outcomes in obese women. How much is enough? Obstet Gynecol 2007; 110:752–758. [II-2]

40. Davies GA, Maxwell C, McLeod L, et al. Obesity in pregnancy. J Obstet Gynaecol Can 2010; 32(2):165–173. [Review]

41. Kramer MS. Energy/protein restriction for high weight-for-height or weight gain during pregnancy. Cochrane Database Syst Rev 2008. [Meta-analysis]

42. Asbee SM, Jenkins TR, Butler JR, et al. Preventing excessive weight gain during pregnancy through dietary and lifestyle counseling – a randomized controlled trial. Obstet Gynecol 2009; 113:305–312. [RCT, $n = 100$]

43. Polley BA, Wing RR, Sims CJ. Randomized controlled trial to prevent excessive weight gain in pregnant women. Intern J Obesity 2002; 26:1494–1502. [RCT, $n = 120$]

44. Siega-Riz AM, Viswanathan M, Moos M-K, et al. A systematic review of outcomes of maternal weight gain according to the Institute of Medicine recommendations: birthweight, fetal growth, and postpartum weight retention. Am J Obstet Gynecol 2009; 201:339.e1–339.e14. [Systematic review of 35 studies from 1990 to 2007]

45. Committee to Reexamine IOM Pregnancy Weight Guidelines, Food and Nutrition Board, and Board on Children, Youth, and Families. Weight gain during pregnancy: reexamining the guidelines. Washington, DC: Institute of Medicine, 2009. [Consensus report]

46. Oken E, Kleinman KP, Belfort MB, et al. Association of gestational weight gain with short- and longer-term maternal and child health outcomes. Am J Epidemiol 2009; 170:173–180. [II-2: project viva, Massachusetts 1999–2002 U.S. observational study, $n = 2012$]

47. Cedergren MI. Optimal gestational weight gain for body mass index categories. Obstet Gynecol 2007; 110(4):759–764. [II-2: Swedish Medical Birth Register, population-based cohort study, $n = 298,648$]

48. Nohr EA, Vaeth M, Baker JL, et al. Pregnancy outcomes related to gestational weight gain in women defined by their body mass index, parity, height, and smoking status. Am J Clin Nutr 2009; 90:1288–1294. [II-2: Danish population-based observational study, $n = 59,147$]

49. Dietz PM, Callaghan WM, Smith R, et al. Low pregnancy weight gain and small for gestational age: a comparison of the association using 3 different measures of small for gestational age. Am J Obstet Gynecol 2009; 201:53.e1–53.e7. [II-2: retrospective cohort study, Pregnancy Risk Assessment Monitoring System (PRAMS), $n = 104,980$]

50. Bianco AT, Smilen SW, Davis Y, et al. Pregnancy outcome and weight gain recommendations for the morbidly obese woman. Obstet Gynecol 1998; 91:97–102. [II-2, U.S. retrospective cohort study, $n = 11,926$]

51. Bech BH, Obel C, Henriksen TB, et al. Effect of reducing caffeine intake on birth weight and length of gestation: randomised controlled trial. BMJ 2007; 334:409. [RCT, $n = 1198$]

52. Shah PS, Ohlsson A. Effects of prenatal multimicronutrient supplementation on pregnancy outcomes: a meta-analysis. CMAJ 2009; 180(12):1188–1189. [Meta-analysis]

53. Haider BA, Bhutta ZA. Multiple-micronutrient supplementation for women during pregnancy. Cochrane Database Syst Rev 2006; (4):CD004905. [Meta-analysis; 9 RCTs, $n = 15,378$]

54. Lumley L, Watson L, Watson M, et al. Periconceptional supplementation with folate and/or multivitamins for preventing neural tube defects. Cochrane Database Syst Rev 2005; (3). [Meta-analysis; 4 RCTs, 6425 women]

55. De-Regil LM, Fernández-Gaxiola AC, Dowswell T, et al. Effects and safety of periconceptional folate supplementation for preventing birth defects. Cochrane Database Syst Rev 2010; (10): CD007950. [Meta-analysis]

56. Wald NJ. Folic acid and the prevention of neural-tube defects. N Engl J Med 2004; 350:101–103. [Editorial]

57. Honein MA, Paulozzi LJ, Mathews TJ, et al. Impact of folic acid fortification of the US food supply on the occurrence of neural tube defects. JAMA 2001; 285:2981–2986. [Observational]

58. Roth C, Magnus P, Schjolberg S, et al. Folic acid supplements in pregnancy and severe language delay in children. JAMA 2011; 306:1566–1573. [II-1]

59. van den Broek N, Dou L, Othman M, et al. Vitamin A supplementation during pregnancy for maternal and new-born outcomes. Cochrane Database Syst Rev 2010; (11): CD008666. [Meta-analysis]

60. Barger MK. Maternal nutrition and perinatal outcomes. J Midwifery Women's Health 2010; 55(6):502–511. [II-3]

61. Thaver D, Saeed MA, Bhutta ZA. Pyridoxine (vitamin B6) supplementation in pregnancy. Cochrane Database Syst Rev 2006; (2):CD000179. [5 RCTS, $n = 1646$]

62. Hillman RW, Cabaud PG, Schenone RA. The effects of pyridoxine supplements on the dental caries experience of pregnant women. Am J Clin Nutr 1962; 10:512–515. [1 RCT, $n = 371$]

63. Rumbold A, Crowther CA. Vitamin C supplementation in pregnancy. Cochrane Database Syst Rev 2005; (2):CD004072. [Meta-analysis; 5 RCTs, $n = 766$]

64. Mahomed K, Gulmezoglu AM. Vitamin D supplementation in pregnancy. Cochrane Database Syst Rev 2009; (1). [Meta-analysis]

65. Rumbold A, Crowther CA. Vitamin E supplementation in pregnancy. Cochrane Database Syst Rev 2005; (2):CD004069. [Meta-analysis; 5 RCTs, $n = 566$]

66. Makrides M, Crowther CA. Magnesium supplementation in pregnancy. Cochrane Database Syst Rev 2001; (4):CD000937. [7 RCTs, $n = 2689$]

67. Hofmeyr JG, Lawrie TA, Atallah AN, et al. Calcium supplementation during pregnancy for preventing hypertensive disorders and related problems. Cochrane Database Syst Rev 2010; (8): CD001059. [13 studies of good quality involving 15,730 women]

68. Pena-Rosas JP, Viteri FE. Effects and safety of preventive oral iron or iron+folic acid supplementation for women during pregnancy. Cochrane Database Syst Rev 2010; (2). [Meta-analysis]

69. Mahomed K, Bhutta ZA, Middleton P. Zinc supplementation for improving pregnancy and infant outcome. Cochrane Database Syst Rev 2007; (2):CD000230. [Meta-analysis; 17 RCTs, $n = >9000$]

70. Rebagliato M, Murcia M, Espada M, et al. Iodine intake and maternal thyroid function during pregnancy. Epidemiology 2010; 21(1):62–69. [II-2]

71. Pearce EN. What do we know about iodine supplementation in pregnancy? J Clin Endocrinol Metab 2009; 94(9):3188–3190. [Review]

72. Hofmeyr JG, Kulier R. Abdominal decompression in normal pregnancy. Cochrane Database Syst Rev 2010; (8). [Meta-analysis]

73. Thinkhamrop J, Hofmeyr GJ, Adetoro O, et al. Prophylactic antibiotic administration in pregnancy to prevent infectious morbidity and mortality. Cochrane Database Syst Rev 2002; (4):CD002250. [Meta-analysis; 6 RCTs, $n =2189$, both low- and high-risk women]

74. McGregor JA, French JI, Richter R, et al. Cervicovaginal micro-flora and pregnancy outcome: results of a double-blind, placebo-controlled trial of erythromycin treatment. Am J Obstet Gynecol 1990; 163:1580–1591. [RCT, *n* = 229]

75. Hodnett ED, Fredericks S, Weston J. Support during pregnancy for women at increased risk of low birthweight babies. Cochrane Database Syst Rev 2010; (6):CD000198. [Meta-analysis; 17 RCTs, *n* = 12,264]

76. Dowswell T, Middleton P, Weeks A. Antenatal day care units versus hospital admission for women with complicated pregnancy. Cochrane Database Syst Rev 2009; (4):CD001803. [Meta-analysis; 3 RCTs, *n* = 504]

77. Dyson L, McCormick F, Renfrew MJ. Interventions for promoting the initiation of breastfeeding. Cochrane Database Syst Rev 2005; (2):CD001688. [Meta-analysis]

78. Palda VA, Guise JM, Wathen CN. Interventions to promote breast-feeding: applying the evidence in clinical. CMAJ 2004; 170(6):976–978. [II-2]

79. Gagnon AJ. Individual or group antenatal education for child-birth/parenthood. Cochrane Database Syst Rev 2005; (3). [Meta-analysis; 6 RCTs, 1443 women]

80. Lassi ZS, Haider BA, Bhutta ZA. Community-based intervention packages for reducing maternal and neonatal morbidity and mortality and improving neonatal outcomes. Cochrane Database Syst Rev 2010; (11):CD007754. [Meta-analysis; 18 cluster-randomized studies]

81. Labrecque M, Marcoux S, Pinault JJ, et al. Prevention of perineal trauma by perineal massage during pregnancy: a pilot study. Birth 1994; 21:20–25. [RCT, *n* = 46]

82. Labrecque M, Eason E, Marcoux S, et al. Randomized controlled trial of prevention of perineal trauma by perineal massage during pregnancy. AJOG 1999; 180:593–600. [RCT, *n* = 1527]

83. Shipman MK, Boniface DR, Tefft ME, et al. Antenatal perineal massage and subsequent perineal outcomes: a randomized controlled trial. BJOG 1997; 104:787–791. [RCT, *n* = 861]

84. Maimburg RD, Vaeth M, Durr J, et al. Randomized trial of structured antenatal training sessions to improve the birth process. BJOG 2010; 117:921–928. [RCT, *n* = 1193]

85. Bergstrom M, Kieler H, Waldenstrom U. Effects of natural childbirth preparation versus standard antenatal education on epidural rates, experience of childbirth and parental stress in mothers and fathers: a randomized controlled trial. BJOG 2009; 116:1167–1176. [RCT, *n* = 1087]

86. Saisto T, Salmela-Aro K, Nurmi J-E, et al. A randomized controlled trial of intervention in fear of childbirth. Obstet Gynecol 2001; 98:820–826. [RCT, *n* = 176]

87. Bonovich L. Recognizing the onset of labour. J Obstet Gynecol Neonatal Nurs 1990; 19(2):141–145. [RCT, *n* = 245; 208 analyzed]

88. Yonkers KA, Wisner KL, Stewart DE, et al. The management of depression during pregnancy: a report from the American Psychiatric Association and the American College of Obstetricians and Gynecologists. Obstet Gynecol 2009; 114(3):703–713. [Review]

89. Lancaster CA, Gold KJ, Flynn HA, et al. Risk factors for depressive symptoms during pregnancy: a systematic review. Am J Obstet Gynecol 2010; 202(1):5–14. [Systematic review]

90. Hirst KP, Moutier CY. Postpartum major depression. Am Fam Physician 2010; 82(8):926–933. [Review]

91. Dennis CL, Creedy D. Psychosocial and psychological interventions for preventing postpartum depression. Cochrane Database Syst Rev 2004; (4):CD001134. [Meta-analysis]

92. Howard LM, Hoffbrand S, Henshaw C, et al. Antidepressant prevention of postnatal depression. Cochrane Database Syst Rev 2005; (2):CD004363. [Meta-analysis]

93. Lawrie TA, Hofmeyr GJ, de Jager M, et al. A double-blind randomised placebo controlled trial of postnatal norethisterone enanthate: the effect on postnatal depression and serum hormones. Br J Obstet Gynaecol 1998; 105:1082–1090. [RCT, *n* = 180]

94. Read MD. A new hypothesis of itching in pregnancy. Practitioner 1977; 218:845–847. [RCT, *n* = 36]

95. Young GL, Jewell D. Creams for preventing stretch marks in pregnancy. Cochrane Database Syst Rev 2010; 2. [Meta-analysis; 2 RCTs, *n* = 130]

96. Young G, Jewell D. Interventions for leg cramps in pregnancy. Cochrane Database Syst Rev 2002; (1):CD000121. [Meta-analysis; 5 RCTs, *n* = 352]

97. Coppin RJ, Wicke DM, Little PS. Managing nocturnal leg cramps-calf-stretching exercises and cessation of quinine treatment: a factorial randomized controlled trial. Br J Gen Pract 2005; 55:186–199. [RCT, *n* = 191 women]

98. Pennick V, Young G. Interventions for preventing and treating pelvic and back pain in pregnancy. Cochrane Database Syst Rev 2007; (2):CD001139. [Meta-analysis; 8 RCTs, *n* = 1805]

99. Jewell D, Young G. Interventions for treating constipation in pregnancy. Cochrane Database Syst Rev 2001; (2):CD001142. [2 RCTs, *n* = 185]

100. Bamigboye AA, Smyth RMD. Interventions for varicose veins and leg oedema in pregnancy. Cochrane Database Syst Rev 2007; (1):CD001066. [Meta-analysis; 3 RCTs, *n* = 159]

101. Quijano CE, Abalos E. Conservative management of symptomatic and/or complicated haemorrhoids in pregnancy and the puerperium. Cochrane Database Syst Rev 2005; (3):CD004077. [Meta-analysis]

102. Dowswell T, Neilson JP. Interventions for heartburn in pregnancy. Cochrane Database Syst Rev 2008; (4):CD007065. [Meta-analysis; 3 RCTs, all different interventions]

103. Gill SK, O'Brien L, Einarson TR, et al. The safety of proton pump inhibitors (PPIs) in pregnancy: a meta-analysis. Am J Gastroenterol 2009; 104:1541–1545. [Meta-analysis]

104. Gill SK, O'Brien L, Koren G. The safety of histamine 2 (H2) blockers in pregnancy: a meta-analysis. Dig Dis Sci 2009; 54 (9):1835–1838. [II-1]

105. Hanson L, VandeVusse L, Roberts J, et al. A critical appraisal of guidelines for antenatal care: components of care and priorities in prenatal education. J Midwifery Women's Health 2009; 54 (6):458–468. [Review]

3

Physiologic changes

Colleen Horan

KEY POINTS

- The normal physiologic changes of pregnancy are several and listed in part in Table 3.1.
- Normal laboratory values for pregnant women are presented in Table 3.2.
- Failure to understand these physiologic changes of pregnancy may result in both undue alarm and costly evaluation of normal symptoms of pregnancy or in the neglect of pathologic conditions whose presentation is dismissed as another "discomfort of pregnancy."
- The physician should carefully address the pregnant patient **keeping in mind the question "how is this presentation affected by the physiology of pregnancy?"**

BACKGROUND

Over the course of human pregnancy, the significance of physiologic changes that occur is such that it often becomes no longer appropriate for the physician to evaluate her according to standards that have been set through the observation and study of men and nonpregnant women. Some of these physiologic changes are advantageous to the growth and survival of the fetus. Others enhance the ability of the maternal system to compensate for demands of pregnancy, prepare for stress of delivery, and recover from delivery. Understanding physiologic changes in pregnancy is important in evaluating common symptoms associated with pregnancy, interpreting laboratory values in the parturient, and understanding pathologic conditions to which pregnant women are susceptible. **Failure to understand the normal physiologic changes of pregnancy may result in both undue alarm and costly evaluation of normal symptoms of pregnancy or in the neglect of pathologic conditions whose presentation is dismissed as another discomfort of pregnancy.** The patient will most likely be better served by the physician who carefully addresses her symptoms while **keeping in mind the questions "how is this presentation affected by the physiology of pregnancy?" and "what pathologic conditions may be represented by this scenario?"** than by the physician who uncritically memorizes laboratory values and makes a diagnosis without considering the interplay between pregnancy and underlying pathophysiology.

Two summary tables are provided. Table 3.1 summarizes the commonly accepted pregnancy-related changes in various physiologic parameters and their importance in the evaluation and management during pregnancy (1). Table 3.2 provides a summary of laboratory values in each trimester of pregnancy versus in the nonpregnant state based on a recent systematic review (2). The reader will note that some values show significant overlap between pregnant and nonpregnant states. Some show little change between pregnant and nonpregnant states. Others show trends that clearly increase

or decrease with pregnancy. In most cases, it is not possible to consider the effect of pregnancy on laboratory values in a simplistic or formulaic way. Rather, it is the understanding of the underlying physiology that these laboratory values reflect that is the most important in their evaluation during pregnancy.

CARDIOVASCULAR/HEMODYNAMIC

An understanding of pregnancy-related hemodynamic changes is crucial in the management of both benign and life-threatening complications of pregnancy ranging from near-syncopal episodes experienced by many pregnant women to hypotension from obstetric hemorrhage and gestational hypertension, both of which are leading causes of maternal intensive care unit admissions and mortality (3). Even the ultimate clinical emergency of cardiac arrest is complicated by hemodynamics that are unique to pregnancy.

Hemodynamic changes in pregnancy that have been well established include an **increase in cardiac output and a decrease in both systemic and pulmonary vascular resistance**. There is an **overall increase in heart rate and a decrease in blood pressure. Blood volume, plasma volume, and erythrocyte volume all increase, with a greater relative increase in plasma volume resulting in a dilution lowering of hematocrit and other blood indices.** There is also a redistribution of cardiac output with an increase in flow to the uterus, kidneys, skin, and breasts (1). The increase in stroke volume and cardiac output creates a more audible physiologic flow murmur and splitting of the S2 sound during pregnancy, which may be striking upon physical exam.

One longitudinal study followed maternal hemodynamics as measured by thoracic electrical bioimpedance monitoring in 50 healthy pregnant women (4). The results showed an increase in mean heart rate from 87 ± 2 beats per minute (bpm) at 10 to 18 weeks to 92 ± 1 bpm at 34 to 42 weeks. Mean arterial pressure (MAP) decreased significantly after 14 weeks and increased after 29 weeks. Systemic vascular resistance (SVR) increased during the last trimester. This study also found a significantly higher mean cardiac output in nulliparous women compared to multiparous women. Mean cardiac output and stroke volume, which show an overall increase during pregnancy, were found to decrease in the third trimester in this study (4). However, the change in cardiac output during the third trimester showed significant individual variation and has not been consistent in other longitudinal studies, demonstrating the need for further research for a more conclusive understanding of how this parameter changes across gestation (5).

A more recent longitudinal study performed serial echocardiography studies on 35 healthy pregnant women from the early second trimester to 6 to 12 weeks postpartum (6). This study showed a significant increase in cardiac output that peaked in the early third trimester and was maintained until

Table 3.1   Summary of Physiologic Adaptations During Pregnancy

Parameter	Expected change	Comments
Cardiovascular system		
Heart size	Increases 12%	Increases diastolic filling and muscle hypertrophy
Murmurs	Physiologic systolic	Ejection murmurs attributable to increased stroke volume usually occur in early or midsystole and are best heard along the left sternal edge
ECG	Positional heart shifts result in changes that resemble ischemia	Heart is pushed upward and forward, deviating electrical axis to the left by 15°–20°, causing flattened or inverted T in lead III
Cardiac output	Increases 1.5 L/min	Greatest increase occurs immediately after delivery with redistribution of blood flow from uterus. Cardiac output then decreases postpartum
Rhythm	Increases atrial and ventricular extrasystole	SVT not infrequent
Heart rate	Increases	Onset of change is first trimester
Stroke volume	Increases	Significant change in second half of pregnancy
Mean arterial pressure	Decreased soon after beginning of pregnancy and midpregnancy (100–110/60–70 mean levels); then returns to prepregnant values by third trimester and term	Supine hypotension—decreased venous return due to compression from gravid uterus; increased blood flow through alternative pathways such as paravertebral-azygous veins
Pulse pressure	Increases	
Venous pressure	Increases in femoral system; unchanged in arms	
Systemic vascular resistance	Decreases	
Pulmonary BP	Unchanged	
Blood flow to uterus	Increases by 500 mL/min	No autoregulation
Blood flow to kidneys	Increases by 400 mL/min	
Blood flow to skin	Increases by 300–400 mL/min	
Blood flow to breasts	Increases by 200 mL/min	
Respiratory system		
Anatomy	Increases subcostal angle from 68° to 103° → 3-cm increase in transthoracic diameter	Increased upper respiratory capillary engorgement can cause increased congestion, epistaxis, and intubation trauma
Tidal volume	Increases by 300 mL or 40%	
Expiratory reserve volume	Decreases by 200 mL	Cephalad displacement of diaphragm
Inspiratory capacity	Increases by 300 mL	
Functional residual volume	Decreases by 500 mL	
Minute volume	Increases by 40% or 3 L/min beginning in first trimester	Increased rate of induction of, and emergence from, inhaled anesthetics
Maximum breathing capacity	Unchanged	
Forced expiratory volume	Unchanged	
Peak expiratory flow rate	Unchanged	
Pulmonary diffusing capacity	Decreases by 4 mL/min/mmHg	
Oxygen requirement	Increases by 30–40 mL/min	
Carbon dioxide output	Increases; expressed as respiratory quotient	
Carbon dioxide pressure	Decreases from 35–40 mmHg to 28–30 mmHg	
Oxygen pressure	Increases	
pH	Mild increase (7.40–7.44 is normal)	Compensated respiratory alkalosis
PCO_2	Decrease (30–31 mmHg is normal)	
PO_2	Mild increase (100–104 mmHg is normal)	
Renal system and homeostasis		
Glomerular filtration rate	Increases from 97 mL/min to 128 mL/min by 10 wk	Increased renal clearance of certain drugs and vitamins
Glucose excretion	Increased	Random glycosuria
Protein excretion	Increased (up to 300 mg/24 hr is normal)	
Renin, angiotensins I and II	Increased	Diminished vascular response causes less pressor effect from angiotensin
Anatomic changes	Dilation of renal calyces and ureters to pelvic brim; "physiologic" hydronephrosis, right > left	Increased risk of pyelonephritis; screen for asymptomatic bacteriuria
Potassium	Increased retention	
Sodium	Increased retention	

(Continued)

Table 3.1 Summary of Physiologic Adaptations During Pregnancy (*Continued*)

Parameter	Expected change	Comments
Renel system and homeostasis (continued)		
Urine output	No significant change	
Vitamin excretion	Increased loss of folate, B12, and ascorbic acid	
Osmolality	Decreases 10 mOsm/kg first trimester, then stable	
Sodium	Decreases 3 mEq/L first trimester, then stable	
Potassium	Decreases 0.5 mEq/L	
Calcium	Decreased total and ionized	Increased intestinal absorption of calcium and increased bone turnover
Magnesium	Decreases 10–20% in first half of pregnancy	
Chloride	Unchanged	
Bicarbonate	Decreases markedly (18–22 mEq/L is normal)	Compensates for decrease in PCO_2
Total protein	Decreases from 72 g/L to 62 g/L	
Albumin	Decreases from 47 g/L to 36 g/L	
Urea, creatinine, and uric acid	Decrease in first trimester; stabilize in second trimester; increase toward term	
Vitamin B6	Decreases	
Blood glucose	Fasting levels **decrease** in first trimester, then unchanged	Postprandial levels remain elevated longer, prolonging return to fasting state. Increased glucose levels allow passive diffusion across placenta to fetus.
Folate	Decreases 50% toward term	
Vitamin B12	Decreases 50% or more	B12 levels in folate-deficient women will increase with folate supplementation alone
Endocrine system		
Pituitary gland	Increases to 50% greater than adult male	Attributable to increase of prolactin-secreting cells in anterior lobe
Prolactin	Increases from 300 mIU/L to 5000 mIU/L	Estrogen stimulates hyperplasia and hypertrophy of pituitary lactotrophs
Follicle-stimulating hormone and luteinizing hormone	Decrease to nearly undetectable	
Melanocyte-stimulating hormone	Increased	Likely responsible for linea nigra, chloasma, and increased areolae pigmentation
Thyroid-stimulating hormone	Normal range is unchanged	May be suppressed during late first to early second trimester due to hCG-mediated increase in TH production—subtle effect may be exacerbated by conditions that increase hCG levels, such as hyperemesis, molar pregnancies, and multiples
Thyroid-binding globulin	Increases—doubles by end of first trimester; triples by term	Due to estrogen effect on liver
Thyroxine (T_4) and triiodothyronine (T_3)	Increased total circulating amount; unchanged free fraction	Fetal thyroid hormone production commences at 18 wk
Reverse T_3	Unchanged in maternal circulation; increased in cord blood	
Cortisol	Increased to 3× nonpregnant values	Episodic pattern of release is maintained.
Aldosterone	Increased twofold by term	
Deoxycorticosterone	Increased by 20–100×	
Testosterone	Increased total amount; decreased free fraction	
Androstenedione	Increases	Tenfold increase rate of transformation to estradiol and estrone
DHEA	Unchanged or small decrease	Precursor for steroid hormone synthesis by placenta
Pancreas	Hypertrophy of islets due to hyperplasia of B cells	
Insulin	Increases fasting levels toward term; hyperplasia of pancreatic B cells	Proportionally less increase of glucagons compared to insulin; so insulin:glucagon ratio is increased
Glucagon	Increases fasting levels	
Glucose	Slight decrease	Especially fasting levels
Parathyroid hormone	Increased during end of pregnancy	Maintains calcium levels in face of increased renal absorption and transfer to fetus
Progesterone	Markedly increases	Production originates in corpus luteum over first 7–8 wk; then placenta takes over.
Estradiol	Markedly increases	
17-Hydroxyprogesterone	Increases	

(Continued)

Table 3.1 Summary of Physiologic Adaptations During Pregnancy (*Continued*)

Parameter	Expected change	Comments
Endocrine system (continued)		
Estriol	Increases	
Human placental lactogen (hPL)	Increases 5000-fold from 0.002 µU/mL to 10 µU/mL	
hCG	Increases to maximum values by 8–10 wk	Peak 93 U/mL; term 14 U/mL
Relaxin	Peaks at 10 wk	
Gastrointestinal system		
Appetite	Increases	
Gastric reflux	Increases	Cardiac sphincter laxity and anatomic displacement; treated during labor and delivery/anesthetic procedures with nonparticulate oral antacids
Gastric secretion	Decreased acidity; increased volume	"Full stomach" effect increases risk of aspiration
Gastric motility	Decreases	
Intestinal absorption	Increased	
Intestinal transit time	Delayed	
Large intestine	Greater absorption; slower transit time	
Gallbladder	Larger due to passive dilation	
Hematologic system		
Plasma volume	40–60% **increase** from 12 to 36 wk; 70–100% increase in multiple gestations	Offsets blood loss at delivery
Total erythrocyte volume	Increases 15–30%	Greater increase with iron supplementation
Hematocrit	Decreases 3–5% by 36 wk	Physiologic anemia due to greater proportionate increase plasma volume compared to erythrocyte volume; less change with iron supplementation
Hemoglobin	Decreases	
Mean corpuscular volume	Unchanged	Best indicator of iron status. Slight increase with iron supplementation
Erythrocyte sedimentation rate	Significantly increased	Provides little diagnostic value; combined with increase in white blood cell (WBC) can cause false suspicion for infection
WBC count	Increases 8% by term and may increase further postpartum	Predominantly due to increase in neutrophils
Serum iron	Decreases 35% by term	
Serum transferrin	Increases by 100% or more by second trimester	Total iron-binding capacity (TIBC) markedly increased
TIBC	Increases by 25–100%	
Serum ferritin	Decreases markedly (even with iron supplementation)	Nadir 30% or less of normal values. Best test to assess iron-deficiency anemia in pregnancy
Erythropoietin	Increases fourfold	
α-Fetoprotein	Increases	Larger increase in neural tube defects, abdominal wall defects, and fetal death
Glutamic-oxaloacetic transaminase and glutamic-pyruvic transaminase	Unchanged	
Alkaline phosphatase	Increases	Heat stable fraction formed by placenta
Lipids	Increase	Triglycerides, cholesterol, phospholipids, and free fatty acids each increase progressively.
Fibrinogen	Increases 2 g/L by term	Overall increased tendency toward thrombosis
Factors VII, VIII, IX, and X	Increase	
Factors XI and XIII	Decrease by about 30%	
Antithrombin III	Decreases	
Fibrin, FDP	Increase progressively	
Protein C	Unchanged	
Protein S	Decreases	Protein S–binding protein levels fluctuate in pregnancy, making screening more reliable in nonpregnant women.

Abbreviations: ECG, electrocardiogram; SVT, supraventricular tachycardia; BP, blood pressure; hCG, human chorionic gonadotropin; TH, thyroid hormone; DHEA, dehydroepiandrosterone; FDP, fibrin degradation products.
Source: From Ref. 1.

Table 3.2 Normal Reference Ranges in Pregnant Women

	Nonpregnant adult	First trimester	Second trimester	Third trimester
Hematology				
Erythropoietin (U/L)	4–27	12–25	8–67	14–222
Ferritin (ng/mL)	10–150	6–130	2–230	0–116
Folate, red blood cell (ng/mL)	150–450	137–589	94–828	109–663
Folate, serum (ng/mL)	5.4–18	2.6–15	0.8–24	1.4–20.7
Hemoglobin (g/dL)	12–15.8	11.6–13.9	9.7–14.8	9.5–15
Hematocrit (%)	35.4–44.4	31–41	30–39	28–40
Iron, total binding capacity (μg/dL)	251–406	278–403		359–609
Iron, serum (μg/dL)	41–141	72–143	44–178	30–193
Mean corpuscular hemoglobin (pg/cell)	27–32	30–32	30–33	29–32
Mean corpuscular volume (μm^3)	79–93	81–96	82–97	81–99
Platelet ($\times 10^9$/L)	165–415	174–391	155–409	146–429
Mean platelet volume (μm^3)	6.4–11	7.7–10.3	7.8–10.2	8.2–7.4
Red blood cell count ($\times 10^6$/mm^3)	4–5.2	3.42–4.55	2.81–4.49	2.71–4.43
Red cell distribution width (%)	<14.5	12.5–14.1	13.4–13.6	12.7–15.3
White blood cell count ($\times 10^3$/mm^3)	3.5–9.1	5.7–13.6	5.6–14.8	5.9–16.9
Neutrophils ($\times 10^3$/mm^3)	1.4–4.6	3.6–10.1	3.8–12.3	3.9–13.1
Lymphocytes ($\times 10^3$/mm^3)	0.7–4.6	1.1–3.6	0.9–3.9	1–3.6
Monocytes ($\times 10^3$/mm^3)	0.1–0.7	0.1–1.1	0.1–1.1	0.1–1.4
Eosinophils ($\times 10^3$/mm^3)	0–0.6	0–0.6	0–0.6	0–0.6
Basophils ($\times 10^3$/mm^3)	0–0.2	0–0.1	0–0.1	0–0.1
Transferrin (mg/dL)	200–400	254–344	220–441	288–530
Transferrin, saturation without iron (%)	22–46		10–44	5–37
Transferrin, saturation with iron (%)	22–46		18–92	9–98
Coagulation				
Antithrombin III, functional (%)	70–130	89–114	88–112	82–116
D-dimer (μg/mL)	0.22–0.74	0.05–0.95	0.32–1.29	0.13–1.7
Factor V (%)	50–150	75–95	72–96	60–88
Factor VII (%)	50–150	100–146	95–153	149–211
Factor VIII (%)	50–150	90–210	97–312	143–353
Factor IX (%)	50–150	103–172	154–217	164–235
Factor XI (%)	50–150	80–127	82–144	65–123
Factor XII (%)	50–150	78–124	90–151	129–194
Fibrinogen (mg/dL)	233–496	244–510	291–538	373–619
Homocysteine (μmol/L)	4.4–10.8	3.34–11	2–26.9	3.2–21.4
International normalized ratio	0.9–1.04	0.89–1.05	0.85–0.97	0.80–0.94
Partial thromboplastin time, activated (sec)	26.3–39.4	24.3–38.9	24.2–38.1	24.7–35
Prothrombin time (sec)	12.7–15.4	9.7–13.5	9.5–13.4	9.6–12.9
Protein C, functional (%)	70–130	78–121	83–133	67–135
Protein S, total (%)	70–140	39–105	27–101	33–101
Protein S, free (%)	70–140	34–133	19–113	20–65
Protein S, functional activity (%)	65–140	57–95	42–68	16–42
Tissue plasminogen activator (ng/mL)	1.6–13	1.8–6	2.4–6.6	3.3–9.2
Tissue plasminogen activator inhibitor-1 (ng/mL)	4–43	16–33	36–55	67–92
Von Willebrand factor (%)	75–125			121–260
Blood chemical constituents				
Alanine transaminase (U/L)	7–41	3–30	2–33	2–25
Albumin (g/dL)	4.1–5.3	3.1–5.1	2.6–4.5	2.3–4.2
Alkaline phosphatase (U/L)	33–96	17–88	25–126	38–229
α1-Antitrypsin (mg/dL)	100–200	225–323	273–391	327–487
Amylase (U/L)	20–96	24–83	16–73	15–81
Anion gap (mmol/L)	7–16	13–17	12–16	12–16
Aspartate transaminase (U/L)	12–38	3–23	3–33	4–32
Bicarbonate (mmol/L)	22–30	20–24	20–24	20–24
Bilirubin, total (mg/dL)	0.3–1.3	0.1–0.4	0.1–0.8	0.1–1.1
Bilirubin, unconjugated (mg/dL)	0.2–0.9	0.1–0.5	0.1–0.4	0.1–0.5
Bilirubin, conjugated (mg/dL)	0.1–0.4	0–0.1	0–0.1	0–0.1
Bile acids, (μmol/L)	0.3–4.8	0–4.9	0–9.1	0–11.3
Calcium, ionized (mg/dL)	4.5–5.3	4.5–5.1	4.4–5	4.4–5.3
Calcium, total (mg/dL)	8.7–10.2	8.8–10.6	8.2–9	8.2–9.7
Ceruloplasmin (mg/dL)	25–63	30–49	40–53	43–78
Chloride (mEq/L)	102–109	101–105	97–109	97–109
Creatinine (mg/dL)	0.5–0.9	0.4–0.7	0.4–0.8	0.4–0.9
γ-Glutamyl transpeptidase (U/L)	9–58	2–23	4–22	3–26
Lactate dehydrogenase (U/L)	115–221	78–433	80–447	82–524
Lipase (U/L)	3–43	21–76	26–100	41–112
Magnesium (mg/dL)	1.5–2.3	1.6–2.2	1.5–2.2	1.1–2.2

(Continued)

Table 3.2 Normal Reference Ranges in Pregnant Women (*Continued*)

	Nonpregnant adult	First trimester	Second trimester	Third trimester
Blood chemical constituents (continued)				
Osmolality (mOsm/kg H_2O)	275–295	275–280	276–289	278–280
Phosphate (mg/dL)	2.5–4.3	3.1–4.6	2.5–4.6	2.8–4.6
Potassium (mEq/L)	3.5–5	3.6–5	3.3–5	3.3–5.1
Prealbumin (mg/dL)	17–34	15–27	20–27	14–23
Protein, total (g/dL)	6.7–8.6	6.2–7.6	5.7–6.9	5.6–6.7
Sodium (mEq/L)	136–146	133–148	129–148	130–148
Urea nitrogen (mg/dL)	7–20	7–12	3–13	3–11
Uric acid (mg/dL)	2.5–5.6	2–4.2	2.4–4.9	3.1–6.3
Metabolic and endocrine tests				
Aldosterone (ng/dL)	2–9	6–104	9–104	15–101
Angiotensin-converting enzyme (U/L)	9–67	1–38	1–36	1–39
Cortisol (μg/dL)	0–25	7–19	10–42	12–50
Hemoglobin A1c (%)	4–6	4–6	4–6	4–7
Parathyroid hormone (pg/mL)	8–51	10–15	18–25	9–26
Parathyroid hormone–related protein (pmol/L)	<1.3	0.7–0.9	1.8–2.2	2.5–2.8
Renin, plasma activity (ng/mL/hr)	0.3–9		7.5–54	5.9–58.8
Thyroid-stimulating hormone (μIU/mL)	0.34–4.25	0.6–3.4	0.37–3.6	0.38–4.04
Thyroxine-binding globulin (mg/dL)	1.3–3	1.8–3.2	2.8–4	2.6–4.2
Thyroxine, free (ng/dL)	0.8–1.7	0.8–1.2	0.6–1	0.5–0.8
Thyroxine, total (μg/dL)	5.4–11.7	6.5–10.1	7.5–10.3	6.3–9.7
Triiodothyronine, free (pg/mL)	2.4–4.2	4.1–4.4	4–4.2	
Triiodothyronine, total (ng/dL)	77–135	97–149	117–169	123–162
Vitamins and minerals				
Copper (μg/dL)	70–140	112–199	165–221	130–240
Selenium (μg/L)	63–160	116–146	75–145	71–133
Vitamin A (retinol) (μg/dL)	20–100	32–47	35–44	29–42
Vitamin B12 (pg/mL)	279–966	118–438	130–656	99–526
Vitamin C (ascorbic acid) (mg/dL)	0.4–1			0.9–1.3
Vitamin D, 1,25-dihydroxy (pg/mL)	25–45	20–65	72–160	60–119
Vitamin D, 24,25-dihydroxy (ng/mL)	0.5–5	1.2–1.8	1.1–1.5	0.7–0.9
Vitamin D, 25-hydroxy (ng/mL)	14–80	18–27	10–22	10–18
Vitamin E (α-tocopherol) (μg/mL)	5–18	7–13	10–16	13–23
Zinc (μg/dL)	75–120	57–88	51–80	50–77
Autoimmune and inflammatory mediators				
C3 complement (mg/dL)	83–177	62–98	73–103	77–111
C4 complement (mg/dL)	16–47	18–36	18–34	22–32
C-reactive protein (mg/L)	0.2–3		0.4–20.3	0.4–8.1
Erythrocyte sedimentation rate (mm/hr)	0–20	4–57	7–47	13–70
Immunoglobulin A (mg/dL)	70–350	95–243	99–237	112–250
Immunoglobulin G (mg/dL)	700–1700	981–1267	813–1131	678–990
Immunoglobulin M (mg/dL)	50–300	78–232	74–218	85–269
Sex hormones				
Dehydroepiandrosterone sulfate (μmol/L)	1.3–6.8	2–16.5	0.9–7.8	0.8–6.5
Estradiol (pg/mL)	<20–443	188–2497	1278–7192	6137–3460
Progesterone (ng/mL)	<1–20	8–48		99–342
Prolactin (ng/mL)	0–20	36–213	110–330	137–372
Sex hormone–binding globulin (nmol/L)	18–114	39–131	214–717	216–724
Testosterone (ng/dL)	6–86	26–211	34–243	63–309
17-Hydroxyprogesterone (nmol/L)	0.6–10.6	5.2–28.5	5.2–28.5	15.5–84
Lipids				
Cholesterol, total (mg/dL)	<200	141–210	176–299	219–349
High-density lipoprotein cholesterol (mg/dL)	40–60	40–78	52–87	48–87
Low-density lipoprotein cholesterol (mg/dL)	<100	60–153	77–184	101–224
Very-low-density lipoprotein cholesterol (mg/dL)	6–40	10–18	13–23	21–36
Triglycerides (mg/dL)	<150	40–159	75–382	131–453
Apolipoprotein A-I (mg/dL)	119–240	111–150	142–253	145–262
Apolipoprotein B (mg/dL)	52–163	58–81	66–188	85–238
Cardiac				
Atrial natriuretic peptide (pg/mL)			28.1–70.1	
B-type natriuretic peptide (pg/mL)	<167		13.5–29.5	
Creatine kinase (U/L)	39–238	27–83	25–75	13–101
Creatine kinase-MB (U/L)	<6			1.8–2.4
Troponin I (ng/mL)	0–0.8			0–0.064 (intrapartum)

(Continued)

Table 3.2 Normal Reference Ranges in Pregnant Women (*Continued*)

	Nonpregnant adult	First trimester	Second trimester	Third trimester
Blood gas				
pH	7.38–7.42 (arterial)	7.36–7.52 (venous)	7.4–7.52 (venous)	7.41–7.53 (venous) 7.39–7.45 (arterial)
PO$_2$ (mmHg)	90–100	93–100	90–98	92–107
PCO$_2$ (mmHg)	38–42			25–33
Bicarbonate (HCO$_3$) (mEq/L)	22–26			16–22
Renal function tests				
Effective renal plasma flow (mL/min)	492–696	696–985	612–1170	595–945
Glomerular filtration rate (GFR) (mL/min)	106–132	131–166	135–170	117–182
Filtration fraction (%)	16.9–24.7	14.7–21.6	14.3–21.9	17.1–25.1
Osmolarity, urine (mOsm/kg)	500–800	326–975	278–1066	238–1034
24-hr albumin excretion (mg/24 hr)	<30	5–15	4–18	3–22
24-hr calcium excretion (mmol/24 hr)	<7.5	1.6–5.2	0.3–6.9	0.8–4.2
24-hr creatinine clearance (mL/min)	91–130	69–140	55–136	50–166
24-hr creatinine excretion (mmol/24 hr)	8.8–14	10.6–11.6	10.3–11.5	10.2–11.4
24-hr potassium excretion (mmol/24 hr)	25–100	17–33	10–38	11–35
24-hr protein excretion (mg/24 hr)	<150	19–141	47–186	46–185
24-hr sodium excretion (mmol/24 hr)	100–260	53–215	34–213	37–149

Source: Adapted from Ref. 2.

term. The detected 46% to 51% increase in cardiac output was attributed to a 15% increase in heart rate and a 24% increase in stroke volume (6). **The changes in heart rate occur early in pregnancy, whereas those of stroke volume occur later, with the net effect of a progressively increasing cardiac output as gestation progresses.** Again, significant variation in cardiac output changes in the late third trimester was attributed to patient factors, precluding confident conclusions regarding the behavior of cardiac output at the very end of pregnancy. Maternal cardiac output was found to correlate with maternal body surface area and with fetal birth weight. Left ventricular mass and left ventricular mass index increased to maximal levels at term but remained well below the cutoff for a diagnosis of left ventricular hypertrophy. This increase corresponded to an increase in mean blood pressure at term as well as to an increase in left atrial size and a decrease in left ventricular diastolic filling value. These changes may explain some of the variations in cardiac output in the third trimester and may be relevant to the vulnerability of pregnant women to pulmonary edema during hypertensive crisis (6).

Perhaps the most common hemodynamic complaint that must be evaluated during pregnancy is that of **syncope or near-syncope**, which provides a useful example of how an understanding of pregnancy physiology is useful in clinical evaluation. Syncope is defined as a transient loss of consciousness and posture, caused by decreased cerebral perfusion that may result from hypotension, changes in heart rate, or changes in blood volume or redistribution. The decreased SVR of pregnancy makes pregnant women particularly susceptible to this condition, with 28.2% of gravidas experiencing at least one episode of presyncope, 10% experiencing recurrent presyncopal episodes, and 4.6% experiencing outright syncope (7). The overwhelming majority of syncopal episodes are benign neurocardiogenic syncope but there are also several potentially dangerous conditions in the differential diagnosis of syncope. An understanding of the vasovagal reflex at the root of most syncopal episodes helps the clinician to manage benign syncopal episodes while being alert for signs and symptoms that may point to a more serious underlying condition. The most common trigger of syncope is venous pooling that results in a drop in venous return and a subsequent

drop in cardiac output. This results in stimulation of arterial baroreceptors which trigger catecholamine stimulation of atria and ventricles. The resultant vigorous cardiac contraction in volume-depleted chambers stimulates cardiac mechanoreceptors or C-fibers which, in susceptible individuals, can result in paradoxical stimulation of the dorsal vagal nucleus. This stimulation is paradoxical because, in the face of low SVR and cardiac output, there is a further decrease in sympathetic tone and an increase in vagal tone causing vasodilation and bradycardia and the clinical presentation of presyncope or syncope (7). The reflex may be initiated by emotional stimuli in some individuals or may be initiated by compression of the inferior vena cava by the gravid uterus causing a decrease in venous return and intracardiac pressure. Less common conditions that may present with symptoms of syncope include cerebrovascular accidents, seizures, cardiac arrhythmias or valvular disease, cardiomyopathy, pericardial tamponade, myocardial infarction, congenital heart defects, thromboembolic phenomenon, anemia, hypoglycemia, or electrolyte disorders (7). Further evaluation for such conditions should be prompted when an apparent syncopal episode is accompanied by focal neurologic findings, prolonged loss of consciousness or postictal confusion, carotid or subclavian bruits, a pathologic cardiac murmur, or electrocardiogram (EKG) or laboratory abnormalities (7).

The above events that are precipitated by a decrease in venous return can also explain the occurrence of **supine hypotension** in pregnancy. The commonly recommended "leftward tilt" position is intended to displace the uterus off of the inferior vena cava, which runs to the right of midline. This position should be used to avoid supine hypotension during bed rest as well as when performing surgery on the parturient. A more extreme application of this physiology comes in the performance of perimortem cesarean section during maternal cardiac arrest. The procedure is purported to not only allow fetal survival but also the evacuation of the uterus may allow an increase in venous return and cardiac output that may increase the chance for maternal survival (8). In order to optimize maternal and fetal survival it is recommended that the procedure should be performed within 4 minutes of cardiac arrest due to the inadequacy of chest compressions in producing adequate cardiac output during pregnancy and the susceptibility of both mother and fetus to anoxic brain injury (8) (see also chaps. 1 and 2 in *Maternal-Fetal Evidence Based Guidelines*).

RESPIRATORY

During pregnancy the respiratory system undergoes alterations that are reflected in pulmonary function tests and in acid-base balance. These are important in the evaluation of dyspnea in pregnancy, the management of pregnancy with coexisting pulmonary diseases such as asthma, and the recognition of acute pulmonary complications of pregnancy.

Pregnancy is associated with a significant increase in ventilatory drive both at rest and during exercise (9). **Minute ventilation increases** mostly due to an **increase in tidal volume** with little or no increase in respiratory rate (3,9,10). Alveolar ventilation increases, along with an **increase in arterial partial pressure of oxygen (PaO$_2$) and alveolar partial pressure of oxygen (PAO$_2$), and a decrease in arterial partial pressure of carbon dioxide (PaCO$_2$), with a compensatory decrease in serum bicarbonate with an overall mild increase in pH, reflecting a state of compensated respiratory alkalosis** (9). These changes occur early in pregnancy and are almost fully established by 7 to 8 weeks' gestation (9). This may be due to stimulation of the ventilatory drive by progesterone and/or estrogen. Ventilatory equivalents for CO$_2$ and O$_2$ are increased both at rest and during exercise throughout pregnancy. The underlying mechanism for the increased ventilatory drive during pregnancy is not fully understood, but theories have included an increased sensitivity to chemoreflexive drives to breathe (due to hypercapnia or hypoxia) versus a hormone-mediated increase in the neural drive to breathe (9).

Uterine enlargement and abdominal distension result in a 4- to 5-cm cephalad displacement of the diaphragm and a 5- to 7-cm increase in thoracic circumference. This results in a **decrease in expiratory reserve volume, residual volume, and functional residual capacity.** There is a compensatory increase in inspiratory capacity, while total lung capacity and vital capacity do not change (9). Chest wall compliance is increased but inspiratory muscle strength is preserved with an overall increase in the oxygen cost of breathing (9). However, it is important to recognize that there is **no significant change in the parameters of forced vital capacity, peak expiratory flow rate (PEFR), or forced expiratory volume in one second (FEV$_1$) during pregnancy**.

Physiologic **dyspnea** of pregnancy, experienced by 60% to 70% of healthy pregnant women, must be clinically distinguished from more serious respiratory conditions. Physiologic dyspnea tends to be an isolated symptom that begins in early pregnancy, plateaus or improves as pregnancy progresses, and does not interfere with daily activities (11). The mechanism for physiologic dyspnea has not been conclusively defined, but pregnant women with dyspnea have been demonstrated to have an increase in minute ventilation and tidal volume and a decrease in end-tidal CO$_2$ pressure compared to pregnant women who do not report dyspnea (11). The perception of physiologic dyspnea during pregnancy has been associated with increased sensitivity to hypoxia and hypercapnia, suggesting an increased chemosensitivity causing an increased central inspiratory drive in pregnant women who experience dyspnea. However, the chemical stimuli of hypoxia and hypercapnia are both reduced in pregnancy, causing others to suggest a neural mechanism (9). In spite of the common symptom

of physiologic dyspnea, **pregnancy has not been found to be associated with a decrease in aerobic work capacity or with an increased perception of breathlessness during exercise** (9).

An understanding of respiratory changes during pregnancy is of utmost importance in the evaluation of the pregnant women with **asthma**, a condition that affects about 4% to 8% of pregnant women (see also chap. 24 in *Maternal-Fetal Evidence Based Guidelines*). As in the nonpregnant patient, the diagnosis of asthma in pregnancy is based on symptoms and spirometry. Asthma in pregnancy has been defined by the National Asthma Education and Prevention Program (NAEPP) 2004 working group as mild intermittent, mild persistent, moderate persistent, or severe based on symptoms and pulmonary function tests (12). Patients with mild-to-moderate asthma generally have excellent pregnancy outcomes, and there is evidence to suggest that improved control of asthma is associated with fewer complications (10). The effect of pregnancy on asthma is variable, with prospective studies showing that some patients have improvement of asthma during pregnancy, some patients have a worsening of asthma, and others have no significant change.

Prevention of asthma exacerbation avoids hypoxic episodes in both mother and fetus. While optimal management of asthma during pregnancy involves avoiding or controlling asthma triggers and using a stepwise approach that uses the least amount of pharmacologic intervention that is needed for each individual patient, it is far safer for both mother and fetus to be treated with appropriate asthma medications than to have asthma symptoms and exacerbations (10). It is important for pregnant patients with asthma to be monitored by PEFR or FEV$_1$ testing during pregnancy (10). While measurement of FEV$_1$ requires a spirometer, measurement of PEFR correlates well with FEV$_1$ and can be measured with a relatively inexpensive spirometer (peak flow meter), which patients can be taught to use at home. Again, these parameters do not change due to pregnancy, so any detected worsening should be treated appropriately and not attributed to pregnancy or to physiologic dyspnea. Patients should be taught to recognize asthma exacerbations at home by changes in symptoms and PEFR and to respond promptly with the use of rescue agents. Prenatal visits should include evaluation of symptoms and pulmonary function (10). In the evaluation of severe acute asthma exacerbations with the potential for impending respiratory arrest, knowledge of physiologic changes of pregnancy is particularly important in the interpretation of blood gases. The normal parturient lives in a state of compensated respiratory alkalosis with a lower partial pressure of carbon dioxide (PCO$_2$) than that of nonpregnant patients. Thus, significant CO$_2$ retention may be present in spite of values that are high normal for nonpregnant patients.

While physiologic dyspnea and asthma exacerbation are two of the most common causes of dyspnea in pregnancy, the obstetrician must also be alert to other pulmonary complications to which the parturient is susceptible such as pulmonary embolism and pulmonary edema. Pulmonary edema may occur as a result of preeclampsia, peripartum cardiomyopathy, or the use of certain tocolytics. It is important that the prevalence of pulmonary symptoms in pregnancy should not be met with complacency by the obstetrician, for it may signify a life-threatening condition for the pregnant woman.

ENDOCRINE

Pregnancy-related endocrine alterations include the production of hormones that are specific to pregnancy, an increase in other reproductive hormones, and alterations in the level and function of nonreproductive hormones, especially of thyroid hormones. There is a significant contribution of steroid hormone secretion by the fetal-placental unit. This section provides a brief description of the changes in reproductive hormones during gestation followed by a more in-depth review of the behavior and clinical application of thyroid hormones during pregnancy.

Pregnancy-specific hormones include human chorionic gonadotropin (hCG) and relaxin. **Relaxin** is detectable in maternal serum by the time of missed menses and peaks at 10 weeks' gestation then declines over the course of the second and third trimesters (13). Relaxin is secreted by the corpora lutea of pregnancy and thought to have an important role in early pregnancy maintenance that has not yet been clearly elucidated (14). hCG also peaks at approximately 10 weeks' gestation. The reproductive hormones **estradiol, progesterone, testosterone, prolactin, and 17-hydroxyprogesterone,** all increase significantly during gestation. Initially the corpus luteum and maternal ovarian tissue make the greatest contribution to steroid hormone concentrations, but as of 9 weeks' gestation aromatization of dehydroepiandrosterone sulfate by the placenta becomes the predominant source of maternal steroids (15). The elevated estradiol levels stimulate increased hepatic production of sex hormone–binding globulin and thyroxin-binding globulin. Estrogen also induces hypertrophy and hyperplasia of pituitary lactotrophs with a resultant increase in prolactin levels corresponding to the increase in estradiol levels throughout gestation (15). Meanwhile, there is a reflexive decrease in follicle-stimulating hormone and luteinizing hormone to almost undetectable levels, as would be expected.

One longitudinal study assayed reproductive hormone levels in the blood of 60 healthy women drawn during the first, second, and third trimesters of uncomplicated pregnancies (15). Mean progesterone levels increased steadily from 49 nmol/L at 5 weeks' gestation to 584 nmol/L at term. Mean 17-hydroxyprogesterone levels are more stable during the first and second trimesters at 12.2 nmol/L but then increase three-fold to 36 nmol/L by term. Mean testosterone increased from 3.3 nmol/L at 5 weeks to 5.7 nmol/L at 40 weeks. Mean serum estradiol levels increased during the first trimester from 1.64 nmol/L at 5 weeks to 11.13 nmol/L at 16 weeks and then increased fivefold to 53.44 nmol/L at 40 weeks. Mean sex hormone–binding globulin levels increase rapidly during the first half of gestation from 71 nmol/L at 5 weeks to 392 nmol/L at 25 weeks, and then remain relatively constant until 40 weeks. Mean levels of dehydroepiandrosterone sulfate decreased from 5.8 μmol/L at 5 weeks to 2.7 μmol/L at midgestation, where they remained rather constant until term. Mean prolactin concentration rose from 294 milli-international units (mIU) to 1106 mIU at 16 weeks. Prolactin levels then continued to increase to a mean of 4092 mIU at 35 weeks and to 4293 mIU at 40 weeks. Mean androstenedione levels increase gradually from 8.1 nmol/L at 5 weeks to 10.6 nmol/L at 40 weeks (15).

Other hormonal alterations include an increase in aldosterone, cortisol, parathyroid hormone, parathyroid-related hormone, and renin (2). Deoxycorticosterone increases. Androstenedione increases with an increase in the transformation to estrone and estradiol (1). Fasting levels of both insulin and glucagon increase (1). There is an increase in melanocyte-stimulating hormone to which can be attributed the pregnancy-related increases in pigmentation seen in the areola, the linea nigra, and in chloasma (1).

The function of the **thyroid gland** is crucial to a healthy gestation (see also chaps. 6 and 7 in *Maternal-Fetal Evidence Based Guidelines*). The interplay between maternal and fetal thyroid function can cause confusion for the obstetrician. Early fetal development is dependent on maternal thyroid function, and both hypothyroidism and hyperthyroidism can have important maternal and fetal effects and risks of thyroid dysfunction extend well into the postpartum period. The effects of subclinical thyroid disease are more controversial. Symptoms of hyperthyroidism and hypothyroidism can mimic symptoms of normal pregnancy. For example, symptoms such as fatigue, muscle cramps, palpitations, thyromegaly, and constipation can be common in normal pregnancy, but progressive symptoms of insomnia, intellectual slowness, or weight loss should be evaluated (16).

Thyroid-binding globulin increases due to stimulation of synthesis by estrogen as well as decreased hepatic clearance. **Total thyroxine (TT_4) and total triiodothyronine (TT_3) both increase while resin triiodothyronine uptake (RT_3U) decreases.** Structural similarities between hCG and thyroid-stimulating hormone (TSH) may result in an hCG-mediated increase in free thyroxine (FT_4) and the free thyroxine index as well as a decrease in TSH in the first trimester. However, these changes, sometimes referred to as gestational transient thyrotoxicosis, are typically self-limited and do not tend to result in values that are outside the normal range for nonpregnant individuals (17) (see also chap. 9 in *Maternal-Fetal Evidence Based Guidelines*).

Iodine requirements during pregnancy increase by greater than 50% due to increased maternal thyroxine production to maintain maternal and fetal euthyroidism and increased renal iodine clearance (18). Plasma iodine levels decrease. This is associated with an increase in the size of the thyroid gland. Longitudinal studies of thyroid ultrasonography in pregnancy show a mean increase in thyroid size of 18%, which is noticeable in most women but not associated with abnormalities in thyroid function tests (17). Iodine supplementation results in a less substantial increase in thyroid gland size (18). While ultrasound or laboratory evaluation is not necessary in the pregnant patient with a mild diffuse increase in thyroid size, a significant goiter or thyroid nodule must be evaluated as in any patient. A woman who is marginally iodine deficient may be able to compensate with increased thyrotropin stimulation of the thyroid to achieve euthyroidism, but become hypothyroid when faced with the increasing iodine requirements of pregnancy (18).

Thyroid homeostasis is important for healthy fetal development. The fetal thyroid begins to concentrate iodide at 10 to 12 weeks. Thyroid hormone necessary for fetal brain development before this time must be provided by the maternal system (16,19). Thyroid hormone synthesis in the fetus is controlled by the fetal pituitary gland by 20 weeks. **Small amounts of T_4 and T_3 pass the placenta but TSH does not cross the placenta. Thyroid-releasing hormone (TRH) and iodide do cross the placenta** (17). Maternal hypothyroidism has been associated with abnormal intelligence quotient testing and pediatric neurodevelopment in offspring, particularly when untreated (19). While severe maternal iodine deficiency can lead to cretinism in the offspring, it is less clear whether mild-to-moderate iodine deficiency leads to more subtle cognitive or neurologic dysfunction. Iodine supplementation in iodine-deficient populations has been found to substantially reduce the relative risk of cretinism and to improve psychomotor and cognitive test scores in the offspring (18).

Subclinical hypothyroidism is defined as an elevated TSH with a normal FT_4 and has been associated with preterm birth and neurodevelopmental problems in offspring (19,20) (see also chap. 6 in *Maternal-Fetal Evidence Based Guidelines*).

Pregnancies in women with subclinical hypothyroidism are more likely to be complicated by placental abruption and preterm birth prior to 34 weeks (20). However, while treatment of overt hypothyroidism has been associated with improved pregnancy outcomes, there is no good evidence that screening and intervention for subclinical hypothyroidism improve outcomes (16,17,19,20). The physiologic basis for fetal effects of subclinical hypothyroidism is unclear since thyroxine levels are normal. Animal studies suggest that it is hypothyroxinemia, not elevated TSH that has adverse implications for fetal brain development (19). Furthermore, it is not clear whether pediatric neurodevelopmental outcomes improve with thyroid hormone treatment. It is also plausible that improvement in iodine supplementation would be of benefit (19). Further evidence is needed before widespread screening and treatment of subclinical hypothyroidism should be initiated.

Inadequately treated maternal **hyperthyroidism** has been associated with increased risk of severe preeclampsia, preterm delivery, low birth rate, fetal loss, and heart failure (17) (see also chap. 7 in *Maternal-Fetal Evidence Based Guidelines*). Thyroid storm is a medical emergency caused by an extreme metabolic state characterized by fever, tachycardia, nervousness, confusion, vomiting, and diarrhea, which has a potentially high mortality in the pregnant patient (17). Thyroid antibodies can cross the placenta and cause fetal thyrotoxicosis, a concern for any pregnant women with a history of Graves' disease (17). The thyroid receptor immunoglobulins, thyroid-stimulating immunoglobulin (TSI), and thyroid-binding inhibitory immunoglobulin (TBII) do pass the placenta. High levels of TSI have been associated with neonatal Graves' disease but the clinical utility of its measurement has been the subject of debate. The risk of immune-mediated thyroid disease in the fetus is not associated with maternal thyroid function (17). **Hyperemesis gravidarum** is associated with elevated levels of hCG, an increase in FT_4, and a decrease in TSH (biochemical hyperthyroidism). However, this is largely transitory and rarely associated with clinical hyperthyroidism. Thus, routine measuring of thyroid function in hyperemesis is not indicated in the absence of other signs of hyperthyroidism such as weight loss or persistent tachycardia (17). Furthermore, treatment of transient hyperthyroidism associated with elevated hCG and hyperemesis should not be undertaken in the absence of evidence of intrinsic thyroid disease (21) (see also chap. 9 in *Maternal-Fetal Evidence Based Guidelines*). A large prospective observational study of 25,765 pregnant women who underwent thyroid screening in pregnancy showed no difference in pregnancy complications or in perinatal morbidity and mortality in women with subclinical hyperthyroidism (22).

The function of the thyroid gland remains important in the postpartum patient. **Postpartum thyroiditis** is an autoimmune inflammation of the thyroid gland that may present as new-onset painless hypothyroidism, transient thyrotoxicosis, or thyrotoxicosis followed by hypothyroidism in the first year postpartum (16,17). Transient thyroiditis occurs in up to 10% of women in the first year after childbirth, with fatigue and palpitations being the most common symptoms. Most women will return to a euthyroid state, but there is a 30% risk of permanent hypothyroidism (16). It is important to consider this diagnosis in patients with postpartum depression or nonspecific systemic complaints in the months following delivery.

HEMATOLOGIC

Pregnancy is characterized by both quantitative and qualitative changes in the hematologic system. These changes can be adaptive to normal pregnancy but can also put the pregnant women at increased risk for certain pathologic conditions. Anemia and thrombocytopenia are commonly diagnosed during pregnancy, as will be discussed below. Measurements of the acute phase response such as erythrocyte sedimentation rate, C-reactive protein, and white blood cell count have been found to increase during pregnancy. This presents a challenge in the evaluation of pregnant women suspected to have various infectious or inflammatory conditions, but careful clinical assessment allows the practitioner to distinguish between physiologic and pathologic abnormalities in these tests. Pregnancy also has important effects on the coagulation system, with the creation of an overall hypercoagulable state. This section also reviews the theories and limitations of the evidence surrounding the diagnosis of thrombophilia during pregnancy.

Anemia is usually defined as a hemoglobin less than 11 g/dL and hematocrit less than 33% in the first trimester, hemoglobin less than 10.5 g/dL and hematocrit less than 32% in the second trimester, and hemoglobin less than 11 g/dL and hematocrit less than 33% in the third trimester (23) (see also chap. 14 in *Maternal-Fetal Evidence Based Guidelines*). Anemia may be caused by decreased production of red blood cells, by increased destruction of red blood cells, or by blood loss. Anemia in pregnancy is complicated by increased iron requirements and an expanded blood volume. Blood volume increases by about 50% while red blood cell mass increases by about 25%, resulting in an anemia of dilution, as measured by hemoglobin and hematocrit, that is physiologic in pregnancy. **Iron requirements increase** in order to support the increase in red blood cell mass, the requirements of the fetus and placenta, and to prepare for blood loss during delivery. **Iron-deficiency anemia** is characterized by microcytosis and hypochromatosis. Iron studies reveal a decrease in total iron and ferritin and an increase in total iron-binding capacity (TIBC). **Ferritin levels** have the highest sensitivity and specificity for iron deficiency, with levels less than 10 to 15 µg/dL being diagnostic of iron deficiency (23). Iron supplementation as well as screening for iron deficiency during pregnancy is recommended by the Centers for Disease Control and Prevention. The typical diet contains 15 mg of elemental iron per day, while the recommended dietary daily allowance during pregnancy is 27 mg/day (23). Iron-deficiency anemia in pregnancy has been associated with an increased risk of low birth weight, prematurity, perinatal mortality, postpartum depression, and poor mental and psychomotor testing in offspring. Severe anemia (less than 6 g/dL) has been associated with abnormal fetal oxygenation, abnormal fetal heart rate patterns, reduced amniotic fluid volumes, cerebral vasodilation, and fetal death. Transfusion may be indicated for fetal indications in the case of anemia of this severity (23). Iron supplementation has been found to decrease the incidence of anemia at delivery, although its effect on healthy, non-iron-deficient women is not clear. Factors that increase the risk for iron deficiency in pregnancy include young maternal age, heavy menses, short interpregnancy interval, low socioeconomic status, and non-Hispanic black race (23). Dietary factors can have a significant effect on iron levels, not only due to levels of consumption of iron-rich foods but also due to consumption of foods that significantly enhance or inhibit iron absorption.

Megaloblastic macrocytic anemia may be caused by deficiency of folic acid and vitamin B12 and by pernicious anemia. Nonmegaloblastic macrocytic anemia may be caused by alcoholism, hypothyroidism, liver disease, aplastic anemia, or increased reticulocyte count. The most common cause of onset of macrocytic anemia during pregnancy in the United States is folic acid deficiency (23). During pregnancy, daily folic acid requirements increase from 50 µg to 400 µg (23). Women who have had gastric surgery and those with Crohn's disease may be at risk of vitamin B12 deficiency in pregnancy (23).

The performance of complete blood counts as a part of routine prenatal screening results in a frequent diagnosis of **thrombocytopenia** in asymptomatic pregnant women. The mean platelet count in pregnant women is lower than in non-pregnant women, with about **8%** of pregnant women meeting criteria for the diagnosis of thrombocytopenia (24). Manifestations of thrombocytopenia include epistaxis, petechiae, and ecchymosis, although frequently there are no clinically significant effects. Clinically significant spontaneous bleeding is rare as long as platelet counts are greater than $10,000/\mu L$ and even excessive bleeding associated with trauma or surgery is unlikely with platelet counts greater than $50,000/\mu L$ (24). **The most common cause of thrombocytopenia in pregnancy is gestational thrombocytopenia,** which is an apparently benign condition whose underlying physiology is not well understood. However, thrombocytopenia in pregnancy may also be caused by more severe underlying conditions such as preeclampsia, human immunodeficiency virus infection, immune thrombocytopenic purpura (ITP), systemic lupus erythematosus, antiphospholipid antibody syndrome, hypersplenism, disseminated intravascular coagulation, thrombotic thrombocytopenic purpura, hemolytic uremic syndrome, congenital thrombocytopenia, or medication effect (24). Most of these conditions can be ruled out by history, physical exam, and exclusion of underlying diagnoses.

The most difficult differential usually comes down to gestational thrombocytopenia versus **ITP**. These conditions cannot be reliably differentiated with antiplatelet antibody testing or any other diagnostic test. Differentiation can be obtained by documenting platelet counts less than $70,000/\mu L$ which suggests ITP, or by documenting a return to normal platelet counts after delivery, suggestive of gestational thrombocytopenia (24). In order to be classified as gestational thrombocytopenia, there are several conditions that must be satisfied. Gestational thrombocytopenia is mild, with platelet counts greater than $70,000/\mu L$. There is no history of significant bleeding and no history of thrombocytopenia prior to pregnancy. Platelet counts generally return to normal within 2 to 12 weeks following delivery, and there is an extremely low risk of fetal or neonatal thrombocytopenia. Many women with ITP have a history of abnormal bleeding prior to pregnancy, although this is not universal. Findings suggestive of ITP include persistent platelet counts less than $100,000/\mu L$, normal or increased megakaryocytes in the bone marrow, absence of splenomegaly, and exclusion of other systemic disorders known to be associated with thrombocytopenia (24).

Women with gestational thrombocytopenia are not at risk for maternal or fetal hemorrhage or bleeding complications (24). Immunologic thrombocytopenia such as ITP and neonatal alloimmune thrombocytopenia (NAIT) have the potential for fetal complications. Both are characterized by increased platelet destruction. Twelve to fifteen percent of neonates born to mothers with ITP may develop platelet counts less than $50,000/\mu L$. This may result in findings such as purpura, ecchymosis, or melena. Less commonly, fetal intracranial hemorrhage may develop, unrelated to mode of delivery. The incidence of serious bleeding complications in neonates of women with ITP is estimated at 3% and the rate of intracranial hemorrhage at 1% (24).

Most intracranial hemorrhage is due to NAIT, the platelet equivalent to hemolytic disease of the newborn (see also chap. 51 in *Maternal-Fetal Evidence Based Guidelines*). NAIT does not have any effects on the mother, and it is typically diagnosed unexpectedly by the finding of severe neonatal thrombocytopenia following an uncomplicated pregnancy. Up to 50% of cases of this potentially life-threatening condition occur in the first liveborn infant. NAIT is associated with a 10% to 20% risk of intracranial hemorrhage in the fetus or neonate, which may be detected by ultrasound when it occurs antenatally. The pathophysiology of NAIT is maternal alloimmunization to fetal platelet antigens. Recurrence risk is related to the zygosity of the father and approaches 100% if the next sibling carries the relevant antigen (24).

Onset of thrombocytopenia during the third trimester should prompt consideration of gestational hypertensive disorders, which are associated with about 20% of maternal thrombocytopenia, and decreasing platelet count is considered a sign of worsening of disorders of this spectrum (see also chap. 1 in *Maternal-Fetal Evidence Based Guidelines*). When combined with hemolytic anemia and elevated liver tests, thrombocytopenia is indicative of the diagnosis of hemolysis, elevated liver enzymes, and low platelet count (HELLP) syndrome. These disorders are associated with an increase in platelet destruction but the underlying physiology is not known. Platelet function may be reduced even if platelet counts are normal, and thrombocytopenia may occur prior to other manifestations of gestational hypertension. Hemorrhage is uncommon in the absence of disseminated intravascular coagulation. Neonatal thrombocytopenia following gestational hypertension is increased in premature infants but not in term infants (24).

Pregnancy is associated with significant alterations in the **coagulation system**. There is a **decrease in protein S levels as well as in coagulation factors XI and XIII. There is an increase in coagulation factors I, VII, VIII, IX, and X. D-dimer and fibrinogen levels** also increase. The overall result is the creation of a hypercoagulable state that is exacerbated by venous stasis and compression of the inferior vena cava and pelvic veins by the enlarging uterus (3,25). This places the pregnant women at increased risk for such phenomena as deep venous thrombosis and pulmonary embolism, which are further elevated when pregnancy is associated with other high-risk states such as obesity, prolonged immobility (bed rest), or surgery (see also chap. 28 in *Maternal-Fetal Evidence Based Guidelines*). Consideration of these risks is important in the evaluation of the pregnant patient with unilateral lower extremity edema or acute dyspnea. They also warrant caution and the responsibility to practice evidence-based medicine when considering the common recommendation of "bed rest" for prevention of treatment of conditions ranging from threatened abortion to preterm contractions to gestational hypertension.

Antiphospholipid syndrome (APS) has been associated with increased risk of thrombosis during pregnancy, recurrent embryonic or fetal loss, preeclampsia, and intrauterine growth restriction (26) (see also chap. 26 in *Maternal-Fetal Evidence Based Guidelines*). Clinical criteria for the diagnosis of APS include vascular thrombosis, unexplained fetal death after 10 weeks, or three or more unexplained embryonic losses prior to 10 weeks' gestation. Premature birth prior to 34 weeks due to preeclampsia or placental insufficiency are also clinical criteria for diagnosis of APS, but it is not yet recommended that women with these disorders be screened for antiphospholipid antibodies (26). For women with APS and a history of thrombosis, anticoagulation with heparin is recommended during pregnancy and postpartum (26). Heparin combined with low-dose aspirin is recommended for patients with antiphospholipid antibodies and a history of recurrent pregnancy loss.

Patients with certain **inherited thrombophilia** (Factor V Leiden, prothrombin gene mutations, and deficiency in activities of antithrombin III, protein S, and protein C) have found to be at increased risk of venous thromboembolism during pregnancy, especially those who have a history of prior thrombosis (25) (see also chap. 27 in *Maternal-Fetal Evidence Based Guidelines*). There has been a great deal of enthusiasm for the theory that such thrombophilias may also increase the risk of uteroplacental thrombosis and thereby lead to adverse pregnancy outcomes such as fetal loss, preeclampsia, fetal growth restriction, and placental abruption (25). Testing for the existence of inherited thrombophilia polymorphisms has increased in response to the occurrence of a range of adverse reproductive outcomes or to a family history of thrombosis. Unfortunately, this represents an area where the use of diagnostic testing has surpassed the knowledge of how abnormal test results should be managed. First, the association of various thrombophilia polymorphisms with adverse reproductive outcomes is largely based on theory and retrospective studies that are subject to publication bias and not confirmed by meta-analysis or prospective studies (25,27,28). Second, treatment trials to support the use of anticoagulation to improve pregnancy outcomes are entirely lacking (25,27,29).

The American College of Obstetricians and Gynecologists currently recommends against screening for inherited thrombophilias in patients with a history of recurrent fetal loss, placental abruption, intrauterine growth restriction, or preeclampsia (25).

GASTROINTESTINAL

Changes in gastrointestinal physiology lead to some of the most commonly described discomforts of pregnancy ranging from nausea and vomiting in early pregnancy to more persistent symptoms of gastroesophageal reflux and constipation. However, gastrointestinal symptoms may reflect coexisting diseases or may even herald life-threatening complications of pregnancy such as severe preeclampsia and HELLP syndrome or acute fatty liver of pregnancy (AFLP). Once again, it becomes crucial for the obstetric care provider to be skilled in recognizing signs and symptoms that result from normal pregnancy physiology and distinguishing those of more serious conditions.

There are several recognizable effects of pregnancy on gastrointestinal function. Gastric secretion acidity declines but volume increases and relaxation of the cardiac sphincter leads to greater esophageal reflux (1). Combined with a **decrease in gastric and intestinal motility,** this leads to the "full stomach" effect that puts pregnant women at increased risk of aspiration. This, combined with increased airway edema, increases the risks of general endotracheal anesthesia during pregnancy. Thus, for anesthesia purposes, all pregnant women are considered to have a full stomach. Precaution to reduce aspiration risk include the use of nonparticulate oral antacids prior to induction of anesthesia, the use of rapid sequence induction methods, and the use of a cuffed endotracheal tube (1).

During pregnancy there is a decrease in colonic motility and an increase in absorption, and **constipation** is a common complaint among pregnant women. A prospective study of constipation in pregnancy found that one in two women reports constipation at some point in pregnancy, with rates of 24%, 26%, 16%, and 24% in first, second, third trimesters, and postpartum, respectively. Constipation is more likely in women with a prior history of constipation and in women

taking iron supplements. The study did not include nonpregnant controls, but historic controls indicate a constipation rate of 7% in a similar age group (30).

The most common gastrointestinal symptom of pregnancy is **nausea and vomiting** (see also chap. 9 in *Maternal-Fetal Evidence Based Guidelines*). As many as 80% of women report nausea during pregnancy and it is also the most common reason for hospitalization in the first trimester (21,31). Nausea is generally considered a normal symptom of early pregnancy, and morning sickness has been associated with improved pregnancy outcomes such as reduced risk of miscarriage, preterm birth, low birth weight, and perinatal death. This is theorized to be due to a placental etiology for nausea and vomiting, which is increased by early development of a healthy and robust placenta (21). However, the exact etiology of this symptomatology is not known. It has been hypothesized that nausea and restricted intake in the mother create an environment that is favorable for early placental development (32) or that it confers an evolutionary advantage by causing the mother to avoid the ingestion of foods that may be dangerous to the developing fetus (21). Numerous psychological theories have also been proposed to explain the phenomenon of nausea and vomiting in pregnancy. Nausea in pregnancy is commonly attributed to hCG levels, but conclusive evidence of the underlying physiology is lacking. Experience of nausea is also correlated with elevated estradiol levels and inversely correlated with prolactin levels (31). Estrogens in oral contraceptive pills have shown a dose-related effect of nausea and vomiting. Smoking decreases both hCG and estrogen, and a reduced rate of nausea and vomiting of pregnancy has been demonstrated in smokers (21). Increased placental mass, as found in multiple gestations and gestational trophoblastic disease, has been found to increase the risk of nausea and vomiting and of hyperemesis gravidarum.

It is important for nausea and vomiting of pregnancy to be distinguished from that resulting from other pathologic conditions. Complacency in the evaluation of pregnant patients with nausea and vomiting may result in undertreatment of distressing symptoms, development of hyperemesis gravidarum, or failure to diagnose a coexisting underlying disease. Nausea and vomiting of pregnancy typically start before 9 weeks' gestation and are not accompanied by fever, abdominal pain, or headache (21). Deviation from this presentation should prompt evaluation for other etiologies. The differential diagnosis includes gastrointestinal disorders such as gastroenteritis, gastroparesis, achalasia, biliary tract disease, hepatitis, intestinal obstruction, peptic ulcer disease, pancreatitis, and appendicitis. Genitourinary conditions that may cause nausea and vomiting include pyelonephritis, uremia, ovarian torsion, kidney stones, and degenerating myoma. Nausea and vomiting may also be due to metabolic disorders such as diabetic ketoacidosis, porphyria, Addison's disease, and hyperthyroidism or neurologic disorders such as pseudotumor cerebri, vestibular lesions, migraines, or central nervous system tumors. Finally, drug-related toxicity, psychologic factors, or pregnancy-related complications such as preeclampsia and AFLP may present with nausea and vomiting (21).

Patients who are taking a multivitamin at the time of conception have reduced rates of nausea and vomiting (21). There is good evidence to support the use of vitamin B6 alone or combined with doxylamine for the treatment of nausea and vomiting in pregnancy. Ginger supplements have also been shown to reduce severity of nausea and vomiting (21,33). Numerous antiemetics have also shown acceptable safety and efficacy against nausea and vomiting. Hospitalization, intravenous fluids, and enteral or parenteral nutrition may be used in cases of continued weight loss in spite of these therapies, but overall, the treatment of nausea and vomiting has been shown to reduce hospitalization rates due to hyperemesis gravidarum, which has been associated with increased risk of low birth weight (21).

RENAL SYSTEM AND HOMEOSTASIS

Pregnancy-related changes in the urinary tract include dilation of calyces, pelvis, and ureters. There are significant increases in renal blood flow and in glomerular filtration rate (GFR) (1). This can have significant effects on renal clearance of vitamins and pharmaceutical agents. There is a lowering of the threshold for glucose excretion, which may result in significant random glucosuria even in the absence of gestational diabetes. A common and challenging application of normal and abnormal renal physiology in pregnancy comes in the evaluation of the patient with proteinuria.

Ureteral dilatation may be present in the first trimester, is present in 90% of gravidas by term, and is often greater on the right. Obstructive and humoral mechanisms have been proposed for this dilatation, with obstruction by the gravid uterus likely causing the dilatation above the pelvic brim that is greater in the right ureter (34). There is also a marked increase in ureteral pressure in the third trimester while standing or sitting that is decreased when in the lateral recumbent position (34). This has implications for collection of 24-hour urine samples, as retention of urine in the dilated collecting system may result in an incomplete sample. This may be alleviated by instructing the patient to lie in the lateral recumbent position for about 45 minutes before the discard void prior to starting the collection and again before the final void of the sample (34).

Abnormal proteinuria may be due to glomerular, tubular, or overflow causes. Proteinuria is considered abnormal if excessive of 150 mg/24 hr in nonpregnant patients. In pregnant patients, levels of proteinuria above 300 mg/24 hr are considered abnormal (34). Increased proteinuria in pregnancy is partially due to the increase in GFR. Maximal GFR is obtained in early pregnancy, but proteinuria may further increase in the third trimester due to increased permeability of the glomerular basement membrane, as will be discussed below. Preeclampsia causes glomerular proteinuria, in which most of the excess urinary protein is albumin. In contrast, tubular disease, such as transplant rejection, causes low–molecular weight proteinuria. Conditions that cause overflow proteinuria, such as leukemia, pancreatitis, and hemolytic disease, also tend to be uncommon in pregnancy (34).

The quantity of glomerular proteinuria is dependent on glomerular plasma flow, the concentration of circulating protein, and the filtrance. There is then significant tubular reabsorption, limiting the amount of protein actually excreted. These factors may change independently of renal disease. Functional proteinuria may occur in response to dehydration, fever, or heavy exercise (34). It is also dependent on posture, with a decrease when supine. The increase in GFR of pregnancy contributes to an increase in proteinuria. Elevations in blood pressure may also result in an increase in proteinuria, even in the absence of progressive renal disease (34). Glomerular filtration is dependent on both size and charge of circulating proteins in comparison to that of the glomerular basement membrane. Glomerular basement membrane integrity is dependent on availability of vascular endothelial growth factor (VEGF). This has been attributed to placental production of antiangiogenic protein sFlt-1, which decreases the amount of VEGF available (34). One theory of the pathogenesis of proteinuria in preeclampsia is that there is an increase in sFlt-1 production and a decrease in the amount of VEGF available, resulting in glomerular endothelial injury (34).

Increased permeability of the glomerular basement membrane in the third trimester may explain why many women with baseline glomerular disease can show a significant increase in proteinuria, even in the absence of other evidence of disease progression. Once abnormal proteinuria develops, maximal tubular reabsorption is likely already occurring, and therefore, small increases in protein filtrance by the glomerulus result in significant increases in proteinuria (34). Appreciation of this underlying physiology is important in making decisions regarding management and delivery of increasing proteinuria in a woman with preeclampsia or preexisting renal disease. Again, it is the overall clinical picture combined with an understanding of the underlying physiology, not the perfunctory reliance on cutoffs in laboratory values, that should guide clinical decision-making.

PHARMACOKINETICS

It may be helpful to conclude with a final clinical topic that illustrates many of the above-described physiologic changes: that of pharmacokinetics. **The four major events involved in pharmacokinetics (absorption, distribution, metabolism, and excretion) are potentially altered by physiologic change of pregnancy in a number of organ systems.** Absorption is affected by changes in gastric pH, gastric emptying, and small intestine motility. Increased cardiac output and heightened blood flow to the stomach and small intestine can increase absorption (35). Changes in plasma volume, body fat, and total body water affect drug distribution, and the proportion of unbound fraction of certain drugs may increase due to a decrease in protein concentration. Metabolism is affected by upregulation or downregulation of various enzymes. For example, liver cytochrome p-450 activities increase while CYP1A2 activity decreases while extrahepatic cholinesterase activity decreases (35). Drug excretion is affected by the increased renal blood flow and elevated GFR of pregnancy as well as by increased respiratory elimination (35). This has important implications for both the maintenance of therapeutic drug levels and the avoidance of toxicity. **Clinical evidence to guide pharmacologic therapy in pregnancy is limited,** in part due to the frequent elimination of women of reproductive age from pharmacokinetic trials. A review of the National Library of Medicine database shows that **there are a very limited quantity of pharmacokinetic data for pregnancy,** and thus evidence-based recommendations for dosing and scheduling of drugs during pregnancy are sparse (35).

REFERENCES

1. Lind T. Maternal Physiology: CREOG Basic Science Monograph in Obstetrics and Gynecology. Washington, DC: CREOG, 1985. [Review]
2. Abbassi-Ghanavati M, Greer L, Cunningham F. Pregnancy and laboratory studies: a reference table for clinicians. Obstet Gynecol 2009; 114(6):1326–1331. [Review]
3. American College of Obstetricians and Gynecologists. ACOG Practice Bulletin No. 100: critical care in pregnancy. Obstet Gynecol 2009; 113:443–450. [Level of Evidence: III]
4. Van Oppen A, Van Der Tweel I, Alsbach GPJ, et al. A longitudinal study of maternal hemodynamics during normal pregnancy. Obstet Gynecol 1996; 88:40–46. [Level of Evidence: II-3]
5. Van Oppen A, Stigter R, Bruinse H. Cardiac output in normal pregnancy: a critical review. Obstet Gynecol 1996; 87:310–318. [Review]

6. Desai D, Moodley J, Naidoo D. Echocardiographic assessment of cardiovascular hemodynamics in normal pregnancy. Obstet Gynecol 2004; 104:20–29. [Level of Evidence: II-2]

7. Yarlagadda S, Poma P, Green L, et al. Syncope during pregnancy. Obstet Gynecol 2010; 115(2 pt 1):377–380. [Review]

8. Katz V, Dotters D, Droegemueller W. Perimortem cesarean delivery. Obstet Gynecol 1986; 68:571–576. [Review]

9. Jensen D, Webb K, O'Donnell D. Chemical and mechanical adaptations of the human respiratory system at rest and during exercise in human pregnancy. Appl Physiol Nutr Metab 2007; 32:1239–1250. [Review]

10. Dombrowski M. Asthma and pregnancy. Obstet Gynecol 2006; 108:667–681. [Review]

11. Garcia-Rio F, Pino J, Gómez L, et al. Regulation of breathing and perception of dyspnea in healthy pregnant women. Chest 1996; 110(2):446–453. [Level of Evidence: II-2]

12. National Institutes of Health, National Heart, Lung, and Blood Institute, National Asthma Education and Prevention Program. Working group report on managing asthma during pregnancy: recommendations for pharmacologic treatment, update 2004. Available at: http://www.nhlbi.nih.gov/health/prof/lung/asthma/astpreg.htm. Retrieved December 2010. [Level of Evidence: III]

13. Bell R, Eddie L, et al. Relaxin in human pregnancy serum measured with homologous radioimmunoassay. Obstet Gynecol 1987; 69:585–589. [Level of Evidence: II-2]

14. Quagliarello J, Steinetz B, Weiss G. Relaxin secretion in early pregnancy. Obstet Gynecol 1979; 53:62–63. [Level of Evidence: II-3]

15. O'Leary P, Boyne P, Flett P, et al. Longitudinal assessment of changes in reproductive hormones during normal pregnancy. Clin Chem 1991; 37(5):667–672. [Level of Evidence: II-3]

16. Casey B, Leveno K. Thyroid disease in pregnancy. Obstet Gynecol 2006; 108(5):1283–1292. [Level of Evidence: III]

17. American College of Obstetricians and Gynecologists. ACOG Practice Bulletin No. 37: thyroid disease in pregnancy. Obstet Gynecol 2002; 100:387–396. [Level of Evidence: III]

18. Zimmermann M. Iodine deficiency in pregnancy and the effects of maternal iodine supplementation in the offspring: a review. Am J Clin Nutr 2009; 89(suppl):668S–672S. [Review]

19. Gyamfi C, Wapner R, D'Alton M. Thyroid dysfunction in pregnancy: the basic science and clinical evidence surrounding the controversy in management. Obstet Gynecol 2009; 113:702–707. [Review]

20. Casey BM, Dashe JS, Wells CE, et al. Subclinical hypothyroidism and pregnancy outcomes. Obstet Gynecol 2005; 105:239–245. [Level of Evidence: II-2]

21. American College of Obstetricians and Gynecologists. ACOG Practice Bulletin No. 52: nausea and vomiting of pregnancy. Obstet Gynecol 2004; 103:803–815. [Level of Evidence: III]

22. Casey BM, Dashe JS, Wells CE, et al. Subclinical hyperthyroidism and pregnancy outcomes. Obstet Gynecol 2006; 107:337–341. [Level of Evidence: II-2]

23. American College of Obstetricians and Gynecologists. ACOG Practice Bulletin No. 95: anemia in pregnancy. Obstet Gynecol 2008; 112:201–207. [Level of Evidence: III]

24. American College of Obstetricians and Gynecologists. ACOG Practice Bulletin No. 6: thrombocytopenia in pregnancy. Obstet Gynecol 1999; reaffirmed 2009. [Level of Evidence: III]

25. American College of Obstetricians and Gynecologists. Practice Bulletin No. 113: inherited thrombophilias in pregnancy. Obstet Gynecol 2010; 116:212–222. [Level of Evidence: III]

26. American College of Obstetricians and Gynecologists. Practice Bulletin No. 118: antiphospholipid antibody syndrome. Obstet Gynecol 2011; 117:192–199. [Level of Evidence: III]

27. Branch D. The truth about inherited thrombophilias and pregnancy. Obstet Gynecol 2010; 115:2–4. [Level of Evidence: III]

28. Said J, Higgins J, Moses EK, et al. Inherited thrombophilia polymorphisms and pregnancy outcomes in nulliparous women. Obstet Gynecol 2010; 115:5–13. [Level of Evidence: II-2]

29. Cleary-Goldman J, Bettes B, Robinson JN, et al. Thrombophilia and the obstetric patient. Obstet Gynecol 2007; 110:669–674. [Level of Evidence: III]

30. Bradley C, Kennedy C, Turcea AM, et al. Constipation in pregnancy: prevalence, symptoms, and risk factors. Obstet Gynecol 2007; 110:1351–1357. [Level of Evidence: II-3]

31. Lagiou P, Tamimi R, Mucci LA, et al. Nausea and vomiting in pregnancy in relation to prolactin, estrogens, and progesterone: a prospective study. Obstet Gynecol 2003; 101:639–644. [Level of Evidence: II-3]

32. Huxley R. Nausea and vomiting in early pregnancy: its role in placental development. Obstet Gynecol 2000; 95:779–782. [Level of Evidence: III]

33. Vutyavanich T, Kraisarin T, Ruangsri R. Ginger for nausea and vomiting of pregnancy: randomized, double-masked, placebo controlled trial. Obstet Gynecol 2001; 97:577–582. [Level of Evidence: I]

34. Lindheimer M, Kanter D. Interpreting abnormal proteinuria in pregnancy: the need for a more pathophysiological approach. Obstet Gynecol 2010; 115:365–375. [Level of Evidence: III]

35. Little B. Pharmacokinetics during pregnancy: evidence-based maternal dose formulation. Obstet Gynecol 1999; 93:858–868. [Level of Evidence: II-2]

4

Ultrasound

Melissa I. March, Suneet P. Chauhan, and Alfred Abuhamad

KEY POINTS

- There is **no evidence that ultrasound examination during pregnancy is harmful**. Prenatal exposure to ultrasound is not associated with adverse influence on school performance and physical or neurological function.
- Ultrasound should be performed by **trained and experienced professionals**, with continuing education and ongoing quality-monitoring programs.
- **Routine use of ultrasound** increases early detection of **multiple pregnancies**, increases **earlier detection of major fetal anomalies** when termination of pregnancy is possible, and increases detection rates of fetal malformations.
- **Ultrasound examination is the best method to estimate gestational age dating in pregnancy**.
- **Ultrasound examination at first prenatal visit (usually** *first trimester*) versus at 18 to 20 weeks **provides more precise estimate of gestational age and may be associated with less women feeling worried about their pregnancy**. First-trimester ultrasound **also allows earlier detection of multiple pregnancies, screening for Down's syndrome with nuchal translucency (NT)**, and **diagnosis of nonviable pregnancies.**
- **All pregnant women should be offered a** *second-trimester* **ultrasound for optimal anatomy evaluation.** Until more evidence accumulates regarding the detection of fetal anomalies on the first-trimester ultrasound, if only one ultrasound will be done in pregnancy, it should be a second-trimester scan at about 18 to 22 weeks.
- In low-risk or unselected populations, routine *third-trimester* **(>24 weeks) pregnancy ultrasound** has **not** been **associated with improvements in perinatal mortality**, though these studies lack sufficient sample size. Routine use of ultrasound in the third trimester significantly **decreases the rate of intrauterine growth restriction (IUGR)**.
- **Routine use of ultrasound reduces** the incidence of **postterm pregnancies** and rates of induction of labor for postterm pregnancy.
- In **low-risk or unselected populations, routine Doppler ultrasound examination**, usually around 28 to 34 weeks, does **not result in reduced perinatal mortality**.
- In **high-risk populations**, such as those with IUGR, umbilical artery Doppler assessment is associated with a **reduction in perinatal deaths and obstetric interventions**.
- Measurement of **cervical length** (CL) by transvaginal ultrasound (TVU) has been shown to be an effective predictor of preterm birth (PTB). When a short CL is detected before 24 weeks, interventions such as vaginal progesterone in singletons without prior PTB (using TVU CL < 21 mm) and cerclage in singletons with prior PTB (using TVU CL < 25 mm) have been associated with decrease in PTB and perinatal morbidity and mortality.

SAFETY OF ULTRASONOGRAPHY

The main concern about the safety of ultrasound is based on tissue temperature elevation from energy transfer and its possible effect of cavitations, or the formation of microbubbles in the tissues exposed to ultrasound waves. The effect of ultrasound on tissues has been studied with animal experimentation and has suggested an adverse effect. In humans, however, the information comes from epidemiological data and population studies. **No epidemiological studies have shown harmful effects in humans.**

There is no consistent evidence that ultrasound examination during pregnancy is harmful. Studies have shown that prenatal exposure to ultrasound is not associated with adverse maternal or perinatal outcome. There is no evidence of an adverse effect on speech, vision, hearing, malignancy in childhood, or mental diseases. There is no adverse influence on school performance up to age 15 to 16 years; however, there may be a weak association between exposure to ultrasound and non-right-handedness in boys (1–4).

Despite the lack of evidence that it has a harmful effect, ultrasound is a form of energy and may produce secondary effects in the tissues it traverses. Current expert consensus is that **ultrasound should be performed only with valid medical indications and with the shortest duration possible and at the lowest settings** to avoid unnecessary exposure to ultrasonic waves. Sonographers and sonologists should familiarize themselves with the mechanical and thermal indices during ultrasound examinations. **Exposing the fetus to ultrasonography with no anticipation of medical benefit is not justified** (5,6).

QUALITY

Ultrasound scanning in pregnancy should be always considered as a medical procedure, with as its goal the examination of the fetus. Levels of expertise vary between different health care centers. Since ultrasound efficiency is operator dependent, **continuing education and ongoing quality-monitoring programs are important** strategies in each center offering ultrasound diagnosis. The ongoing risks of "false-negative" tests and/or misinterpretation of the images obtained (either false-positives or wrong diagnoses) can be minimized if those examinations are carried out and interpreted by **trained and experienced professionals**. Sensitivity of ultrasound screening for pregnancy varies widely. **Appropriate accreditation, documentation, and continuous careful quality control are essential** (5,6).

INFORMED CONSENT AND PATIENTS' EXPECTATIONS

Even though a formal written informed consent is not always needed **before the examination, every pregnant woman should be informed on expectations about the obstetric** ultrasound, as well as its benefits and risks. The patients should know that ultrasound evaluation is a screening test with wide variations in detection rates for fetal anomalies, and that all ultrasound diagnoses, especially false-positive and false-negative ones, can put both mother and fetus at risk.

Whether the sex of the fetus should be revealed or not to the patient with a singleton gestation should be addressed. It may be harmful for the physician-patient relationship to withhold this information, especially if the patient previously requested it. Although a moral conflict may exist in some cultures around the world where this information is used by the patient for voluntary abortions based on sex selection and sex preferences, in general disclosing fetal gender during ultrasound can benefit not only the doctor-patient relation but also parent-child relationship (7).

ROUTINE VS. SELECTIVE USE OF ULTRASOUND

Routine (i.e., performed on every pregnant woman) ultrasound examination is associated with the following, compared to selective ultrasound examination (i.e., performed only on women with specific indications) (1):

1. Increases the early detection of multiple pregnancies
2. Increases earlier detection of major fetal anomalies when termination of pregnancy is possible (8)
3. Increases detection rates of fetal malformations
4. Significantly decreases the likelihood of growth-restricted newborns, though it significantly increases antenatal intervention (9)
5. Reduces the incidence of postterm pregnancies and rates of induction of labor for postterm pregnancy by allowing a more precise estimation of exact gestational age
6. No significant differences are detected for clinical outcomes such as perinatal mortality or health service use by mothers or babies. The effect of ultrasound on perinatal mortality is dependent on the detection rate of fetal malformations and on the uptake of pregnancy termination in the population at study

If one routine ultrasound examination is done, it is usually performed at 18 to 22 weeks (<24 weeks). Earlier examination provides more accurate assessment of gestational age; later examination (e.g., between 18 and 22 weeks) allows more full inspection of fetal anatomy (see later in this chapter).

GESTATIONAL AGE DATING IN PREGNANCY

Precise estimation of gestational age is extremely important for optimal obstetric care, including evaluation of fetal growth, interpretation of maternal screening markers, choosing the appropriate gestational age to perform interventions, and management of preterm and postterm pregnancies.

For gestational age estimation, cardinal numbers should be preferred to ordinal numbers to avoid confusion. So week 0 is 1 to 7 days after last menstrual period (LMP), week 2 is 8 to 14 days, etc. In medicine, weeks are used to estimate dating, and not months. If a lay person asks "How many months am I?," then 6 weeks of gestation can be equated approximately to 1 month, etc., and 38 weeks = 9 months. Some other definitions (not uniformly accepted, with variation in literature) include the following: first trimester: 0 to 13 6/7 weeks; second trimester: 14 to 27 6/7 weeks; third trimester: 28 weeks to delivery; term: 37 to 41 6/7 weeks; preterm: 20 to 36 6/7 weeks; and postterm: 42 weeks to delivery.

Ultrasound examination is the best method to estimate gestational age dating in pregnancy (10). The first day of the LMP should be asked of all pregnant women for calculating the approximate date when the dating ultrasound should be performed. Compared with LMP, ultrasound-based gestational age is more precise. The error, even with certain LMP, is due often to late ovulation (>14 days after LMP). Some have stated that there is no reason to use LMP for dating when adequate ultrasound data is available by 24 weeks (10,11).

Ultrasound-based gestational age estimates are lower than LMP-based gestational age estimates and generate a higher rate of PTB and lower rate of postterm birth. The Naegele's rule (add 7 days to first day of LMP, add 1 year, take back 3 months), manual assessment of uterine size, quickening, etc. should not be used unless ultrasound dating is unavailable.

In general, the earlier the ultrasound is obtained in the pregnancy, the more accurate the dating will be. Multiple parameters and equations have been evaluated to estimate gestational age. The crown-rump length (CRL) is associated with the most accurate estimation, with an error of around 2.1 days, and most accurate in assessing gestational age at about 8 to 12.5 weeks. For biparietal diameter (BPD), the error is around 2.8 days, and is most accurate between 12 and 14 weeks. For pregnancies in the second trimester, beyond 14 weeks' gestation, the head circumference appears to be the best predictor of gestational dating. Combining three or more parameters improved dating slightly over single biometric parameter (12). A combination of BPD, abdominal circumference (AC), and fetal length (FL) is commonly used for dating by ultrasound in the second and third trimesters (11). Repeated examinations improve the prediction only marginally, and the estimated date of confinement (EDC) should always be set by the earliest ultrasound, as the earlier the examination is made the smaller is the prediction error. While prediction of gestational age by ultrasound can be very accurate, prediction of date of delivery remains less accurate, with an error of usually ≥7 to 8 days, given other biologic factors.

The transcerebellar diameter (TCD) is an accurate predictor of gestational age and can be used between 14 and 28 weeks reliably with the use of normograms (13). There is some reliability in gestational age prediction even up to 35 weeks, and TCD is spared effects from IUGR, so can be used to assess pregnancies at risk for this complication. The presence of epiphyses in lower extremities usually signifies a gestational age of >32 weeks.

Gestational age determination can generally follow simple suggestions (11) (Table 4.1). The first day of the LMP should be

Table 4.1 Gestational Age Determination

- IVF pregnancies should be dated by the date of embryo transfer minus 14 days to obtain LMP, and then EDC by Naegele's rule. There is no need to ever change dating in these pregnancies.
- First trimester (0–13 6/7 wk): If LMP and ultrasound-based dating differ by ≥7 days, preference should be given to the ultrasound-based date.
- Early second trimester (14–20 6/7 wk): If LMP and ultrasound-based dating differ by ≥10 days, preference should be given to the ultrasound-based date.
- Late second trimester (21–27 6/7 wk): If LMP and ultrasound-based dating differ by ≥14 days, preference should be given to the ultrasound-based date.
- Third trimester (28–42+ wk): If LMP and ultrasound-based dating differ by ≥21 days, preference should be given to the ultrasound-based date.

Abbreviations: IVF, in vitro fertilization; LMP, last menstrual period; EDC, estimated date of confinement.

asked of all pregnant women. They should be asked if they have regular menses, have taken oral contraceptive pills within the last 2 months, or have had any unusual bleeding in the first trimester. The women should be asked if they are certain of their LMP (but this is still not precise). Ultrasound dating is best and often corrects dating by even a "sure" LMP (Table 4.1).

ULTRASOUND EXAMINATIONS BY TRIMESTER
First Trimester

Ultrasonographic evaluation in the first trimester (0–13 6/7 weeks) is the most accurate method to determine exact gestational age, as discussed above. **Ultrasound examination at first prenatal visit versus at 18 to 20 weeks provides more precise estimate of gestational age and may be associated with less women feeling worried about their pregnancy.** High feedback (women can see the monitor screen and receive detailed visual and verbal explanations) ultrasound may not reduce maternal anxiety but may influence positive health behaviors such as decrease in smoking and alcohol use as compared to low feedback (women cannot see the monitor screen and women are given only a summary statement of the scan) (1,14). First-trimester ultrasound also allows **earlier detection of multiple pregnancies, screening for Down's syndrome with NT, and diagnosis of nonviable pregnancies** (1,6). No other important maternal or perinatal outcome differences are detected, with insufficient data to accurately assess some rare outcomes such as perinatal mortality.

Transvaginal scanning is preferred in cases of a pregnancy resulting from ovulation induction or other assisted reproductive technologies, first-trimester bleeding, or increased risk of aneuploidy, and should be used if transabdominal examination is inconclusive for diagnosis. First-trimester screening for congenital defects by TVU is an option for pregnant women who meet certain criteria and should be done by experienced sonographers and confirmed at 18 to 22 weeks.

NT is measured at the area of the back of the fetal neck and is to be performed between weeks 10 6/7 and 13 6/7 of gestation. Increase in nuchal thickness has been associated with chromosomal and anatomical abnormalities in the fetus. Screening permits choosing earliest definitive diagnostic procedures like chorionic villus sampling, allowing women to prepare for a child with health problems, and also providing the option to terminate the pregnancy earlier (6) (see chap. 5).

Indications by American College of Obstetricians and Gynecologists (ACOG) and American Institute of Ultrasound in Medicine (AIUM) for first-trimester ultrasound are shown in Table 4.2, and essential elements of first-trimester ultrasound are in Table 4.3 (5,6).

Ultrasound Diagnosis of Missed Abortion/Embryonic Demise
Anembryonic pregnancy (also called blighted ovum): mean gestational sac size of ≥20 mm and no embryonic pole, or absence of a visible yolk sac with a mean sac diameter of 13 mm, by TVU.

Embryonic demise (also called missed abortion): CRL of ≥5 mm and no heart beat, by TVU.

If the beta human chorionic gonadotropin (BHCG) is >1500, a gestational sac should be visualized by TVU; if the gestational sac is not seen in the uterus, suspect ectopic pregnancy (see also chap. 29).

Prognostic ability: The presence of normal embryonic cardiac activity in the uterine cavity in the first trimester has a >90% prediction for a live birth in both symptomatic and asymptomatic pregnancies.

Table 4.2 Indications for First-Trimester Ultrasound

- To confirm the presence of an intrauterine pregnancy
- To evaluate suspected ectopic pregnancy
- To define the cause of vaginal bleeding
- To evaluate pelvic pain
- To estimate gestational age
- To diagnose or evaluate multiple gestations
- To confirm cardiac activity and identify nonviable pregnancies
- As an adjunct to chorionic villus sampling, embryo transfer, and localization and removal of an intrauterine device
- To evaluate maternal pelvic masses and/or uterine anomalies
- To evaluate suspected hydatidiform mole
- To screen for certain anomalies such as anencephaly in patients at high risk
- To measure nuchal translucency when part of a screening program for fetal aneuploidy

Source: From Refs. 5, 6.

Table 4.3 Essential Elements of First-Trimester Ultrasound

- Gestational sac (location, mean diameter)
- Yolk sac (diameter)
- Crown-rump length (CRL)[a] of embryo
- Development of fetal anatomy in early pregnancy
- Fetal viability (cardiac activity should be seen in embryo >5 mm)
- Fetal number (amnionicity and chorionicity has to be reported for multiples)
- Ultrasound features of early pregnancy failure, for example, ectopic pregnancy and hydatidiform mole
- Uterus, adnexa, and cul de sac
- If possible, the appearance of the nuchal region should be assessed, and specific measurement of NT measured as part of desired screening.
- Any other abnormalities (e.g., leiomyomata)

[a]CRL is a more accurate indicator of gestational age than gestational sac size.
Abbreviation: NT, nuchal translucency.
Source: From Refs. 5, 6.

Precautions and Pitfalls
Physiologic midgut herniation at 7 to 11 weeks (resolve ≥12 weeks): do not confound with omphalocele. The rhomboencephalon can look as a cystic mass up until 8 to 10 weeks and should not be confused with a central nervous system (CNS) anomaly; ventriculomegaly cannot be assessed well in the first trimester. The amnion and chorion are expected to be fused by 14 weeks.

Second Trimester (Aka "Anatomy," or "Standard" Ultrasound)

The best timing for just one ultrasound screening of the fetal anatomy and dating is the early to mid second trimester (18–22 weeks) (1), not only to obtain an accurate estimation of gestational age or a satisfactory inspection of the fetal anatomy but also as a tool to detect anomalies so as to allow the patients to choose about whether or not to proceed with their pregnancies. This is therefore usually called the anatomy, or standard ultrasound examination (nomenclature such as Level I, II, etc. ultrasound is controversial and less descriptive). Given the benefits highlighted above, **all pregnant women should be offered a second-trimester ultrasound**, whether or not they have had a first-trimester ultrasound. At least two aspects are important about early fetal anomalies detection with ultrasound: first, the estimated sensitivity to detect anomalies

Table 4.4 Indications for Second-Trimester Ultrasound[a]

- Estimation of gestational age
- Evaluation of fetal growth
- Vaginal bleeding
- Abdominal and pelvic pain
- Cervical insufficiency
- Determination of fetal presentation
- Suspected multiple gestation
- Adjunct to amniocentesis
- Significant discrepancy between uterine size and clinical dates
- Pelvic mass
- Suspected hydatidiform mole
- Adjunct to cervical cerclage placement
- Suspected ectopic pregnancy
- Suspected fetal death
- Suspected uterine abnormality
- Evaluation of fetal well-being (e.g., BPP)
- Suspected amniotic fluid abnormalities
- Suspected placental abruption
- Adjunct to external cephalic version
- Premature rupture of membranes or premature labor
- Evaluation of abnormal biochemical markers
- Follow-up evaluation of fetal anomaly
- Follow-up evaluation of placental location for suspected placenta previa
- History of previous congenital anomaly
- Evaluation of fetal condition in late registrants for prenatal care
- To assess findings that may increase the risk of aneuploidy
- To screen for fetal anomalies

[a]If not performed in second trimester, a third-trimester ultrasound is indicated.
Abbreviation: BPP, biophysical profile.
Source: From Refs. 5, 6.

Table 4.5 Essential Elements for Second-Trimester Ultrasound[a]

- Fetal cardiac activity (abnormal heart rate or rhythm should be reported).
- Fetal number (multiple pregnancies require additional information: chorionicity, amnionicity, comparison of fetal sizes, estimation of amniotic fluid volume at each side of the membranes, and fetal gender).
- Presentation.
- A qualitative or semiquantitative assessment of amniotic fluid (e.g., amniotic fluid index, single deepest pocket, and 2-diameter pocket) (see chap. 56 in *Maternal-Fetal Evidence Based Guidelines*).
- The placental location, appearance, and relationship to the internal cervical os should be recorded.[b]
- Transvaginal ultrasound may be offered for detection of short cervical length (see chap. 16 in *Maternal-Fetal Evidence Based Guidelines*).
- Gestational age assessment.[c]
- Fetal weight estimation can be calculated by obtaining measurements, such as biparietal diameter, head circumference, abdominal circumference, and femoral length.[d]
- Evaluation of the maternal uterus and adnexal structures should be performed.
- Fetal anatomy survey: Fetal anatomy is best assessed by ultrasound $\geq$18 wk. Essential elements of a standard examination are as follows:
  - Head and neck: cerebellum, choroid plexus, cisterna magna, lateral cerebral ventricles, midline falx, cavum septi pellucidi, and upper lip
  - Chest: the basic cardiac inspection includes a four-chamber view of fetal heart. An attempt should be made, if technically feasible, to view the outflow tracts
  - Abdomen: stomach (presence, size, and situs), kidneys, bladder, and umbilical cord (insertion site into fetal abdomen and vessel number)
  - Spine: cervical, thoracic, lumbar, and sacral spine
  - Extremities: legs and arms (presence or absence)
  - Gender: for evaluation of multiple gestations

[a]If not performed in second trimester, a third-trimester ultrasound is indicated.
[b]The apparent position early in pregnancy may not correlate well with its location at the time of delivery. Therefore, if low-lying placenta or placenta previa are suspected early in gestation, a transvaginal ultrasound is indicated, with verification in the third trimester by a transvaginal ultrasound if previa or placental edge within 20 mm of internal os is found.
[c]First-trimester CRL measurement is the most accurate means for sonographic dating.
[d]None of the several equations for estimating fetal weight based on such fetal biometric measurements is superior to others; ideally, the equations should be derived by actual fetal weights of the local or institutional population. Results can be compared to fetal weight percentiles from published normograms. Consecutive ultrasound examinations for growth evaluation should typically be performed no less than 3 weeks apart.
Abbreviation: CRL, crown-rump length.
Source: From Refs. 5, 6.

varies widely, with higher rates of detection for major anomalies than for the minor anomalies, and some organs (e.g., neural tube defect) versus others (e.g., heart). A **"genetic"** **ultrasound** can be performed with the aim to detect anomalies or markers associated with fetal aneuploidy.

The best time for detection of most malformations is around 20 to 24 weeks even in specialized centers; however, it is important for the woman to obtain this information as early as possible. In some circumstances more than one second-trimester ultrasound is necessary, especially if the first second-trimester ultrasound is performed at 18 to 19 weeks. Experts have suggested indications (Table 4.4) and essential elements (Table 4.5) for second-trimester ultrasound (5,6).

There can be other types of ultrasounds, not necessarily needing all elements. **Limited ultrasound examination** is performed when a specific question requires investigation. For example, to assess amniotic fluid volume, to verify fetal life or death, to evaluate fetal biophysical profile (BPP), to guide amniocentesis, to localize the placenta in antepartum bleeding, to evaluate fetal position, etc. It is appropriate generally only if a prior complete standard ultrasound examination has been done. A **specialized** (aka detailed or targeted) **ultrasound examination** should be considered for a patient who, by history, clinical evaluation, or prior scanning evaluation, is suspected to have an anatomic or physiological abnormality in the fetus. This ultrasound examination must be done by personnel with expertise in obstetric ultrasonography and maternal and fetal disease. Other specialized examinations might include fetal Doppler, three-dimensional (3D), BPP, fetal echocardiography, or others (see below).

Third Trimester

The potential benefit of a third-trimester ultrasound examination greatly depends on how many and how accurate the prior (if any) ultrasounds have been. If the first and only ultrasound is in the third trimester, it probably has similar benefits as the routine second-trimester ultrasound, except early detection and accurate dating are not possible. Assuming prior accurate second-trimester ultrasound(s) have been done, ultrasound evaluations in the third trimester involve assessments of fetal growth, amniotic fluid volume, and placenta, trying to identify a compromised or malformed fetus, etc. Indications for third-trimester ultrasound and essential elements of the ultrasound are the same as second-trimester ultrasound (Tables 4.3 and 4.4) (5,6).

In low-risk women, ultrasound examinations at 30 to 32 weeks and at 36 to 37 weeks **significantly decrease the likelihood of newborns with growth restriction**, though they do increase the rate of antenatal intervention (9). This randomized control trial had 1998 women, and investigators calculate over 30,000 women are required for a trial to show a significant decrease in neonatal mortality (9). In a meta-analysis, there was no difference in antenatal, obstetric, and neonatal intervention or in women screened with >24 weeks (late) ultrasound versus those not screened. There was a slightly higher cesarean section rate in women screened with late ultrasound, but this difference did not reach statistical significance. Routine late pregnancy ultrasound was not associated with improvements in overall perinatal mortality (15). There is insufficient data about the potential psychological effects of routine ultrasound in late pregnancy, and limited data about its effects on both short- and long-term neonatal and childhood outcome. **Placental grading as an adjunct to third-trimester ultrasound examination was associated with a significant reduction in the stillbirth rate in one trial** (16). **More research is needed in placental grading for prediction of poor perinatal outcome for routine recommendation.**

DOPPLER
Fetal and Umbilical Artery

In low-risk or unselected populations, routine Doppler ultrasound examination, usually of the umbilical artery and fetal vessels at around 28 to 34 weeks, does not result in increased antenatal, obstetric, and neonatal interventions, and no overall differences are detected for substantive short-term clinical outcomes such as perinatal mortality (17). However, the use of umbilical artery Doppler ultrasound in high-risk pregnancy (poor growth, diabetes, and hypertension) is associated with a reduction in perinatal deaths and obstetric interventions (18) (see chap. 44 in *Maternal-Fetal Evidence Based Guidelines*).

Fetal middle cerebral artery (MCA) peak systolic velocity (PSV) Doppler has been used to evaluate fetal anemia in cases of maternal red cell alloimmunization from Rhesus disease. Fetal MCA Dopplers are considered a screening test that requires a confirmatory test for diagnosis (fetal blood sampling) at the initiation of therapy (transfusion). MCA-PSV is regarded as the best noninvasive screening for fetal anemia (19) (see chap. 52 in *Maternal-Fetal Evidence Based Guidelines*).

Uterine Artery

Current evidence has not shown a benefit to performing routine midpregnancy uteroplacental Doppler ultrasound for prediction and prevention of preeclampsia, IUGR, or adverse pregnancy outcome (20) (see chap. 44 in *Maternal-Fetal Evidence Based Guidelines*). Studies are currently under way and the utility of uterine Doppler in association with other parameters for the screening of preeclampsia will need to be reevaluated.

BIOPHYSICAL PROFILE

A fetal BPP is a specialized obstetric ultrasound consisting of monitoring of fetal movements, tone and breathing, and assessment of amniotic fluid volume, with or without fetal heart rate monitoring. BPP has been used to identify babies

that may be at high risk of poor pregnancy outcome. Available evidence does not support the use of BPP as the best and only test of fetal well-being in high-risk pregnancies, though it should be acknowledged that the size of the study was insufficient to find clinically significant differences (21) (see chap. 55 in *Maternal-Fetal Evidence Based Guidelines*).

CERVICAL LENGTH

TVU for the measurement of CL has been shown to be predictive of spontaneous PTB in all populations studied so far and can be effective in evaluating the need for such interventions as cervical cerclage or progesterone supplementation. Measurement of CL has been shown to be an effective predictor of spontaneous preterm delivery (<35 weeks) in women hospitalized for preterm labor and women at high risk for preterm delivery, as well as asymptomatic patients with singleton gestations at routine second-trimester ultrasound (22). The recommended threshold is usually <20 mm or <25 mm to identify such patients. CL measurement may also be a good predictor of spontaneous PTB in asymptomatic women with twin pregnancies (23). Cervical funneling (specifically U-shaped funnels) in women with short cervix has also been associated with earlier birth (24), but CL is the one measurement that is most accurate and reproducible for prediction of PTB. Currently, we suggest obtaining **TVU CL at 18 to 24 weeks** (time of second-trimester ultrasound) **in all singleton gestations**. In those without a prior spontaneous PTB, a CL <21 mm should prompt offering vaginal progesterone. In those with a prior spontaneous PTB, a CL <25 mm should prompt offering cerclage (see chap. 16 in *Maternal-Fetal Evidence Based Guidelines*).

3D ULTRASOUND

3D ultrasound examination is not considered a required modality for all pregnant women at this time (4), but it can add accuracy in the assessment of the fetus identified to have anomalies (especially facial anomalies, neural tube defects, and skeletal malformations) by 2D ultrasound. 3D ultrasound allows the acquisition of volume measurements, which can depict topographic anatomy that cannot be seen on 2D scanning. It has not been shown to have a clear clinical advantage over traditional ultrasound (6).

Routine 3D ultrasound (vs. the traditional 2D ultrasound) among low-risk women has not shown a significant impact on maternal-fetal bonding (25). Additionally, 3D/4D ultrasound in women at risk for having a fetus with congenital anomalies does not reduce maternal anxiety compared to conventional 2D ultrasound alone (26).

REFERENCES

1. Whitworth M, Bricker L, Neilson JP, et al. Ultrasound for fetal assessment in early pregnancy. Cochrane Database Syst Rev 2010; (4):CD007058. [Meta-analysis: 11 RCTs, n = >37,505]
2. Newnham JP, Doherty DA, Kendall GE, et al. Effects of repeated prenatal ultrasound examinations on childhood outcome up to 8 years of age: follow-up of a randomized trial. Lancet 2004; 364:2038–2044. [Follow-up at 8 years of RCT of 5 vs. 1 ultrasounds in pregnancy]
3. Stalberg K, Axelsson O, Haglund B, et al. Prenatal ultrasound exposure and children's school performance at age 15–16: follow-up of a randomized controlled trial. Ultrasound Obstet Gynecol 2009; 34:297–303. [RCT, n = 4458]
4. Torloni MR, Vedmedovska N, Merialdi M, et al. Safety of ultrasonography in pregnancy: WHO systematic review of the

literature and meta-analysis. Ultrasound Obstet Gynecol 2009; 33:599–608. [Meta-analysis: RCT, n = 16]

5. American Institute of Ultrasound in Medicine. AIUM practice guideline for the performance of antepartum obstetric ultrasound examination. J Ultrasound Med 2010; 29:157–166. [Review]

6. American College of Obstetricians and Gynecologists. ACOG Practice Bulletin No. 101: ultrasonography in pregnancy. Washington, DC: American College of Obstetricians and Gynecologists, 2009. [Review]

7. Raphael T. Disclosing the sex of the fetus: a view from the UK. Ultrasound Obstet Gynecol 2002; 20:421–424. [Review]

8. Saltvedt S, Almström H, Kublickas M, et al. Detection of malformations in chromosomally normal fetuses by routine ultrasound at 12 or 18 weeks of gestation—a randomized controlled trial in 39,572 pregnancies. BJOG 2006; 113(6):675–682. [RCT, n = 39,572]

9. McKenna D, Tharmaratnam S, Mahsud S, et al. A randomized trial using ultrasound to identify the high-risk fetus in a low-risk population. Obstet Gynecol 2003; 101(4):626–632. [RCT, n = 1998]

10. Gardosi J. Dating of pregnancy: time to forget the last menstrual period. Ultrasound Obstet Gynecol 1997; 9(6):367–368. [Review]

11. Taipale P, Hilesmaa V. Predicting delivery date by ultrasound and last menstrual period in early gestation. Obstet Gynecol 2001; 97:189–194. [II-2]

12. Chervenak FA, Skupski DW, Romero R, et al. How accurate is fetal biometry in the assessment of fetal age? Am J Obstet Gynecol 1998; 178(4):678–687. [II-2]

13. Chavez MR, Ananth CV, Smulian JC, et al. Fetal transcerebellar measurement with particular emphasis on the third trimester: a reliable predictor of gestational age. AJOG 2004; 191:979–984. [II-2]

14. Nabhan AF, Faris MA. High feedback versus low feedback of prenatal ultrasound for reducing maternal anxiety and improving maternal health behaviour in pregnancy. Cochrane Database Syst Rev 2010. [Meta-analysis: 2 RCTs, n = 346]

15. Bricker L, Neilson JP, Dowswell T. Routine ultrasound in late pregnancy (after 24 weeks' gestation). Cochrane Database Syst Rev 2009; (3). [Meta-analysis: 8 RCTs, n = 27,024]

16. Proud J, Grant AM. Third trimester placental grading by ultrasonography as a test of fetal well-being. BMJ 1987; 294:1641–1644. [RCT, n = 2000]

17. Alfirevic Z, Stampalija T, Gyte GM. Fetal and umbilical Doppler ultrasound in normal pregnancy. Cochrane Database Syst Rev 2010; (8):CD001450. [Meta-analysis: 5 RCTs, n = 14,185]

18. Alfirevic Z, Stampalija T, Gyte GM. Fetal and umbilical Doppler ultrasound in high-risk pregnancies. Cochrane Database Syst Rev 2010; (1):CD007529. [Meta-analysis: 18 RCTs, n = 10,000+]

19. Pretlove SJ, Fox CE, Khan KS, et al. Noninvasive methods of detecting fetal anaemia: a systematic review and meta-analysis. BJOG 2009; 116:1558–1567. [Meta-analysis: 9 RCTs, n = 675]

20. Stampalija T, Gyte GM, Alfirevic Z. Utero-placental Doppler ultrasound for improving pregnancy outcome. Cochrane Database Syst Rev 2010; (9):CD008363. [Meta-analysis: 2 RCTs, n = 4993]

21. Lalor JG, Fawole B, Alfirevic Z, et al. Biophysical profile for fetal assessment in high risk pregnancies. Cochrane Database Syst Rev 2009; (3). [Meta-analysis: 5 RCTs, n = 2974]

22. Domin CM, Smith EJ, Terplan M. Transvaginal ultrasonographic measurement of cervical length as a predictor of preterm birth. Ultrasound Q 2010; 26(4):241–248. [Meta-analysis: 23 RCTs, n = 26,792]

23. Conde-Agudelo A, Romero R, Hassan SS, et al. Transvaginal sonographic cervical length for the prediction of spontaneous preterm birth in twin pregnancies: a systematic review and metaanalysis. AJOG 2010; 203:128.e1–128.e12. [Meta-analysis: 21 RCTs, n = 3523]

24. Mancuso MS, Szychowski JM, Owen J, et al. Cervical funneling: effect on gestational length and ultrasound-indicated cerclage in high-risk women. AJOG 2010; 203:259.e1–259.e5. [RCT, n = 301]

25. Lapaire O, Alder J, Peukert R, et al. Two versus three dimensional ultrasound in the second and third trimester of pregnancy: impact on recognition and maternal-fetal bonding. A prospective pilot study. Arch Gynecol Obstet 2007; 276:475–479. [RCT, n = 60]

26. Leung KY, Ngai CSW, Lee A, et al. The effects on maternal anxiety of two-dimensional versus two-plus three-/four-dimensional ultrasound in pregnancies at risk of fetal abnormalities: a randomized study. Ultrasound Obstet Gynecol 2006; 28:249–254. [RCT, n = 124]

5

Prenatal diagnosis and screening for aneuploidy

Dawnette Lewis and Thomas M. Jenkins

KEY POINTS

- **All women should be offered aneuploidy screening,** ideally starting in the first trimester. Population screening should have **genetic counseling services available** to discuss the different modalities, advantages and disadvantages, and the time frame for each test prior to screening. All women should have counseling available if desired or if an "abnormal" result occurs. The difference between a screening and a diagnostic test should be clearly explained before any testing.
- Issues of **sensitivity, specificity, and positive and negative predictive values** are vital to the interpretation of a screening test. Positive predictive value of a screening test is greatly influenced by **prevalence** rates in the population tested.
- **The performance of a screening test depends on** the **age of the women** screened (which determines prevalence of trisomies), **women's preference** of screening methods, their **choice of invasive testing,** and their **attitudes toward pregnancy termination.** There is as of now **no definitive noninvasive prenatal diagnostic test. The only diagnostic tests are invasive, that is, chorionic villus sampling (CVS) and amniocentesis.**
- Compared to a Down's screening policy of amniocentesis for age ≥35 years and universal ultrasound at 18 weeks, a policy of **nuchal translucency (NT) screening is associated with similar numbers of Down's neonates born and a decrease in invasive tests.**
- **First-trimester screening (FTS) includes NT, pregnancy-associated plasma protein-A (PAPP-A), and beta human chorionic gonadotropin (B-HCG) and can be performed at 10 3/7 to 13 6/7 weeks, with the best detection rate achieved at 11 weeks.** The overall detection rate (sensitivity) is about **84% to 87%** [false-positive rate (FPR)—5%]. FTS should be offered only if
  - appropriate training and ongoing quality-monitoring programs are in place for both ultrasound (NT) and laboratory assays of analytes;
  - sufficient information and resources are available to provide comprehensive counseling to women regarding the different options and limitations of these tests; and
  - access to an appropriate diagnostic test (i.e., CVS) is available when screening results are positive.

  Compared to management using second-trimester screening (STS), management using FTS is also associated with a significant reduction in induction for postterm pregnancy because of better dating with first-trimester ultrasound.

- Analyte screening **(quadruple marker screen)** can **detect approximately 70% to 81%** of affected pregnancies **(FPR 5%).**
- **Integrative screening** has the **best detection rate for Down's syndrome (95%), with a low (1–4%) FPR,** but results are available **only in the second trimester. Stepwise or contingent sequential screening** offers **the same 95% detection rate, a reasonable 5% FPR, and availability of results in the first trimester.**
- **Second-trimester "genetic" ultrasound** has an impact, among other things, on dating, induction rates, and anatomic evaluation of the fetus. As a modality for genetic screening, the data are more limited compared to other available tests. Major anomalies (e.g., congenital cardiac defects and duodenal atresia) and some markers (especially nuchal thickening, short humerus or femur, and echogenic bowel) are associated with a significantly higher risk for Down's syndrome.
- **Second-trimester amniocentesis is safer than transcervical (TC) CVS or early amniocentesis (<15 weeks). Early amniocentesis should never be performed. With expert operators (>400 CVS), CVS by any route may be as safe as second-trimester amniocentesis.**
- If **earlier diagnosis** is required, **transabdominal (TA) CVS is preferable to early amniocentesis or TC CVS.** In circumstances where TA CVS may be technically difficult, the preferred options are TC CVS in the first trimester with expert operator, or second-trimester amniocentesis, per patients' preference.

DEFINITION

Prenatal diagnosis: Prenatal diagnosis incorporates screening for fetal aneuploidies and anomalies, with many different modalities, including population screening, individual risk assessment, genetic counseling, and diagnostic testing.

SCREENING VS. DIAGNOSTIC TESTS

Prior to screening a population with an available test, test specifics should be assessed. **Issues of prevalence, sensitivity, specificity, and positive and negative predictive values are vital to the interpretation of a screening test** and are a large part of the problem that exists in interpreting the value of a test by either practitioners or the public. Sensitivity of a screening test can also be called detection rate. Table 5.1 lists the characteristics of an ideal perinatal screening test. High sensitivity and specificity are preferable; however, the prevalence of a condition (based upon the population tested) will ultimately determine the value of a positive or negative result (Fig. 5.1). With lower prevalence, the chance of a particular "positive" test to be a true finding is much less. For example, based upon the numbers from Figure 5.1, if all the women with a positive test from group "A" had a CVS, there would be one positive result for every 55 CVS performed. If all the women in "B" had a CVS, one out of every 2.4 tests would yield a positive result.

The performance of a screening test depends on the age of the women screened (which determines prevalence of

Table 5.1   Ideal Perinatal Screening Test

Identify common or important fetal disorder.
Be cost-effective.
High detection rate; low false-positive rate.
Be reliable and reproducible.
Diagnostic test exists.
Be positive early in pregnancy.
Possible intervention if screening test is positive.

trisomies), **women's preference** of screening methods, their **choice of invasive testing**, and their **attitudes toward pregnancy termination. There is as of now no definitive non-invasive prenatal diagnostic test.** The only **diagnostic tests are invasive, that is, CVS and amniocentesis.**

PRETEST GENERAL COUNSELING

There is no treatment for aneuploidy, so the woman must be aware that the **main aims of screening for aneuploidy** are the **possibility of termination**, and the **knowledge of the diagnosis**, with no definite proof that this knowledge will improve outcome. Similarly, there are usually minimal, experimental, and often no treatments for fetal anomalies, so the woman

must be aware that the main aims of screening for anomalies are (similarly) the possibility of termination, and the knowledge of the diagnosis, with no definite proof that this knowledge will improve outcome. Down's syndrome is the most frequent chromosomal disorder among live-born infants, with an expected prevalence of about 1/600 to 1/800 livebirths, and the most common identifiable cause of mental retardation, with a life expectancy of almost 50 years (see chap. 6).

While complicated, discussion of sensitivity (detection rates) at 5% FPR of main screening tests (highlighted in Table 5.2) is necessary. Specific resources (time, expertise, plus the availability of genetic counseling) are paramount. Continuing education of health care providers is necessary. Some couples might prefer a screening approach with earliest detection even with a higher, for example, 5%, FPR (e.g., FTS). Some other couples might prefer highest detection with lowest FPR (e.g., integrative screening). Most women who present in first trimester and opt for aneuploidy screening in centers of excellence choose sequential screening, such as stepwise or contingent screening.

No matter the sensitivity of available tests, for women undergoing screening, particularly those in a higher risk group, **detailed discussions regarding the advantages and disadvantages of screening versus diagnostic testing should occur.** After such counseling, each woman can make the most

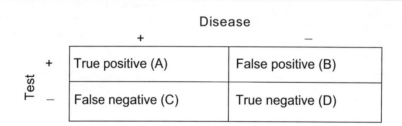

Sensitivity = A/A+C

Specificity = D/B+D

Positive predictive value (PPV) = A/A+B

Negative predictive value (NPV) = D/C+D

Effect of prevalence

N = 100,000
Sensitivity 90%
False positive = 5%

A. Prevalence = 0.1%

90	5,000
10	94,900

PPV = 1.8%
NPV = 99.9%

B. Prevalence = 4%

3600	5,000
400	91,000

PPV = 41.9%
NPV = 99.5%

Figure 5.1   Screening test concepts and effect of prevalence.

Table 5.2 Screening Tests for Down's Syndrome

Test	FPR (%)	Sensitivity (%)
Age	5	25–30
First trimester (11–14 wk)		
NT	5	65–80
PAPP-A and β-HCG	5	60–80
Age, NT, PAPP-A, and β-HCG (FTS)	5	85
Age, NT, PAPP-A, and HCG (FTS)	5	80–85
Second trimester (15–21 wk)		
Age, MSAFP, HCG, and uE$_3$ (TS)	5	60–70
Age, MSAFP, HCG, uE$_3$, and inhibin (QS)	5	70–81
Integrative (nondisclosure of FTS)		
Integrated (NT, PAPP-A, and QS)	4	95
Serum integrated (PAPP-A and QS)	5	85–90
Sequential (disclosure of FTS)		
Independent	11	95
Stepwise	5	95
Contingent	5	88–94
Genetic ultrasound	5	50–70
Extended ultrasound[a]	5	80–85

[a]Genetic ultrasound and serum screening (QS).
Abbreviations: NT, nuchal translucency; PAPP-A, pregnancy-associated plasma protein-A; HCG, human chorionic gonadotropin; MSAFP, maternal serum α-fetoprotein; uE$_3$, unconjugated estriol; FTS, first-trimester screening; TS, triple screen; QS, quadruple screen.

informed and best choice for her situation. **Since screening tests will never detect 100% of disease, the option of diagnostic testing in higher risk populations can be offered.** Several studies have shown that **most pregnant women prefer early (vs. later) screening** for Down's syndrome.

Many women still believe that the whole purpose behind screening for aneuploidy is that a couple can terminate a pregnancy prior to viability. While it is true that couples faced with the reality of an aneuploid pregnancy may opt for termination, **the purpose of prenatal diagnosis and screening is to provide information**. If an abnormality is found, depending on the specifics, couples can be provided with specific information regarding their situation. When a couple decides to carry an abnormal pregnancy to term, the antenatal, intrapartum, and postpartum care can be performed under more ideal circumstances, hopefully altering the outcome. Also, one can not underestimate the effect that preparation can have for the individuals involved.

ANTENATAL SCREENING FOR DOWN'S SYNDROME (TABLE 5.2)
History
Langdon Down, in 1866, reported that the skin of individuals with trisomy 21 appears enlarged. In the 1970s, data became available on the relationship with maternal age and increased risk for aneuploidy. A statistically relevant difference was seen between the 30- to 34-year-old group and the 35- to 39-year-old group, so that this difference led to the offering of women 35 years of age diagnostic evaluation for karyotype. Maternal serum α-fetoprotein (MSAFP) was originally found to be elevated in women carrying fetuses with neural tube defects (NTDs); then in 1984 a low MSAFP was associated with a higher risk of Down's syndrome. NT first-trimester ultrasound screening was introduced in the early 1990s (1). While livebirths to women >35 years of age continue to increase, due to better, more diffuse screening, the number of Down's neonates is decreasing.

Principles
All women should be offered aneuploidy screening, ideally in the first trimester. There is presently a general consensus in the United States that invasive testing for Down's syndrome be offered to those with a second-trimester risk of 1:270 or higher (live-born risk of 1:380). The cutoff level and subsequent public policy were determined over 30 years ago and based on a maternal age risk of 35 years at delivery. Factors considered in determining this value included the prevalence of disease, a perceived significant increase in the trisomy 21 risk after this age, the risk of invasive testing, the availability of resources, and a cost-benefit analysis. Since that time, a number of additional screening tests for Down's syndrome have become available that challenge the validity of maternal age as a single indication for invasive testing. There are a limited amount of randomized-control trials for the evaluation of different tests. Most data come from cohort studies or cross-sectional analysis.

Age
The risk of fetal trisomy 21 increases with maternal age but decreases with the gestational age at assessment in determining the risk, secondary to in utero death rates (Table 5.3) (2).

Women greater than 35 years of age have a higher individual risk than younger women; however, the vast majority of Down's syndrome pregnancies are born to the <35-year-old age group. Screening programs have developed to try and detect affected pregnancies in both the "higher" and "lower" risk groups.

First Trimester Screening: Nuchal Translucency
NT is elevated in fetuses with Down's syndrome at **10 3/7 to 13 6/7 weeks** [crown-rump length (CRL) about 36–86 mm]. The NT measurement is obtained in a midsagittal plane with the neck of the fetus in a neutral position. The amnion should be seen separately from the neck. The image should be enlarged >75% of the screen. The measurement is obtained from the inner to inner aspect of the NT, and multiples of the medians (MoMs) are used to calculate the Down's syndrome risk via computer software. An increased NT is >70% sensitive for trisomy 21, trisomy 18, and trisomy 13 (Table 5.2) (1). Rigorous training, certification, and ongoing quality control are necessary to achieve the detection rates published in the literature

Table 5.3 Risk for Down's Syndrome Based on Maternal and Gestational Age

Maternal age	Gestational age (wk)			Live-born
	12	16	20	
20	1/1068	1/1200	1/1295	1/1527
25	1/946	1/1062	1/1147	1/1352
30	1/626	1/703	1/759	1/895
31	1/543	1/610	1/658	1/776
32	1/461	1/518	1/559	1/659
33	1/383	1/430	1/464	1/547
34	1/312	1/350	1/378	1/446
35	1/249	1/280	1/302	1/356
36	1/196	1/220	1/238	1/280
37	1/152	1/171	1/185	1/218
38	1/117	1/131	1/142	1/167
39	1/89	1/100	1/108	1/128
40	1/68	1/76	1/82	1/97
42	1/38	1/43	1/46	1/55
44	1/21	1/24	1/26	1/30
45	1/16	1/18	1/19	1/23

(www.fetalmedicine.com; www.ntqr.org). The optimal time to perform NT for Down's screening is about 11 weeks.

Compared to a Down's screening policy of amniocentesis for age ≥35 years and ultrasound at 18 weeks, a policy of NT screening is associated with similar numbers of Down's neonates born (a nonsignificant 37.5% decrease) and a significant 82% decrease in invasive tests (3). One explanation for the small nonsignificant difference in Down's neonates born alive may be that NT screening certainly identifies better Down's fetuses, but the majority of these identified Down's fetuses are those that would have miscarried without intervention.

Biochemistry

The maternal serum analytes measured are B-HCG and PAPP-A. **B-HCG** normally decreases in pregnancy but is *increased* in fetuses affected with trisomy 21. **Free** B-HCG performs better than **total HCG** as an independent marker, but there does not appear to be a clinically significant difference in sensitivity when either is combined with NT and PAPP-A for FTS (4). **PAPP-A** normally increases in pregnancy but is *decreased* in fetuses affected with trisomy 21. B-HCG discrimination is greatest at 13 weeks, while PAPP-A's is greatest at 10 weeks, making 11 weeks the optimal time for first-trimester analyte screening.

First Trimester Screening

FTS consists of measurement of the **NT** combined with maternal serum screening (**PAPP-A and B-HCG**). Over 20 studies in over 200,000 women have been performed to assess the sensitivity of this screening test, making this the best studied screening test in pregnancy (4–7). The gestational age for FTS is about **10 3/7 to 13 6/7 weeks** (about 73–98 days; CRL about 36–86 mm). The usual cutoff risk is 1:270. The detection rate (sensitivity) is about **84% to 87%** (95% CI 80–90%). **The best detection rate is achieved at 11 weeks.**

FTS should be offered only if the following criteria can be met (4–7):

1. Appropriate training and ongoing quality-monitoring programs are in place for both ultrasound (NT) and laboratory assays of analytes.
2. Sufficient information and resources are available to provide comprehensive counseling to women regarding the different options and limitations of these tests.
3. Access to an appropriate diagnostic test (i.e., CVS) is available when screening results are positive.

The Maternal-Fetal Medicine Foundation (www.mfmf.org) and the Fetal Medicine Foundation (www.fetalmedicine.com) both provide nuchal translucency education and quality review programs. There is sufficient evidence to support implementing FTS for Down's syndrome provided the above three requirements are met. Almost 85% of women in the United States present for care within 12 weeks and can be offered FTS. FTS can provide high detection, early reassurance, more time/diagnostic options, and earlier completion of aneuploidy screening.

Compared to management using STS, management using FTS is associated also with a significant reduction in induction for postterm pregnancy because of better dating with first-trimester ultrasound (8).

Nasal Bone

Over 12 studies in over 18,000 women demonstrated that nasal bone when imaged at 11 to 14 weeks is absent in approximately 70% of Down's fetuses, and in only 1.5% of unaffected fetuses. When added to FTS (NT, PAPP-A, and B-HCG), it can increase the detection rate to about 95%, decreasing the FPR to 2%. Possibly given to the difficulty of this exam, these data have not been confirmed in all studies. Abnormal ductus venosus Doppler flow and tricuspid regurgitation have also been found to be >70% sensitive for trisomy 21, but there are insufficient prospective data for any increase in accuracy over FTS alone.

Second Trimester Screening

Maternal analyte screening had the first reported association with Down's syndrome with low **MSAFP** (MoM 0.75), followed by the association of high **human chorionic gonadotropin (hCG)** (MoM 2.3) and a low **unconjugated estriol** (MoM 0.7) to form the "**triple screen.**" The detection rate for women under the age of 35 with a triple screen ranges between 57% and 74%, with a constant 5% FPR (3,5). For women above the age of 35 (using similar cutoff values), the sensitivity increases to 87%, but the FPR also balloons to 25% (9). **Inhibin** was added to analyte screening [**quadruple screen (QS)**], but, since levels correlate somewhat with hCG, it is not an independent predictor like the other markers, and the increase in detection is more limited (7–11 percentage points). Approximately 70% to 81% of cases are detected in the majority of studies, holding the FPR at 5% (4,6). This screening test can be performed between 15 and 22 weeks, with best results obtained at 16 to 18 weeks. Values need to be adjusted, as needed, for diabetes, obesity, and other factors.

Other combinations of markers have been assessed; however, with the addition of extra markers, the potential benefit versus the cost must be balanced. With each additional marker, costs to society reach into the millions secondary to the numbers of pregnancies tested each year. The relative cost and value of raising the sensitivity or lowering the FPR a few percentage points is an ongoing debate.

Combining Both First- and Second-Trimester Tests

Combined screening programs in the first trimester (using both ultrasound assessments of the NT and maternal analytes) and the second trimester (using maternal analytes) have been described. Patterns of testing include sequential testing (results given after each test) and integrated testing (delaying reporting until both tests have been completed).

Integrative Screening
This involves performance of screening tests at different times during pregnancy with a single result provided to the patient only after all tests have been completed. A protocol for integrated screening for Down's syndrome is based upon tests performed during the first and second trimesters (NT, PAPP-A, MSAFP, hCG, estriol, and inhibin). Mathematical models calculated that >85% of affected pregnancies would be detected with an FPR of only 0.9%. The first- and second-trimester evaluation of risk (FASTER) trial performed integrated screening in 33,557 women (84 with Down's syndrome) (6). Cutoff values for the different tests varied (first-trimester combined test cutoff 1:150; second-trimester "quad screen," 1:300). The authors report a sensitivity of 86% with FTS (FPR 5%), 85% with STS (FPR high at 8.5%), and, when combined, a 94% detection of Down's syndrome cases. If results are revealed after STS, the FPR is only 4.9%, with the **best**

sensitivity. If NT is not available, an "integrated serum screening test" has a detection rate of 85% with 3.9% FPR (4). Disadvantages of integrative screening include the lack of early diagnosis, the physical and psychological ramifications created if an abnormality is found and the woman opts for termination (compared to the first trimester), the increase in costs (compared to either FTS or STS), the perception of "hiding" abnormal results, as well as the limitations it places on multiple gestations if discordant karyotypes are found.

Sequential Screening

It involves performance of different screening tests at different times during pregnancy with results provided to the patient after each test. There are three approaches to sequential testing: independent, stepwise, and contingent.

Independent. This approach involves the independent interpretation of FTS and STS. While the sensitivity is as exemplary with this approach as with integrative screening (94–95%), combining screening tests and revealing the results after each increase the chance for false-positive results. The FASTER trial's (6) FPR was 10.8% with sequential independent screening, far too high for population-based usage. As a high FPR means higher loss rates due to more invasive testing, independent sequential screening is the least efficient risk assessment strategy and should *not* be used.

Stepwise. Both FTS and STS (usually QS) are performed, with results revealed after FTS: If FTS risk is above a certain cutoff, invasive testing (i.e., CVS) is offered; if FTS is below a certain cutoff, STS is recommended with a final risk revealed at that point. In the FASTER trial, such an approach (low cutoff 1:150; high cutoff 1:300) had a **detection rate of 95% with an FPR of 4.9%** (6). The advantages of this approach are a very high detection rate (as with integrative screening), with the option of early results in first trimester for the highest risk women. **This is currently the most common way to perform screening for aneuploidy in women presenting in the first trimester** in centers with adequate expertise and facilities. With FTS and such low FPRs, there has also been a decrease in the number of women requesting invasive prenatal diagnosis.

Contingent. Both FTS and STS (usually QS) are performed, with results revealed after FTS: If FTS risk is above a certain cutoff (e.g., 1/150), invasive testing (i.e., CVS) is offered; if FTS is below a certain cutoff (e.g., 1/300), no further screening is necessary; and if FTS is in between, STS is recommended with a final risk revealed at that point. Careful determination of risk cutoffs is necessary. This strategy has not been studied prospectively.

Genetic Ultrasound Screening for Down's Syndrome

An ultrasound of the fetus performed at **18 to 24 weeks** is associated with several important benefits (see chap. 4). One of the benefits is the antenatal detection of anomalies. The identification of a fetus with an issue allows for directed counseling and optimization of antepartum, intrapartum, and postpartum care. Whether routine or targeted anatomic assessment is being performed, it should be done by experienced centers with ongoing quality assessment to increase detection of anomalies and limit false-positive results.

The in utero diagnosis of Down's syndrome can be suspected when anomalies or physical features that occur more frequently in Down's syndrome than in the general population are noted on an ultrasound examination. Certain

of these major structural congenital anomalies, such as atrioventricular canal or duodenal atresia, strongly suggest the possibility of Down's syndrome and are independent indications to offer invasive testing. Although, when present, there is a high risk of trisomy 21, these anomalies have low sensitivity and, thus, are not useful in screening. For example, when **duodenal atresia** is identified, there is approximately a 40% risk of Down's syndrome, yet it is seen in only 8% of affected fetuses. About 50% of Down's fetuses have **congenital heart defects.**

Physical characteristics that are not structural anomalies but occur more commonly in fetuses with Down's syndrome are called **markers**. By comparing the prevalence of markers in Down's syndrome fetuses to their prevalence in the normal population, a likelihood ratio (LR) can be calculated, which can be used to modify risk. This is the basis for ultrasound screening for Down's syndrome. In order for a marker to be useful for Down's syndrome screening, it should be sensitive (i.e., present in a high proportion of Down's syndrome pregnancies), specific (i.e., not commonly seen in normal fetuses), easily imaged in standard sonographic examination, and present early enough in the second trimester that diagnostic testing can be performed so that results are available when pregnancy termination remains an option. A list of presently available markers and LRs are seen in Tables 5.4 and 5.5, respectively (10–12). Markers commonly sought to assess the risk of Down's syndrome include the following:

Increased nuchal fold: About 35% of Down's syndrome fetuses, but only 0.7% of normal fetuses, have a nuchal skin fold measurement ≥6 mm (some studies use ≥5 mm). When an increased nuchal fold is an isolated finding, the LR is strong at 10 to 17. Thus, the presence of an increased nuchal fold alone is usually an indication to offer invasive testing.

Increased echogenicity of the fetal bowel: When brighter than the surrounding bone, this marker has a Down's syndrome LR of 3.0 to 6.7. This finding can also be seen with fetal cystic fibrosis, congenital cytomegalovirus (CMV) infection, swallowed bloody amniotic fluid, and severe fetal growth restriction (FGR).

Short humerus and, in a lesser degree, short femur: These markers in the second trimester are associated with Down's syndrome, relative to the length expected from their biparietal diameter (BPD). This can be used to identify at-risk

Table 5.4 Selected Ultrasound Findings Associated with Down's Syndrome

Major anomalies
Congenital heart defects
Duodenal atresia

Major markers
Increased nuchal thickness
Hyperechoic bowel
Shortened humerus
Shortened femur
Echogenic intracardiac focus
Renal pyelectasis

Minor markers
Shortened or absent nasal bone
Foot length
"Sandal gap" of the foot
Widened ischial spine angle
Hypoplasia of the mid-phalynx of the fifth digit
Brachycephaly

Table 5.5 Likelihood Ratios and 95% Confidence Limits for Isolated Ultrasound Markers

Isolated sonographic marker	Nyberg et al. (10) LR (95% CI)	Smith-Bindman et al. (11) LR (95% CI)	Nicolaides et al. (12) LR
Nuchal fold/Thickening	11 (5.2–22)	17 (8–38)	9.8
Hyperechoic bowel	6.7 (2.7–16.8)	6.1 (3–12.6)	3.0
Short humerus	5.1 (1.6–16.5)	7.5 (4.7–12)	4.1
Short femur	1.5 (0.8–2.8)	2.7 (1.2–6)	1.6
EIF	1.8 (1.0–3)	2.8 (1.5–5.5)	1.1
Pyelectasis	1.5 (0.6–3.6)	1.9 (0.7–5.1)	1.0

Abbreviations: LR, likelihood ratio; CI, confidence interval; EIF, echogenic intracardiac focus.

pregnancies by calculating a ratio of observed to expected (O/E) femur/humerus length based on the fetus' BPD. An O/E ratio for femur length of <0.91 has a reported LR of 1.5 to 2.7 when present as an isolated finding. A short humerus is more strongly related to Down's syndrome, with reported LRs ranging from 4.1 to 7.5.

Pyelectasis: This marker is defined as a renal anteroposterior (AP) diameter of ≥4 to 5 mm and has an LR that ranges from 1.1 to 1.9 as an isolated marker. This has been found by some not to be significantly more frequent in Down's syndrome pregnancies than in normals (low specificity) (12).

Echogenic intracardiac foci: This marker occurs in up to 5% of normal pregnancies and in approximately 13% to 18% of Down's syndrome gestations. The LR for Down's syndrome when an echogenic focus is present as an isolated marker has ranged from 1.0 to 2.8. This has been found by most investigators not to be significantly more frequent in Down's syndrome pregnancies than in normals (low specificity) (12). The risk does not seem to vary if the focus is in the right or left ventricle or if it is unilateral or bilateral but may be affected by ethnicity.

Other markers described include a hypoplastic fifth middle phalanx of the hand, short ears, a sandal gap between the first and second toes, an abnormal iliac wing angle, an altered foot-to-femur ratio, short or absent nasal bone, and others. These markers are inconsistently used because of the time and expertise required to obtain them. Mild ventriculomegaly (10–15 mm) can be an indication for invasive prenatal diagnosis, since it is associated with 1% to 2% risk of aneuploidy if isolated. If the karyotype is normal, mild ventriculomegaly is still associated with about 8% structural anomalies, 3% perinatal death, and 10% to 20% abnormal neurodevelopment.

Except for major anomalies and increased nuchal thickness, isolated genetic ultrasound markers should, in general, not be used as the sole indication for invasive testing. As with other screening modalities, genetic ultrasound can be used to alter the a priori risk in either direction. A positive LR can be used to increase estimated risk. The magnitude of the increase depends upon the marker(s) or anomalies seen. While most of the clinical prospective data justifying this approach have come from a baseline age-related risk, some have advocated using these LRs to adjust whichever baseline risk, even that derived by other screening tests (e.g., FTS and/or QS, or even integrative or consecutive approaches). A benign second-trimester scan having none of the known markers and no anomalies has been suggested to have an LR of 0.4 to 0.5, assuming the image quality is satisfactory when the genetic ultrasound is normal. It is doubtful that the same sensitivity can be achieved in every center.

ULTRASOUND SCREENING FOR OTHER CHROMOSOMAL ABNORMALITIES

Fetal aneuploidy other than Down's syndrome can be suspected based on ultrasound findings (13). The rates reported are usually in high-risk populations and may overestimate the strength of the association when such findings are noted on a screening examination.

Trisomy 18

FTS and STS with MSAFP, hCG, and unconjugated estriol and inhibin (QS) have a high detection rate for trisomy 18. Second-trimester ultrasound also has a high detection rate for trisomy 18.

Choroid plexus cysts (CPC) have a very weak association with trisomy 18 and should not be the sole indication for invasive testing if isolated. The presence of CPC should be an indication for a detailed second-trimester ultrasound for trisomy 18 major anomalies, such as cardiac, central nervous system (CNS), and hands defects.

POSITIVE SCREENING FOR ANEUPLOIDY BUT NORMAL KARYOTYPE
NT

An NT above the 95th percentile for gestational age, and especially ≥3.5 mm at 10 3/7 to 13 6/7 weeks, is associated with an increased risk of other anomalies and syndromes, with the risk directly proportional to the increase in NT (14) (Table 5.6). The list of anomalies is long (14), and a detailed second-trimester ultrasound is recommended. The incidence of cardiac anomalies is ≥3.7% for NT ≥3.5 mm, so that a fetal cardiac ultrasound by experienced operator is recommended.

First-Trimester PAPP-A and B-HCG

Low PAPP-A in FTS in the presence of a normal karyotype is associated with several adverse pregnancy outcomes, including fetal loss, preterm birth (PTB), and FGR. Low free B-HCG is associated with fetal loss. There are no randomized trials assessing any type of intervention or treatment for patients with abnormal serum markers (15).

Second Trimester Screening

High MSAFP is associated with NTDs, as well as abdominal wall defects and several other fetal abnormalities. High MSAFP, negative acetylcholinesterase (AChE), and normal ultrasound can be associated with congenital nephrosis or other syndromes, or normal pregnancy. Unexplained high MSAFP is associated with mild increases in the incidence of preeclampsia, abruption, placental ischemia, PTB, fetal demise,

Table 5.6 Risk of Chromosome Abnormalities and (If Normal Karyotype) of Fetal Death or Anomalies According to Nuchal Translucency

NT	Chromosomal defects (%)	Fetal death (%)	Normal karyotype		
			Major fetal anomalies (%)	Alive and well (%)	Cardiac defects (%)
<95th centile	0.2	1.3	1.6	97	0.6
95th–99th centiles	3.7	1.3	2.5	93	0.6
3.5–4.4	21.1	2.7	10.0	70	3.7
4.5–5.4	33	3.4	18.5	50	6.7
5.5–6.4	50	10	24	30	13
≥6.5	65	19	46	15	20

Abbreviation: NT, nuchal translucency.

low birth weight, and sudden infant death syndrome (SIDS). No trials have assessed specific management to prevent these complications (15).

Low unconjugated estriol is associated with steroid sulfatase deficiency, Smith–Lemli–Optitz, or other conditions when very low (usually <0.3) MoM (15).

MSAFP Screening for NTD

Elevated (usually ≥2.5 MoM) MSAFP between 14 to 21 weeks is associated with a ≥90% to 95% sensitivity for NTDs (false-negative rate 5%). Given that ultrasound is also ≥95% sensitive for NTDs, the routine use of MSAFP screening is most important for pregnancies that will not have a detailed second-trimester ultrasound.

NON-INVASIVE SCREENING FOR ANEUPLOIDIES IN TWINS

NT is accurate in estimating Down's syndrome risk in dizygotic twins, using each NT separately for each fetus. In monochorionic twins, the average NT is the most effective screening method. Detection rates comparable to singletons can be achieved. Detection rates of FTS or STS tests are usually lower than in singletons, with higher rates of false-positive and false-negative results. Chorionicity does not seem to affect serum analytes in FTS or STS (see chap. 43 in *Maternal-Fetal Evidence Based Guidelines*).

DIAGNOSTIC TESTS
CVS and Amniocentesis

Selected common indications for invasive prenatal diagnosis of fetal aneuploidy are listed in Table 5.7. Both CVS and amniocentesis have been performed for many years and can fairly safely diagnose a karyotypic or genetic abnormality. Both procedures have been studied extensively. Differences in technique, as well as timing of the procedure, affect loss rates. To fairly compare procedure-induced loss rates between the two procedures, adjustments must be made for the higher background frequency of pregnancy loss earlier in gestation.

Second-Trimester Amniocentesis

One study in a low-risk population (*n* = 4606) with a background pregnancy loss of around 2% found that a second-

Table 5.7 Selected Common Indications for Invasive Prenatal Diagnosis

- Abnormal first- or second-trimester aneuploidy screen
- Abnormal ultrasound findings
- Parental concern/anxiety

trimester amniocentesis increases total pregnancy loss by another 1% compared to no amniocentesis (RR 1.41; 95% CI 0.99–2.00) (16). **Compared to no amniocentesis, second-trimester amniocentesis is associated with a 0.8% increase in spontaneous miscarriage** (2.1% vs. 1.3%; RR 1.60; 95% CI 1.02–2.52), but similar incidence of perinatal deaths (0.4% vs. 0.7%) (16,17).

There is insufficient data to assess the effect of polymerase chain reaction (PCR) testing [fluorescence in situ hybridization (FISH)]. In a small trial, reporting karyotype in 3 days with PCR did not affect maternal anxiety level compared to about 3 weeks later in Chinese women with an abnormal screening test for Down's syndrome (18). Another study compared median trait- and state-anxiety scores and found no difference between the two groups (19). Therefore, there is insufficient evidence that, while waiting for the full karyotype following amniocentesis, issuing results from a rapid analysis reduces maternal anxiety. The limited evidence from the two trials does not help resolve the dilemma about whether full karyotyping should be abandoned in favor of limited rapid testing for women undergoing Down's syndrome screening. This choice rests on clinical arguments and cost-effectiveness rather than impact on anxiety (20).

Early Amniocentesis

Early amniocentesis (<15 weeks) is not a safe early alternative to second-trimester amniocentesis, because it is associated with increased pregnancy loss (7.6% vs. 5.9%; RR 1.29; 95% CI 1.03–1.61), and higher incidence of talipes (1.8% vs. 0.2%) compared to CVS (RR 4.61; 95% CI 1.82–11.66) (17,21).

CVS

CVS before 10 weeks is associated with an unacceptably high incidence of limb deficiencies and should not be performed. The optimal time for CVS is 10 to 12 weeks, with trials of safety performed only in this gestational age. TA CVS can also be performed after 12 weeks (called usually placental biopsy) in cases in which placental karyotype is needed, but there are no trials on this "late" CVS.

Compared to second-trimester amniocentesis, CVS in general (TA and TC combined) is associated with a slight increased incidence of pregnancy losses and spontaneous miscarriages (17).

Compared to second-trimester amniocentesis, TC CVS is associated with a higher risk of pregnancy loss (14.5% vs. 11%) **and higher** (12.9% vs. 9.4%) **risk in spontaneous miscarriage**, although the results are quite heterogeneous and certainly operator- and experience-dependent (17).

Compared to second-trimester amniocentesis, TA CVS is associated with similar risk of pregnancy loss (6.3% vs.

7.0%) **and spontaneous miscarriage** (3.0% vs. 3.9%) in one study (17,22).

A systemic review of procedure-related losses for CVS and amniocentesis revealed pooled loss rates for CVS at 14 days, 30 days, and prior to 24 weeks of 0.7%, 1.3%, and 1.3%, respectively. The pooled loss rates for amniocentesis for the same time period were 0.6%, 0.8%, and 0.9% (23). Since CVS and amniocentesis are performed at different time periods, it is difficult to compare these procedures due to the higher background loss rate for the time period when CVS is performed. The benefit of earliest diagnosis with CVS compared to amniocentesis should not be underestimated. With the advent of FTS, prenatal diagnosis has moved more to the first trimester. While the total miscarriage rate is higher following first-trimester CVS because of the higher background rate in early pregnancy, for experienced centers, the rates of procedure-induced losses secondary to CVS are similar to those of second-trimester amniocentesis.

The learning curve for TA and TC CVS has been estimated to exceed 400 cases, with postprocedure loss rates for operators having performed less than 100 cases being two to three times higher when compared to more experienced operators. **The importance of operator experience cannot be overemphasized**, particularly for route of CVS, with TC CVS requiring more experience.

TC versus TA CVS: Compared to TA CVS, TC CVS is associated with similar pregnancy loss rates (9.0% vs. 7.4%) **and similar spontaneous miscarriages** (7.9% vs. 4.5%) (17). The results related to comparative pregnancy loss between TA and TC CVS are inconclusive, with significant heterogeneity between studies (17).

TC CVS technical instrument: There is some evidence to support the use of **small forceps** compared to cannulas for TC CVS. When different types of cannulas are compared, Portex cannula is more likely to result in an inadequate sample and a difficult or painful procedure when compared with either the silver or aluminum cannula, respectively. The evidence is not strong enough to support change in practice for clinicians who have become familiar with aspiration cannulas, and no recent studies have been performed (24).

CGH and Other Genetic Tests: Present and Future

Advances in technology have demonstrated many new avenues for **noninvasive** diagnostic testing in utero (i.e., fetal cells from maternal circulation or cervical sampling, free fetal DNA in the maternal circulation, etc.). While different groups have demonstrated capability with these techniques, practicality for population testing is still not yet available.

Array comparative genomic hybridization (aCGH) is instead a new technique (based on **invasive** prenatal samples such as CVS and amniocentesis), which has found clinical use. It can query the entire human genome for copy number changes such as aneuploidy, deletions, duplications, and unbalanced translocations. Unlike traditional cytogenetics that requires dividing cells, aCGH does not (25–30). Conventional karyotype remains the principal cytogenetic tool for prenatal diagnosis, but the indications for aCGH are as follows:

- Abnormal ultrasound findings with normal karyotype
- Intrauterine fetal demise with congenital anomalies and culture failure with conventional karyotype (31)

We eagerly await the results of the ongoing study by the National Institute of Child Health and Human Development (NICHD) regarding the clinical utility of aCGH in prenatal diagnosis.

REFERENCES

1. American College of Obstetricians and Gynecologists. ACOG Practice Bulletin No. 77: screening for fetal chromosome anomalies. Obstet Gynecol 2007; 109:217–227. [Review]
2. Hook, EB. Rates of chromosome abnormalities at different maternal ages. Obstet Gynecol 1981; 58(3):282–285. [II-1]
3. Salvedt A, Almstrom H, Kublickas M, et al. Screening for Down's syndrome based on maternal age or fetal nuchal translucency: a randomized controlled trial in 39,572 pregnancies. Ultrasound Obstet Gynecol 2005; 25:537–545. [RCT, *n* = 39,572]
4. Wald NJ, Rodeck C, Hackshaw AK, et al. SURUSS Research Group. First and second trimester antenatal screening for Down's syndrome: the results of the serum, urine and ultrasound screening study. Health Technol Assess 2003; 7: 1–77. [II-3]
5. Nicolaides KH, Spencer K, Avgidou K, et al. Multicenter study of first-trimester screening for trisomy 21 in 75,821 pregnancies: results and estimation of the potential impact of individual risk-orientated two-stage first-trimester screening. Ultrasound Obstet Gynecol 2005; 25:221–226. [II-3]
6. Malone FD, Canick JA, Ball RH, et al., for the First-and-Second Trimester Evaluation of Risk (FASTER) Research Consortium. First-trimester or second-trimester screening, or both, for Down syndrome. N Engl J Med 2005; 353:2001–2011. [II-3]
7. Wapner R, Thom E, Simpson JL, et al., for the First Trimester Maternal Serum Biochemistry and Fetal Nuchal Translucency Screening (BUN) Study Group. First-trimester screening for trisomies 21 and 18. N Engl J Med 2003; 349:1405–1413. [II-3]
8. Bennett KA, Crane JMC, O'Shea P, et al. First trimester ultrasound screening is effective in reducing postterm labor induction rates: a randomized controlled trial. Am J Obstet Gynecol 2004; 190:1077–1081. [RCT, *n* = 218]
9. Haddow JE, Palomaki GE, Knight GJ, et al. Reducing the need for amniocentesis in women 35 years of age or older with serum markers for screening. N Engl J Med 1994; 330(16):1114–1118. [II-2]
10. Nyberg DA, Resta RG, Luthy DA, et al. Isolated sonographic markers for detection of fetal Down syndrome in the second trimester of pregnancy. J Ultrasound Med 2001; 20(10):1053–1063. [II-2]
11. Smith-Bindman R, Hosmer W, Feldstein VA, et al. Second-trimester ultrasound to detect fetuses with Down syndrome: a meta-analysis. JAMA 2001; 285(8):1044–1055. [II-2]
12. Nicolaides KH, Snijders RJM, Sebire N, eds. The 11–14 Week Scan: the Diagnosis of Fetal Anomalies. 2nd ed. Carnforth, Lancs: Parthenon Press, 2004. [Review]
13. Snijders R, Nicolaides K. Ultrasound Markers for Fetal Markers for Chromosomal Defects. New York, NY: Parthenon Publishing Group, 1996. [II-2]
14. Souka AP, von Kaisenberg CS, Hyett JA, et al. Increased nuchal translucency with normal karyotype. AJOG 2005; 192:1005–1021. [Review]
15. Dugoff L, for the Society for Maternal–Fetal Medicine. First- and second-trimester maternal serum markers for aneuploidy and adverse obstetric outcomes. Obstet Gynecol 2010; 115:1052–1061. [Review]
16. Tabor A, Madsen M, Obel EB, et al. Randomised controlled trial of genetic amniocentesis in 4606 low-risk women. Lancet 1986; 1:1287–1293. [RCT, *n* = 4606]
17. Alfirevic Z, Mujezinovic F, Sundberg K. Amniocentesis and chorionic villus sampling for prenatal diagnosis. Cochrane Database Syst Rev 2003; (3):CD003252. [Meta-analysis; 16 RCTs, *n* = >5000]
18. Leung WC, Lam YH, Wong Y, et al. The effect of fast reporting by amnio-PCR on anxiety levels in women with positive biochemical screening for Down's syndrome—a randomized controlled trial. Prenat Diag 2002; 22:256–259. [RCT, *n* = 60]
19. Hewison J, Nixon J, Fountain J, et al. A randomised trial of two methods of issuing prenatal test results: the ARIA (amniocentesis results: investigation of anxiety) trial. BJOG 2007; 114(4):462–468. [RCT, *n* = 226]
20. Mujezinovic F, Prosnik A, Alfirevic Z. Different communication strategies for disclosing results of diagnostic prenatal testing.

Cochrane Database Syst Rev 2010; (11):CD007750. [Meta-analysis; 2 RCTs, $n = 286$]

21. Collaborative. The Canadian Early and Mid-trimester Amniocentesis Trial (CEMAT) Group. Randomised trial to assess safety and fetal outcome of early and midtrimester amniocentesis. Lancet 1998; 351(9098):242–247. [RCT, $n = 4334$]

22. Smidt-Jensen S, Permin M, Philip J, et al. Randomized comparison of amniocentesis and transabdominal and transcervical chorionic villus sampling. Lancet 1992; 340:1237–1244. [RCT, $n = 2234$]

23. Mujezinovic F, Alfirevic Z. Procedure-related complications of amniocentesis and chorionic villus sampling: a systemic review. Obstet Gynecol 2007; 110:687–694. [Meta-analysis]

24. Alfirevic Z, von Dadelszen P. Instruments for chorionic villus sampling for prenatal diagnosis. Cochrane Database Syst Rev 2003; (1):CD000114. [Meta-analysis; 5 RCTs, $n = 472$]

25. Schaeffer AJ, Chung J, Heretis K, et al. Comparative genomic hybridization-array analysis enhance the detection of aneuploidies and submicroscopic imbalances in spontaneous miscarriages. Am J Hum Genet 2004; 74:1168–1174. [II-3]

26. Oostlander AE, Meijer GA, Yistra B. Microarray-based comparative genomic hybridization and its applications in human genetics. Clin Genet 2004; 66:488–495. [II-3]

27. Schaffer LG, Bui T-H. Molecular cytogenetic and rapid aneuploidy detection methods in prenatal diagnosis. Am J Med Genet 2007; 145C:87–98. [Review]

28. Van den Veyver IB, Patel A, Shaw CA, et al. Clinical use of array comparative genomic hybridization (aCGH) for prenatal diagnosis in 300 cases. Prenat Diag 2009; 29:29–39. [II-3]

29. Fruhman G, Van den Veyver IB. Applications of array comparative genomic hybridization in obstetrics. Obstet Gynecol Clin N Am 2010; 37:71–85. [Review]

30. Park JH, Woo JH, Shim SH, et al. Application of a target array comparative genomic hybridization to prenatal diagnosis. BMC Med Genet 2010; 11:102. [II-3]

31. American College of Obstetricians and Gynecologists. ACOG Practice Bulletin No. 446: array comparative genomic hybridization in prenatal diagnosis. Obstet Gynecol 2009; 114:1161–1163. [Review]

6

Genetic screening

Adele Schneider and Nancy W. Hendrix

KEY POINTS
- **Basic genetic counseling should be available to every pregnant woman.** This counseling is even more beneficial if performed **preconception**.
- There are no trials to assess any intervention for genetic screening and testing in pregnancy.
- Appropriate counseling regarding prognosis, possible complications, long-term issues, and follow-up should be provided to every couple with a pre- or postnatal diagnosis of aneuploidy or other genetic defects.
- **Trisomy 21** is the most common trisomy at birth, and its incidence increases with increasing maternal age.
- **Cystic fibrosis** (CF) testing should be offered to women with a family history of CF, reproductive partners of individuals with CF, and couples in whom one or both partners are Caucasian and planning a pregnancy or are seeking prenatal care. **It is reasonable to offer CF screening to all patients.**
- Prenatal testing for **fragile X syndrome** should be offered to known carriers of the fragile X premutation or full mutation. Women with a family history of fragile X–related disorders, unexplained mental retardation or developmental delay, autism, or premature ovarian insufficiency are candidates for genetic counseling and fragile X premutation carrier screening.
- Preconception and prenatal screening for spinal muscular atrophy (SMA) is not recommended in the general population at this time.
- Carrier screening for Tay–Sachs disease (TSD) (enzyme and DNA), Canavan disease, CF, and familial dysautonomia should be offered to **Ashkenazi Jewish (one Jewish grandparent)** individuals before conception or during early pregnancy. At least 15 other disorders common in this population can be discussed for screening.

BACKGROUND
Screening for aneuploidy, prenatal diagnosis (see chap. 5), and ultrasound (see chap. 4) screening have been reviewed in previous chapters. There are no trials to assess any intervention for genetic screening and testing in pregnancy although the incidence of TSD in the Ashkenazi Jewish population has decreased by 90% since screening was initiated.

GENETIC COUNSELING
Basic genetic counseling should be available to every pregnant woman. This counseling is even more beneficial if performed **preconception**. All couples should have a basic screen for family history of genetic disorders, with a pedigree to at least the second prior generation (three-generation pedigree). Questions should also involve history of recurrent spontaneous pregnancy loss and history of a previous fetus or child

who was affected by a genetic disorder. Those patients belonging to an ethnic group at increased risk for a recessive condition (e.g., sickle cell—African-American; TSD and others—Jewish; TSD in Irish, Cajun, and French Canadian; α-thalassemia—Southeast Asian; and β-thalassemia—Mediterranean) should be offered specific screening (see chaps. 14 and 15 in *Maternal-Fetal Evidence Based Guidelines*). Women with a specific indication for genetic testing should be referred for genetic counseling and a discussion of options available for prenatal diagnosis. **Responsibilities of clinicians** (e.g., ob-gyns, family medicine specialists, and nurse midwives) caring for pregnant women regarding genetic screening are shown in Table 6.1 (1). **Possible indications for genetic consultation** for preconception and prenatal patients are shown in Table 6.2 (2). Possible indications for genetic consultation for adult patients are shown in Table 6.3 (2).

DIRECT-TO-CONSUMER GENETIC TESTING
Direct-to-consumer (DTC) genetic testing differs from traditional genetic testing in that consumers order tests and receive test results without an independent medical provider serving as an intermediary. Some DTC companies offer genetic counseling (generally by telephone), whereas others do not. These tests are typically advertised and sold over the Internet. DTC is permitted in about half the states in the United States and is subject to little oversight at the federal level. Internationally, several countries have issued reports cautioning against its use, and **several European countries have banned or are considering banning it entirely**. The American Society of Human Genetics has issued guidelines for transparency, provider education, and test and laboratory quality on DTC genetic testing (3). The American College of Medical Genetics (ACMG) suggests the following regarding DTC genetic testing (www.acmg.net):

- A knowledgeable professional should be involved in the process of ordering and interpreting a genetic test.
- The consumer should be fully informed regarding what the test can and cannot say about his or her health.
- The scientific evidence on which a test is based should be clearly stated.
- The clinical testing laboratory must be accredited by Clinical Laboratory Improvement Amendments (CLIA), the State, and/or other applicable accrediting agencies.
- Privacy concerns must be addressed.

COMMON KARYOTYPE ABNORMALITIES
Trisomy 21 (Down Syndrome)
Historic notes: First complete description in 1846 was by Seguin. Report by Down in 1866 established the name of the

Table 6.1 Responsibilities of Clinicians Caring for Pregnant Women Regarding Genetic Screening

1. Clinicians should be able to identify patients within their practices who are candidates for genetic testing and should maintain competence in the face of increasing genetic knowledge.
2. Obstetrician-gynecologists should recognize that geneticists and genetic counselors are an important part of the health care team and should consult with them and refer as needed.
3. Discussions with patients about the importance of genetic information for their kindred, as well as a recommendation that information be shared with potentially affected family members as appropriate, should be a standard part of genetic counseling.
4. Obstetrician-gynecologists should be aware that genetic information has the potential to lead to discrimination in the workplace and to affect an individual's insurability adversely.[a] In addition to including this information in counseling materials, physicians should recognize that their obligation to professionalism includes a mandate to prevent discrimination.

[a]In the United States, Title II of the Genetic Information Nondiscrimination Act (GINA) of 2008 prohibits genetic information discrimination in employment. It is illegal to discriminate against employees or applicants because of genetic information. Title II of GINA prohibits the use of genetic information in making employment decisions; restricts employers and other entities covered by Title II (employment agencies, labor organizations, and joint labor management training and apprenticeship programs— referred to as "covered entities") from requesting, requiring, or purchasing genetic information; and strictly limits the disclosure of genetic information.
Source: From Ref. 1.

Table 6.2 Possible Indications for Genetic Consultation for Preconception and Prenatal Patients

Either member of the couple with:	Reason to consider consultation
A positive carrier screening test for a genetic condition such as cystic fibrosis	Discuss additional testing strategies and inheritance, testing of partner and siblings
A personal history of stillbirths, previous child with hydrops, recurrent pregnancy losses, or a child with sudden infant death syndrome (SIDS)	Rule out a chromosomal, metabolic, or syndromic diagnosis associated with an unexplained neonatal death or SIDS
A progressive neurologic condition known to be genetically determined such as progressive ataxia	Discuss a potential diagnosis, the differential diagnosis, inheritance, and testing options
A statin-induced myopathy	Discuss a potential mitochondrial disorder, inheritance, and testing options
Either member of the couple with a family or personal history of:	Reason to consider consultation
A birth defect such as cleft lip	Discuss recurrence risks and testing options
A chromosomal abnormality such as translocation	Discuss risks to the fetus and testing options
Significant hearing or vision loss thought to be genetically determined	Discuss risks to the fetus and testing options
Mental retardation or autism	Discuss risks to the fetus and testing options

Source: From Ref. 2.

syndrome. In 1959, LeJeune and Jacobs independently described that Down syndrome was caused by trisomy 21.

Definition: Down syndrome is **trisomy 21**, or the presence of an extra chromosome #21, either as three #21s or as a translocation between 21 and another chromosome, usually an acrocentric in a Robertsonian translocation.

Epidemiology/Incidence: About **1 in 800 live births**. This is the most common trisomy at birth. Incidence increases with increasing maternal age (see chap. 5).

Embryology: The Down syndrome critical region on chromosome 21 is being studied extensively to identify the genes involved in the Down **syndrome phenotype**. However, this region is not one small isolated spot, but most likely several areas on chromosome 21 that are not necessarily side by side.

Genetics/Inheritance: Error in cell division at the time of conception (**nondisjunction**) is responsible for 92% of Down syndrome resulting in **full trisomy 21**. Approximately 90% of nondisjunction occurs in the eggs. The cause of the nondisjunction error is not known, but there is definitely a connection with maternal age. The recurrence risk is empirically 1% or the age-related risk as a woman gets older. Three to four percent of all cases of trisomy 21 are due to a **Robertsonian translocation** usually between chromosomes #14 and #21. In the balanced state the individual is healthy and has 45 chromosomes with a #21 stuck on #14, or another acrocentric chromosome (15, 21, or 22). An individual with Down syndrome due to a translocation has 46 chromosomes, but one is actually a combination of #21 and another acrocentric like #14. Translocations resulting in

trisomy 21 may be inherited, so parental chromosomes must be checked. A female carrier of a balanced Robertsonian translocation has about a 12% risk of recurrence of Down syndrome in future pregnancies, while a male carrier has approximately a 3% risk of recurrence. **Mosaic trisomy 21** occurs when there is a mixture of cell lines, some of which have normal chromosomes and another cell line with trisomy 21. It is impossible to know how the normal and trisomy 21 cells are distributed in the different organs; therefore, the percentage of mosaic to normal cells in the peripheral blood cannot be used to predict outcome. Another tissue can be examined to help determine the level of mosaicism, usually skin.

Teratology: None.

Classification: Full trisomy 21, translocation trisomy 21, and mosaic trisomy 21.

Risk factors/Associations: Advanced maternal age. Individuals who are carriers of balanced Robertsonian translocations involving #21 have an increased risk unrelated to age.

Pregnancy Management

Screening (nonultrasound and/or ultrasound): First- and second-trimester ultrasound, first-trimester screen, second-trimester multiple-marker screening, or combinations are described in chapter 5.

Ultrasound findings in fetus:

- Thickened nuchal translucency (NT) at 11 to 14 weeks (80%) (at times cystic hygroma—10%)
- Thickened nuchal fold ($\geq$6 mm) at 16 to 23 weeks
- Congenital heart disease (CHD) (40–50%)

Table 6.3 Possible Indications for Genetic Consultation for Adult Patients

Personal history of:	Reason to consider consultation
Abnormal sexual maturation or delayed puberty	Rule out an intersex condition, chromosomal abnormality, or syndromic diagnosis
Recurrent pregnancy losses (more than two)	Rule out a chromosomal rearrangement such as a balanced translocation with karyotype
Tall or short stature for genetic background	Rule out a skeletal dysplasia, chromosomal or syndromic diagnosis
One or more birth defects	Rule out a chromosomal or syndromic diagnosis, and provide genetic counseling
Six or more café-au-lait macules >1.5 cm in diameter	Rule out neurofibromatosis type 1
Statin-induced myopathy	Rule out a mitochondrial disorder

Personal or family history of:	Reason to consider consultation
A cancer or cancers known to be associated with specific genes or mutations in the context of a compelling family history: young age at onset, bilateral lesions, and familial clustering of related tumors	Rule out an identifiable mutation in a gene such as BRCA1; rule out a cancer syndrome (MEN2); discuss surveillance, treatment, testing options, and inheritance
Cardiovascular problems known to be associated with genetic factors such as cardiomyopathy	Rule out a mutation in a causative or contributory gene; discuss surveillance, treatment, testing options, and inheritance
Suspected genetic disorder affecting connective tissue	Rule out a syndromic diagnosis (Marfan syndrome); discuss surveillance, treatment, testing options, and inheritance
Hematologic condition associated with excessive bleeding or excessive clotting	Confirm or rule out genetic condition; discuss treatment, testing options, and inheritance
Progressive neurologic condition known to be genetically determined such as unexplained myopathy	Confirm or rule out suspected diagnosis; discuss surveillance, treatment, testing options, and inheritance
Visual loss known to be associated with genetic factors such as retinitis pigmentosa	Rule out a syndromic diagnosis (Stickler syndrome); discuss testing options, if applicable, and inheritance
Early-onset hearing loss	Rule out a syndromic or nonsyndromic genetic form of hearing loss; discuss surveillance, testing options, and inheritance
Recognized genetic disorder including a chromosomal or single-gene disorder	Confirm the diagnosis, discuss prognosis, medical management, and inheritance
Mental illness such as schizophrenia	Discuss diagnosis, inheritance, recurrence risks, and identify syndromes, when possible
A close relative with a sudden, unexplained death, particularly at a young age	Rule out a genetic condition associated with this history

Source: From Ref. 2.

- Duodenal atresia (2%)
- Omphalocele (2%)
- Ventriculomegaly
- Hydrops or some hydropic changes (pleural effusion, ascites, etc.)
- Several "soft markers," such as short humerus and femur, echogenic bowel, renal pyelectasis, cardiac (usually left ventricular) echogenic focus, short middle phalanx fifth digit, "sandal foot," iliac crest >90° angle, and short ear length
- Biometry may reveal symmetric fetal growth restriction (FGR) by the third trimester.
- **Amniotic fluid:** polyhydramnios [if gastrointestinal (GI) obstruction or macroglossia present]
- **Placenta:** normal
- **Biometry/Measurement data:** symmetric FGR
- **When detectable:** at 11 to 14 weeks if increased NT is detected

Ultrasound after 14 weeks only detects approximately 50% of fetuses with Down syndrome. Choroid plexus cysts do not increase the risk. Screening provides the mother and family with a risk for Down syndrome, but true diagnosis can only be achieved with chorionic villus sampling (CVS) or amniocentesis.

Diagnosis: CVS or amniocentesis achieves the diagnosis by a study of the fetal chromosomes, which reveal trisomy 21. In the neonate, usually peripheral blood is cultured and karyotyped.

Counseling: The major abnormalities are increased risk of FGR, congenital heart defects, fetal and postnatal death, and developmental delay, with average IQ 50 to 75. Congenital heart defects are major contributors to mortality.

Workup/Investigations and consultations: A **fetal echocardiogram** is recommended. Depending on the lesions detected, specific pediatric subspecialty consultation can be offered. Genetic counseling can be offered as well. Care in a tertiary care center is indicated if there are significant associated anomalies, or if they cannot be ruled out adequately.

Fetal intervention: None available.

Termination issues: Termination can be offered as sole intervention as regulated by local law (usually legal <24 weeks).

Fetal monitoring/Testing: No specific trials. Nonstress tests (NSTs) weekly at ≥32 weeks can be offered. Nonreassuring fetal heart rate tracing (NRFHT) is common.

Delivery/Anesthesia: Mode and management of delivery should not be affected by the diagnosis of Down syndrome. NRFHT is common.

Neonatology Management

Resuscitation: Providing life support as needed as in any other infant is generally appropriate.

Transport: Indicated if counseling, general care, and/or major anomalies cannot be assessed and treated adequately at the birth institution.

Testing and confirmation: Karyotype is usually confirmed by blood lymphocyte culture.

Nursery Management
Neonatal echocardiogram and physical exam to assess any anomaly. **Surgery** may need to be scheduled for GI or cardiac anomalies. Down syndrome presents with a wide variety of features and characteristics. There is a wide range of intellectual disability and developmental delay noted among children with Down syndrome. There is a great deal of variability in the presence of other anomalies such as CHD and GI and hematological problems in these children. Hypothyroidism occurs in a high percentage of individuals with Down syndrome and should be monitored closely for their lifetime. **Early intervention** and specialized help with education and home rearing have improved the outcome in children with Down syndrome. Many young adults with Down syndrome move in to community living arrangements and work regular jobs or in sheltered workshops.

Future Pregnancy Preconception Counseling
With full trisomy 21, the recurrence risk is empirically 1% or the age-related risk as a woman gets older. With Robertsonian translocation, parental chromosomes should be checked, with genetic counseling regarding specific future risks. There are other rare translocations leading to Down syndrome. One is a Robertsonian translocation between two chromosomes 21, reported as t(21;21); this has a 100% risk for Down syndrome when transmitted by a carrier parent. Also rare is a non-Robertsonian translocation formed by the union of two 21s such that the translocation forms a mirror image of the normal 21. There is some literature that suggests that in some families where there have been recurrent trisomies, a relationship exists with their methylenetetrahydrofolate reductase (MTHFR) status. This has not been proven in large studies.

Helpful Websites
General: http://www.ds-health.com/
        Health care guidelines for care of individual with Down syndrome: http://www.denison.edu/collaborations/dsq/health96.html

Trisomy 18 (Edward Syndrome)
Historic notes: Trisomy 18 was independently described by Edwards et al. and Smith et al. in 1960.
        Definition: Edward syndrome is **trisomy 18**, or the presence of an extra chromosome #18.
        Epidemiology/Incidence: Incidence of 1 in 6600 live births in United States and United Kingdom. This is the second most common trisomy at birth. Incidence increases with increasing maternal age.
        Embryology: Extra chromosome #18 affects development of all organs.
        Genetics/Inheritance/Recurrence: Extra chromosome #18 is usually (95%) secondary to de novo **meiotic nondisjunction** associated with advanced maternal age. In approximately 90% of cases, the extra chromosome is maternal in origin, with meiosis II errors occurring twice as frequently as meiosis I errors. Other human trisomies have a higher frequency of nondisjunction in maternal meiosis I. Approximately 80% of nondisjunctions occur in females. **Mosaicism** occurs in approximately 10% and is due to postzygotic nondisjunction or anaphase lag. The causes of meiotic and mitotic nondisjunction are unknown. **Translocations** may also result in trisomy or partial trisomy 18 with varying phenotype due to monosomy of another chromosome and variable size of piece

of chromosome #18 involved. The smallest extra region necessary for expression of serious anomalies of trisomy 18 appears to be 18q11-q12.
        Teratology: None.
        Classification: Trisomy 18 (95%), mosaic trisomy 18, and variable partial trisomy 18 related to translocations.
        Risk factors/Associations: Advanced maternal age and translocation carriers have increased risk. Recurrence risk approximately 1% for full trisomy 18.

Pregnancy Management
Screening: NT has a sensitivity of >80%; first-trimester screening has a sensitivity of >90%, second-trimester multiple-marker screening has typically low α-fetoprotein (AFP), low human chorionic gonadotropin (hCG), and low estriol with a sensitivity of about >80%. Accurate ultrasound is usually >90% sensitive for trisomy 18 (see chap. 5).
        Ultrasound findings in fetus:

- Thickened NT at 11 to 14 weeks (80%) (at times cystic hygroma—15%)
- Thickened nuchal fold (≥6 mm) at 16 to 23 weeks
- CHD (90%)
- Omphalocele (25%)
- Neural tube defects (20%)
- Clenched hands with overlapping fingers
- Choroid plexus cysts (25%) (most commonly isolated and seen in normal fetuses; karyotyping not indicated if isolated)
- Enlarged (>1 cm) cisterna magna
- Single umbilical artery
- Micrognathia
- Cleft lip or palate
- Hydrops or some hydropic changes (pleural effusion, ascites, etc.)
- Biometry may reveal FGR by the third trimester.
    - **Amniotic fluid:** polyhydramnios (25%)
    - **Placenta:** normal
    - **Biometry/Measurement data:** symmetric FGR (>50%); microcephaly in third trimester
    - **When detectable:** at 11 to 14 weeks if increased NT is detected

Diagnosis: CVS or amniocentesis.
        Counseling (4,5): Approximately 95% of conceptuses with trisomy 18 die in embryonic or fetal life. Five to ten percent of affected children born alive survive beyond the first year of life. In utero, there are decreased fetal movements. Clinical findings the parents should be informed about include severe psychomotor and growth delay, microcephaly, microphthalmia, malformed ears, micrognathia or retrognathia, microstomia, distinctively clenched fingers, rocker-bottom feet, and other congenital malformations. **CHD occurs in 90%**, with ventricular septal defect (VSD) and polyvalvular heart disease (pulmonary and aortic valve defects) common. Renal anomalies and GI and brain malformations are common. It is associated with classical dermatoglyphics with digital arch patterns on finger and toe tips and distal palmar triradius with hypoplastic finger tips and small nails. Central apnea is a frequent cause of death, along with cardiac, central nervous system (CNS), and renal malformations.
        If diagnosed prenatally, recommend discussion with parents about how to proceed in labor and delivery allowing "nature to take its course" without monitoring, or level of intervention desired by parents including the extent of

resuscitation after delivery. Indication for C-section for fetal indications may be futile. **Parents need to be counseled that some children with trisomy 18 do survive and require life-long complete care**, but never achieve any independence. Few milestones are reached. There is an increased incidence of Wilms' tumor in trisomy 18 children who survive. Cardiac surgery is controversial. In first weeks it may be considered a heroic measure, but if the child is surviving it may make life more comfortable (comfort care). Apnea is a common cause of death, and can happen at home; there is the need to understand "nobody's fault" if this happens.

Workup/Investigations and consultations required: A fetal echocardiogram is recommended. Genetic counseling can be offered. **Neonatal consultation** is extremely important to help the couple decide regarding neonatal management; usually just comfort care for the baby and psychological support for the parents are most appropriate.

Fetal intervention: None available.

Termination issues: Termination can be offered as sole intervention as regulated by local law (usually legal <24 weeks).

Antepartum testing: As NRFHT is very common, and prognosis poor, fetal testing is not recommended. Many pregnancies continue without spontaneous labor until postterm (>42 weeks).

Delivery/Anesthesia: Fetal heart monitoring is usually declined, and not indicated. Every attempt should be made to maximize the chances of vaginal delivery to minimize maternal morbidity given frequently fatal neonatal prognosis. Cesarean delivery for fetal indications is not recommended and should be discussed.

Neonatology Management
Resuscitation: Comfort care only. Allow parents to grieve appropriately. Providing life support is usually not appropriate.

Transport: Not indicated.

Testing and confirmation: Karyotype is usually confirmed by blood lymphocyte culture.

Future Pregnancy Preconception Counseling
Test parents if due to translocation.

Helpful Websites
http://www.emedicine.com/ped/topic652.htm

Trisomy 13
Historic notes: Patau first identified in laboratory in 1960 noting three of the group 13 to 15 chromosomes.

Definition: Patau syndrome is **trisomy 13**, or the presence of an extra chromosome #13.

Epidemiology/Incidence: 1/10,000 live births. Incidence increases with increasing maternal age. Approximately 1% of all first-trimester spontaneous losses are due to trisomy 13.

Embryology: Extra chromosome #13 affects development of all organs.

Genetics/Inheritance: Extra #13 chromosome resulting in **full trisomy 13** (80% of cases). This is due to maternal nondisjunction usually in meiosis I. About 15% of cases are due to **translocation**, mostly Robertsonian translocation t(13q14). In 5%, translocation is familial with recurrence risk of 5% and risk of spontaneous abortion (SAB) of 20%. The other cases are due to **mosaicism** (5%) with trisomy 13 and a normal cell line. Mosaicism cases may have milder phenotype.

Teratology: None.

Classification: Trisomy 13, mosaic trisomy 13, and translocation trisomy or partial trisomy 13.

Risk factors/Associations: Advanced maternal age. Individuals who are carriers of balanced Robertsonian translocations involving chromosome #13 have an increased risk.

Pregnancy Management
Screening: First-trimester ultrasound (with NT). First-trimester screen and second-trimester multiple-marker screening are not sensitive and clinically useful for detecting trisomy 13. Accurate ultrasound is usually 90% sensitive for trisomy 13.

Ultrasound findings in fetus:

- Thickened NT at 11 to 14 weeks (>70%) (at times cystic hygroma—20%)
- Thickened nuchal fold (≥6 mm) at 16 to 23 weeks
- CHD (80%) [atrial septal defect (ASD) and VSD most common, but also often complex CHD]
- Holoprosencephaly (40%)
- Cleft lip and palate (45%)
- Hypotelorism/Microphthalmia
- Polydactyly
- Rocker-bottom feet
- Omphalocele (10%)
- Polycystic kidneys (30%)
- Enlarged (>1 cm) cisterna magna (15%)
- Neural tube defects
- Hydrops or some hydropic changes (pleural effusion, ascites, etc.)
- Biometry may reveal symmetric FGR by the third trimester.
  - **Amniotic fluid:** polyhydramnios or oligohydramnios
  - **Placenta:** normal
  - **Biometry/Measurement data:** symmetric FGR (50%)
  - **When detectable:** at 11 to 14weeks if increased NT is detected

Diagnosis: CVS or amniocentesis achieves the diagnosis by a study of the fetal chromosomes, which reveals trisomy 13. In the neonate, usually peripheral blood is cultured and karyotyped.

Counseling (4,5): Most trisomy 13 conceptions result in SABs. Median survival is fewer than 3 days. Mean life expectancy is 130 days with most dying in first month of life, 95% die within 6 months. Apnea is a common cause of death, and can happen at home; there is the need to understand nobody's fault if this happens. Family needs to be prepared for intense care needs and possible sudden death. Most common causes of death are cardiopulmonary arrest, 69%; CHD, 13%; and pneumonia, 4%.

Some infants do survive and those need complete care and achieve few milestones. Survival depends on associated medical problems. Survivors with trisomy 13 have severe intellectual disability and developmental delays. For survivors there are specific growth charts available for monitoring growth. Children with trisomy 13 are irritable, do not achieve milestones beyond smiling, and most need to be fed by tube.

If diagnosed prenatally, recommend discussion with parents about how to proceed, usually allowing nature to take its course given the grim prognosis. Parents need to be counseled that some children with trisomy 13 do survive and require lifelong complete care; and never achieve any independence.

Workup/Investigations and consultations: A fetal echocardiogram is recommended. Genetic counseling can be offered. **Neonatal consultation** is extremely important, to help the couple decide regarding neonatal management;

usually just comfort care for the baby and psychological support for the parents are most appropriate.

Fetal intervention: None available.

Termination issues: Termination can be offered as sole intervention as regulated by local law (usually legal <24 weeks).

Antepartum testing: As NRFHT is very common, and prognosis poor, fetal testing is not recommended. Many pregnancies continue without spontaneous labor until postterm (>42 weeks).

Delivery/Anesthesia: Fetal heart monitoring is usually declined, and not indicated. Every attempt should be made to maximize the chances of vaginal delivery to minimize maternal morbidity given almost universally fatal neonatal prognosis.

Cesarean delivery for fetal indications is not recommended and should be discussed.

Neonatology Management

Resuscitation: Comfort care only. Allow parents to grieve appropriately. Providing life support is usually not appropriate.

Transport: Not indicated.

Testing and confirmation: Karyotype is usually confirmed by blood lymphocyte culture.

Long-term care: Feeding issues and gastrostomy; irritability; chronic infections and aspiration pneumonia; heart failure; frequent hospitalizations; seizures; blindness and hearing loss; few milestones achieved (smile and laugh); and parental stress.

Future Pregnancy Preconception Counseling

With full trisomy 13, the recurrence risk is empirically 1% or the age-related risk as a woman gets older. With Robertsonian translocation, parental chromosomes should be checked, with genetic counseling regarding specific future risks. There are other rare translocations leading to trisomy 13. In rare translocation of t(13q13q), the risk of recurrence or SAB is 100%.

Helpful Website

http://www.emedicine.com/ped/topic1745.htm

Turner Syndrome

Historic notes: In 1938 Turner described the combination of sexual infantilism, webbed neck, and cubitus valgus. Ford showed in 1959 that this combination of findings was associated with a missing X chromosome.

Definition: Turner syndrome is the **presence of single X chromosome**, or **any karyotype with Xp missing** such as isochromosome Xq, ring X, or deletion Xp. Also called 45X0 or 45X syndrome.

Epidemiology/Incidence: 1/2500 female births (**1/5000** total births). Ninety-eight to ninety-nine percent of Turner fetuses are spontaneously aborted; about 20% of all SABs are due to Turner syndrome.

Embryology: Lymphedema usually due to congenital hypoplasia of lymphatic channels.

Genetics/Inheritance:

The **presence of single X chromosome**, or **any karyotype with Xp missing** such as isochromosome Xq, ring X, or deletion Xp. The presence of a single X chromosome results from chromosomal nondisjunction. **Mosaicism** is common (40%) and may include a 46,XY karyotype associated with ambiguous genitalia. Since features of Turner syndrome are seen in other syndromes, karyotype is essential to make the diagnosis. Chromosome studies on more than one tissue may be needed to detect mosaicism. Not associated with advanced maternal age.

Teratology: None.

Classification: 45,X in 50%. 46,X,i(Xq) in 17%, and mosaicism in 40%.

Risk factors/Associations: *Not* associated with advanced maternal age. Different from Noonan syndrome by karyotype that is normal in Noonan syndrome.

Pregnancy Management

Screening: First-trimester screen with NT measurement. Biochemical screening is usually not sensitive enough for clinical use.

Ultrasound findings in fetus:

- Cystic hygroma
- Thickened nuchal fold (≥6 mm) at 16 to 23 weeks
- CHD (20%) (usually left side: coarctation, aortic stenosis, bicuspid aortic valve, and left hypoplastic heart)
- Renal anomalies (60%)
- Hydrops or some hydropic changes (pleural effusion, ascites, etc.)
  - **Amniotic fluid:** occasionally oligohydramnios
  - **Placenta:** normal
  - **Biometry/Measurement data:** usually normal
  - **When detectable:** at 10+ weeks if cystic hygroma detected

Diagnosis: CVS or amniocentesis achieves the diagnosis with a study of the fetal chromosomes, which reveals 45,X or missing Xp. In the neonate, usually peripheral blood is cultured and karyotyped.

Counseling: 45,X conceptions frequently (>95%) end in SAB. **The presence of a cystic hygroma with the diagnosis of Turner syndrome is >99% fatal.** If cystic hygroma is not present or resolves, and fetus is still alive >20 weeks, many survive until birth. Female infants with Turner syndrome have excess nuchal skin and edema of the hands and feet (80%) due to lymphedema. CHD, if present, usually most affects prognosis, requires surgery and long-term care. In childhood short stature is apparent. Teenagers have delayed puberty and primary amenorrhea (>90%), with infertility (>99%). Other clinical findings include shield-shaped chest with widely spaced nipples; low posterior hair line with webbing or shortness of neck; renal anomalies (60%); cubitus valgus; short fourth metacarpal; narrow, hyper convex, and deep set nails; hearing loss; and thyroid dysfunction. Some girls with Turner syndrome have learning difficulties including difficulty with math and reading maps related to a deficit in spatial ability. Intelligence and verbal skills are usually within the normal range. Mosaicism with a normal female cell line may result in a milder phenotype and spontaneous puberty with fertility but often early menopause. If there is a deleted X but the X-inactive-specific transcript (XIST) locus is intact, normal random X-inactivation may occur and the phenotype may be milder. If XIST is not present in a small X chromosome marker, the phenotype may be more severe. In mosaic 45X/46,XY individuals clitoral enlargement may be present and virilization may occur. In these cases there is an increased risk of gonadoblastoma and the gonad should be removed. Psychological impact of short stature, infertility, and learning difficulties needs to be discussed.

Workup/Investigations and consultations: A **fetal echocardiogram** is recommended. Depending on the lesions detected, specific pediatric subspecialty (in particular for cardiac anomalies) consultation can be offered. Genetic counseling can be offered as well. Care in a tertiary care center is indicated if there are significant associated anomalies, or if they cannot be ruled out adequately. Endocrine follow-up is indicated.

Fetal intervention: None available.

Termination issues: Termination can be offered as sole intervention as regulated by local law (usually legal <24 weeks).

Fetal monitoring/Testing: No specific trials. NSTs weekly at ≥ 32weeks can be offered.

Delivery/Anesthesia: Mode and management of delivery should not be affected by the diagnosis of Turner syndrome.

Neonatology Management
Resuscitation: Providing life support as needed as in any other infant is generally appropriate.

Transport: Indicated if counseling, general care, and/or major anomalies cannot be assessed and treated adequately at the birth institution.

Testing and confirmation: Karyotype is usually confirmed by blood lymphocyte culture.

Nursery Management
Neonatal echocardiogram, renal ultrasound, and physical exam are indicated to assess any anomaly. **Surgery** may need to be scheduled for cardiac anomalies. **Early intervention** and specialized help with education have improved the outcome in children with Turner syndrome.

Long-term care: Thyroid studies annually; hearing test if otitis and not done before; speech evaluation, if needed; blood pressure checks routinely (hypertension a complication); annual echocardiogram to measure aortic root; annual urinalysis and culture if renal anomaly; use Turner growth curve after 2 years old; monitor diet (calories and calcium); ophthalmology follow-up as indicated; psychological support; individualized education program (IEP) at school if indicated; refer to endocrinologist in infancy, discuss growth hormone (GH) and hormone replacement therapy (HRT): GH treatment can improve growth and influence a girl's final adult height. HRT helps the girl with Turner syndrome develop the physical changes of puberty. In vitro fertilization can make it possible for some women with Turner syndrome to become pregnant using a donor egg. It is important to discuss at what age to inform the child of her diagnosis and its implications.

Future Pregnancy Preconception Counseling
Recurrence risk in 45,X is not increased over population risk. There is an increased risk if associated with a translocation.

Klinefelter Syndrome
Historic notes: In 1942, Dr Harry Klinefelter described males who had enlarged breasts, sparse facial and body hair, small testes, and azospermia. By the late 1950s these findings were associated initially with an extra Barr body, and later the extra X chromosome was identified with the karyotype 47,XXY.

Diagnosis/Definition: Chromosome study 47,XXY. There are no specific phenotypic features to identify Klinefelter syndrome in an infant.

Epidemiology/Incidence: 1/500 to 1/1000 male births.

Genetics/Inheritance/Recurrence/Future prevention: Advanced maternal age slightly increases the risk for the XXY. Recent studies have shown that half the time, the extra chromosome comes from the father.

Risk factors/Associations: Advanced maternal age.

Screening: No phenotypic features noted prenatally.

Clinical features: Occasional breast enlargement, lack of facial and body hair, and a female-type body configuration. Small testes. Taller than others in their family. Delayed speech occurs in >50%. Poor gross motor coordination is present in

approximately 27%. School difficulties are relatively common, and many boys with 47,XXY need assistance at school. Many are shy and somewhat passive and easy babies to care for. The average IQ is 90, verbal IQ higher than performance IQ. XXY boys enter puberty normally, without any delay of physical maturity. But as puberty progresses, they fail to keep pace with other males. Most XXY boys benefit from receiving an injection of testosterone every 2 weeks, beginning at puberty.

Counseling: Regular injections of the male hormone testosterone, beginning at puberty, can promote strength and facial hair growth—as well as bring about a more muscular body type.

Psychological support and therapy can help with self-esteem issues and interaction with peers. Depression also may be a problem in adults.

Boys with 47,XXY have a slightly increased risk of auto-immune disorders such as type I (insulin-dependent) diabetes, autoimmune thyroiditis, and lupus erythematosus. XXY males with enlarged breasts have the same risk of breast cancer as do women—roughly 50 times the risk of XY males. XXY males who do not receive testosterone injections may have an increased risk of developing osteoporosis in later life.

It is unnecessary to share this diagnosis outside of medical providers as diagnosis may be misunderstood.

Rare/Related: Variations include the XY/XXY mosaic who may have enough normally functioning cells in the testes to allow them to father children. Males with two or even three additional X chromosomes have also been reported in the medical literature. In these individuals, the classic features of Klinefelter syndrome may be exaggerated, with low IQ or moderate to severe mental retardation also occurring. Testosterone injections may not be appropriate for all of them.

Helpful Website
http://www.nichd.nih.gov/publications/pubs/klinefelter.htm#xwhat

47,XXX
Diagnosis/Definition: Karyotype shows 47,XXX.

Epidemiology/Incidence: 1/1000 newborn females.

Genetics/Inheritance/Recurrence: Sporadic, increased by advanced maternal age.

Risk factors/Associations: Advanced maternal age.

Screening: No identifying physical features. Must have karyotype to make diagnosis.

Clinical features: Girls with 47,XXX are usually tall. Pubertal development is usually normal and fertility is probably normal, but there may be an increased incidence of offspring with chromosome abnormalities.

Counseling: Girls with 47,XXX are shy and may demonstrate immaturity. The support of a loving and understanding family can improve the outcome for these girls. Many have learning difficulties (math and reading) but they are not intellectually disabled. The IQ of a girl with 47,XXX may be a few points lower than that of her siblings. Those diagnosed on amniocentesis or CVS with normal ultrasound, where indication is advanced material age, have better prognosis than those diagnosed postnatally because a problem has been noted.

OTHER COMMON GENETIC DISORDERS
Cystic Fibrosis
CF is an autosomal-recessive disorder. The most common mutation is △F508, but >1700 other mutations have been described (Table 6.4) (6). The mutation leads to faulty chloride

Table 6.4 Recommended Core Mutation Panel for General Population Cystic Fibrosis Carrier Screening

107delT	711+1G>T	R117H
1717-1G>A	A455E	xR334W
1898+G>A	DeltaF508	R347P
2184delA	DeltaI507	R553X
2789+5G>A	G542X	R560T
3120+1G>A	G551D	W1282X
3659delC	G85E	
3849+10kbC>T	I148T	
621+G>T	N1303K	

Table 6.5 Cystic Fibrosis Carrier Rate by Racial and Ethnic Group, Before and After Screening

Racial or ethnic group	Incidence of CF	Carrier frequency	%△F508
Caucasians	1/3,300	1/29	70
Hispanics	1/8,000–9,000	1/46	46
African-Americans	1/15,300	1/62	48
Asian-Americans	1/32,000	1/90	30

Source: From Ref. 7.

Table 6.6 Incidence and Carrier Risk for CF Based on Race or Ethnicity

Racial or ethnic group	Detection rate (%)	Estimated carrier risk before test	Estimated carrier risk after a (−) test
Ashkenazi Jewish	97	1/29	~1/930
European Caucasian	80	1/29	~1/140
Hispanic American	57	1/46	~1/105
African-American	69	1/65	~1/207
Asian-American	–	1/90	–

transport, increased sweat chloride levels, and increased thick mucus in lungs, pancreas, biliary tree, and intestines. This is the most common life-limiting genetic disorder in Caucasians (Tables 6.5 and 6.6) (6).

It is reasonable to offer CF screening to all patients (6). It is generally more cost-effective and practical to initially perform CF carrier screening for the patient only (6). Nonetheless, screening can be concurrent or sequential, and both strategies are acceptable alternatives.

Concurrent screening:

- Both partners tested simultaneously
- Both partners' results revealed
- Assesses couple's risk
- Identifies couples at risk more rapidly
- More precise

Sequential screening:

- Initial screening of one partner
- Other partner tested if first partner is positive
- Low-risk racial/ethnic groups
- Other partner not available

Interpretation of Results

- Both partners negative (−/−)—prenatal diagnostic testing not indicated
- One partner carrier (−), one not screened: Intermediate risk—prenatal diagnostic testing not indicated
- One partner carrier (+), one carrier (−): Prenatal diagnostic testing not recommended
- One partner carrier (+), one untested: Partner should be tested if possible Genetic counseling Availability/Limitations of prenatal testing
- Both partners carrier (+): 25% chance of having an affected offspring Genetic counseling Prenatal diagnosis offered (CVS, amniocentesis) Counseling regarding continuation versus termination of pregnancy for affected pregnancies

Risk of affected offspring depends also on prevalence of carrier status in the specific ethnic group (Table 6.7).

Fragile X Syndrome

Diagnosis/Definition: Most common inherited cause of intellectual disability; caused by expansion of a repetition of the cytosine-guanine-guanine (CGG) trinucleotide segment of the fragile X mental retardation 1 (FMR-1) gene that is located on the X chromosome at Xq27.3.

The diagnosis is based on molecular genetic analysis. Most laboratories use a combination of two approaches: (*i*) Southern blot analysis to measure the degree of methylation and (*ii*) polymerase chain reaction to discriminate small differences in the intermediate and premutation sizes. Fragile X syndrome occurs when expansion of the CGG repeat occurs.

Epidemiology/Incidence: Both males and females can be affected. The prevalence is 1 in 4000 males and 1 in 6000 females.

Genetics/Inheritance/Recurrence: The FMR-1 gene is typically comprised of a limited number of CGG repeats. This region is usually stable, relatively small (<40 repeats), and passes from one generation to the next. However, during meiosis in oocytes, the region can expand, reaching either intermediate (41 to 60 repeats) or premutation (61 to 200 repeats) lengths. As repeat size increases, stability decreases and further increases in the number of repeats become likely. Once the premutation reaches expansion to >90 repeats, the

Table 6.7 Risk of Offspring Having Cystic Fibrosis

Racial or ethnic group	No test	One partner −, one untested	One partner +, one −	One partner +, one untested	Both partners −
Ashkenazi Jewish	1/3,300	1/107	1/3720	1/116	1/3,459,600
European Caucasian	1/3,300	1/16	1/560	1/116	1/3,459,600
Hispanic American	1/8464	1/19	1/420	1/184	1/78,400
African-American	1/16,900	1/53	1/828	1/260	1/44,100
Asian-American	1/32,000	1/53	–	1/360	1/171,396

Table 6.8 Fragile X: Risk of Full Mutation (and Therefore Affected Child) Based on Number of Maternal Repeats

Maternal repeats	% Risk expansion to full mutation
55–59	0–13
60–69	5–21
70–79	17–58
80–89	50–73
90–99	80–100
100–200	75–99

Source: From Ref. 8.

likelihood of expansion to a full mutation is at least 80% (Table 6.8) (8).

Only women with a premutation FMR-1 can pass the full mutation to their offspring. Fathers with premutations usually pass the gene in a stable fashion to all of their daughters and none of their sons and will have affected grandsons. Premutation male and female carriers are at risk for fragile X–associated tremor/ataxia syndrome (FXTAS) usually after age 50 years (8).

Screening: Prenatal testing for fragile X syndrome should be offered to known carriers of the fragile X premutation or full mutation. Women with a family history of fragile X–related disorders, FXTAS, unexplained mental retardation or developmental delay, autism, or premature ovarian insufficiency are candidates for genetic counseling and fragile X premutation carrier screening (9). General population screening is not recommended. A careful assessment of the family history for males with cognitive impairment related through females should be performed to identify individuals at sufficient likelihood of premutation or full mutation carrier status to warrant screening.

Women who accept fragile X premutation screening should be offered FMR-1 DNA mutation analysis after genetic counseling about the risks, benefits, and limitations of screening (9). All identified carriers should be referred for follow-up genetic counseling. Diagnostic modalities for prenatal diagnosis (including CVS and amniocentesis) should be discussed.

Clinical features:

Males: Wide range of behavioral and cognitive manifestations and often subtle physical manifestations, but never asymptomatic. The behavioral phenotype is characterized by autism spectrum behaviors such as attention deficit/hyperactivity, expressive delay, tactile defensiveness, perseverative speech, and echolalia as well as social anxiety and avoidance of eye contact. The cognitive phenotype generally is **moderate to severe mental impairment**. Ten to twenty percent have seizures. Physical characteristics are more readily identifiable around puberty. Findings similar to a connective tissue disorder including hyperextensible joints; soft, smooth skin; flat feet; and mitral valve prolapse may be present. The facial appearance is often described as long and narrow with prognathism and large ears. Macrocephaly may be present. Most develop macroorchidism, and height tends to be below average.

Females: Tend to have fewer and milder abnormalities than males. More likely to have relatively normal cognitive development.

Spinal Muscular Atrophy

Diagnosis/Definition: SMA refers to a group of diseases that affect the motor neurons of the spinal cord and brainstem, which are responsible for supplying electrical and chemical signals to muscle cells. Without proper signals, muscle cells do not function properly and thus become much smaller (atrophy). This leads to muscle weakness. Individuals affected with SMA have progressive muscle degeneration and weakness, eventually leading to death.

Incidence: 1/10,000 infants.

Genetics/Classification: There are several forms of SMA, depending on the age of onset and the severity of the disease. Two genes, SMN1 and SMN2, have been linked to SMA types I, II, III, and IV. Type I is the most severe form of SMA and characterized by muscle weakness present from birth, often manifested by difficulties with breathing and swallowing, and death usually by age 2 to 3 years. Type II has onset of muscle weakness after 6 months of age and can obtain some early physical milestones like sitting without support. Type III is a milder form of SMA, with onset of symptoms after 10 months of age. Individuals with Type III SMA often achieve the ability to walk but may have frequent falls and difficulty with stairs. The weakness is more in the extremities and affects the legs more than the arms. Type IV is the mildest form and is characterized by adult onset of muscle weakness.

SMA is most often caused by a deletion of a segment of DNA, in exon 7 and exon 8, in the SMN1 gene located on chromosome #5. Rarely, SMA is caused by a point mutation in the SMN1 gene.

Screening: Preconception and prenatal screening for SMA is not recommended in the general population at this time (10). Carrier testing for SMA measures the number of copies of the deleted segment in the SMN1 gene. A noncarrier is expected to have two copies present (no deletion), while a carrier will have only one copy present (a deletion of one copy). However, carrier testing will not identify carriers of point mutations. Approximately 90% of SMA carriers in the Ashkenazi Jewish population can be identified with this testing method. It is estimated that 1 in 41 individuals, including Ashkenazi Jews, is a carrier for SMA.

DiGeorge Syndrome (22q11.2 Deletion Syndrome)

Historic notes: DiGeorge syndrome, described in 1965, and velo-cardio-facial syndrome, described in 1978, are different manifestations of the same deletion of chromosome 22q11.2.

Diagnosis/Definition: Fluorescence in situ hybridization (FISH) study reveals an interstitial deletion of chromosome 22p11.2. Can be detected on microarray.

Epidemiology/Incidence: 1/2000 to 1/4000 births.

Embryology: Defects occur in the third and fourth pharyngeal pouches, which later develop into the thymus and parathyroid glands. Developmental abnormalities may also occur in the fourth branchial arch.

Genetics/Inheritance/Recurrence/Future prevention: Autosomal-dominant inheritance. In 6% of affected individuals one of the parents is affected. Expression is very variable so both parents of an affected child should be tested for the deletion.

Risk factors/Associations: Other conditions have been noted to be associated with de 22q11.2 including conotruncal anomaly face syndrome (CAFS) (Japan) and sometimes Opitz G/BBB syndrome, CHARGE association, and Cayler-cardio-facial syndrome.

Screening: All women with a fetus or neonate with a diagnosis of congenital heart defect, especially if conotruncal, can be offered testing (usually FISH) for this deletion. Testing is available from amniocytes or chorionic villi.

Clinical features: Characteristic facies; cardiovascular defects in 85%, most are VSD; cleft of secondary palate, may be submucous cleft or velopharyngeal incompetence; nasal reflux in infants; transient neonatal hypocalcemia; hypotonia; immune system dysfunction; postnatal growth delay; developmental delay, learning disability, and psychological problems especially in adolescence; and hypernasal speech.

Counseling (prognosis, complications, and pregnancy considerations): Clinical features should be reviewed. Early death due to congenital heart defects before 6 months of age in 8%. Early intervention for speech and motor delays. Special education for older children. Chance of psychiatric disorders in 10%. Very variable phenotype, not predictable from laboratory result.

5p– (Cri-Du-Chat Syndrome)

Historic notes: In 1963, Lejeune et al. described a syndrome of multiple congenital anomalies, developmental delay, microcephaly, dysmorphic features, and a high-pitched, cat-like cry in infants with deletion of a B group chromosome (Bp–), later identified as 5p–.

Diagnosis/Definition: 5p– syndrome is characterized at birth by a high-pitched cat-like cry, low birth weight, poor muscle tone, and microcephaly. The cry is caused by abnormal laryngeal development. The cry disappears by age 2 years in about one-third children with 5p–.

A karyotype is needed for the diagnosis. The size of the deletion of the short arm of chromosome 5 is variable, and a very small deletion may be missed using conventional G-banding. High-resolution studies may be needed or a FISH study using a specific probe for the small deleted area of 5p that is essential for this diagnosis. Microarray would identify this deletion.

Epidemiology/Incidence: Estimated prevalence is about 1 in 50,000 live births. Up to 1% of profoundly retarded individuals have 5p–.

Genetics/Inheritance/Recurrence/Future prevention: May be sporadic (80–85%) if both parents have normal chromosomes with a recurrence risk of less than 1%. In rare cases, gonadal mosaicism in one parent may result in a recurrence. If one parent carries a balanced translocation (10–15%) involving 5p, the recurrence risk is substantially higher.

Most cases have a terminal deletion of 5p. The cat-like cry maps to 5p15.3, and the cri-du-chat critical region of 5p15.2 is associated with all the clinical features of the syndrome. The deletion is paternal in origin in 80% of cases.

Affected females are fertile and have a 50% chance of passing on the deletion to their offspring although none is documented to have reproduced.

Risk factors/Associations: Increased risk if translocation carrier involving 5p.

Screening: Amniocentesis, CVS, and ultrasound.

Counseling: Early feeding problems are common because of swallowing difficulties; poor suck with resultant failure to thrive. Death occurs in 6% to 8% of the overall population with cri-du-chat due to pneumonia, aspiration pneumonia, and congenital heart defects. Survival to adulthood is possible. Children who are raised at home with early intervention and schooling do better than those described in the early literature. Almost all individuals with 5p– have significant cognitive, speech, and motor delays (IQ rarely above 35). Many children can develop some language and motor skills. They may also become independent in self-care skills. Physical features include microcephaly, growth retardation, hypertelorism, epicanthal folds, downslanting palpebral fissures, round face with full cheeks, flat nasal bridge, downturned corners of mouth, micrognathia, low-set ears, and variable cardiac defects. Renal anomalies have been described as have cleft lip and palate, talipes equinovarus, and gut malrotation. Treatment is symptomatic.

Helpful Websites
http://www.emedicine.com/ped/topic504.htm

ASHKENAZI JEWISH ANCESTRY GENETIC SCREENING
Who to Screen

The family history of individuals considering pregnancy, or who are already pregnant, should **determine whether either member of the couple is of Eastern European (Ashkenazi) Jewish ancestry (one grandparent is Ashkenazi Jewish) or has a relative with one or more of the following genetic conditions**: TSD, Canavan disease, CF, familial dysautonomia, Fanconi anemia group C, Niemann–Pick disease type A, mucolipidosis IV, Bloom syndrome, and Gaucher disease (11).

What to Screen for

Carrier screening for **TSD, Canavan disease, CF, and familial dysautonomia** should be offered to Ashkenazi Jewish individuals before conception or during early pregnancy so that a couple has an opportunity to consider prenatal diagnostic testing options. If the woman is already pregnant, it may be necessary to screen both partners simultaneously so that the results are obtained in a timely fashion to ensure that prenatal diagnostic testing is an option.

Individuals of Ashkenazi Jewish descent may inquire about the availability of carrier screening for other disorders. Carrier screening is available also for **mucolipidosis IV, Niemann–Pick disease type A, Fanconi anemia group C, Bloom syndrome, and Gaucher disease**. The ACMG recommends screening also for these five disorders, for a total of nine (12). ACMG provides criteria for adding new diseases to the panel of Jewish genetic diseases based on significant burden of the disorder, carrier rate >1/100 and/or test sensitivity >90%. Patient education materials can be made available so that interested patients can make an informed decision about having additional screening tests. Some patients may benefit from genetic counseling.

There are currently 19 diseases that are being made available for screening on Jewish genetic disease panels. In addition to those mentioned above, the following diseases are included in the new panels: maple syrup urine disease, glycogen storage disease type 1a, dihyrolipoamide dehydrogenase (DLD) deficiency, familial hyperinsulinism, Joubert syndrome, nemaline myopathy, SMA, Usher syndrome type 1F, Usher syndrome type III, and Walker–Warburg syndrome.

How to Screen

All the disorders on the Ashkenazi Jewish genetic disease panel are autosomal recessive. A carrier is unaffected but if two carriers of a mutation in the same gene have a child together, they have a 25% risk with each pregnancy of having an affected child (Fig. 6.1).

When only one partner is of Ashkenazi Jewish descent, that individual should be screened first. If it is determined that this individual is a carrier, the other partner should be offered screening for that disorder. However, the couple should be informed that the carrier frequency and the

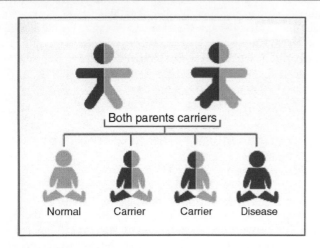

Figure 6.1 Autosomal recessive inheritance.

detection rate in non-Jewish individuals are unknown for many of these disorders. Therefore, it is difficult to accurately predict the couple's risk of having a child with the disorder, and gene sequencing may be necessary to determine if a non-Jewish partner is a carrier. Referral to a genetic counselor is recommended in these cases.

Individuals with a positive family history of one of these disorders should be offered carrier screening for the specific disorder (and others for this group) and may benefit from genetic counseling.

When both partners are carriers of one of these disorders, they should be referred for genetic counseling and offered prenatal diagnosis. Carrier couples should be informed of the disease manifestations, range of severity, and available treatment options. Prenatal diagnosis by DNA-based testing can be performed on cells obtained by CVS and amniocentesis.

When an individual is found to be a carrier, his or her relatives are at risk for carrying the same mutation. The patient should be encouraged **to inform his or her relatives of the risk and the availability of carrier screening**. The provider does not need to contact these relatives because there is no provider-patient relationship with the relatives, and confidentiality must be maintained (11).

SELECTED DISORDERS
Tay–Sachs Disease
Carrier frequency is 1 in 25.

Clinical features: The most well-known of these diseases. An apparently healthy child begins to lose skills around 4 to 6 months of age, and there is a progressive neurological decline leading to blindness, seizures, and unresponsiveness. Death usually occurs by the age of 4 to 6.

Familial Dysautonomia
Carrier frequency is 1/32 with disease incidence of 1/3700.

Clinical features: Causes the autonomic and sensory nervous system to malfunction, affecting the regulation of body temperature, blood pressure, and stress response, and causes decreased sensitivity to pain. Frequent pneumonia and poor growth may occur. Survival into adulthood is possible but with careful medical care.

Testing: Carrier testing for one major mutation and one other mutation accounts for 99.5% of carriers.

Canavan Disease
Carrier frequency is 1/40 with a disease incidence of 1/3000 to 1/6000.

Clinical features: Appear normal at birth; then progressive loss of skills, hypotonia, macrocephaly, and spasticity. Most die within first year of life but may survive to second decade.

Testing: Carrier testing detects 98% carriers.

Bloom Syndrome
Carrier frequency is 1/102 with a disease incidence of 1/48,000.

Clinical features: Short stature, a sun-sensitive skin rash, an increased susceptibility to infections and higher incidence of leukemia and other cancers, infertility, and immunodeficiency.

Testing: Carrier testing detects 95% to 97% of carriers.

Fanconi Anemia Type C
Carrier frequency is 1/89 with disease incidence of 1/32,000.

Clinical features: Associated with short stature, bone marrow failure, and a predisposition to leukemia and other cancers. Some children have limb, heart, or kidney abnormalities and learning difficulties.

Treatment: Pancytopenia can be treated with stem cell transplantation.

Testing: Carrier testing.

Gaucher Disease
Carrier rate is 1/15 with disease incidence of 1/900.

Clinical features: A variable condition both in age of onset and symptoms. It may present with a painful, enlarged spleen, anemia, and low white blood cell count. Bone deterioration is a major cause of pain and disability.

Treatment: Treatment is available.

Carrier testing: Seven mutations account for >96% mutations.

Mucolipidosis Type IV
Carrier frequency is 1/122.

Clinical features: A progressive neurological disorder with variable symptoms beginning in infancy. Characteristics include muscle weakness, mental retardation, and eye problems—both corneal clouding and retinal abnormalities develop.

Glycogen Storage Disease, Type 1a
Carrier frequency is 1 in 71.

Clinical features: A metabolic disorder that causes poor blood sugar maintenance with sudden drops in blood sugar, growth failure, enlarged liver, and anemia.

Treatment: Disease management involves lifelong diet modification.

Maple Syrup Urine Disease
Carrier frequency is 1 in 81.

Clinical features: A variable disorder of amino acid metabolism. Named for the characteristic maple syrup smell of urine in those with the disorder.

Treatment: With careful dietary control, normal growth and development are possible. If untreated, it can lead to poor feeding, lethargy, seizures, and coma.

Niemann–Pick Disease Type A

Carrier frequency is 1 in 90.

Clinical features: A progressive neurodegenerative disease characterized by hepatosplenomegaly, leading to death by age 2 to 4 years.

Dihyrolipoamide Dehydrogenase Deficiency (DLD Deficiency)

Carrier frequency is 1 in 96.

Clinical features: Presents in early infancy with poor feeding, frequent episodes of vomiting, lethargy, and developmental delay. Affected individuals develop seizures, enlarged liver, blindness, and ultimately suffer an early death.

Familial Hyperinsulinism

Carrier frequency is 1 in 66.

Clinical features: Characterized by hypoglycemia that can vary from mild to severe. It can be present in the immediate newborn period through the first year of life with symptoms such as seizures, poor muscle tone, poor feeding, and sleep disorders.

Joubert Syndrome

Carrier frequency is 1 in 92.

Clinical features: Characterized by structural mid- and hindbrain malformations. Affected individuals have mild to severe motor delays, developmental delay, decreased muscle tone, abnormal eye movements, and characteristic facial features.

Nemaline Myopathy

Carrier frequency is 1 in 108.

Clinical features: Most common congenital myopathy. Infants are born with hypotonia and usually have problems with breathing and feeding. Later some skeletal problems may arise, such as scoliosis. In general, the weakness does not worsen during life but development is delayed.

Usher Syndrome Type 1F

Carrier frequency is 1 in 141.

Clinical features: Characterized by profound hearing loss, which is present at birth, and adolescent-onset retinitis pigmentosa, a disorder that significantly impairs vision.

Usher Syndrome Type III

Carrier frequency is 1 in 107.

Clinical features: Causes progressive hearing loss and vision loss. Hearing is often normal at birth with progressive hearing loss typically beginning during childhood or early adolescence. Often leads to blindness by adulthood.

Walker–Warburg Syndrome

The carrier frequency in the Ashkenazi population for one Ashkenazi founder mutation is 1 in 149.

Clinical features: It is a muscle, eye, and brain syndrome. It is a severe condition that presents with muscle weakness, feeding difficulties, seizures, blindness, brain anomalies, and delayed development. Life expectancy is below 3 years.

REFERENCES

1. American College of Obstetricians and Gynecologists. ACOG committee Opinion No. 410: ethical issues in genetic testing. Obstet Gynecol 2008; 111:1495–1502. [Review]
2. Pletcher BA, Toriello HV, Noblin SJ, et al. Indications for genetic referral: a guide for healthcare providers. Genet Med 2007; 9:385–389. [Review]
3. American Society of Human Genetics. ASHG statement on direct-to-consumer genetic testing in the United States. Am J Hum Genet 2007; 81:635–637. [Review]
4. Baty BJ, Blackburn BL, Carey JC. Natural history of trisomy 18 and trisomy 13: I. Growth, physical assessment, medical histories, survival, and recurrence risk. Am J Med Genet 1994; 49(2):175–188. [Review]
5. Baty BJ, Jorde LB, Blackburn BL. Natural history of trisomy 18 and trisomy 13: II. Psychomotor development. Am J Med Genet 1994; 49(2):189–194. [Review]
6. American College of Obstetrics and Gynecology. ACOG Committee Opinion No. 486: Update on carrier screening for cystic fibrosis. Obstet Gynecol 2011; 117:1028–1031. [Review]
7. American College of Obstetrics and Gynecology. Preconception and Prenatal Carrier Screening for Cystic Fibrosis: Clinical and Laboratory Provider Guidelines. Washington, DC: ACOG, 2001. [Review]
8. Nolin SL, Lewis FA III, Ye LL, et al. Familial transmission of the FMR 1 CGG repeat. Am J Hum Genet 1996; 59:1252–1261. [Review]
9. American College of Obstetrics and Gynecology. ACOG Committee Opinion No. 469: Carrier screening for fragile X syndrome. Obstet Gynecol 2010; 116:1008–1010. [Review]
10. American College of Obstetrics and Gynecology. ACOG Committee Opinion No. 432: Spinal muscular atrophy. Obstet Gynecol 2009; 113:1194–1196. [Review]
11. American College of Obstetricians and Gynecologists. ACOG Committee Opinion No. 442: Preconception and prenatal carrier screening for genetic disease in individuals of Eastern European Jewish descent. Obstet Gynecol 2009; 114:950–953. [Review]
12. Gross SJ, Pletcher BA, Monaghan KG; for the Professional Practice and Guidelines Committee. Carrier screening in individuals of Ashkenazi Jewish descent. Genet Med 2008; 10(1):54–56. Available at: www.acmg.net. [Review]

7

Before labor and first stage of labor

Vincenzo Berghella

KEY POINTS

- **Before labor**
  - **If nonvertex** presentation, perform **cesarean delivery (CD)**.
  - **If ≥41 weeks**, start **induction.**
  - **Antenatal training to prepare for labor and delivery** is associated with **arriving to** labor and delivery **(L&D) ward more often in active labor, less visits to the labor suite**, and **using less epidural analgesia.**
  - **Pelvimetry should not be performed** as it is associated with no benefits, and it increases incidence of CDs.
- **There is limited evidence to assess the safety and efficacy of planned home birth for low-risk pregnant women.** Compared to planned hospital birth, **planned home birth is associated with a higher risk of neonatal deaths (0.2% vs. 0.09%). The hospital is the safest setting for labor and delivery.**
- A birth center in the hospital is a safe location for birth. The trend for a 67% higher perinatal mortality should be weighted against the significant 4% increase in spontaneous vaginal delivery (SVD) and 96% higher satisfaction, during counseling.
- **Most women (those without risk factors) should be offered midwife-led models of care, and women should be encouraged to ask for this option.**
- **Training of traditional birth assistants in developing countries is associated with a trend for less maternal mortality and significantly less perinatal mortality.**
- **Delayed hospital admission** until active labor (regular painful contractions and cervical dilatation >3 cm) **is associated with less time in the labor ward, less intrapartum oxytocics,** and **less analgesia.**
- Admission tests such as fetal heart rate (FHR) tracing and amniotic fluid assessment have not been associated with any benefit.
- Routine enema is not recommended.
- Perineal shaving is not recommended.
- Vaginal chlorhexidine irrigation is not recommended.
- **Universal prenatal maternal screening with anovaginal specimen at 35 to 37 weeks and intrapartum antibiotic treatment** are the most efficacious of the current strategies for prevention of neonatal early-onset group B streptococcus (GBS) disease.
- **All women should have continuous, one-on-one support throughout labor and birth**, as it is associated with less intrapartum analgesia, cesarean birth, operative birth, and dissatisfaction with the childbirth experiences, and more spontaneous vaginal birth.
- There is insufficient evidence for providing nutritional recommendations for women in labor. **There is little justification for the restriction of fluids and food in labor for women at low risk of complications.**

- There is insufficient evidence for need or rate of IV fluids in labor.
- **Upright positions** (either standing, sitting, kneeling, or walking around) in the first stage of labor **reduce the length of labor** by approximately **1 hour** and are associated with **less epidural analgesia**. Since walking does not seem to have a beneficial or detrimental effect on labor and delivery, **women can choose freely to walk or lay in bed, preferably upright, during labor, whichever is more comfortable for them.**
- **Water immersion** during the *first stage* of labor **reduces the use of analgesia and by about 30 minutes the duration of the first stage of labor,** without adverse maternal or neonatal outcomes.
- Routine early (or even late) **amniotomy cannot be recommended as part of standard labor management and care.**
- **The use of the partogram cannot be recommended as a routine intervention in labor.**
- There are no trials to evaluate the frequency of cervical exams in labor per se. Most studies, including those with active management, perform cervical exams every 2 hours in active labor, but the risk of chorioamnionitis increases with increasing number of exams.
- **For women making slow progress in the first stage of spontaneous labor,** the use of **oxytocin augmentation** is associated with a **reduction in the time to delivery of approximately 2 hours.**
- The individual interventions that are part of **active management of labor** should be studied separately, and only those that are beneficial (e.g., support by doula) implemented.
- **Dystocia cannot be diagnosed unless rupture of membranes (ROM) has occurred, and adequate oxytocin to** achieve at least 3 to 5 adequate contractions per hour has been instituted. Dystocia also **cannot be diagnosed reliably before the first stage of labor has entered the active phase, which has been defined, especially in nulliparous with epidurals in place, as at least 6 cm of cervical dilatation. Before performing a CD for active phase labor arrest, labor should be arrested for a minimum of 4 hours [if uterine activity is greater than 200 Montevideo units as documented with intrauterine pressure catheter (IUPC)] or 6 hours (if greater than 200 Montevideo units could not be sustained).**

INTRODUCTION

For management of induction, meconium, oligo/polyhydramnios, intrapartum monitoring (including amnioinfusion for variables), operative vaginal delivery, shoulder dystocia, trial of labor after cesarean (TOLAC), intrauterine growth restriction (IUGR), macrosomia, abnormal third stage, etc., **see**

appropriate distinct guidelines in this book and its companion, *Maternal-Fetal Evidence Based Guidelines*.

ASSOCIATIONS

There is no strong association between changes in barometric pressure and onset of labor (1). Diurnal rhythms seem to show a higher rate of starting labor in the evening and night hours.

BEFORE LABOR
Antenatal Classes

Antenatal classes to improve the birth process have been studied in at least three RCTs.

Compared to no such training, 9 hours of antenatal training to prepare for labor and delivery are associated with **arriving to L&D ward more often in active labor** (RR 1.45, 95% CI 1.26–1.65) and **using less epidural analgesia** (RR 0.84, 95% CI 0.73–0.97) (2).

Compared to no such education, antenatal education focusing on natural childbirth preparation with training in breathing and relaxation techniques is not associated with any effects on maternal or perinatal outcomes, including similar incidences of epidural analgesia, childbirth, or parental stress, in nulliparous women and their partners (3).

In a small RCT, **specific antenatal education program is associated with a reduction in the mean number of visits to the labor suite before the onset of labor** (4). It is unclear whether this results in fewer women being sent home because they are not in labor.

Nonvertex Presentation

If **nonvertex presentation** is detected, CD is recommended (see chap. 22).

≥41 weeks

Induction advised at **≥41 weeks** (see chap. 24).

Pelvimetry

There is not enough evidence to support the use of X-ray pelvimetry in women whose fetuses have a cephalic or non-cephalic presentation. **Women undergoing X-ray pelvimetry are more likely to be delivered by cesarean section** (5). No significant impact is detected on perinatal outcome, but numbers are small, insufficient for meaningful evaluation (e.g., perinatal mortality 1% vs. 2%). The results are similar for women with or without a prior CD.

SITE OF LABOR MANAGEMENT
Planned Home Birth

There is limited evidence to assess the safety and efficacy of planned home birth for low-risk pregnant women as there is only 1 RCT with only 11 women ever published (6,7). In healthy low-risk women, compared to planned hospital birth, **planned home birth is associated with a higher risk of neonatal deaths (0.2% vs. 0.09%)** in a meta-analysis of nonrandomized studies including over 500,000 births (8). This means, therefore, that the **hospital is the safest setting for labor and delivery** (9). A home birth service ought to be backed up by a modern hospital system. There are diverging opinions even in Western countries, with about 30% of Dutch births occurring at home, versus <1% of U.S. births. In the United States, about 75% of home births are delivered by **noncertified** midwives. In the Netherlands, travel time of

>20 minutes from home to hospital is associated with increased risk of perinatal mortality and other adverse outcomes (10). **Women with risk factors for abnormal outcome should deliver in a hospital setting.** All women should be aware of possible maternal and fetal risks, including severe morbidity and mortality, associated with labor and delivery even in low-risk women, and should be aware of the **absence of intensive care and operative capabilities in the home setting** (6). Inference from results of "home-like" versus conventional ward setting (see below) should warn against home birth.

Ethical experts agree that hospital birth is safer. Some medical ethics experts emphasize that physicians should counsel strongly against home birth (11). Some other medical ethics experts argue instead that, given the increased risk of perinatal mortality is about 1 to 2/1000 in home compared to hospital birth, women should be counseled on these absolute numbers and allowed a choice based on autonomy (12).

Freestanding Birth Center

There are no RCTs of freestanding birth centers, and therefore the evidence is insufficient to recommend this setting (13).

Planned Hospital Birth: Alternative Setting (Home-Like) Vs. Conventional Ward Setting

Several RCTs have evaluated the option of "alternative" setting" versus conventional hospital ward setting for L&D. For alternative setting, most trials included care by midwives in a location in the hospital, close to the regular L&D ward, that did not look like a usual L&D setting. Some RCTs randomized women in labor, while others at the beginning of pregnancy. So continuity of care was usually higher in the alternative setting group. **Usually about 40% to 50% of patients randomized to alternative setting** (often about 60% for nulliparous women, 20–30% for multiparous women) **need to be moved in labor to the conventional L&D ward**.

Compared to conventional hospital ward, allocation to an alternative hospital setting **increased the likelihood of the following: no intrapartum analgesia/anesthesia** (RR 1.17, 95% CI 1.01–1.35); **SVD** (RR 1.04, 95% CI 1.02–1.06); **breastfeeding at 6 to 8 weeks** (RR 1.04, 95% CI 1.02–1.06); and **very positive views of care** (RR 1.96, 95% CI 1.78–2.15). Allocation to an alternative setting **decreased the likelihood of epidural analgesia** (RR 0.82, 95% CI 0.75–0.89); **oxytocin augmentation** of labor (RR 0.78, 95% CI 0.6–0.91); and **episiotomy** (RR 0.83, 95% CI 0.77–0.90). There was no apparent effect on maternal morbidity and mortality, serious perinatal morbidity/mortality (RR 1.17, 95% CI 0.51–2.67), perinatal mortality (RR 1.67, 95% CI 0.93–3.00), other adverse neonatal outcomes, or postpartum hemorrhage. The 4% increase in SVD may be secondary to less epidural anesthesia, which may in turn be secondary to less availability in home-like settings, and/or to less intrapartum monitoring. **The trend for a 67% higher perinatal mortality should be weighted against the significant 4% increase in SVD and 96% higher satisfaction, during counseling.** Episiotomy should be avoided in general (see chap. 8). No firm conclusions can be drawn regarding the effects of variations in staffing, organizational models, or architectural characteristics of the alternative settings (13). **A birth center in the hospital is a safe location for birth** (9).

PROVIDER
Midwife-led Care

In many parts of the world, midwives are the primary providers of care for childbearing women. Elsewhere it may be medical doctors or family physicians who have the main responsibility for care, or the responsibility may be shared. The underpinning philosophy of midwife-led care is normality, continuity of care, and being cared for by a known and trusted midwife during labor. There is an emphasis on the natural ability of women to experience birth with minimum intervention (14).

The effect of midwife-lead care compared to physician-led care or to other provider-led care has been evaluated mostly for the whole pregnancy, including together both antepartum care and care during labor and delivery (see also chap. 2). Therefore it is difficult to assess the effect of midwife-led care just on labor and delivery.

From the evidence from both antepartum and labor and delivery care, **most women should be offered midwife-led models of care and women should be encouraged to ask for this option**. Caution should be exercised in applying this advice to women with substantial medical or obstetric complications. In a meta-analysis, women, the vast majority low-risk, who had midwife-led models of care, were **less likely to experience antenatal hospitalization** (RR 0.90, 95% CI 0.81–0.99), **regional analgesia** (RR 0.81, 95% CI 0.73–0.91), **episiotomy** (RR 0.82, 95% CI 0.77–0.88), and **instrumental delivery** (RR 0.86, 95% CI 0.78–0.96), and were **more likely to experience no intrapartum analgesia/anesthesia** (RR 1.16, 95% CI 1.05–1.29), **spontaneous vaginal birth** (RR 1.04, 95% CI 1.02–1.06), **feeling in control during childbirth** (RR 1.74, 95% CI 1.32–2.30), **attendance at birth by a known midwife** (RR 7.84, 95% CI 4.15–14.81), and **initiate breastfeeding** (RR 1.35, 95% CI 1.03–1.76), although there were no statistically significant differences between groups for cesarean births (RR 0.96, 95% CI 0.87–1.06). Women who were randomized to receive midwife-led care were **less likely to experience fetal loss before 24 weeks' gestation** (RR 0.79, 95% CI 0.65–0.97), although there were no statistically significant differences in fetal loss/neonatal death of at least 24 weeks (RR 1.01, 95% CI 0.67–1.53) or in fetal/neonatal death overall (RR 0.83, 95% CI 0.70–1.00). In addition, their babies were more likely to have a **shorter length of hospital stay** [mean difference (MD) −2.00, 95% CI −2.15 to −1.85] (14) (see also subsection "Continuous Support in Labor").

Training of Birth Assistants
Training of traditional birth assistants **in developing countries is associated with a trend for less maternal mortality and significantly less perinatal mortality (15)**. There are no trials in the developed world.

Teamwork Training
There is **insufficient evidence** to assess the effects of training and teamwork education for labor and delivery personnel. Quality and safety initiatives are probably beneficial but have not been sufficiently studied in RCTs. Compared to no such training, a standardized teamwork training curriculum based on crew resource management that emphasized communication and team structure was not associated with significant effect on adverse maternal and perinatal outcomes in one RCT (16).

ADMISSION
Delayed Vs. Early Hospital Admission
Labor assessment programs, which aim to **delay hospital admission until active labor**, may benefit women with term pregnancies. Active labor was defined as regular painful contractions and cervical dilatation >3 cm. In one RCT, compared to direct admission to hospital, delayed admission until active labor is associated with **less time in the labor ward, less intrapartum oxytocics**, and **less analgesia** (17). Women in the labor assessment and delayed admission group report **higher levels of control during labor**. CD rates are similar, with a nonsignificant 30% decrease. A 30% to 40% decrease in CD has been reported in retrospective studies with delayed versus direct admission. There is insufficient evidence (a larger trial needed) to assess true effects on rate of CD and other important measures of maternal and neonatal outcome. Potential risks of delayed admission include unplanned out-of-hospital births and the potentially harmful effects of withholding caregiver support and attention to women in early or latent phase labor.

In another RCT, compared to no use of algorithm, use of an algorithm by midwives to assist in their diagnosis of active labor (painful, regular contractions with at least one of the following: 3 cm dilated, ROM, or "show") was associated with more women being discharged after their first labor ward assessment, and no effect of oxytocin augmentation and other medical interventions in labor (18).

Suggested criteria for admission based on these studies are a cervix of at least 3 to 4 cm dilatation and regular painful contractions. Pregnant women should be informed of these data during prenatal care.

Fetal Assessment Tests upon Admission
FHR Tracing for 20 Minutes
FHR tracing for 20 minutes upon admission followed by auscultation is not associated with any benefits compared to intermittent auscultation, including similar neonatal morbidity and mortality (19,20).

Amniotic Fluid Volume Index
Obtaining an AFI in early labor is associated with a higher incidence of CD, and similar neonatal outcomes, compared to no AFI (21).

Neither a 2×1 pocket (abnormal in 8%) nor an AFI (abnormal in 25%) upon admission for labor identifies a pregnancy at risk for adverse outcome such as nonreassuring fetal heart rate tracing (NRFHT) or CD for NRFHT (22).

Other Tests
There is insufficient evidence to support the use of vibroacoustic stimulation or Doppler ultrasound as fetal admission tests.

Enemas
Enemas do not have a significant beneficial effect on infection rates such as perineal wound infection or other neonatal infections and women's satisfaction. Compared to no enema, enema in labor is associated with no significant differences for infection rates in puerperal women (RR 0.66, 95% CI 0.42–1.04) or newborn children (RR 1.12, 95% CI 0.76–1.67). No significant differences are found in the incidence of neonatal lower or upper respiratory tract infections.

One RCT described labor to be significantly shorter (50 minutes) with enema versus no enema. A second RCT found labor to be significantly longer (112 minutes) with enema compared to no enema. No significant differences in the duration of labor were found in the third RCT that scored as having a low risk of bias and was adjusted for parity. One RCT that researched women's views found no significant differences in satisfaction between groups. **The routine use of enemas during labor should be discouraged** (23). This intervention (enema) generates discomfort in women and increases the costs of delivery.

Perineal Shaving

There is **no support for routine perineal shaving** (shaving with a razor) for women prior to or in labor. In a very old trial, 389 women were alternately allocated to receive either skin preparation and perineal shaving or clipping of vulvar hair only. In the second old trial, which included 150 participants, perineal shaving was compared with the cutting of long hairs for procedures only. In the third trial, 500 women were randomly allocated to shaving of perineal area or cutting of perineal hair. Compared to no shaving, shaving was associated with as similar incidence of maternal febrile morbidity (OR 1.16, 95% CI 0.70–1.90), perineal wound infection (OR 1.52, 95% CI 0.79–2.90), and perineal wound dehiscence (OR 0.13, 95% CI 0.00–6.70). In the smaller trial, fewer women who had not been shaved had gram-negative bacterial colonization compared with women who had been shaved (OR 0.43, 95% CI 0.20–0.92). There were no differences in maternal satisfaction immediately after birth (24). The potential for complications (redness, multiple superficial scratches and burning and itching of the vulva, and embarrassment and discomfort afterward when the hair grows back), which often occur later, suggests that **shaving should not be part of routine clinical practice.** The first two trials are old (1922 and 1965) and included the clipping of long hairs in their control groups to aid in operative procedures, which is itself usually unnecessary and can lead to complications.

FIRST STAGE
Chlorhexidine

Compared to placebo sterile water irrigation, vaginal chlorhexidine irrigation during labor is associated with **similar incidences of maternal and neonatal infections,** including similar chorioamnionitis, postpartum endometritis, neonatal sepsis, and perinatal mortality (25).

Compared to saline wipes, chlorhexidine wipes of maternal vagina while in labor and infant by 6 hours of age are not associated with significant effects in maternal and perinatal mortality and neonatal sepsis in Pakistan (26). The effectiveness of vaginal chlorhexidine might depend on the concentration and volume of the solution used. Chlorhexidine solution is safe, not expensive, and vaginal irrigation is easy to perform, but apparently not beneficial.

GBS Prophylaxis

Universal prenatal maternal screening with anovaginal specimen at 35 to 37 weeks and intrapartum (ampicillin first line) **antibiotic treatment** are the most efficacious of the current strategies for prevention of early-onset GBS disease (27). It is >50% more effective than a risk factor–based strategy. There is no prevention of late-onset GBS sepsis. **Women with GBS bacteriuria** in the current pregnancy or who had a **prior infant with GBS sepsis** are candidates for **intrapartum antibiotics prophylaxis** and should be the only two groups **not screened.** **Intrapartum treatment for chorioamnionitis is recommended regardless of GBS maternal status** (see chap. 37 in *Maternal-Fetal Evidence Based Guidelines*).

Continuous Support in Labor
Definition

For support, it is generally intended emotional support (continuous presence, reassurance, and praise), information about labor progress and advice regarding coping techniques, comfort measures (comforting touch, massage, warm baths/showers, promoting adequate fluid intake and output), and advocacy (helping the woman articulate her wishes to others) (28).

Mechanism of Action

Anxiety during labor is associated with high levels of the stress hormone epinephrine in the blood, which may in turn lead to abnormal FHR patterns in labor, decreased uterine contractility, a longer active labor phase with regular well-established contractions, and low Apgar scores. One example of possible mechanisms of action for support to reduce complications of labor and delivery is decreased anxiety (28). This in turn can lead to a beneficial "chain-reaction": for example, if continuous support leads to reduced use of epidural analgesia, then several complications associated with regional anesthesia (see chap. 11) can be prevented.

Types of Support

Family member or friend (not part of hospital staff) or hospital-based (part of hospital staff). Doula (a Greek word for "handmaiden") is a support person with the sole job of providing support to the laboring woman. They are usually not part of the hospital staff. This member of the caregiver team may also be called a labor companion, birth companion, labor support specialist, labor assistant, or birth assistant.

Effectiveness

Continuous support during labor has clinically meaningful benefits for women and infants and no known harm. **All women should have support throughout labor and birth.** Women allocated to continuous support are more likely to have a **spontaneous vaginal birth** (RR 1.08, 95% CI 1.04–1.12) and **less likely to have intrapartum analgesia** (RR 0.90, 95% CI 0.84–0.97) **or to report dissatisfaction** (RR 0.69, 95% CI 0.59–0.79). In addition their labors are about **1-hour shorter** (MD −0.58 hours, 95% CI −0.86 to −0.30), they are **less likely to have a cesarean** (RR 0.79, 95% CI 0.67–0.92) or **instrumental vaginal birth** (RR 0.90, 95% CI 0.84–0.96), or a **baby with a low 5-minute Apgar score** (RR 0.70, 95% CI 0.50–0.96). There is no apparent impact on other intrapartum interventions, maternal or neonatal complications, or on breastfeeding. **Continuous support is most effective when provided by a woman who is neither part of the hospital staff nor the woman's social network, and in settings in which epidural analgesia is not routinely available.** No conclusions could be drawn about the timing of onset of continuous support. **Hospitals should permit and encourage women to have a companion of their choice during labor and birth, and administrators and policymakers should ensure that these services are available to every pregnant woman** (28) (see also subsection "Midwife-led Care").

It may be possible to increase access to one-to-one continuous labor support worldwide by encouraging women to invite a family member or friend to commit to being present at the birth and assuming this role. The mother selects her doula during pregnancy; they establish a relationship (which is likely to involve the woman's partner, if any) and discuss the mother's and partner's preferences and concerns before labor. The doula brings her experience and training (often to the level of certification) to the labor support role during childbirth, and the mother and doula frequently have telephone and/or face-to-face contact in the early postpartum period. Other models of support, for which there are little or no data, include support by a female family member and support by the husband/partner (28).

Aromatherapy

There **is insufficient evidence** to assess the effects of aromatherapy in labor. Compared to no such intervention, administration of selected essential oils during labor is not associated with significant effects on CD, instrumental delivery, or use of oxytocin. While maternal pain perception in nulliparous women was decreased in one RCT on this intervention, this RCT was also not blind (29).

Nutrition in Labor

Since the evidence shows no benefits or harms, **there is little justification for the restriction of fluids and food in labor for women at low risk of complications**. All studies looked at women in active labor and at low risk of potentially requiring a general anesthetic. One study looked at complete restriction versus giving women the freedom to eat and drink at will; two studies looked at water only versus giving women specific fluids and foods; and two studies looked at water only versus giving women carbohydrate drinks.

When comparing any restriction of fluids and food versus women given some nutrition in labor (three RCTs), the meta-analysis was dominated by one study undertaken in a highly medicalized environment. There were no statistically significant differences identified in the following: cesarean section (RR 0.89, 95% CI 0.63–1.25), operative vaginal births (RR 0.98, 95% CI 0.88–1.10), and Apgar scores <7 at 5 minutes (RR 1.43, 95% CI 0.77–2.68), nor in any of the other outcomes assessed. Women's views were not assessed. The pooled data were insufficient to assess the incidence of Mendelson syndrome (bronchopulmonary reaction following aspiration of gastric contents during anesthesia), an extremely rare outcome (30).

A carbohydrate (mean intake 44 g in 350 mL) drink in early labor is associated with an increased risk of CD compared to placebo in women allowed to drink "at will" (31), but a carbohydrate (25 g) drink in late (8–10 cm) labor is associated with similar rates of CD compared to placebo (32). Umbilical cord studies revealed lactate transport to the fetal circulation with potential (but not observed) fetal academia (31,32). These results should be interpreted with caution as the sample size was small, and there is conflicting evidence on the effects of these carbohydrate drinks.

No studies looked specifically at women at increased risk of complications; hence, there is no evidence to support restrictions in this group of women (30).

Ice chips to moisten the mouth and sips of clear liquids are the only oral intake recommended by U.S. authorities (33). Some experts allow also sport drinks, yogurt, or sherbet. In the Netherlands women in labor are allowed to eat and drink. The reason for avoiding solid food is risk of aspiration ("Mendelson syndrome"), which is rare (about 15/10,000 CDs) (34). When there is increased gastric volume, there is increased risk of vomiting and therefore aspiration. Airway precautions in labor and delivery are paramount to avoid aspiration.

Acid Prophylaxis Drugs

There is **no good evidence to support** the routine administration of acid prophylaxis drugs in normal labor to prevent gastric aspiration and its consequences (35). Giving such drugs to women once a decision to give general anesthesia is made is discussed in chapter 11.

IV Fluids (or not), Rate

There are **no trials comparing IV fluids to no IV fluids in labor**. The data on IV fluids type and infusion rate are insufficient for a strong recommendation.

Compared to 125 mL/hr, an infusion rate of IV fluids (lactated Ringers or normal saline) of **250 mL/hr in early labor** (2–5 cm) of term nulliparous women with vertex presentation is associated with **less labors lasting >12 hours** (36). Other outcomes (length of labor for vaginal deliveries, use of oxytocin, and successful vaginal delivery) are not significant but trended for benefit of 250 mL/hr, for example, in a 71-minute shorter labor, in particular first stage (36). While the data in pregnancy are limited to one trial, the benefits are substantiated by the fact that several trials in nonpregnant adults demonstrate that increased fluid intake improves exercise performance.

Compared to normal saline without dextrose, normal saline with **5% dextrose**, both given IV at 125 mL/hr in early labor (3–5 cm), is associated with a **shorter (by about 70 minutes) duration of labor** from initiation of IV infusion to delivery. The incidence of labor lasting >12 hours was decreased from 22% to about 10% (37). Five percent dextrose has also been associated with less umbilical cord acidemia compared to lactated Ringer's solution (38).

Maternal Position

Upright positions (either standing, sitting, kneeling, or walking around) **in the first stage of labor reduce the length of labor** and do not seem to be associated with increased intervention or negative effects on mothers' and babies' well-being. Compared to recumbent positions, the first stage of labor is approximately **1 hour shorter** for women randomized to upright positions. Women randomized to upright positions are **less likely to have epidural analgesia** (RR 0.83, 95% CI 0.72–0.96). There are no differences between groups for other outcomes including length of the second stage of labor, mode of delivery, or other outcomes related to the well-being of mothers and babies. For women who had epidural analgesia there were no differences between those randomized to upright versus recumbent positions for any of the outcomes examined in the review. Little information on maternal satisfaction was collected, and none of the studies compared different upright or recumbent positions. A woman semireclining or lying down on the side or back during the first stage of labor may be more convenient for staff and can make it easier to monitor progression and check the baby. Fetal monitoring, epidurals for pain relief, and use of IV infusions also limit movement. **Women should be encouraged to take up whatever position they find most comfortable in the first stage of labor** (39).

Ambulation

Compared to remaining in bed, walking in labor is associated with similar length of first stage of labor, use of oxytocin, use of analgesia, need for forceps vaginal delivery, or CD, and also similar neonatal outcomes in women at term with cephalic presentation starting at 3 to 5 cm of dilatation (40) or in other groups of women (39,41–44). Since walking does not seem to have a beneficial or detrimental effect on labor and delivery, **women can choose freely to walk or stay upright** (see subsection "Maternal Position") **in bed during labor, whichever is more comfortable for them**.

Immersion in Water

Compared to controls (labor not in water), water immersion **during the first stage of labor reduces by 10% the use of epidural/spinal analgesia** (RR 0.90, 95% CI 0.82–0.99) **and by**

about 30 minutes the duration of the first stage of labor. There is **no difference in other outcomes**: assisted vaginal deliveries (RR 0.86, 95% CI 0.71–1.05), cesarean sections (RR 1.21, 95% CI 0.87–1.68), use of oxytocin infusion (RR 0.64, 95% CI 0.32–1.28), perineal trauma or maternal infection, Apgar score <7 at 5 minutes (RR 1.58, 95% CI 0.63–3.93), neonatal unit admissions (RR 1.06, 95% CI 0.71–1.57), or neonatal infection rates (RR 2.00, 95% CI 0.50–7.94). There is limited information for other outcomes related to water use during the first and second stages of labor, due to intervention and outcome variability. There is no evidence of increased adverse effects to the fetus/neonate or woman from laboring in water. Laboring in water is usually linked to midwifery care, which is associated with its own benefits (see subsection "Midwife-led Care"). For water birth and immersion in water in the second stage, see chapter 8. There are no trials evaluating different baths/pools, immersion in water during pregnancy, or during the third stage of labor.

Stripping in Labor

There are no trials to evaluate stripping during spontaneous labor (see also chap. 24 for stripping before labor).

Early Artificial Rupture of Membranes (AROM) (aka Amniotomy)

Compared to no amniotomy, amniotomy is not associated with significant differences in length of the first stage of labor (MD −20.43 minutes, 95% CI −95.93 to 55.06), cesarean section (RR 1.27, 95% CI 0.99–1.62), maternal satisfaction with childbirth experience, or low Apgar score <7 at 5 minutes (RR 0.57, 95% CI 0.31–1.06). Other maternal and perinatal outcomes are also not different. There is no consistency between RCTs regarding the timing of amniotomy during labor in terms of cervical dilatation. An association between early amniotomy and CD for NRFHT is noted in one large trial (45). Therefore, routine early (or even late) **amniotomy cannot be recommended as part of standard labor management and care**. Women should be counseled regarding these results, and make an informed decision regarding the option of this intervention (45). Early amniotomy may be possibly reserved for women with slow labor progress.

Use of Partogram

A partogram is a preprinted form, the aim of which is to provide a pictorial overview of labor to plot progress in labor and to alert health professionals to any problems with the mother or baby. The general intervention with the partogram is early use of oxytocin as soon as the cervical dilatation falls to the right of the partogram, usually on the 2-hour cervical exams.

The use of the partogram cannot be recommended as a routine intervention in labor. Compared to no partogram, the use of the partogram is **not associated with significant effects** on cesarean section (RR 0.64, 95% CI 0.24–1.70); instrumental vaginal delivery (RR 1.00, 95% CI 0.85–1.17), or Apgar score <7 at 5 minutes (RR 0.77, 95% CI 0.29–2.06).

Compared to a 4-hour action line, women in the 2-hour action line group are more likely to require oxytocin augmentation (RR 1.14, 95% CI 1.05–1.22). When the 3- and 4-hour action lines are compared, cesarean section rate is lowest in the 4-hour action line group (RR 1.70, 95% CI 1.07–2.70) (45–48).

Frequency of Cervical Exams

There are **no trials to evaluate the frequency of cervical exams in labor per se**. Most studies, including those with active management, perform cervical exams every 2 hours in labor. The risk of chorioamnionitis though increases with increasing number of exams (49).

Oxytocin Augmentation

There are **no trials to evaluate the timing and dosing of oxytocin in labor in women making normal progress in labor.**

For women making slow progress in the first stage of spontaneous labor, treatment with oxytocin as compared with no treatment or delayed oxytocin treatment does not result in any discernable difference in the number of cesarean sections performed, in one meta-analysis. In addition there are no detectable adverse effects for mother or baby (50). The use of oxytocin is associated with a **reduction in the time to delivery of approximately 2 hours**, which might be important to some women. However, if the primary goal of this treatment is to reduce cesarean section rates, then doctors and midwives may have to look for alternative options. Two comparisons were made in this meta-analysis: (*i*) the use of oxytocin versus placebo or no treatment and (*ii*) the early use of oxytocin versus its delayed use. There were no significant differences in the rates of cesarean section or instrumental vaginal delivery in either comparison. Early use of oxytocin resulted in an increase in uterine hyperstimulation associated with fetal heart changes. However, the early use of oxytocin versus its delayed use resulted in no significant differences in a range of neonatal and maternal outcomes. Use of early oxytocin resulted in a statistically significant reduction in the mean duration in labor of approximately 2 hours but did not increase the normal delivery rate in both this meta-analysis (50) and a recent RCT (51).

In a different meta-analysis, early oxytocin was associated with a 9% significant increase in the probability of SVD, but also a tripling of the rate of hyperstimulation, without apparent perinatal consequences (52).

In summary, **oxytocin augmentation in women making slow progress in the first stage seems to be associated with a 2-hour shortening of labor**. The effect on mode of delivery is still uncertain.

There is insufficient evidence to assess how to best use (i.e., dosing issues) oxytocin for augmentation of labor. There are four variables to assess: (*i*) type of dilution; (*ii*) initial dose; (*iii*) incremental increase; and (*iv*) maximum dose (53). In a meta-analysis, a higher initial dose (e.g., 2 mU/min) of oxytocin and incremental dose (e.g., 4 mU/min or more) was associated with a significant reduction in length of labor reported from one trial (MD −3.50 hours, 95% CI −6.38 to −0.62, 1 RCT, *n* = 40). There was a decrease in rate of cesarean section (RR 0.53, 95% CI 0.38–0.75, 4 RCTs, *n* = 650) and an increase in the rate of spontaneous vaginal birth (RR 1.37, 95% CI 1.15–1.64, 2 RCTs, *n* = 350). There were no significant differences for neonatal mortality, hyperstimulation, chorioamnionitis, epidural analgesia; or neonatal outcomes of Apgar scores, umbilical cord pH, or admission to special care baby unit. Many outcomes were not evaluated, such as perinatal mortality, women's satisfaction, instrumental vaginal birth, uterine rupture, postpartum hemorrhage, abnormal cardiotocography, women's pyrexia, dystocia, and neonatal neurological morbidity (54). Based mostly on physiologic studies, an oxytocin dilution of 10 mU/mL, and initial dose of 2 mU/min (12 mL/hr), incremental increase of 2 mU (12 mL) every 30 to 45 minutes until adequate labor, and maximum dose of 16 mU/min (up to 24 mU) have been proposed (53).

For use of oxytocin in induction, see chapter 20.

Active Management of Labor

Active management of labor was originally devised to prevent prolonged labor. Its components have varied somewhat in the literature but generally include antenatal classes, admission not before premature rupture of membranes (PROM) or 2 cm dilatation and full effacement (active labor), early amniotomy, support by doula, use of partogram, and vaginal exams every 2 hours, with oxytocin started for rate of progress off the partogram or <1 cm/hr. Oxytocin rate is started at 4 to 6 mU/min, increased by 4 to 6 mU every 15 minutes to reach contractions every 2 to 3 minutes (but not more than 7/15 minutes) or 40 mU/min. Early amniotomy and early use of high-dose oxytocin are the two most characteristic interventions of active management of labor.

Compared to "routine" care (no active management), active management of labor is associated with a trend for a slightly lower incidence of CD (RR 0.88, 95% CI 0.77–1.01). However, in one study there were a large number of post-randomization exclusions. On excluding this study, **CD rates in the active management group were statistically significantly lower than in the routine care group** (RR 0.77, 95% CI 0.63–0.94). **More women in the active management group had labors lasting less than 12 hours**, but there was wide variation in length of labor within and between trials. The **reduced duration of labor** is about 50 to 100 minutes, mostly in the first stage. There were no differences between groups in use of analgesia, rates of assisted vaginal deliveries, or maternal or neonatal complications. Only one RCT examined maternal satisfaction; the majority of women (over 75%) in both groups were very satisfied with care (55–59). The shorter labor is probably due to the early amniotomy [see subsection "Early Artificial Rupture of Membranes (AROM) (aka Amniotomy)"]. The effects on incidence of CD may be due to the fact that some aspects of active managements, that is, support by doula, decrease CD rate, but some others (i.e., early amniotomy) may increase it. It is recommended that **the individual interventions that are part of active management of labor should be studied separately, and only those that are beneficial (e.g., support by doula) implemented.**

Use of Continuous Vs. Intermittent Monitoring, Amnioinfusion for Variables, Scalp Sampling, Etc.

See chapter 10.

Bladder Catheterization

There are **no trials** to evaluate the necessity, timing, and frequency of bladder catheterization in labor per se.

Epidural or Other Anesthesia

See chapter 11.

Use of Ultrasound During Labor

There is insufficient evidence to assess the effect of using ultrasound during labor and delivery. There are several potential uses, including as an aid to the diagnosis of dystocia, but none have been tested by RCTs (60).

Use of Intrauterine Pressure Catheter

The IUPC can measure more objectively than external toco-monitor the intensity of uterine contractions. It necessitates ROM. Intensity is usually calculated by Montevideo units, that is, sum of peak pressures above baseline of all contractions in 10 minutes.

Several RCTs have assessed the effect of IUPC on labor outcomes. In the largest RCT, compared to no IUPC, IUPC use is associated with **no effect** in rate of operative deliveries, maternal or fetal infection, or other maternal or perinatal recorded outcome (61) (see also section "Criteria for Diagnosis of Failure to Progress in First Stage").

CRITERIA FOR DIAGNOSIS OF FAILURE TO PROGRESS IN FIRST STAGE

Abnormal progression of labor, including terms such as dystocia, dysfunctional labor, failure to progress, cephalopelvic disproportion, and others, is the most common problem in labor, and the **reason for the majority of CDs** (62). Risk factors for dystocia are, among others, as follows: obesity, induction, Bishop <5 at start of labor, station higher than −2, persistent occiput posterior, macrosomia, epidural anesthesia, etc.

In term women in spontaneous active labor not on oxytocin and with no epidural, the fifth percentile rates of dilatation for nulliparous and parous women are 1.2 cm/hr and 1.5 cm/hr, respectively (63,64). In term women in labor *necessitating oxytocin* and *with epidural*, the fifth percentile rate for dilatation is about 0.5 cm/hr for both nulliparous and parous women (65).

In term women with epidural, labor may take more than 6 hours to progress from 4 to 5 cm, and more than 3 hours to progress from 5 to 6 cm of dilation (66).

Dystocia cannot be diagnosed unless ROM has occurred, and adequate oxytocin to achieve at least 3 to 5 adequate contractions per hour has been instituted. Dystocia also **cannot be diagnosed reliably before the first stage of labor has entered the active phase, which has been defined, especially in nulliparous with epidurals in place, as at least 6 cm of cervical dilatation** (66). The majority (>60%) of women who experience 2 hours of labor arrest despite a sustained uterine contraction pattern of at least 200 Montevideo units in the first stage of labor will achieve a vaginal delivery if oxytocin is continued (67). **Before performing a CD for active phase labor arrest, labor should be arrested for a minimum of 4 hours (if uterine activity is greater than 200 Montevideo units as documented with IUPC) or 6 hours (if greater than 200 Montevideo units could not be sustained)** (67). These data are not from an RCT, and there was a significant higher risk of shoulder dystocia among parturient who had arrest for 4 hours or more. Vaginal birth after cesarean (VBAC) and diabetics were not included in this study. Please see chapter 8 for additional evidence on dystocia.

In women at term with singleton gestations and requiring oxytocin by obstetrician because of "dystocia" at 4 to 6 cm, **meperidine 100 mg IV does not affect operative delivery rates and worsens neonatal outcomes compared to placebo** (68) (see also chap. 8).

REFERENCES

1. Noller KL, Resseguie LL, Voss V. The effect of changes in atmospheric pressure on the occurrence of the spontaneous onset of labor in term pregnancies. Am J Obstet Gynecol 1996; 174:1192–1199. [II-2]
2. Maimburg RD, Vaeth M, Durr J, et al. Randomized trial of structured antenatal training sessions to improve the birth process. BJOG 2010; 117:921–928. [RCT, *n* = 1193]
3. Bergstrom M, Kieler H, Waldenstrom U. Effects of natural childbirth preparation versus standard antenatal education on epidural rates, experience of childbirth and parental stress in mothers and fathers: a randomized controlled trial. BJOG 2009; 116:1167–1176. [RCT, *n* = 1087]

4. Bonovich L. Recognizing the onset of labour. J Obstet Gynecol Neonatal Nurs 1990; 19(2):141–145. [RCT, *n* = 245; 208 analyzed]

5. Pattinson RC, Farrell E. Pelvimetry for fetal cephalic presentations at or near term. Cochrane Database Syst Rev 2005; (4): CD003514. [Meta-analysis: 4 RCTs (all used X-ray pelvimetry; all not of good quality), *n* = 895]

6. Dowswell T, Thornton JG, Hewison J, et al. Should there be a trial of home versus hospital delivery in the United Kingdom? Measuring outcomes other than safety is feasible. BMJ 1996; 312:753. [RCT, *n* = 11]

7. Olsen O, Jewell D. Home versus hospital birth. Cochrane Database Syst Rev 1998; (3):CD000352. [Meta-analysis: 1 RCT, *n* = 11]

8. Wax JR, Lucas FL, Lamont M, et al. Maternal and newborn outcomes in planned home birth vs planned hospital births: a metaanalysis. Am J Obstet Gynecol 2010; 203:243.e1–243.e8. [Meta-analysis on non-RCTs]

9. American College of Obstetricians and Gynecologists. ACOG Committee Opinion No. 476: planned home birth. Obstet Gynecol 2011; 117:425–427. [Review]

10. Ravelli ACJ, Jager KJ, de Groot MH, et al. Travel time from home to hospital and adverse perinatal outcomes in women at term in the Netherlands. BJOG 2010; 118(4):457–465. [II-2]

11. Chervenak FA, McCullough LB, Arabin B. Obstetric ethics: an essential dimension of planned home birth. Obstet Gynecol 2011; 117(5):1183–1187. [Review]

12. Ecker J, Minkoff H. Home birth. What are physicians' ethical obligations when patient choices may carry increased risk? Obstet Gynecol 2011; 117:1179–1182. [Review]

13. Hodnett ED, Downe S, Walsh D, et al. Alternative versus conventional institutional settings for birth. Cochrane Database Syst Rev 2010; (9):CD000012. [Meta-analysis: 9 RCTs, *n* = 10,684]

14. Hatem M, Sandall J, Devane D, et al. Midwife-led versus other models of care for childbearing women. Cochrane Database Syst Rev 2008; (4):CD004667. [11 RCTs, *n* = 12,276]

15. Jokhio AH, Winter HR, Cheng KK. An intervention involving traditional birth attendants and perinatal and maternal mortality in Pakistan. NEJM 2005; 352:2091–2099. [1 RCT, *n* = 20,557]

16. Nielsen PE, Goldman MB, Mann S, et al. Effects of teamwork training on adverse outcomes and process of care in labor and delivery: a randomized controlled trial. Obstet Gynecol 2007; 109:48–55. [RCT, *n* = 1307 personnel, 28,536 deliveries]

17. McNiven PS, Williams, JI, Hodnett E, et al. An early labour assessment program: a randomised, controlled trial. Birth 1998; 25(1):5–10. [RCT, *n* = 209]

18. Cheyne H, Hundley V, Dowding D, et al. Effects of algorithm for diagnosis of active labour: cluster randomized trial. BMJ 2008; 337:a2396. [RCT, *n* = 4503]

19. Impey L, Reynolds M, MacQuillan K, et al. Admission cardiotocography: a randomized controlled trial. Lancet 2003; 361:466–470. [RCT, *n* = 8580]

20. Blix E, Reinar LM, Klovning A, et al. Prognostic value of the labour admission test and its effectiveness compared with auscultation only: a systematic review. BJOG 2005; 112:1595–1604. [Meta-analysis: 3 RCTs, *n* = 11,259]

21. Chauhan SP, Washburne JF, Magann EF, et al. A randomized study to assess the efficacy of the amniotic fluid index as a fetal admission test. Obstet Gynecol 1995; 86:9–13. [RCT, *n* = 883]

22. Moses J, Doherty DA, Magann EF, et al. A randomized clinical trial of the intrapartum assessment of amniotic fluid volume: amniotic fluid index versus the single deepest pocket technique. Am J Obstet Gynecol 2004; 190:1564–1570. [RCT, *n* = 499]

23. Reveiz L, Gaitán HG, Cuervo LG. Enemas during labour. Cochrane Database Syst Rev 2007; (4):CD000330. [Meta-analysis; 4 RCTs, *n* = 1917]

24. Basevi V, Lavender T. Routine perineal shaving on admission in labour. Cochrane Database Syst Rev 2000; (4):CD001236. [Meta-analysis, 3 RCTs]

25. Lumbiganon P, Thinkhamrop J, Thinkhamrop B, et al. Vaginal chlorhexidine during labour for preventing maternal and neonatal infections (excluding Group B Streptococcal and HIV). Cochrane Database Syst Rev 2004; (4):CD004070. [3 RCTs, *n* = 3012]

26. Saleem S, Rouse D, McClure EM, et al. Chlorhexidine vaginal and infant wipes to reduce perinatal mortality and morbidity. Obstet Gynecol 2010; 115:1225–1232. [RCT, *n* = 5008]

27. Schrag S, Gorwitz R, Fultz-Butts K, et al. Prevention of perinatal group B streptococcal disease. MMWR Recomm Rep 2002; 51 (RR-11):1–24. [Review/Guideline; www.cdc.gov/groupbstrep]

28. Hodnett ED, Gates S, Hofmeyr GJ, et al. Continuous support for women during childbirth. Cochrane Database Syst Rev 2011; (2): CD003766. [Meta-analysis: 21 RCTs; *n* = 15,061]

29. Burns E, Zobbi V, Panzeri D, et al. Aromatherapy in childbirth: a pilot randomized controlled trial. BJOG 2007; 114:838–844. [RCT, *n* = 513]

30. Singata M, Tranmer J, Gyte GML. Restricting oral fluid and food intake during labour. Cochrane Database Syst Rev 2010; (1): CD003930. [Meta-analysis: 5 RCTs, *n* = 3130]

31. Scheepers HCJ, Thans MCJ, de Jong PA, et al. A double-blind, placebo controlled study on the influence of carbohydrate solution intake during labor BJOG 2002; 109:178–181. [RCT, *n* = 201]

32. Scheepers HCJ, de Jong PA, Essed GGM, et al. Carbohydrate solution intake during labour just before the start of the second stage: a double-blind study on metabolic effects and clinical outcome. BJOG 2004; 111:1382–1387. [RCT, *n* = 2021]

33. Practice guidelines for obstetrical anesthesia. A report by the American Society of Anesthesiologist Task Force on Obstetrical Anesthesia. Anesthesiology 1999; 90:600–611. [Review]

34. Olsson GL, Hallen B, Hambreas-Jonzon K. Aspiration during anaesthesia: a computer aided study of 185358 anaesthetics. Acta Anaesthesiol Scand 1986; 30:84–92. [II-2]

35. Gyte GML, Richens Y. Routine prophylactic drugs in normal labour for reducing gastric aspiration and its effects. Cochrane Database Syst Rev 2006; (3):CD005298. [Meta-analysis; 3 RCTs, *n* = 2465]

36. Garite TJ, Weeks J, Peters-Phair K, et al. A randomized controlled trial of the effect of increased intravenous hydration on the course of labor in nulliparous women. AJOG 2000; 183:1544–1548. [RCT, *n* = 195]

37. Shrivastava VK, Garite TJ, Jenkins SM, et al. A randomized, double-blinded controlled trial comparing parenteral normal saline with and without dextrose on the course of labor in nulliparas. Am J Obstet Gynecol 2009; 200:379.e1–379.e6. [RCT, *n* = 300]

38. Fisher AJ, Huddleston JF. Intrapartum maternal glucose infusion reduces umbilical cord academia. Am J Obstet Gynecol 1997; 177:765–769. [RCT, *n* = 106]

39. Lawrence A, Lewis L, Hofmeyr GJ, et al. Maternal positions and mobility during first stage labour. Cochrane Database Syst Rev 2009; (2):CD003934. [Meta-analysis: 21 RCTs, *n* = 3706]

40. Bloom SL, McIntire DD, Kelly MA, et al. Lack of effect of walking on labor and delivery. NEJM 1998; 339:76–79. [RCT, *n* = 1067]

41. McManus TJ, Calder AA. Upright posture and the efficiency of labour. Lancet 1978; 1:72–74. [RCT, *n* = 40]

42. Flynn AM, Kelly J, Hollins G, et al. Ambulation in labour. BMJ 1978; 2:591–593. [RCT, *n* = 68]

43. Read JA, Miller FC, Paul RH. Randomized trial of ambulation versus oxytocin for labor enhancement: a preliminary report. Am J Obstet Gynecol 1981; 139:669–672. [RCT, *n* = 14]

44. Hemminki E, Saarikoski S. Ambulation and delayed amniotomy in the first stage of labor. Eur J Obstet Gynecol Reprod Biol 1983; 15:129–139. [RCT, *n* = 630]

45. Smyth RMD, Alldred SK, Markham C. Amniotomy for shortening spontaneous labour. Cochrane Database Syst Rev 2007; (4): CD006167. [Meta-analysis: 15 RCTs, *n* = 5583]

46. Lavender T, Hart A, Smyth RMD. Effect of partogram use on outcomes for women in spontaneous labour at term. Cochrane Database Syst Rev 2008; (4):CD005461. [Meta-analysis: 5 RCTs, *n* = 6187]

47. Pattison RC, Howarth GR, Mdluli W, et al. Aggressive or expectant management of labour: a randomized clinical trial. BJOG 2003; 110:457–461. [RCT, *n* = 694]

48. World Health Organization Maternal Health and Safe Motherhood Programme. World Health Organization partograph in the management of labour. Lancet 1994; 343:1399–1404. [RCT, $n = 35{,}484$]

49. Soper DE, Mayhall CG, Dalton HP. Risk factors for intraamniotic infection: a prospective epidemiologic study. Am J Obstet Gynecol 1989; 161:562–566; discussion 566–568. [II-2]

50. Bugg GJ, Siddiqui F, Thornton JG. Oxytocin versus no treatment or delayed treatment for slow progress in the first stage of spontaneous labour. Cochrane Database Syst Rev 2011; (7): CD007123. [Meta-analysis: 8 RCTs, $n = 1338$]

51. Dencker A, Berg M, Bergqvist L, et al. Early versus delayed oxytocin augmentation in nulliparous women with prolonged labor-a randomized trial. BJOG 2009; 116:530–536. [RCT, $n = 630$]

52. Wei S-Q, Luo Z-C, Xu H, et al. The effect of early oxytocin augmentation in labor—a meta-analysis. Obstet Gynecol 2009; 114:641–649. [Meta-analysis: 9 RCTs, $n = 1983$]

53. Hayes EJ, Weinstein L. Improving patient safety and uniformity of care by a standardized regimen for the use of oxytocin. Am J Obstet Gynecol 2008; 198(6):622.e1–622.e7. [Review]

54. Mori R, Tokumasu H, Pledge D, et al. High dose versus low dose oxytocin for augmentation of delayed labour. Cochrane Database Syst Rev 2011; (10):CD007201. [Meta-analysis: 4 RCTs, $n = 660$]

55. Brown HC, Paranjothy S, Dowswell T, et al. Package of care for active management in labour for reducing caesarean section rates in low-risk women. Cochrane Database Syst Rev 2008; (4): CD004907. [Meta-analysis: 7 RCTs, $n = 5370$]

56. Lopex-Leno JA, Peaceman AM, Adashek JA, et al. A controlled trial of a program for the active management of labor. NEJM 1992; 326:450–454. [RCT, $n = 705$]

57. Frigoletto FD, Leiberman E, Lang JM, et al. A clinical trial of active management of labor. NEJM 1995; 333:745–750. [RCT, $n = 1915$]

58. Rogers R, Gilson GJ, Miller AC, et al. Active management of labor: does it make a difference? AJOG 1997; 599–605. [RCT, $n = 405$]

59. Sadler LC, Davison T, McCowan LME. A randomized controlled trial and meta-analysis of active management of labour. BJOG 2000; 107:909–915. [RCT, $n = 651$]

60. Vintzileos AM, Chavez M, Kinzler WL. Use of ultrasound in labor and delivery. J Matern Fet Neo Med 2010; 23:469–475. [Review]

61. Bakker JJH, Verhoeven MS, Janssen PF, et al. Outcomes after internal versus external tocodynamometry for monitoring labor. NEJM 2010; 362:306–313. [RCT, $n = 1456$]

62. Ness A, Goldberg J, Berghella V. Abnormalities of the first and second stages of labor. Obstet Gynecol Clin N Am 2005; 32:201–220. [Review]

63. Friedman EA. Primigravid labor: a graphicostatistical analysis. Obstet Gynecol 1955; 6:567–589. [II-3]

64. Friedman EA. Labour: Clinical Evaluation and Management. 2nd ed. New York: Appleton-Century-Croft, 1978. [II-3]

65. Rouse DJ, Owen JO, Hauth JC. Active-phase labor arrest: oxytocin augmentation for at least 4 hours. Obstet Gynecol 1999; 93:323–328. [II-3]

66. Zhang J, Landy HJ, Branch DW, et al. Contemporary patterns of spontaneous labor with normal neonatal outcomes. Obstet Gynecol 2010; 116(6):1281–1287. [II-1]

67. Rouse DJ, Owen JO, Savage KG, et al. Active-phase labor arrest: revisiting the 2-hour minimum. Obstet Gynecol 2001; 98:550–554. [II-3]

68. Sosa CG, Balaguer E, Alonso JG, et al. Meperidine for dystocia during the first stage of labor: a randomized controlled trial. AJOG 2004; 191:1212–1218. [RCT, $n = 407$]

8

Second stage of labor

Geoffrey Bowers

KEY POINTS

- **Prophylactic intrapartum maternal oxygen in the second stage of normal labor should not be used**, since it is associated with more frequent low (<7.20) cord blood pH values than the control group.
- **Prophylactic intrapartum betamimetics in the second stage of normal labor should not be used**, since their use is associated with an increase in forceps deliveries.
- **Women should be encouraged to give birth in the position they find most comfortable, which is usually upright.** Use of any **upright or lateral position**, compared with supine or lithotomy positions, is associated, **in women without epidural analgesia**, with **reduction in duration of second stage of labor; reduction in assisted deliveries; reduction in episiotomies; increase in second-degree perineal tears; increase in estimated blood loss >500 mL; reduction in reporting of severe pain during second stage of labor; and reduction in abnormal fetal heart rate patterns.** In women with epidural anesthesia, the evidence is limited and insufficient to make a recommendation.
- **There is insufficient evidence to recommend water immersion in second stage of labor, and risks have not been adequately assessed.**
- In women at term with **epidural** analgesia and a singleton, cephalic fetus, **delayed pushing** (waiting 1–3 hours or until "urge to push") is associated with **similar rate of operative vaginal** delivery and of cesarean delivery (CD), but **higher incidence of spontaneous vaginal delivery** compared with early (immediate upon entering second stage) pushing (8). The duration of the second stage is **longer by about 60 minutes**, the duration of pushing is similar, as are all other studied maternal and perinatal outcomes. **Careful monitoring of mother and fetus is necessary** to allow labor to continue safely.
- In women without epidural anesthesia, compared with encouraging a woman's own urge to push (open glottis), **pushing using the Valsalva maneuver (closed glottis) is associated with shorter (by 19 minutes) duration of labor; similar incidences of operative vaginal deliveries, need for perineal repair, and postpartum hemorrhage; and similar neonatal outcomes.** Labor attendant should counsel women in labor regarding these data and probably **support the parturient in her own choice of either technique.**
- **Coaching during pushing may shorten the second stage of labor, but lack of available coaching support does not adversely affect labor outcomes.**
- **Use of a dental support device has been associated with a shorter second stage of labor and reduction in the number of failures to descend requiring operative intervention.**
- **Both manual and belt fundal pressures** to aid in vaginal delivery have not been associated with effect on maternal and perinatal outcomes, except for **decreased maternal satisfaction**.
- **Perineal massage and stretching of the perineum with a water-soluble lubricant** in the second stage of labor is associated with **similar rates of intact perineum** compared with the control group. The incidence of **third-degree lacerations is decreased.**
- Use of **perineal warm packs in the second stage of labor is associated with a reduction in third- and fourth-degree tears, as well as a reduction in pain on postpartum day 1 and 2.**
- Routine use of the Ritgen's maneuver does not appear to be associated with any benefits.
- **"Hands-poised" is preferred to the "hands-on" method**, since they are associated with similar incidences of perineal and vaginal tears, but the hands-on method is associated with higher incidence of episiotomies.
- **Routine episiotomy should not be performed**, as restricting episiotomy use is associated with less posterior perineal trauma, less suturing, and fewer healing complications.
- There is insufficient evidence to determine when the second stage is prolonged, and associated with enough complications with continuing labor so as to justify either operative vaginal delivery or CD.

PROPHYLACTIC INTERVENTIONS
Maternal Oxygen

Prophylactic intrapartum maternal oxygen in the second stage of normal labor is **associated with more frequent low (<7.20) cord blood pH** values than the control group (1). There are no other statistically significant differences between the groups. There is a tendency toward reduced cord arterial blood oxygen content and oxygen saturation in mothers treated with oxygen compared with controls. Therefore, **routine maternal oxygenation throughout the second stage should not be performed**. Short-term oxygenation may be beneficial and long-term oxygenation harmful.

Prophylactic Tocolysis

There is no evidence to support the prophylactic use of betamimetics to prevent nonreassuring fetal heart rate tracing (NRFHT) during the second stage of labor. Compared with placebo, prophylactic betamimetic therapy is **associated with an increase in forceps deliveries**. The trial protocol required forceps to be used if the second stage of labor exceeded 30 minutes, in both groups. There are no clear effects on postpartum hemorrhage, neonatal irritability, feeding slowness, umbilical arterial pH values, or Apgar scores at 2 minutes (2).

Therefore, **routine prophylactic tocolysis should not be performed in the second stage of labor.**

Prophylactic Positioning to Prevent Shoulder Dystocia
See chapter 23.

MANAGEMENT
Maternal Position
There are several benefits for upright posture [sitting (obstetric chair/stool); semirecumbent (trunk tilted backward 30° to the vertical); kneeling; squatting (unaided or using squatting bars); and squatting (aided with Birth cushion)] during the second stage of labor.

Use of any **upright or lateral position**, compared with supine or lithotomy positions, is associated, **in women without epidural analgesia**, with a **small (4 minutes) reduction in duration of second stage of labor**; a 20% **reduction in assisted deliveries**; a 17% **reduction in episiotomies**; a 23% **increase in second-degree perineal tears**; a 63% **increase in estimated blood loss >500 mL**; a 23% **reduction in reporting of severe pain during second stage of labor**; and a 69% **reduction in abnormal fetal heart rate patterns** (3). Use of the birth stool showed no effect and results with the birth chair were variable. Estimation of blood loss in the upright group may have been influenced by the fact that blood loss in the birth chair is collected in a receptacle. Physiological advantages for non-recumbent or upright labor may include the effects of gravity, lessened risk of aortocaval compression and improved acid-base outcomes in the neonates, stronger and more efficient uterine contractions, improved alignment of the fetus for passage through the pelvis ("drive angle"), and radiological evidence of larger anteroposterior and transverse pelvic outlet diameters, resulting in an increase in the total outlet area in the squatting and kneeling positions (3).

In women with epidural anesthesia, the evidence is limited and insufficient to make a recommendation. In a small RCT, compared with a supported sitting position, lateral position was associated with a lower chance of an instrumental vaginal delivery (4). Kneeling and sitting upright are associated with similar duration of second stage and other outcomes, except for a more favorable maternal experience and less pain associated with kneeling (5).

Women without epidural anesthesia **should be encouraged to give birth in the upright position**, which is also the position they usually find most comfortable. The evidence is insufficient for a recommendation on women with epidural anesthesia.

Epidural or Other Anesthesia
See chapter 11.

Water Immersion
Although there is some evidence that water immersion in the first stage of labor may reduce the need for epidural/spinal anesthesia and length of first stage of labor (see chap. 7), **immersion during the second stage has been insufficiently studied** and may be best avoided given lack of sufficient safety data. Of the three trials that compared water immersion during the second stage with no immersion, one trial showed a significantly higher level of satisfaction with the birth experience (RR 0.24, 95% CI 0.07–0.70). There are reports of neonatal water aspirations from birth (end of second stage) in water (6,7). **In summary, there is insufficient evidence to recommend water immersion in second stage of labor, and risks have not been adequately assessed.**

Pushing
Delayed Vs. Early Pushing
In women at term with **epidural** analgesia and a singleton, cephalic fetus, **delayed pushing** (waiting 1–3 hours or until urge to push) is associated with **similar rate of operative vaginal delivery and of CD**, but **higher incidence of spontaneous vaginal delivery** compared with early (immediate upon entering second stage) pushing (8). The duration of the second stage is longer by about 60 minutes, the duration of pushing is similar, as are all other studied maternal outcomes. The neonatal outcomes are also similar, including incidence of admission to neonatal intensive care unit (NICU). Women should be counseled regarding these data. The longer duration of second stage with delayed pushing has not been associated with detrimental effects on the fetus, but **careful monitoring of both mother and fetus is necessary to allow labor to continue safely** (see also section "Criteria for Diagnosis of Prolonged Second Stage").

Pushing Method: Valsalva Vs. Spontaneous
Most women spontaneously choose to Valsalva in the second stage of labor. In women without epidural anesthesia, compared with encouraging a woman's own urge to push (open glottis), **pushing using the Valsalva maneuver (closed glottis: taking a deep breath, holding it, and pushing for as long and hard as possible, that is, 2 to 3 times during each contractions) is associated with shorter (by 19 minutes) duration of labor; similar incidences of operative vaginal deliveries, need for perineal repair, and postpartum hemorrhage; and similar neonatal outcomes** (9). Urodynamics 3 months after delivery are worse in the closed glottis group, but long-term outcome has not been studied (9). Labor attendant should counsel women in labor regarding these data and probably **support the parturient in her own choice of either technique.**

Coached Pushing
Although **coached pushing confers the benefit of a slightly shorter second stage**, coached maternal pushing confers no other advantages and withholding such coaching is not detrimental to maternal or fetal outcomes (10).

Use of a Dental Support Device
Wearing a dental support device (mouthguard) is associated with a shorter second stage (19 minutes) in one RCT. In addition, less operative interventions were used in the intervention group. Further research into optimizing maternal expulsive efforts is needed to evaluate overall benefit (11).

Fundal Pressure
In the second stage of labor, fundal pressure has been evaluated either as just manual pressure or with an obstetric belt wrapped around the woman's abdomen above the level of the uterine fundus. **Manual and belt fundal pressures** to aid in vaginal delivery have both not been associated with effect on maternal and perinatal outcomes, except for **decreased maternal satisfaction.**

Compared with no manual fundal pressure, **manual fundal pressure (Kristeller maneuver) concomitant with each contraction while patient had urge to push during the** second stage is associated with **no significant changes in duration of labor, or other maternal and perinatal outcomes** in one RCT (12).

The belt evaluated for fundal pressure inflates with each contraction to a maximum of 200 mmHg for 30 seconds. Compared with no belt, the **inflatable obstetric belt is associated with similar incidence of spontaneous vaginal delivery** in nulliparous women with singleton term pregnancies and an epidural at term. All other maternal and neonatal outcomes are similar, but **women with no belt have greater satisfaction** (13).

Perineal Massage

Perineal massage has been evaluated for decrease in perineal lacerations. Perineal massage has not been associated with complications. For perineal massage during pregnancy and before labor, see chapter 2. Perineal massage and stretching of the perineum with a water-soluble lubricant in the second stage of labor are associated with **similar rates of intact perineum** compared with the control group. The incidence of **third-degree lacerations is decreased** (14). In another RCT, perineal massage with lubricant was associated with similar incidence of genital tract trauma compared with either no touching, or to warm compresses (15).

Perineal Warm Packs

Although no difference was seen in minor perineal trauma or requirement for suturing, **application of perineal warm packs during the second stage was associated with less severe (third- or fourth-degree) tears** than was standard management. In addition, **pain scores were less** on postpartum days 1 and 2 in the intervention group. After 3 months, a trend toward decreased symptoms of urinary incontinence was seen in the intervention group (16). In another RCT, warm compresses were associated with similar incidence of genital tract trauma compared with either no touching, or to perineal massage (15).

Manual Rotation

Persistent fetal occiput posterior position is a risk factor for prolonged labor and higher rate of CD. **There is insufficient evidence (no trials) to evaluate the efficacy of manual rotation in labor.** In a retrospective cohort study, in women with a fetus in persistent occiput posterior or transverse position in the second stage of labor, manual rotation was associated with lower rates of CD, perineal lacerations, postpartum hemorrhage, and chorioamnionitis, but a higher rate of cervical lacerations (17). Another prospective (but not randomized) study of singletons with occiput posterior position reported an increase in fetuses delivered in occiput anterior position (93% vs. 15%) and in spontaneous vaginal delivery (77% vs. 27%) compared with no manual rotation, using historic controls (18) (see also chap. 22).

Ritgen's Maneuver

Ritgen's maneuver (originally described by Ritgen in 1855) involves reaching for the fetal chin when this has reached the plane between the maternal anus and the coccyx, and pulling it anteriorly, while using the fingers of the other hand on the fetal occiput to control speed of delivery and keep flexion of the fetal neck. Its aim is usually to protect the perineum from lacerations. Compared with no Ritgen's maneuver, Ritgen's maneuver performed for delivery of fetal head during uterine contractions is not associated with any effect on the incidence of perineal tears, or other reported maternal or perinatal outcomes. The length of second stage and several perinatal outcomes were not reported in this RCT (19). **In summary, Ritgen's maneuver does not appear to be associated with any benefits.**

"Hands-on" Vs. "Hands-poised"

The hands-on method (also described by Ritgen) usually involves pressure on the infant's head upon crowning, and support with the other hand of the perineum, with the aim of protecting for lacerations. In the hands-poised method, the fetal head and perineum are not touched or supported by the delivering personnel. These two methods are associated with **similar incidences of perineal and vaginal tears, but the hands-on method is associated with higher incidence of episiotomies** (20). A policy of hands-poised has also been supported by a quasi-randomized study, reporting less third-degree tears compared with hands-on (21). Therefore, **the hands-on method should not be employed in labor.**

Episiotomy

Routine episiotomy should not be performed, as restrictive episiotomy policies have a number of benefits compared with routine episiotomy policies. In the most recent meta-analysis of RCTs, 75% of women had episiotomies in the routine episiotomy group, while the rate in the restrictive episiotomy group was 28%. Compared with routine use, **restrictive episiotomy is associated with less severe perineal trauma** (RR 0.67, 95% CI 0.49–0.91), **less suturing** (RR 0.71, 95% CI 0.61–0.81), **and fewer healing complications** (RR 0.69, 95% CI 0.56–0.85) (22). Restrictive episiotomy is associated with **more anterior perineal trauma** (RR 1.84, 95% CI 1.61–2.10). There was no difference in severe vaginal/perineal trauma (RR 0.92, 95% CI 0.72–1.18); dyspareunia (RR 1.02, 95% CI 0.90–1.16); urinary incontinence (RR 0.98, 95% CI 0.79–1.20), or several pain measures. Results for restrictive versus routine mediolateral versus midline episiotomy were similar to the overall comparison (22). There is insufficient evidence to evaluate if there are (if any) indications for any use of episiotomy, such as assisted delivery (forceps or vacuum), preterm delivery, breech delivery, predicted macrosomia, and presumed imminent tears. **Episiotomy should be avoided if at all possible**, but, if used, it is unknown which episiotomy technique (mediolateral or midline) provides the best (or worst) outcome.

CRITERIA FOR DIAGNOSIS OF PROLONGED SECOND STAGE

There is insufficient evidence to determine when the second stage is prolonged, and associated with enough complications with continuing labor so as to justify either operative vaginal delivery or CD. Some have proposed the criteria in Table 8.1 for the diagnosis of prolonged second stage (also named at times criteria for dystocia or failure to progress), but these are not based on level 1 evidence (23–25). Clinically, the start of the second stage is imprecise and begins when the subjectively timed cervical exam reveals complete (10 cm) cervical dilation. It is also important to realize that, based on data above, women often do not begin to push until more than 1 hour after complete dilation has been ascertained.

Several non-level-1 studies have compared maternal and perinatal outcomes between women with shorter versus "prolonged" second stage. In a review of all studies up to 2004, a

Table 8.1 Proposed Criteria for Prolonged Second Stage

Maternal characteristics	Suggested upper limit of length of second stage (hr)
Nulliparous, epidural	3
Nulliparous, no epidural	2
Multiparous, epidural	2
Multiparous, no epidural	1

Source: From Refs. 23–24.

strong **association between prolonged second stage and operative delivery** was noted (26). The definition of prolonged second stage was inconsistent across studies. In addition, significant associations with maternal outcomes such as **postpartum hemorrhage, infection, and severe obstetric lacerations** were reported, but methods varied widely. From other data, urinary incontinence may also be increased with prolonged second stage (25). Instead, anal incontinence does not seem to be affected (27). Perhaps most importantly, **no clear associations between prolonged second stage and adverse neonatal outcomes were reported** (26). The length of the second stage is not associated with poor neonatal outcome, as long as reassuring fetal testing is present.

The problem with the evidence above is that these maternal detriments of prolonged second stage occur when these women are compared with women without prolonged second stage. It is evident that a planned cesarean before labor might decrease some of these complications (e.g., bleeding, infection, lacerations, and incontinence). **The clinical issue is different, though. Once a woman has prolonged second stage, should she be delivered operatively or should she continue labor?** CD performed after prolonged second stage has been associated with longer surgery time, increased postoperative fevers, maternal intraoperative trauma including higher risk of extensions of the uterine incision, higher composite maternal morbidity, but similar perinatal outcomes, compared with CD performed before prolonged second stage (28).

There are **no such trials** to evaluate the management of prolonged second stage and best diagnosis of dystocia. Operative intervention is not warranted just because a set number of hours have elapsed in the second stage. **If there are no signs of infection (maternal or fetal), no maternal exhaustion, and reassuring fetal testing, labor can be allowed to continue beyond these limits** (Table 8.1) **as long as some progress has been made.** If contractions are adequate, the chance of vaginal delivery decreases progressively after 3 to 5 hours of pushing in the second stage.

Mandatory second opinion is associated with 22 fewer intrapartum CDs per 1000 deliveries, without affecting maternal or perinatal outcomes (29) (see chap. 13).

REFERENCES

1. Fawole B, Hofmeyr GJ. Maternal oxygen administration for fetal distress. Cochrane Database Syst Rev 2005; (4). [2 RCTs, $n = 245$]
2. Campbell J, Anderson I, Chang A, et al. The use of ritodrine in the management of the fetus during the second stage of labour. Aust NZ J Obstet Gynaecol 1978; 18:110–113. [RCT, $n = 100$. Normal obstetric women selected during the first stage of labor. Infusion of ritodrine 5 μg/kg/min starting when the second stage of labor is diagnosed, compared with placebo infusion (dextrose water)]
3. Gupta JK, Hofmeyr GJ. Position in the second stage of labour for women without epidural anaesthesia. Cochrane Database Syst Rev 2005; (3). [Meta-analysis: 20 RCTs; $n = 6135$. Variable trial quality, inconsistencies within trials, and heterogeneity of subjects]
4. Downe S, Gerrett D, Renfrew MJ. A prospective randomized trial on the effect of position in the passive second stage of labour on birth outcome in nulliparous women using epidural anesthesia. Midwifery 2004; 20:157–168. [RCT, $n = 107$]
5. Ragnat I, Altman D, Tyden T, et al. Comparison of the maternal experience and duration of labour in two upright delivery positions—a randomized controlled trial. BJOG 2006; 113:165–170. [RCT, $n = 271$]
6. Cluett ER, Burns E. Immersion in water in labour and birth. Cochrane Database Syst Rev 2009; (2):CD000111. [Meta-analysis: 12 RCTs, $n = 3243$]
7. Mammas IN, Thiagarajan P. Water aspiration at birth: report of 2 cases. J Matern Fetal Neonatal Med 2009; 22:365–367. [Case report]
8. Roberts CL, Torvaldsen S, Cameron CA, et al. Delayed versus early pushing in women with epidural analgesia: a systematic review and meta-analysis. BJOG 2004; 111:1333–1340. [Meta-analysis: 9 RCTs; $n = 2953$]
9. Prins M, Boxem J, Lucas C, et al. Effect of spontaneous pushing versus Valsalva pushing in the second stage of labour on mother and fetus: a systematic review of randomized trials. BJOG 2011; 118(6):662–670. [Meta-analysis: 3 RCTs, $n = 425$]
10. Bloom SL, Casey BM, Schaffer JI, et al. A randomized trial of coached versus uncoached maternal pushing during the second stage of labor. Am J Obstet Gynecol 2006; 194:10–13. [RCT, $n = 320$]
11. Matsuo K, Mudd JV, Kopelman JN, et al. Duration of the second stage in labor while wearing a dental support device: a pilot study. J Obstet Gynaecol Res 35(4):672–678. [RCT, $n = 64$]
12. Api O, Blacin ME, Ugurel V, et al. The effect of uterine fundal pressure on the duration of the second stage of labor: a randomized controlled trial. Acta Obstet Gynecol 2009; 88:320–324. [RCT, $n = 197$]
13. Cox J, Cotzias CS, Siakpere O, et al. Does an inflatable obstetric belt facilitate spontaneous vaginal delivery in nulliparae with epidural analgesia? BJOG 1999; 106:1280–1286. [RCT, $n = 500$]
14. Stamp G, Kruzins G, Crowther C. Perineal massage in labour and prevention of perineal trauma: randomized controlled trial. BMJ 2001; 322:1277–1280. [RCT, $n = 1340$]
15. Albers LL, Sedler KD, Bedrock EJ, et al. Midwifery care measures in the second stage of labor and reduction of genital tract trauma at birth: a randomized trial. J Midwifery Women Health 2005; 50:365–372. [RCT, $n = 1211$]
16. Dahlen HG, Homer CS, Cooke M, et al. Perineal outcomes and maternal comfort related to the application of perineal warm packs in the second stage of labor: a randomized controlled study. Obstet Gynecol Surv 2008; 63(5):286–287. [RCT, $n = 717$]
17. Shaffer BL, Cheng YW, Vargas JE, et al. Manual rotation to reduce caesarean delivery in persistent occiput posterior position. J Matern Fetal Neonatal Med 2010; 24:65–72. [II-2]
18. Reichman O, Gdanski E, Latinsky B, et al. Digital rotation from occipito-posterior to occipito-anterior decreases the need for cesarean section. Eur J Obstet Gynecol Reprod Biol 2008; 136:25–28. [II-2]
19. Jonsson ER, Elfaghi I, Rydhstrom H, et al. Modified Ritgen's maneuver for anal sphincter injury at delivery. Obstet Gynecol 2008; 112:212–217. [RCT, $n = 1623$]
20. McCandlish R, Bower U, Van Asten, et al. A randomized controlled trial of care of the perineum during second stage of normal labor. BJOG 1998; 105:1262–1272. [RCT, $n = 5471$]
21. Mayerhofer K, Bodner-Adler B, Bodner K, et al. Traditional care of the perineum during birth: a prospective, randomized, multicenter study of 1,076 women. J Reprod Med 2002; 47:477–482. [Quasi-RCT, $n = 1076$]
22. Carroli G, Mignini L. Episiotomy for vaginal birth. Cochrane Database Syst Rev 2009; (1):CD000081. [Meta-analysis: 8 RCTs, $n = 5541$]
23. American College of Obstetricians and Gynecologists. ACOG Practice Bulletin No. 17: Operative vaginal delivery. Washington, DC: American College of Obstetricians and Gynecologists, 2000. [Review]
24. Royal College of Obstetricians and Gynaecologists. NICE Guideline No. 26: Operative vaginal delivery. London: RCOG Press, Revised 2005. [Review]

25. Brown SJ, Gartland D, Donath S, et al. Effects of prolonged second stage, method of birth, timing of cesarean section and other obstetric risk factors on postnatal urinary incontinence: an Australian nulliparous cohort study. BJOG 2011; 118:991–1000. [II-2]

26. Altman MR, Lydon-Rochelle MT. Prolonged second stage of labor and risk of adverse maternal and perinatal outcomes: a systematic review. Birth 2006; 33(4):315–322. [Systematic review of PubMed, Cochrane Library, and CINAHL from 1980 until 2005]

27. Badiou W, Bousquet P-J, Prat-Pradal D, et al. Short vs long second stage of labour: is there a difference in terms of postpartum anal incontinence? Eur J Obstet Gynecol Reprod Biol 2010; 152:168–171. [II-2]

28. Sung JF, Daniels KI, Brodzinsky L, et al. Cesarean delivery outcomes after a prolonged second stage of labor. Am J Obstet Gynecol 2007; 197:306. [II-1]

29. Althabe F, Belizan JM, Villar J, et al. Mandatory second opinion to reduce rates of unnecessary caesarean sections in Latin America: a cluster randomized controlled trial. Lancet 2004; 363:1934–1940. [RCT, $n = 149,276$]

9

Third stage of labor and its complications

Elizabeth Brass and Jorge E. Tolosa

PART 1—NORMAL THIRD STAGE OF LABOR
Key Points

- **Oxytocin is the prophylactic uterotonic of choice at delivery** as it reduces blood loss and has less side effects compared with other agents such as ergot alkaloids and prostaglandins, including misoprostol. Oxytocin 5 to 10 IU IM or 10 to 20 IU IV in 500 to 1000 cc normal saline (NS) or lactated Ringer's (LR) bolus should be routinely administered after delivery of the anterior shoulder or immediately after delivery of the neonate.
- **Active management of the third stage of labor (AMTSL),** including routine, prophylactic use of an **oxytocic agent (oxytocin preferred), early cord clamping and cutting, cord traction, and uterine massage,** shortens the third stage and reduces blood loss and postpartum hemorrhage (PPH), compared with expectant management.
- **Delayed cord clamping in preterm neonates by 30 to 60 (maximum 120) seconds** is associated with fewer transfusions, less hypotension, and intraventricular hemorrhage.
- Vaginal and perineal **lacerations** should be **repaired with one continuous absorbable synthetic suture,** including continuous subcuticular skin repair.
- Rectal NSAIDs, topical Epifoam, and therapeutic ultrasound each decrease perineal pain and need for additional pain therapy.

Definitions and Duration

Third stage of labor is defined as the interval between delivery of the neonate and expulsion of the placenta. Mean length of time of the third stage is about 6 minutes. An interval of 30 minutes is the 97th percentile, and represents the definition of prolonged third stage.

Pathophysiology

The third stage involves separation of the placenta with capillary hemorrhage and shearing of the placental surface when the uterus contracts after delivery of the infant. **Signs of separation include a gush of blood, cord lengthening, and anterior cephalic movement of the uterine fundus becoming more globular and firm.**

Risk Factors

Preterm deliveries are associated with prolongation of the third stage of labor with increased risk of retained placenta. Longer third stage of labor is associated with increased maternal blood loss.

Complications

- Postpartum hemorrhage—excessive bleeding >500 cc after vaginal birth or 1000 cc after cesarean delivery
- Retained placenta—placenta not expelled ≥30 minutes after infant delivery
- Uterine inversion—collapse of uterine fundus into the endometrial cavity

See part 2 of this chapter for further details.

MANAGEMENT

An algorithm including uterotonics and active management of placenta delivery is shown in Figure 9.1.

Uterotonics

Common types of uterotonics include oxytocin, ergot alkaloids like methergine, syntometrine, and prostaglandins (Table 9.1).

Oxytocin (Syntocinon®)

Oxytocin binds to specific uterine receptors with immediate action causing increasing strength and frequency of contractions. The mean half-life is 3 minutes with the plateau reached after 30 minutes. It can either be given as intravenous (IV) or intramuscular (IM), though IM injection has time of onset of 3 to 7 minutes and clinical effect is longer, lasting 30 to 60 minutes. It is metabolized by the liver and kidneys with a known 5% antidiuretic effect of vasopressin. If given in large volumes, greater than 40 to 50 cc/min, and high concentration, or when given without dilution, it may result in hyponatremia and syndrome of inappropriate antidiuretic hormone hypersecretion (SIADH) with symptoms of headache, vomiting, drowsiness, and convulsions.

Oxytocin is the **prophylactic uterotonic** of choice in the third stage of labor. Compared with no uterotonics, prophylactic oxytocin reduces blood loss >500 cc after vaginal delivery and the need for therapeutic oxytocics with blood loss >1000 cc (1). There are similar incidences of manual removal of the placenta, and rates of blood transfusions with the use of oxytocin compared to no uterotonic.

Compared with ergot alkaloids [methergine or erogometrine (ergonovine)], oxytocin is associated with less manual removals of the placenta and does not increase maternal blood pressure (1).

Compared with oxytocin alone, ergometrine in addition to oxytocin is associated with increased side effects with only modest benefits. Benefits include a statistically significant reduction in the risk of PPH when compared to oxytocin alone for blood loss of 500 ml or more. There is no difference in PPH for blood loss >1000 cc. In addition, there are no differences in blood transfusion, retained placenta, or other neonatal outcomes. Unfortunately, adverse side effects are significant including nausea, vomiting, and hypertension, from the ergometrine added to oxytocin (2).

As part of AMTSL, oxytocin is routinely administered after delivery of the anterior shoulder or immediately after

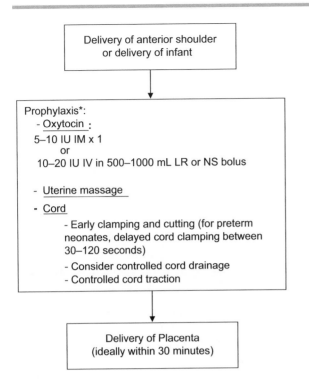

IU, international units; LR, lactated Ringer's solution;
NS, normal saline; IM, intramuscular.

*To decrease the incidence of postpartum hemorrhage and retained placenta

Figure 9.1 Algorithm for active management of the third stage of labor. *Abbreviations*: IU, international units; LR, lactated Ringer's solution; NS, normal saline; IM, intramuscular.

infusion, usually of 10 to 20 IU in 500 to 1000 cc of NS or LR solution, given as a bolus. This IV infusion bolus has not been quantified well in RCTs, so there is insufficient evidence to recommend a rate of infusion.

Intraumbilical injection is not superior to IV administration (5).

Side effects are rare but may include hyponatremia (Table 9.1).

Oxytocin agonists
There is insufficient evidence that 100 µg of carbetocin IV is as effective as oxytocin to prevent PPH. Three out of 4 RCTs are on cesarean delivery. In comparison to oxytocin, carbetocin is associated with reduced need for additional uterotonic agents, and uterine massage. There is limited comparative evidence on adverse events (6,7). Compared with syntometrine, carbetocin has similar efficacy, but less side effects, in two other trials evaluating its prophylactic use in vaginal delivery (8).

Ergot alkaloids (Methergine® or ergometrine)
Methylergonovine and its parent compound ergometrine result in sustained tonic contraction of uterine smooth muscle by stimulation of α-adrenergic myometrial receptors. Compared with oxytocin, ergot alkaloids used as a prophylactic uterotonic have similar benefits, but worse side effects, making oxytocin preferable as the first-line prophylactic agent (see above) (9). Methergine can instead be used as a second-line agent for treatment of PPH (Fig. 9.2) (see below). Administration is commonly intramuscular although intravenous administration is an option but associated with more severe side effects.

Nausea and vomiting are common side effects although the most concerning side effect is vasoconstriction of the vascular smooth muscle. This results in elevation of central venous pressure and systemic blood pressure leading to possible pulmonary edema, stroke, or myocardial infarction.

Dose is 0.2 mg IM injection or PO with a mean elimination half-life of 3.39 hours (range 1.5 to 12.7 hours).

Contraindications include cardiac disease, autoimmune diseases associated with Raynaud's phenomena, peripheral vascular disease, arteriovenous shunts, hypertension, preeclampsia, and eclampsia.

Syntometrine (oxytocin plus ergometrine)
This combination is **not recommended over oxytocin** for prophylaxis.

Dose is oxytocin 5 IU in combination with ergometrine 0.5 mg IM. Side effects are significant, including nausea, vomiting, and hypertension.

delivery of the neonate. Blood loss and retained placenta rates are similar with oxytocin administration before and after placental delivery (3,4). Nonsignificant trends for less PPH but more retained placenta are associated with oxytocin given before compared with after placental separation (3).

Many different ways of administering oxytocin for prophylaxis in the third stage of labor have been used, including IM, IV (either undiluted or as a diluted infusion), and intraumbilical. The two routes of administration best supported by RCTs for safety and efficacy are, in order, IM and IV diluted infusion. The IM dose is 5 to 10 IU, and we use 10 IU at the delivery of the anterior shoulder, or soon after, before delivery of the placenta. Oxytocin can also be used as a continuous IV

Table 9.1 Common Uterotonics (Usually for Management of PPH)

	Usual route/dose	Continuing	Maximum dose	Contraindications/Precautions
Oxytocin	IV 20–40 IU in 1 L LR/NS	IV infuse 20 IU	80–100 IU	1. Do not give undiluted IV bolus 2. Hyponatremia
Ergometrine/ Methergine	IM 0.2 mg PO 0.2 mg	Every 15 minutes	5 doses 1 mg	1. Preeclampsia 2. Hypertension 3. Cardiac disease
Prostaglandin F2α (Hemabate)	IM 0.25 mg Intramyometrial 0.25 mg	Every 15 minutes	8 doses 2 mg	1. Asthma 2. Cardiac disease
Misoprostol	PO, PR, PV, sublingual 200–1000 µg	Information not available	Information not available	Caution in febrile patients

Abbreviations: PPH, postpartum hemorrhage; IV, intravenous; IM, intramuscular; PO, orally; PR, per rectum; PV, per vagina.

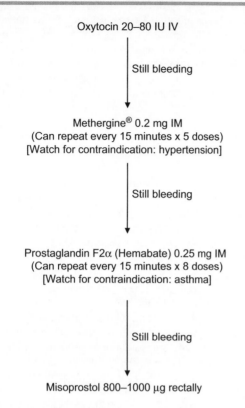

Oxytocin 20–80 IU IV

↓ Still bleeding

Methergine® 0.2 mg IM
(Can repeat every 15 minutes x 5 doses)
[Watch for contraindication: hypertension]

↓ Still bleeding

Prostaglandin F2α (Hemabate) 0.25 mg IM
(Can repeat every 15 minutes x 8 doses)
[Watch for contraindication: asthma]

↓ Still bleeding

Misoprostol 800–1000 µg rectally

Figure 9.2 Suggested management protocol of uterotonic agents for primary postpartum hemorrhage (with continued use of uterine massage).

Prostaglandins

Misoprostol is a synthetic analog of prostaglandin E1 and is metabolized in the liver. The tablet can be given orally, vaginally, or rectally and does not require sterile needles and syringes for administration. It is inexpensive, heat and light stable, making it more accessible and beneficial in low-income countries.

There is a limited role for prophylactic prostaglandins like misoprostol in the routine management of the third stage of labor. Compared with no uterotonics, oral misoprostol does not reduce the rate of PPH, other measures of blood loss, and has more side effects in a meta-analysis (10), but was associated with a significant 24% reduction in PPH compared with placebo in a recent large trial in Pakistan, with delivery performed by birth assistants (11). Compared with oxytocin, oral misoprostol 600 µg shows significantly more blood loss <1000 cc. Side effects include shivering, elevated body temperature >38°C, and gastrointestinal (GI) upset with nausea, vomiting, and pain. Rectal misoprostol given prophylactically showed similar results (10). Despite its side effect profile, misoprostol may be a reasonable option in low-income countries, given ease of storage and administration, if oxytocin is not available.

Misoprostol can be used as a second-line agent for treatment of PPH (see below and Fig. 9.2).

Prostaglandin F2α (Hemabate/carboprost) causes contraction of uterine smooth muscle cells. **Hemabate has been established as a second-line treatment for PPH unresponsive to oxytocin.** Administration is either 0.25 mg IM or as a direct injection into the myometrium. It may be repeated every 15 to 20 minutes for a maximum of 8 doses or 2 mg. Side effects are secondary to smooth muscle constriction causing bronchocon-

striction, venoconstriction, and constriction of GI smooth muscle. Common side effects are nausea, vomiting, diarrhea, pyrexia, bronchospasm, and case reports of hypotension and intrapulmonary shunting with arterial oxygen desaturation. It is **contraindicated in patients with cardiac and pulmonary disease**. Prostaglandin F2α can be used as a second-line agent for treatment of PPH (see below and Fig. 9.2).

Tranexamic acid

There is insufficient evidence to recommend tranexamic acid for prevention of PPH. In two small RCTs of suboptimal quality, tranexamic acid decreased postpartum blood loss after vaginal birth and after cesarean section (12).

Summary

Oxytocin (5 to 10 IU IM or 10 to 20 IU IV in 500 to 1000 cc NS or LR bolus) should be routinely administered either before placental separation with delivery of the anterior shoulder or before delivery of the neonate (or after placental separation), in all pregnancies as prophylaxis to prevent PPH. Methergine, prostaglandin F2α, and misoprostol should generally not be used for prophylaxis in normal third stage of labor, unless oxytocin is unavailable. Instead, Methergine, prostaglandin F2α, and misoprostol are best used for treatment of PPH (see below and Fig. 9.2).

Umbilical Cord

Cord gases

Cord gases are stable in a clamped segment of cord for 60 minutes and in a heparinized syringe for 60 minutes. Umbilical artery pH, pCO2, and base deficit may be helpful in indicating timing of insult and can be collected in cases of nonreassuring fetal heart rate tracings (NRFHTs), meconium, low APGAR scores (defined as below 7 at 5 minutes), growth restriction, preterm birth, or any sentinel event including cord prolapse, uterine rupture, or placental abruption. Umbilical vein pH may be helpful in cases of uteroplacental problems like growth restriction, placental abruption, asthma, and hypertension. Routine sending of umbilical cord gases is not necessary or recommended for normal labor, delivery, and APGAR scores without risk factors.

Cord blood collection

Cord blood is routinely sent for Rh status of the infant, especially in Rh-negative women.

Cord blood collection for stem cells has increased in popularity in recent years. **Obstetricians should support public banking of cord blood** (13). Public banking is recommended over private banks secondary to more stringent FDA guidelines, given its increased legal responsibilities, cost-effectiveness, and greater access to cord blood by the general population. The chance of a child requiring a transplant of its own cord blood is rare at about 1/2700. Directed donation of cord blood when there is a disease in the family amenable to stem cell transplantation can be arranged through many public banks with other applications not yet proven.

Timing of cord clamping

In preterm neonates, delayed cord clamping by about 30 to 60 seconds (120 maximum) is associated with **fewer transfusions for anemia, less hypotension, and less intraventricular hemorrhage** than early clamping at <30 seconds (14). In addition, delayed cord clamping has been shown to be safe and does not compromise the preterm infant (15). There are no clear differences in other outcomes including respiratory distress, death, initial adaptation phase, or long-term outcomes. There is no current recommendation on positioning of the preterm infant during delayed cord clamping secondary to insufficient data. No randomized trials have assessed the influence of gravity on placental transfusion at either vaginal or cesarean delivery (16).

Milking of cord has been evaluated in two small RCTs in preterm neonates, so there is insufficient evidence for recommendation, even if it appears as beneficial as delayed cord clamping. Compared with no milking, milking of cord has been associated with less need for blood transfusions and less need for circulatory and respiratory support (17). Compared with 30-second delayed cord clamping, milking of cord four times achieved a similar amount of placento-fetal blood transfusion (18).

In term neonates, timing of cord clamping has not been adequately studied. Compared with early clamping, delayed cord clamping for at least 2 to 3 minutes seems not to increase the risk of PPH (19). The possible increased risk of neonatal jaundice requiring phototherapy must be weighed against the physiological benefit of greater hemoglobin and iron levels up to 6 months of age conferred by delayed cord clamping in term infants, which may be of clinical value particularly in infants where access to good nutrition is poor (19).

Placenta

Cord drainage and traction

Compared with no drainage and traction, **cord drainage and traction is associated with shorter third stage and less decrease in maternal hemoglobin** when no uterotonics are used in the largest trial on this issue (20). **Cord traction alone has been associated with lower mean blood loss and shorter third stage in a very small trial** (21,22). In another small trial, cord drainage was associated with a statistically significant 5-minute reduction in the length of third stage of labor (23). There is insufficient evidence regarding the effect of cord drainage on PPH and retained placenta.

Massage of the uterus

There is limited evidence to evaluate the effect of massage of uterus alone. In one trial, compared to no uterine massage, the numbers of women with blood loss >500 mL was small, with wide confidence intervals and no statistically significant difference (RR 0.52, 95% CI 0.16–1.67). There were no cases of retained placenta in either group. The mean blood loss was less in the uterine massage group at 30 minutes [mean difference (MD) −41 mL] and 60 minutes after enrollment (MD, −77 mL). The need for additional uterotonics was reduced in the uterine massage group (RR 0.20, 95% CI 0.08–0.50). Two blood transfusions were administered in the control group (24). This intervention has also been evaluated with the other interventions of the AMTSL, and found to be beneficial in prevention of prolonged third stage and PPH. Therefore, **uterine massage after delivery of the placenta is recommended.**

Injection of oxytocin in umbilical cord

Injection of oxytocin into the umbilical cord is not superior to IV oxytocin for prophylaxis (25,26). **Umbilical vein injection of saline solution with oxytocin compared with saline solution alone showed a significant reduction in manual removal of the placenta, less blood loss, and shorter duration of the third stage** (27) in women managed with prophylactic IV oxytocin and controlled cord traction. Likewise, umbilical vein injection of saline solution with prostaglandin showed significant reduction in manual removal of the placenta compared with injection of saline solution alone. There were no differences detected in length of third stage of labor, blood loss, hemorrhage, blood transfusion, curettage, infection, fever, hospital stay, or oxytocin augmentation (25,26).

Active Management of the Third Stage

AMTSL usually consists of (28)

- **Prophylactic oxytocin at delivery of the anterior shoulder or after delivery of the baby**
- **Uterine massage**
- **Early cord clamping and cutting**
- **Controlled cord traction**

Expectant management usually consists of

- No uterotonics
- No uterine massage or early cord clamping, cutting, and traction
- Using gravity and maternal expulsive efforts for placenta delivery

AMTSL reduces the risk of PPH and should be offered and recommended to all women. Compared with expectant management, active management is associated with reduced risk of maternal primary hemorrhage of blood loss >1000 cc and of maternal hemoglobin <9 g/dL following birth (28,29). Adverse effects were identified including increases in maternal diastolic blood pressure, increased use of analgesia or after-pains, more women returning to the hospital with bleeding, and decrease in the baby's birth weight, reflecting the lower blood volume from interference with placental transfusion if early cord clamping is performed. Each element of AMTSL should be assessed separately. Unfortunately, there is confusion in the literature stemming from different definitions being used for AMTSL. We have used the one utilized for evaluation of the existing RCTs of AMTSL by the Cochrane collaboration (28), which is different from the one used by WHO.

Repair of Laceration

Closure and repair

Compared with nonclosure, **closure of first- and second-degree perineal lacerations after vaginal delivery is associated with better healing seen at 10 days and 6 weeks and similar pain scores** (30–32). The **continuous** suturing techniques, compared with the interrupted, are associated with less short-term pain in second-degree and episiotomy repairs (33). Furthermore, approximation (end-to-end) and overlap technique for third- and fourth-degree laceration repair are associated with similar outcomes (34,35). One small randomized trial showed that use of antibiotics at the time of third- and fourth-degree repairs decreased wound complications and wound infection rates (36).

Suture

Absorbable synthetic materials should be used for all layers of the repair. Compared with catgut (plain or chromic), **absorbable synthetic sutures** (e.g., Vicryl) used for perineal repair decreased women's experience of short-term (3 day) pain, less need for analgesia, reduced rate of suture dehiscence up to day 10, and less need for resuturing at <3 months. There is no significant difference in long-term pain or dyspareunia experienced by women (37). More women with catgut sutures required resuturing compared with synthetic sutures, while more women in the standard synthetic suture group required suture removal compared with the rapidly absorbed group. Clinical experience has shown suture removal is necessary <5% of the time when using **3–0 or finer sutures and performing subcuticular skin closures** (37). **Polyglactin (Vicryl)** and polydioxanone (PDS) have similar outcomes (38).

Anal ultrasound
Anal endosonography with clinical examination immediately after delivery in nulliparous women with second-degree lacerations detected more sphincter tears than clinical examination. Anal endosonography with immediate repair of these tears is associated with less severe fecal incontinence at 1 year compared with clinical examination only (39).

Perineal Pain Control
NSAIDS
There are no RCTs to accurately assess the effectiveness of oral NSAIDs for perineal pain control. However, clinical experience shows a reduction in perineal pain. Rectally administrated NSAIDs appear to provide effective pain relief in postpartum women. Rectal indomethacin or diclofenac are associated with less pain up to 24 hours after birth and less requirement for additional analgesia in the first 24 hours and 48 hours postpartum (40). No information is available on pain experienced >72 hours after birth or other outcomes of importance such as the impact on daily activities, resumption of sexual intercourse, and the impact on the mother-baby relationship. More studies are needed to assess the acceptability of this route of administration and comparison to oral NSAIDs.

Topical anesthetics
Compared with placebo, topical anesthetics applied to the perineum are associated with similar pain relief up to 24 hours to 72 hours postpartum, but women are more satisfied (41). Epifoam (1% hydrocortisone acetate and 1% pramaxine hydrochloride in the mucoadhesive foam base) use is associated with less additional analgesia, while lignocaine/lidocaine showed no difference with regard to additional analgesia use compared with placebo (41). Compared with indomethacin vaginal suppositories, topical anesthetics have similar mean pain scores.

Therapeutic ultrasound for perineal pain
There is insufficient evidence to evaluate the use of ultrasound in treating perineal pain and/or dyspareunia following vaginal delivery. Women treated with active ultrasound for acute perineal pain are more likely to report improvement in pain, less pain at 10 days and 3 months, but more likely to have bruising at 10 days compared with placebo (42). Additionally, women with persistent perineal pain or dyspareunia treated with ultrasound are less likely to report pain with sexual intercourse (42).

Anesthesia
Epidural is commonly used during labor for pain control. Spinal, epidural, paracervical block, or general anesthesia may be used if complications arise in the management of retained placenta, intractable PPH, uterine inversion, or assisted vaginal deliveries.

Breastfeeding
Hypertension and headache are associated with misoprostol and ergotamine use. There are no other known complications with breastfeeding after use of other uterotonics. There are no differences in breastfeeding or onset of jaundice with AMTSL.

Delivery Note
If a complicated delivery occurs with possible fetal compromise, a detailed note should address the pertinent and immediate

neonatal status, including APGAR scores, umbilical cord pH and base deficit (if obtained), and assessment of fetal heart testing prior to delivery (see chap. 28).

PART II—ABNORMAL THIRD STAGE OF LABOR
Key Points

- The most common complications of the third stage of labor are PPH, retained placenta, and uterine inversion.
- Adequate physical exam, IV access, anesthesia, and nursing support are important for the management of third-stage complications.
- In cases of PPH, perform **uterine massage, explore for and repair any vaginal or cervical lacerations**, and **manually explore the uterus.**
- Oxytocin (at higher doses, up to 80 IU IV) can be used as uterotonic for PPH.
- **Methergine** (except in women with hypertension) and **prostaglandin F2α** (except in women with asthma) **are beneficial in the treatment of PPH.**
- **Misoprostol**, in particular rectally, is helpful as treatment of primary PPH.
- There is insufficient evidence with RCTs to assess all other interventions for PPH.
- Interventions for retained placenta, such as umbilical vein injection of oxytocin, have not been associated with increase in delivery of the placenta in high-quality trials.
- There is insufficient evidence to assess interventions for uterine inversion.

POSTPARTUM HEMORRHAGE
Definitions
Primary PPH is defined as blood loss within 24 hours of delivery exceeding >500 cc for vaginal deliveries and 1000 cc for cesarean delivery. Secondary PPH is defined as excessive blood loss after 24 hours and <12 weeks postpartum.

Incidence
Approximately 3% of all deliveries are complicated by PPH.

Etiology
Etiologies include the following:
Common:

- Uterine atony—lack of efficient uterine contraction (most common, about 80%)
- Retained parts of the placenta
- Genital tract trauma—vaginal, cervical, vulvar lacerations, and hematomas

Less common:

- Uterine rupture
- Uterine inversion
- Consumptive coagulopathy
- Inherited or acquired bleeding disorders

Risk Factors
At term, the uteroplacental circulation has a blood supply of 600 to 800 cc/min. Most major hemorrhage occurs within the first hour postpartum. The blood volume expansion of 1.5 to 2.0 L in pregnant women provides a physiologic reserve for blood loss at delivery.

Cessation of placental site blood flow is due mostly to effective myometrial contractions. Risk factors that contribute to decreased myometrial contractions include the following:

- Maternal factors:
  - First pregnancy
  - Maternal obesity
  - Previous PPH—10% recurrence risk
  - High parity
- Antepartum bleeding—previa, abruption
- Chorioamnionitis
- Uterine fibroids
- Overdistension—macrosomia, multiples, polyhydramnios
- Uterine relaxing drugs—magnesium, nitroglycerin, anesthetic gas
- Labor factors:
  - Precipitous delivery
  - Prolonged labor—first stage >24 hours
  - Prolonged oxytocin use, and/or maximum of $\geq$40 to 50 cc/min

Complications

The most reliable estimates of global mortality for mothers in childbirth are reported to be between 250,000 and 300,000 annually (43). This number has decreased significantly over the past decade. Many of these deaths result from complications of the third stage of labor (43). Ninety-nine percent of maternal deaths occur in the developing countries. **In low-income countries, maternal mortality remains unacceptably high. In sub-Saharan Africa, the risk of maternal death is very high at 1:31, with at least 25% of those deaths due to hemorrhage** (44), **while in high income countries a woman's lifetime risk of dying during or following pregnancy is 1:4300.** Secondary PPH is a significant contributor to maternal death mainly, but not only, in low income countries. PPH has other serious complications including hypovolemic shock, disseminated intravascular coagulopathy (DIC), renal failure, hepatic failure, and adult respiratory distress syndrome (ARDS).

Management

Primary PPH. The management of PPH begins with **obtaining help** in a multidisciplinary fashion, including obstetricians, nurses (including charge nurse), anesthesia, and blood bank. Common accepted approach to PPH includes:

Logistics:

- Obtain help
- Ensure adequate IV access with large bore access (may need two sites)
- Consider placing Foley catheter to empty bladder and monitor urine output
- Obtain laboratory tests—complete blood count with platelets, blood type, antibody screen, fibrinogen, fibrin split products, prothrombin time, and partial prothrombin time

Treatment:

- Vigorous **uterine massage** until firm
- **Explore and repair any vaginal or cervical lacerations**
- **Manually explore the uterus**
  - Administer **uterotonic drugs** (Figs. 9.2 and 9.3)
  - Oxytocin 40 to 80 IU in 1000 cc of NS, fast IV drip
  - Methergine 0.2 mg IM every 15 minutes to 4 hours—watch for contraindications including hypertension
  - Prostaglandin F2α (carboprost tromethamine, Hemabate) 0.25 mg IM every 15 to 90 minutes up to 8 doses

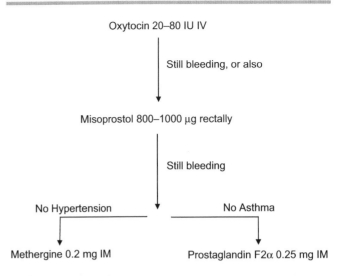

Figure 9.3 Alternative management of uterotonic agents for postpartum hemorrhage.

(maximum 2 mg) —watch for contraindications including asthma
- Misoprostol 800 to 1000 µg rectally

Little evidence exists to base a protocol in respect to the order of administration of uterotonics for the treatment of PPH (Figs. 9.2 and 9.3). There are very few specific trials on oxytocin, methergine, Hemabate, versus placebo or versus each other for treatment of PPH. Studies comparing misoprostol to ergot alkaloids have demonstrated conflicting results and the studies are small and heterogeneous. The addition of misoprostol (e.g., 600 µg sublingually) has not been associated with benefits when added to the combination of oxytocin and ergometrine alone (or other injectable uterotonics) for the treatment of primary PPH (45,46). Traditionally, oxytocin and ergot alkaloids (e.g., methergine) are initially used with prostaglandin F2α employed as adjunctive therapy (Fig. 9.2). There is no compelling data to suggest any alternation at this time. However, rectal misoprostol may be a useful "first-line" drug for the treatment of PPH (Fig. 9.3), especially in the setting of no IV access, patients with contraindications to other uterotonics, or in low-income countries. Rectal misoprostol is associated with a statistically significant reduction in the number of women who continued to bleed after the intervention and those who required medical co-interventions to control bleeding (47–49). There is insufficient evidence to evaluate the effects of misoprostol on maternal morbidity or hysterectomy rates in women with PPH. In addition, compared with visual estimation of postpartum blood loss, the use of a collector bag after vaginal delivery did not reduce the rate of severe PPH (50).

Other possible therapies:

- Uterine curettage if retained placental products cannot be removed
- Transfusion of blood and blood products as necessary
- *Stable*—consider pelvic arterial embolization done by interventional radiology (IR)
- *Unstable*—there are no randomized trials on the following techniques
  - Uterine tamponade—packing, Bakri tamponade balloon catheter, or Foley catheter

- Laparotomy—suture bleeding sites, uterine artery ligation, B-Lynch stitch for compression
- Hysterectomy
- Aortic compression (temporary)
- Pelvic packing
- Hemostatic drugs—Factor VIIa, tranexamic acid
- LifeWrap—nonpneumatic anti-shock garment (NASG) is a giant wetsuit that is Velcro fastened around a woman who is hemorrhaging to reduce bleeding and reverse shock, buying time to get her to a higher level treatment facility (32).

Secondary PPH. There is insufficient evidence to make recommendations for management of secondary PPH (51). Management similar to that for PPH can be suggested, with high suspicion for retained placenta. Ultrasound is unfortunately though not very specific for identifying retained products of conception.

RETAINED PLACENTA
Definition
Placenta undelivered ≥30 minutes after infant delivery.

Incidence
Between 0.5% and 1–2%.

Complications
Hemorrhage, infection, and genital tract trauma.

Etiology
- Preterm birth—inversely proportional to gestational age
- Cord avulsion—incidence up to 3% with controlled cord traction, especially in inexperienced operators
- Placenta accreta (see chap. 25)

Management
- Umbilical vein injection of oxytocin (10–20 IU in 1–2 cc NS)
- Consider alternative uterotonics (Hemabate, sulprostone)
- Persistent retained placenta despite above, then obtain adequate anesthesia
- **Attempt manual extraction**
  - Consider ultrasound to ascertain all placental tissue has been removed
- Palpate and massage the fundus until firm
- Proceed to operating room for curettage if unsuccessful extraction
- Consider diagnosis of placenta accreta

Umbilical vein injection
Compared with expectant management, umbilical vein injection (UVI) of saline solution alone does not show any significant difference in the incidence of need for manual removal of the placenta (RR 0.99, 95% CI 0.84–1.16). Compared with expectant management, UVI of oxytocin solution is associated with no reduction in the need for manual removal (RR 0.87, 95% CI 0.74–1.03) (26,27).

Compared with UVI of saline solution, UVI of oxytocin solution shows a reduction in need for manual removal of the placenta, but this was not statistically significant (RR 0.91, 95% CI 0.82–1.00). When only high-quality studies are assessed,

there was no statistical difference (RR 0.92, 95% CI 0.83–1.01). There were no differences in any of the other outcomes including length of third stage of labour, blood loss, haemorrhage, haemoglobin, blood transfusion, curettage, infection, hospital stay, fever, or oxytocin augmentation. Therefore, **while UVI of oxytocin solution is an inexpensive and simple intervention, high-quality randomized trials show that it has little or no effect** (26,27).

There is insufficient and limited information on the use of other UVI interventions. Compared with UVI of plasma expander, UVI of oxytocin solution showed no statistically significant difference in the outcomes assessed by only one small trial. Prostaglandin solution compared with saline solution alone was associated with a statistically significant lower incidence in manual removal of placenta (RR 0.42, 95% CI 0.22–0.82) but no difference in the other outcomes was seen. Prostaglandin plus saline solution showed a statistically significant reduction in manual removal of placenta when compared with oxytocin plus saline solution (RR 0.43, 95% CI 0.25–0.75), and there was also a small reduction in time from injection to placental delivery (MD −6.00, 95% CI −8.78 to −3.22).

Prostaglandins. Prostaglandin F2α (Hemabate) and prostaglandin E2 (sulprostone) are alternative uterotonics to consider. In a small trial, Hemabate 20 mg in 20 cc of saline was more effective than even 30 IU of oxytocin in preventing the need for manual placental removal, but no difference was observed in blood loss, fever, abdominal pain, and oxytocin augmentation (52). Sulprostone can be given 250 μg IV and reduce the need for manual removal of the placenta by 49%, with retained placenta expelled in 52% of sulprostone cases versus 18% of placebo controls (52). The major disadvantage is the need to administer the dose over 30 minutes.

Retained placenta commonly occurs in preterm pregnancies. In women undergoing termination of pregnancy at 13 to 28 weeks, if the placenta had not delivered spontaneously within 10 minutes of the fetus/neonate, misoprostol 200 μg orally given every hour for a maximum of 3 doses does not reduce the time to complete spontaneous placental delivery in a small trial (53).

Tocolytics. There is insufficient evidence to recommend the use of tocolytics for the management of retained placenta. In a very small trial, sublingual nitroglycerin, given when oxytocin fails, seems to reduce both the need for manual removal of placenta and blood loss during the third stage of labor when compared with placebo (54).

Antibiotics The benefit of antibiotic use at the time of manual extraction of the placenta has not been well estimated. However, WHO recommends single-dose penicillin or first-generation cephalosporin (55).

UTERINE INVERSION
Definition
The collapse of the uterine fundus into the endometrial cavity.

Incidence
Approximately 1 in 2500 deliveries.

Risk Factors
- Excess cord traction
- Fundal pressure
- Fundal cord insertions
- Abnormal placentations

Management

There are no randomized trials to determine the optimal management for uterine inversion. Suggested management may include the following:

- Obtain assistance from other obstetricians or experienced providers, nursing staff and anesthesia
- Provide large IV bore access
- IV fluid therapy
- Withhold uterotonic agents
- Avoid separating the placenta to decrease bleeding
- **Consider uterine relaxing agents**
  - Magnesium sulfate IV bolus
  - Terbutaline IV 0.25 SQ
  - Nitroglycerin 50 to 500 µg orally or anesthesia
- **Manual manipulation of the uterus**
  - Reposition the portion of the uterus that inverted last
  - Grab the uterus with palm and fingers posteriorly and thumbs anteriorly
  - Do not use a fist
- Surgical intervention—laparotomy (rarely needed)
  - Huntington procedure—clamps are placed on the round ligaments 2 cm deep in the inversion and gentle upward traction applied. Repeat clamping as necessary.
  - Haultain procedure—incision is made in the posterior portion of the inversion ring to increase its size and to reposition the uterus
  - Uterotonic agents when uterus repositioned
- If present, treat PPH or retained placenta as mentioned above

PART III—CARE OF THE JEHOVAH'S WITNESS PREGNANT WOMAN
Key Points

- Members of the Jehovah's Witness faith refuse blood transfusions due to their beliefs that **accepting them violates God's law,** and would lead to excommunication and eternal damnation.
- Refusal of blood can lead to an **increased risk of maternal** (and at times therefore fetal) **death**, especially in cases of obstetric hemorrhage.
- All obstetrical providers are responsible to **ask *each* woman at her first prenatal visit** (or preconceptionally) **if she has any objection to receiving any blood product in case of necessity**.
- The woman's wishes should be **respected,** following the principle of **autonomy.**
- After counseling, the patient should be asked to sign the **consent for blood products**, as well as the **Health Care Power of Attorney.**
- The third stage should be managed actively, and PPH prevented as much as possible. The use of cell saver is safe and effective in pregnancy.

Historic

"That is why I have said to the sons of Israel: 'No soul of you must eat blood and no alien resident who is residing as an alien in your midst should eat blood.'" (Holy Bible: Leviticus 17:12). Charles Russell started the Jehovah's Witness Christian sect in Pennsylvania in 1872.

Members of the Jehovah's Witness faith **refuse blood transfusions** due to their beliefs that prohibit use of blood products, because they believe that **accepting them violates God's law,** and would lead to excommunication and eternal damnation, as they take literally the statement reported in the Bible.

Complications

The risk of **obstetric hemorrhage** is approximately 6% in Jehovah's Witness women (56). The risk of **maternal death** is about 0.5%, a 44-fold increase compared with non-Jehovah's Witness controls (56).

Management

There are no trials to assess the efficacy of interventions specifically in women who are Jehovah's witnesses. Refer to the guidelines of third stage and abnormal third stage for general recommendations.

Preconception Counseling
Counsel regarding complications, and management in pregnancy.

Prenatal Care
All obstetrical providers are responsible to ask *each* woman at her first prenatal visit (or preconceptionally) if she has any objection to receiving any blood product in case of necessity. The woman who states she would decline blood transfusion even if medically necessary and/or is a Jehovah's Witness should be managed as follows:

- Counsel the woman and any family member present regarding the reasons and the risks of blood product refusal, including the possibility of maternal and fetal death. The counseling should be documented on the medical record. The patient might want to consult with the "elders" before signing informed refusal. **Her wishes should be respected, following the principle of autonomy.** A physician has the right of refusing to provide care for a Jehovah's Witness only if an alternative caregiver agrees to accept and care for the patient (57).
- After counseling, the patient should be asked to sign the **consent for blood products** (Fig. 9.4), as well as the **Health Care Power of Attorney** (57). These two consents should be kept in the medical record chart and available at labor and delivery. Approximately 39% of Jehovah's Witness pregnant women accept a variety of donated blood products, and 55% accept either intraoperative normovolemic hemodilution or transfusion of their own blood obtained by a cell saver (58).
- Consider including a copy of this guideline in the medical record, for reference.
- Selected high-risk patients, for example, those with hemoglobin <9 mg/dL, may be considered for appropriate replacement of iron, folic acid, and erythropoietin, which can be coordinated by a maternal-fetal medicine and/or a hematologist specialist.
- A routine consult with the Maternal-Fetal Medicine service is not required, but can be considered.
- A routine ethics consult is not indicated, but can be considered in specific cases.

Antepartum Testing

No specific antepartum testing is indicated.

Delivery

- Consents: Upon admission and prior to the surgery/delivery, all Jehovah's Witness patients should have

I hereby consent to the blood products marked below:

- ____Whole Blood
- ____Fresh Frozen Plasma
- ____Cryoprecipitate
- ____Albumin
- ____Erythropoietin
- ____Immune globulins (blood fraction, Rh immunoglobulin)
- ____Clotting factors
- ____PolyHeme (human hemoglobin), Hemopure products (bovine hemoglobin).
- ____Recombinant Factors (VII, VIIa, VIII, IX)
- ____Platelet cell fractions (Platelet Gel)
- ____Other surgical procedures, medical tests, or current therapy using my own blood, i.e. tagged red cells, white cells, blood patching
- ____Hemodialysis equipment (nonblood primed)
- ____Intraoperative blood salvage ("cell saver")
- ____Intraoperative hemodilution

_____

Patient's name—please print

_____

Patient's Signature

_____

Date

Figure 9.4   Blood product consent for Jehovah's Witness patients.

signed a consent form as shown in Figure 9.4 and the previously mentioned health care power of attorney. If consents have not been previously signed or are not available, the patient should be recounseled and consents signed.

- **The third stage should be managed actively, and PPH prevented as much as possible** (see third-stage and abnormal third-stage guidelines). Oxytocin, methylergonovine, 15-methyl-prostaglandin F2α, misoprostol, and other medical and, if necessary, surgical therapies should be employed (59).
- If an operative delivery or bleeding disorder is anticipated, if the patient has a history of a low-lying placenta or a placenta previa, or if an operative delivery is to occur, a **cell saver** can be on standby in labor and delivery throughout the patient's labor and delivery. Use of the cell saver is safe in obstetrics (60).

Anesthesia

An anesthesiology consult should be obtained. The anesthesiologist will review the patient's medical record and consents, including consent or refusal for blood products.

REFERENCES

1. Cotter AM, Ness A, Tolosa JE. Prophylactic oxytocin for the third stage of labour. Cochrane Database Syst Rev 2010; (2):CD001808. [Meta-analysis: vs. no oxytocics: 7 RCTs, n = >3000; vs. ergot-alkaloids: 6 RCTs, n = >2800; 5 RCTs, n = >2800—total 16 RCTs]
2. McDonald SJ, Abbott JM, Higgins SP. Prophylactic ergometrine-oxytocin versus oxytocin for the third stage of labour. Cochrane Database Syst Rev 2009; (3):CD000201. [Meta-analysis: 6 RCTs; n = 9332].
3. Soltani H, Hutchon DR, Poulose TA. Timing of prophylactic uterotonics for the third stage of labour after vaginal birth. Cochrane Database Syst Rev 2010; (8):CD006173. [Meta-analysis: 3 trials, n = 1671]
4. Jackson KW Jr., Allbert JR, Schemmer GK, et al. A randomized controlled trial comparing oxytocin administration before and after placental delivery in the prevention of postpartum hemorrhage. Am J Obstet Gynecol 2001; 185:873. [RCT, n = 1486]
5. Porter KB, O'Brien WF, Collins MK, et al. A randomized comparison of umbilical vein and intravenous oxytocin during the puerperium. Obstet Gynecol 1991; 78:254. [RCT, n = 104]
6. Su LL, Chong YS, Samuel M. Oxytocin agonists for preventing postpartum haemorrhage. Cochrane Database Syst Rev 2007; (3): CD005457. [Meta-analysis: 4 RCTs, n = 1037]
7. Leung SW, Ng PS, Wong WY, et al. A randomized trial of carbetocin versus syntometrine in the management of the third stage of labor. BJOG 2006; 113:1459–1464. [RCT, n = 329]
8. Lu SS, Rauff M, Chan YH, et al. Carbetocin versus syntometrine for the third stage of labor following vaginal delivery. BJOG 2009; 116:1461–1466. [RCT, n = 370]
9. Liabsuetrakul T, Choobun T, Peeyananjarassri K, et al. Prophylactic use of ergot alkaloids in the third stage of labour. Cochrane Database Syst Rev 2007; (2):CD005456. [Meta-analysis: 6 RCTs, n = 3941]
10. Gulmezoglu AM, Forna F, Villar J, et al. Prostaglandins for prevention of postpartum haemorrhage. Cochrane Database Syst Rev 2008; (4):CD000494. [Meta-analysis: 24 RCT misoprostol: 5 RCTs-oral misoprostol vs. no uterotonics/placebo; 8 RCTs IM prostaglandins]
11. Mobeen N, Durocher J, Zuberi NF, et al. Administration of misoprostol by trained traditional birth assistants to prevent postpartum hemorrhage in homebirths in Pakistan: a randomized placebo-controlled trial. BJOG 2010; 118(3):353–361. [RCT, n = 1119]
12. Novikova N, Hofmeyr GJ. Tranexamic acid for preventing postpartum haemorrhage. Cochrane Database Syst Rev 2010; (7): CD007872. [Meta-analysis: 2 RCTs, 365]
13. Moise KJ. Umbilical cord stem cells. Obstet Gynecol 2005; 106:1393–1407. [Review]
14. Rabe H, Reynolds G, Diaz-Rossello J. Early versus delayed umbilical cord clamping in preterm infants. Cochrane Database of Syst Rev 2010; (3). [7 RCTs, n = 297. All are small trials]
15. Rabe H, Reynolds G, Diaz-Rossello J. A systemic review and meta-analysis of a brief delay in clamping the umbilical cord of preterm infants. Neonatology 2007; 93:138–144. [Meta-analysis]
16. Airey RJ, Farrar D, Duley L. Alternative positions for the baby at birth before clamping the umbilical cord. Cochrane Database Syst Rev 2010; (10):CD007555. [37 studies excluded no studies met inclusion criteria]
17. Hosono S, Mugishima H, Fijita H, et al. Umbilical cord milking reduces the need for red blood cell transfusions and improves neonatal adaptation in infants born at less than 29 weeks' gestation: a randomized controlled trial. Arch Dis Child Fetal Neo Ed 2008; 93:F14–F19. [RCT, n = 40]
18. Rabe H, Jewison A, Fernadez Alvarez R, et al. Milking compared to delayed cord clamping to increase placental transfusion in preterm neonates. Obstet Gynecol 2011; 117:205–211. [RCT, n = 58]
19. McDonald SJ, Middleton P. Effect of timing of umbilical cord clamping of term infants on maternal and neonatal outcomes. Cochrane Database Syst Rev 2008; (2):CD004074. [Meta-analysis: 11 RCTs, n = 2989]
20. Giacalone PL, Vignal J, Daures JP, et al. A randomized evaluation of two techniques of management of the third stage of labor in women at low risk of postpartum hemorrhage. BJOG 2000; 107:396. [RCT, n = 477]
21. Kinmond S, Aitchison TC, Holland BM, et al. Umbilical cord clamping and preterm infants: a randomized trial. BMJ 1993; 306:172–175. [RCT, n = 36]
22. Soltani H, Dickinson F, Symonds IM. Placental cord drainage after spontaneous vaginal delivery as part of the management of the third stage of labour. Cochrane Database Syst Rev 2005; (4): CD004665. [Meta-analysis: 2 RCTs, n = 624]

23. Razmkhah N, Kordi M, Yousophi Z. The effects of cord drainage on the length of third stage of labour. Sci J Nurs Midwifery Mashad Univ 1999; 1:10–14. [RCT, $n = 177$]

24. Hofmeyr GJ, Abdel-Aleem H, Abdel-Aleem MA. Uterine massage for preventing postpartum haemorrhage. Cochrane Database of Syst Rev 2008; (3). [Meta-analysis: 1 RCT, $n = 200$]

25. Kovasarach E, Rojsangruang S. Effect of umbilical vein oxytocin injection on the third stage of labor: a randomized controlled study. J Med Ass Thailand 1998; 81:693–697. [RCT, $n = 50$]

26. Nardin JM, Weeks A, Carroli G. Umbilical vein injection for management of retained placenta. Cochrane Database of Systematic Reviews 2011; (5). [15 RCTs; $n = 1704$]

27. Gungorduk K, Asicioglu O, Besimoglu B, et al. Using intraumbilical vein injection of oxytocin in routine practice with active management of the third stage of labor. Obstet Gynecol 2010; 116:619–624. [RCT, $n = 412$]

28. Begley CM, Gyte GML, Murphy DJ, et al. Active versus expectant management in the third stage of labour. Cochrane Database Syst Rev 2010; (7):CD007412. [Meta-analysis: 5 RCTs; $n = 6486$]

29. Jangsten E, Mattson L-A, Lyckestam I, et al. A comparison of active management and expectant management of the third stage of labour: a Swedish randomized controlled trial. BJOG 2011; 118:362–369. [RCT, $n = 1902$]

30. Fleming VEM, Hagen S, Niven C. Does perineal suturing make a difference? The SUNS trial. BJOG 2003; 110:684–689. [RCT, $n = 74$]

31. Lunquist M, Olsson A, Nissen E, et al. Is it necessary to suture all lacerations after vaginal delivery? Birth 2000; 27:79–85. [RCT, $n = 78$]

32. Gordon B, Mackrodt C, Fern E, et al. The Ipswich childbirth study: 1. A randomized evaluation of two stage postpartum perineal repair leaving the skin unsutured. BJOG 1998; 105:435–440. [RCT, $n = 1780$]

33. Kettle C, Hills RK, Ismail KMK. Continuous versus interrupted sutures for repair of episiotomy or second degree tears. Cochrane Database Syst Rev 2009; (1):CD00947. [Meta-analysis: 7 RCTs, $n = 3822$]

34. Fitzpatrick M, Behan M, O'Connell PR, et al. A randomized clinical trial comparing primary overlap with approximation repair of third degree obstetric tears. Am J Obstet Gynecol 2000; 183:1220–1224. [RCT, $n = 112$]

35. Williams A, Adams EJ, Tincello DG, et al. How to repair an anal sphincter injury after vaginal delivery: results of a randomized controlled trial. BJOG 2006; 113:201–207. [RCT, $n = 112$]

36. Buppasira P, Lumbiganon P, Thinkhamrop J, et al. Antibiotic prophylaxis for third and fourth degree perineal tear during vaginal delivery. Cochrane Database of Syst Rev 2010; (11). [1 RCT, $n = 147$]

37. Kettle C, Dowswell T, Ismail KMK. Absorbable suture materials for primary repair of episiotomy and second degree tears. Cochrane Database Syst Rev 2010; (6):CD000006. [18 RCTs, $n = 10,171$]

38. Dencker A, Lundgren I, Sporrong T. Suturing after childbirth—a randomized controlled study testing a new monofilament material. BJOG 2006; 113:114–116. [RCT, $n = 1139$]

39. Flatin DL, Boulvain M, Floris LA, Irion O. Diagnosis of anal sphincter tears to prevent fecal incontinence. Obstet Gynecol 2005; 106:6–13. [RCT, $n = 752$]

40. Hedayati H, Parsons J, Crowther CA. Rectal analgesia for pain from perineal trauma following childbirth. Cochrane Database Syst Rev 2009; (4):CD003931. [Meta-analysis: 3 RCTs, $n = 249$]

41. Hedayati H, Parsons J, Crowther CA. Topically applied anaesthetics for treating perineal pain after childbirth. Cochrane Database Syst Rev 2009; (4):CD004223. [Meta-analysis: 8 RCTs, $n = 976$]

42. Hay-Smith, EJC. Therapeutic ultrasound for postpartum perineal pain and dyspareunia. Cochrane Database Syst Rev 2009; (4): CD00495. [Meta-analysis: 4 RCTs, $n = 459$]

43. Lozano R, Wang H, Foreman K, et al. Progress towards Millennium Development Goals 4 and 5 on maternal and child mortality: an updated systemic analysis. The Lancet 2011; 378 (9797):1139–1165. [II–1]

44. Hogan MC, Foreman KJ, Naghavi M. Maternal mortality of 181 countries, 1980-2008: a systemic analysis of progress towards Millennium Development Goals 5. Lancet 2010; 375(9726):1609–1623. [Review]

45. Mousa HA, Alfirevic Z. Treatment for primary postpartum haemorrhage. Cochrane Database Syst Rev 2007; (1):CD003249. [Meta-analysis: 3 RCTs, $n = 462$]

46. Widmer M, Blum J, Hofmeyr GJ, et al. Misoprostol as an adjunct to standard uterotonics for treatment of postpartum hemorrhage: a multicenter, double-blind randomized trial. Lancet 2010; 375:1808–1813. [RCT, $n = 1422$, used sublingual misoprostol]

47. Alfirevic Z, ed. Postpartum haemorrhage. Best Practice & Research Clinical Obstetrics and Gynaecology. Vol. 22, No. 6. Elsevier, 2008:1057–1074. [Review]

48. Lokugamage AU, Sullivan KR, Niculescu I, et al. A randomized study comparing rectally administered misoprostol versus syntometrine combined with an oxytocin infusion for the cessation of primary post partum hemorrhage. Acta Obstet Gynecol Scand 2001; 80(9):835–839. [RCT, $n = 64$ women with PPH > 500 mL]

49. Royal College of Obstetricians and Gynaecologists. Postpartum Haemorrhage, Prevention and Management (Green-top 52). 2009. Available at: http://www.rcog.org.uk/womens-health/clinical-guidance/prevention-and-management-postpartum-haemorrhage-green-top-52. [Review]

50. Zhang WH, Deneux-Tharaux C, Brocklehurst P, et al.; EUPHRATES Group. Effect of a collector bag for measurement of postpartum blood loss after vaginal delivery: cluster randomised trial in 13 European countries. BMJ 2010; 340:c293.

51. Alexander J, Thomas PW, Sanghera J. Treatments for secondary postpartum haemorrhage. Cochrane Database Syst Rev 2002; (1): CD002867. [Meta-analysis: no RCTs]

52. van Beekhuizen HJ, de Groot ANJA, Boo TD, et al. Sulprostone reduces the need for manual removal of the placenta in patients with retained placenta: a randomized controlled trial. Am J Obstet Gynecol 2006; 194:446–450. [RCT, $n = 103$]

53. Leader J, Bujnovsky M, Carla SJ, et al. Effect of oral misoprostol after second trimester delivery: a randomized, blinded study. Obstet Gynecol 2002; 100:689–694. [RCT, $n = 118$]

54. Abdel-Aleem H, Abdel-Aleem MA, Shaaban OM. Tocolysis for management of retained placenta. Cochrane Database Syst Rev 2011; (1):CD007708. [Meta-analysis: 1 RCTs, $n = 24$]

55. World Health Organization (WHO). WHO Guidelines for the Management of Postpartum Haemorrhage and Retained Placenta. France: WHO, 2009. [Review]

56. Singla AK, Lapinski RH, Berkowitz RL, et al. Are women who are Jehovah's witnessess at risk of maternal death? Am J Obstet Gynecol 2001; 185:893–895. [II-2; $n = 332$]

57. Gyamfi C, Gyamfi MM, Berkowitz RL. Ethical and medicolegal considerations in the obstetric care of a Jehovah's Witness. Obstet Gynecol 2003; 102:173–180. [Review]

58. Gyamfi C, Berkowitz RL. Responses by pregnant Jehovah's Witnesses on health care proxies. Obstet Gynecol 2004; 104:541–544. [II-3]

59. Singla AK, Berkowitz RL, Saphier CJ. Obstetric hemorrhage in Jehovah's witnesses. Conteporary Obstet Gynecol 2002; 4:32–43. [Review]

60. Catling S, Joels L. Cell salvage in obstetrics: the time has come. BJOG 2005; 112:131–132. [Review]

10

Intrapartum fetal monitoring

Nancy W. Hendrix, Brittany L. Anderson, and Suneet P. Chauhan

KEY POINTS

- Compared with intermittent auscultation (IA), the **use of continuous electronic fetal heart rate (FHR) monitoring significantly increases the rate of operative interventions** [vacuum, forceps, and cesarean delivery (CD)] for nonreassuring patterns, **but it does decrease the likelihood of neonatal seizures and perinatal mortality secondary to hypoxia**.
- With some persistent category II or III patterns, **intrauterine resuscitation with maternal oxygen, change in maternal position, discontinuation of labor stimulation and/or tocolytics, or amnioinfusion (if variable decelerations) reduce the need to proceed with emergent CD but do not reduce the likelihood of asphyxial injury.**
- The labor of **women at risk** for poor peripartum outcomes **should be monitored with continuous electronic FHR tracing**.
- Reinterpretation of the FHR tracing, especially knowing the neonatal outcome, should be avoided.
- There is **insufficient evidence** to assess **computerized FHR monitoring**.
- **ST analysis is not associated with significant perinatal benefits** in women with nonreassuring FHR (NRFHR) on continuous monitoring. No benefit from ST analysis is observed with proper use of fetal scalp sampling.
- **Fetal pulse oximetry (FPO) is not associated with significant maternal or neonatal benefits** compared to continuous FHR monitoring alone.

BACKGROUND

Electronic FHR monitoring during labor is the most common obstetric procedure in the United States (1). Between 1997 and 2003 in the Unites States, monitoring was utilized in 84% (23,273,458) of the over 27 million births (1). For admission tests at the beginning of labor, see chapter 7. For meconium, see chapter 21.

FHR DEFINITIONS

Adapted from the 2008 National Institute of Child Health and Human Development Workshop (2), the definitions of FHR pattern are described in Table 10.1 and depicted in Figures 10.1 to 10.3. The definitions were developed for intrapartum monitoring but may be applicable to antepartum monitoring. No distinction is made between short- and long-term variability (2). Accelerations, decelerations, bradycardia, and tachycardia can be quantified by describing the nadir/zenith and the duration in minutes and seconds of the FHR change. A **recurrent deceleration** occurs with ≥50% of uterine contractions in any 20-minute period.

A three-tier system for categorization of FHR patterns has now been recommended (2). According to this classification, category I tracing is predictive of normal fetal acid-base status at the time of observation and may be followed in a routine manner. Category II tracings are indeterminate and not predictive of abnormal fetal acid-base status but require evaluation and continued surveillance and reevaluation. Category III tracings are abnormal and predictive of abnormal fetal acid-base status (Table 10.2, Figs. 10.4–10.6). These tracings require prompt evaluation and should include efforts to expeditiously resolve the abnormal pattern. It is noteworthy that a full description of an electronic fetal monitoring (EFM) tracing requires a qualitative and quantitative description of the following: (i) uterine contractions, (ii) baseline FHR, (iii) baseline FHR variability, (iv) presence of accelerations, (v) periodic or episodic decelerations, and (vi) changes or trends of FHR patterns over time (2).

In relation to uterine activity, **tachysystole** is defined as >5 contractions in 10 minutes averaged over 30 minutes, whether the contractions are spontaneous or stimulated. The terms hyperstimulation and hypercontractility should be abandoned. Terms such as "asphyxia," "hypoxia," and "fetal distress" should not be used in the interpretation of FHR tracing.

pH DEFINITIONS
Acidemia: increased concentration of hydrogen ions in blood
Acidosis: a pathologic condition marked by increased concentration of hydrogen ions in tissue
Hypoxemia: decreased oxygen content in blood
Hypoxia: a pathologic condition marked by decreased level of oxygen in tissue
Asphyxia: acidemia, hypoxia, and metabolic acidosis; must have all of the following: (i) umbilical arterial pH < 7.00; (ii) Apgar ≤ 3 at >5 minutes; and (iii) neonatal neurologic sequelae (e.g., seizures, coma, and hypotonia) (3). This term should be used with caution and never before birth (see also chap. 28).

INCIDENCE
The prevalence of CD for NRFHR tracing is about 3% or more, and it is increasing (4).

RISK FACTORS AND PREDICTORS OF ABNORMAL FHR
The risk of CD for NRFHR is >20% in patients with moderate/severe asthma, severe hypothyroidism, severe preeclampsia, postterm, or fetal growth restriction (FGR) with abnormal Doppler studies (4).

Use of likelihood ratio suggests that fetal movement count, abnormal FHR on admission, vibroacoustic stimulation, amniotic fluid index, contraction stress test, and modified and completed biophysical profile are poor diagnostic tests to identify which patients will require emergent CD for NRFHR (4). Umbilical artery systolic/diastolic ratio, however, is a reliable test to predict the need for CD for NRFHR.

Table 10.1 Definitions of Fetal Heart Rate Patterns

	Definitions
Baseline FHR	The mean FHR rounded to increments of 5 bpm during a 10-min period (excluding accelerations, decelerations, and periods of marked variability)
	The baseline must be for a minimum of 2 min.
	May need to compare the previous 10-min segment to determine the baseline
	Bradycardia—baseline FHR <110 bpm
	Tachycardia—baseline FHR >160 bpm
	Sinusoidal pattern—visually apparent, smooth, sine-wave-like undulating FHR baseline pattern with cycle frequency 3–5/min, persisting ≥20 min
Baseline FHR variability	Fluctuations in the baseline FHR that are irregular in amplitude and frequency (excluding accelerations and decelerations)
	Variability is quantitated as the amplitude of peak-to-trough in bpm
	Absent—amplitude range undetectable
	Minimal—amplitude range ≤5 bpm
	Moderate (normal)—amplitude range 6–25 bpm
	Marked—amplitude range >25 bpm
Acceleration	An abrupt (peak within 30 sec) increase in the FHR from baseline
	Acme is ≥15 bpm above baseline, lasting for 15 sec or more and <2 min from the onset to return to baseline
	Before 32 wk, acceleration is acme ≥10 bpm over the baseline and lasting at least 10 sec but <2 min.
	Prolonged acceleration if it lasts >2 min but <10 min
	If the acceleration is >10 min, then it is a baseline change.
Deceleration	An abrupt or gradual decrease in FHR as characterized below:
	Recurrent—occur with ≥50% contractions in 20 min
	Intermittent—occur with <50% contractions in 20 min
	Prolonged—visually apparent decrease in FHR ≥15 bpm, lasting ≥2min but <10 min
Early deceleration (Fig. 10.1)	In association with a uterine contraction, a visually apparent, usually symmetrical and gradual (onset to nadir ≥30 sec) decrease in FHR with return to baseline.
	Onset, nadir, and recovery of deceleration occur at same time as beginning, peak, and ending of contraction, respectively.
Late deceleration (Fig. 10.2)	In association with a uterine contraction, a visually apparent, gradual (onset to nadir ≥30 sec) decrease in FHR
	Onset, nadir, and recovery of deceleration occur after the beginning, peak, and end of the contraction, respectively.
Variable deceleration (Fig. 10.3)	An abrupt (onset to nadir <30 sec) decrease in FHR
	The decrease in FHR is at least 15 bpm, lasting ≥15 sec but <2 min.
	Onset, depth, and duration vary with contractions.

Abbreviation: bpm, beats per minute; FHR, fetal heart rate.
Source: Adapted from Ref. 2.

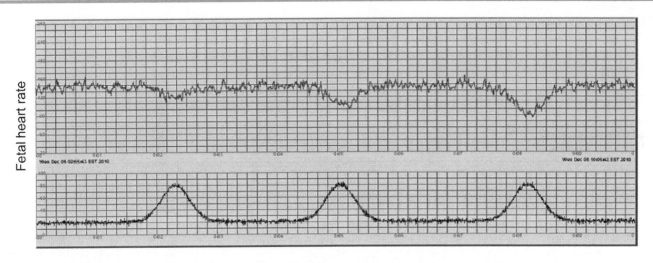

Figure 10.1 Early decelerations of 15, 30, and 45 BPM, respectively. *Abbreviation*: BPM, beats per minute.

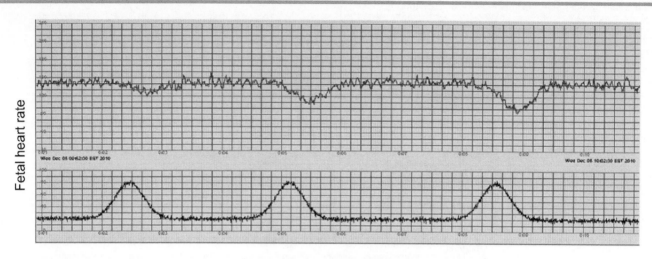

Figure 10.2 Late decelerations of 15, 30, and 45 BPM, respectively. *Abbreviation*: BPM, beats per minute.

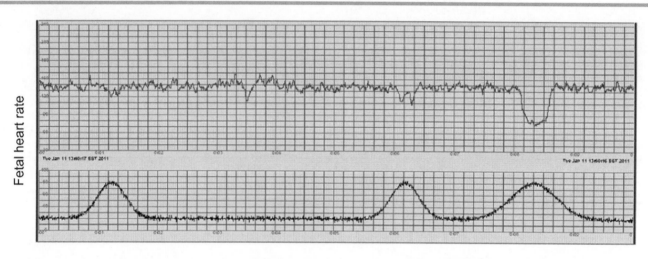

Figure 10.3 Variable decelerations of 15, 40, 30, and 60 BPM respectively. *Abbreviation*: BPM, beats per minute.

Table 10.2 Three-Tier FHR Interpretation System

	Baseline	Variability	Acceleration	Deceleration
Category I (Fig. 10.4A–C)	110–160 bpm	Moderate	Possible, not necessary	Possible early; no variable or late
Category II (includes those not in category I or III; Fig. 10.5A–I)	1. Bradycardia without absent variability 2. Tachycardia	1. Minimal 2. Absent without recurrent decelerations 3. Marked	After fetal stimulation	1. Recurrent variable with minimal to moderate variability 2. Prolonged 3. Recurrent late with moderate variability 4. Variable with other characteristics (i.e., slow return to baseline, overshoots, or shoulders)
Category III (Fig. 10.6A–C)	1. Bradycardia 2. Sinusoidal	Absent		1. Recurrent late 2. Recurrent variable

Abbreviations: FHR, fetal heart rate; bpm, beats per minute.
Source: Adapted from Ref. 2.

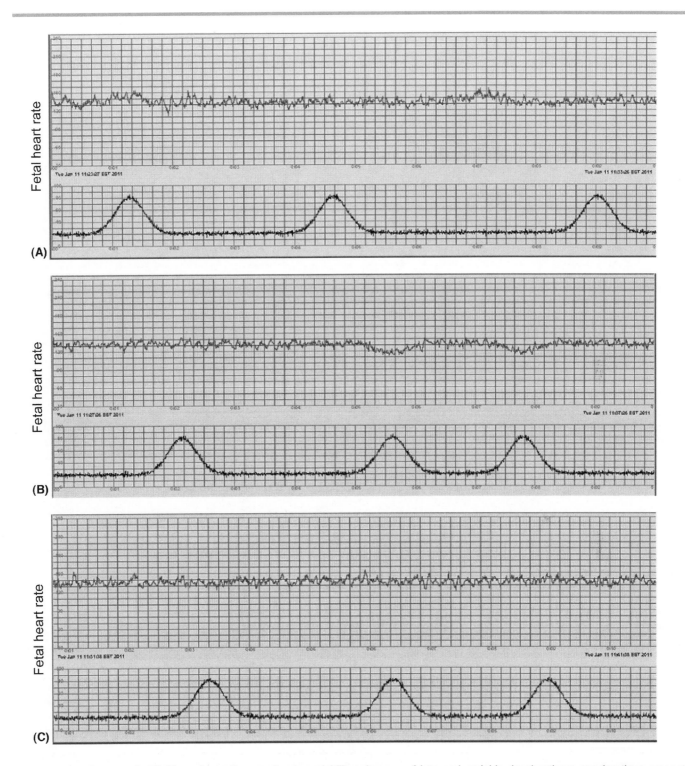

Figure 10.4 Category I. (**A**) Normal baseline, moderate variability, absence of late and variable decelerations, accelerations present. (**B**) Normal baseline, moderate variability, absence of late and variable decelerations, early decelerations present. (**C**) Normal baseline, moderate variability, absence of late and variable decelerations.

CONTINUOUS ELECTRONIC FHR MONITORING VS. INTERMITTENT AUSCULTATION

Despite the ubiquitous use, there are concerns about the efficacy of EFM. As noted by the American College of Obstetricians and Gynecologists (ACOG) practice bulletin (5), the efficacy of monitoring is adjudicated by comparing the neonatal and infant morbidity, including seizure and cerebral palsy, or mortality averted versus the unnecessary interventions (operative vaginal delivery or CD) undertaken. Since all the randomized clinical trials (RCTs) with EFM compare it to IA, the efficacy is determined by calculating the relative risks (RR) of interventions, neonatal seizures, cerebral palsy, or death. **Compared with IA, continuous EFM is associated with a significantly increased likelihood of operative vaginal**

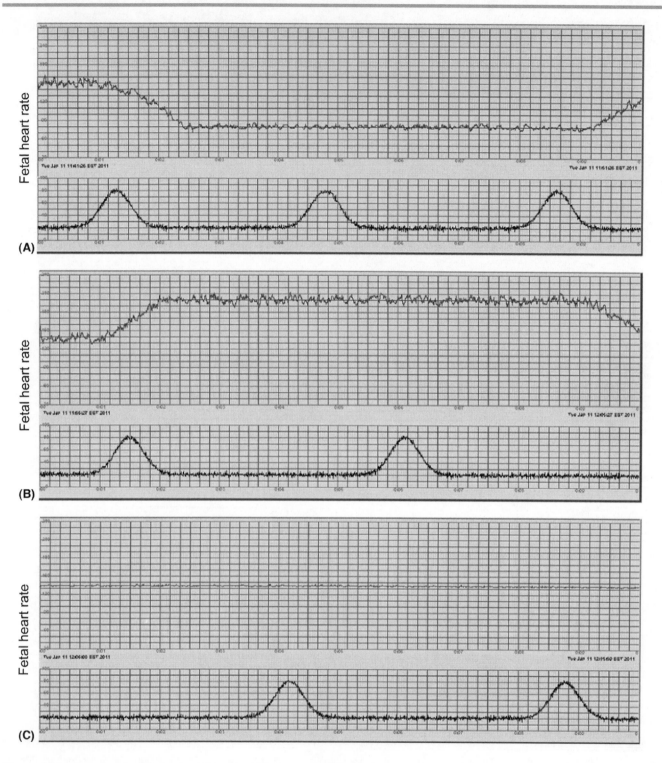

Figure 10.5 Category II. (**A**) Bradycardia with moderate variability. (**B**) Tachycardia. (**C**) Minimal variability. (**D**) Absent variability. (**E**) Marked variability. (**F**) Recurrent variable decelerations, minimal variability. (**G**) Prolonged deceleration. (**H**) Recurrent late decelerations, moderate variability. (**I**) Variable decelerations.

delivery, overall CD, as well as CD for NRFHR tracing or fetal acidosis. The use of continuous EFM has been associated with a **significant 50% decrease in the incidence of neonatal seizures**, but it has not been shown to lower the risk of cerebral palsy or neonatal death (5,6). EFM is associated with 1 additional CD for every 58 women monitored continuously;

661 women need to have EFM during labor to prevent one neonatal seizure (6).

While the efficacy of EFM is debated, it is noteworthy that there are concerns regarding the 12 RCTs, which are sampled over 37,000 women, on continuous FHR monitoring versus IA (6). Only two of these trials were of high quality

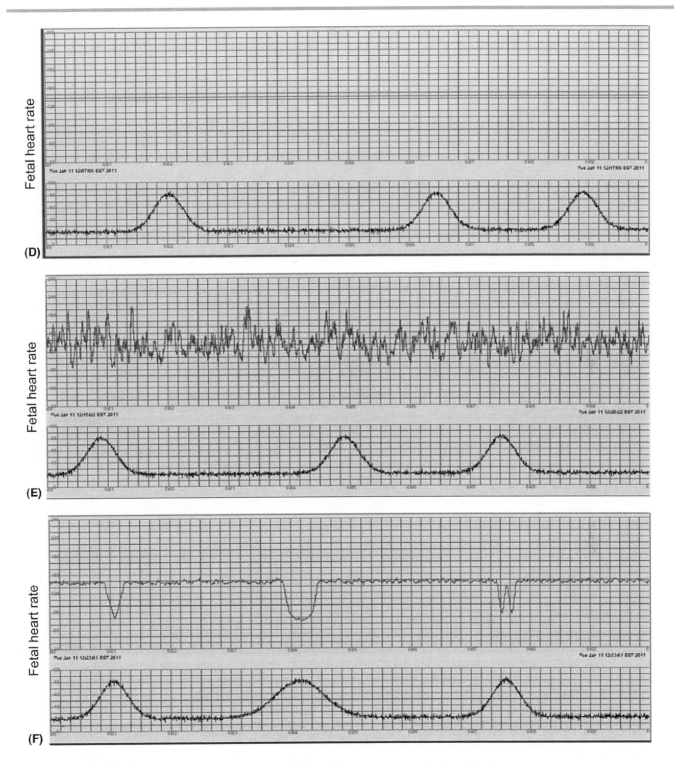

Figure 10.5 (Continued)

(7,8), and only three trials reported data in low-risk women (7–9). The risk of cerebral palsy was examined by one trial (10), which randomized women at <32 weeks. Only one trial (11) provided data on hypoxic-ischemic encephalopathy with a combined sample size insufficient to determine if EFM can significantly lower neonatal mortality. The authors of the meta-analysis on this subject (6) noted that to test the hypoth-esis that continuous monitoring can prevent 1 death in 1000 births, more than 50,000 women would have to be random-ized. Additionally, there are concerns that the meta-analysis combines results from RCTs published prior to the introduc-tion of the Consolidated Standards of Reporting Trials (CON-SORT) guidelines (12), and that inadequate study size may not reflect the outcomes in contemporary obstetrical practice (13).

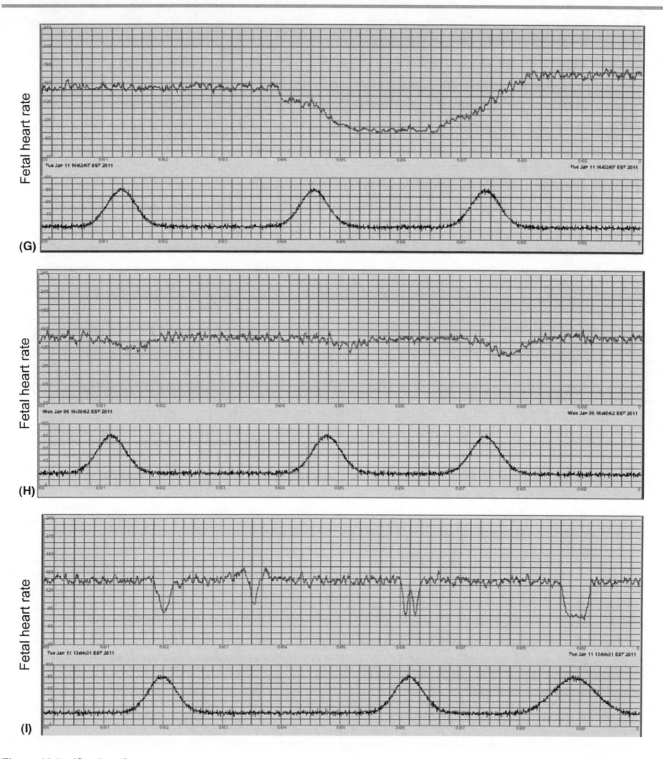

Figure 10.5   (Continued)

Thus, if IA is available on the labor and delivery, it is reasonable to discuss the options with the patients (14). Admittedly both patients and clinicians prefer FHR monitoring as the method to evaluate the fetus during labor (15). The explanations for the preference include the ease of use, the reassurance women derive from hearing the heart beat during labor, and the different value patients and clinicians place on the route of delivery and neonatal outcomes. Compared with pregnant patients and mothers, obstetricians overestimate the burden posed by cesarean, and, contrary to obstetricians, women value a newborn with permanent neurologic handicap over neonatal death (15).

Clinicians choosing to utilize IA should be aware of some of the problems associated with its use. **Continuous electronic FHR monitoring has a significantly better ability to detect acidemia** (umbilical arterial pH < 7.15 in this study)

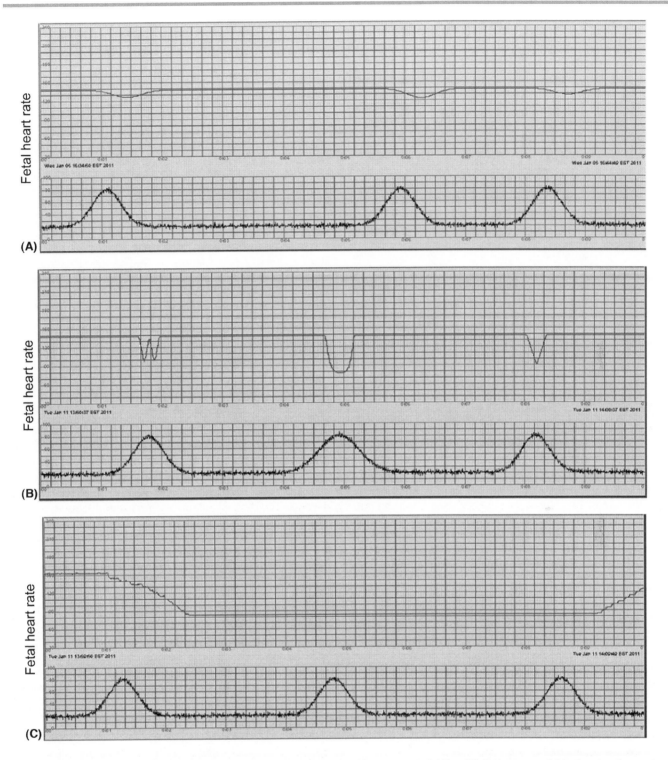

Figure 10.6 Category III. (**A**) Recurrent late decelerations, absent fetal heart rate variability. (**B**) Recurrent variable decelerations, absent fetal heart rate variability. (**C**) Bradycardia, absent fetal heart rate variability.

than IA: a sensitivity of 97% versus 34% and a higher positive predictive value of 37% versus 22%, respectively (16). Continuous tracing of the FHR was not only superior with detection of respiratory and mixed acidosis but metabolic as well. It is possible that the ominous FHR patterns are poorly assessed by IA. Logistically **it may not be feasible to adhere to guidelines**

of how frequently the heart rate should be auscultated with IA. One prospective study noted that the protocol for IA was successfully completed with only 3% of the cases (17).

Even though the use of continuous electronic monitoring of the FHR does not decrease the prevalence of cerebral palsy, it assists in determining if the injury occurred during the ante- or intrapartum periods. Review of the FHR tracing of neurologically injured newborns indicates that the majority of them had an abnormal pattern consistent with asphyxial injury **prior** to the onset of labor (18). Moreover, a pregnancy with chronic fetal distress may develop superimposed acute asphyxia, in which case the impairment may be more severe than if the sentinel event and injury occurred during labor.

Not all pregnancies should be monitored with IA because **those at risk for adverse outcomes like cerebral palsy, neonatal encephalopathy, and perinatal death should be monitored with continuous FHR tracing during labor** (19). Thus, high-risk pregnancies that underwent antepartum surveillance should not be evaluated with IA, nor should those who are likely to have CD for an NRFHR pattern (4). These include FGR, oligohydramnios, polyhydramnios, placenta previa, postterm (≥42 weeks), multiple gestation, isoimmunized pregnancy, prior intrauterine fetal demise (IUFD), or maternal renal disease, diabetes, preeclampsia, collagen disorders, hemoglobinopathies, and cardiovascular disease. Additionally, parturients should be monitored with continuous tracing of the FHR if they have been induced or augmented, or have dysfunctional labor, tocolytics administered more than once/hr, suspected FHR abnormalities with auscultation, abnormal fetal presentation, regional anesthesia, abruption, infection, preterm labor, prior CD [vaginal birth after cesarean (VBAC) attempt], hypertonic uterus, and meconium staining of the amniotic fluid (20).

FHR monitoring should be continued until delivery. If CD is performed, internal scalp monitoring can be continued until delivery, while external monitoring can be discontinued when the abdominal preparation begins.

REVIEWING ELECTRONIC FHR MONITORING

When EFM is utilized during labor, the nurses or physicians should review it frequently. If the patient is at low-risk pregnancy, the FHR tracing should be reviewed every 30 minutes in the first stage of labor and every 15 minutes during the second stage. The corresponding frequency for high-risk parturients is 15 and 5 minutes, respectively. The maternal pulse should be taken to make sure the FHR is indeed fetal, and not maternal. **Health care providers should document** that they have reviewed the tracing by a narrative note or use of comprehensive flow sheets or by placing one's initials on the monitor strip, if it is reassuring (20). Among low-risk patients, it is more feasible to confirm that the strips are reviewed according to the guidelines, whereas among high-risk patients, compliance during active phase, and especially during second stage of labor, is more demanding and difficult. The FHR tracing, as a part of the medical chart, should be labeled and available for review if the need arises. Alternatives like computer storage of the FHR tracing that do not permit overwriting or revisions are reasonable, as are microfilm recordings (20).

Due to the **inter- and intraobserver variability**, FHR tracing should be interpreted cautiously and preferably without knowing the neonatal outcome (21–23). When four obstetricians, for example, examined 50 cardiotocograms, they agreed in only 22% of the cases. Two months later, during the second review of the same 50 tracings, the clinicians interpreted 21% of the tracings differently than they did during the first evaluation (22). Factors that influence the interpretation of cardiotocograms include the clinician's experience, whether the tracing is normal versus equivocal or ominous with greater agreement if the tracing is reassuring, and the time of the day, with possibly greater error at night. With retrospective reviews, the fore-knowledge of neonatal outcome alters the impressions of the

tracing. Given the same intrapartum tracing but opposite neonatal outcomes, the reviewer is more likely to find evidence of fetal hypoxia and criticize the obstetrician's management if the outcome was supposedly poor versus good (23).

The positive predictive value of NRFHR for cerebral palsy is about 0.1% (7). The **false-positive rate is extremely high** (99%) for FHR tracing and abnormal neonatal outcome, especially cerebral palsy (24).

EXTERNAL VS. INTERNAL FHR MONITORING

External FHR monitoring is accomplished via a Doppler ultrasound device applied to the maternal abdomen. Internal scalp electrode ("scalp lead") for FHR monitoring measures the R-R interval between consecutive beats. This provides an accurate representation of FHR variability. There are no RCTs comparing these two monitoring techniques. Internal monitoring is used, in general, for an FHR that cannot be consistently assessed by external monitoring. Contraindications to internal monitoring include maternal infections such as HIV, active hepatitis B or C, and fetal thrombocytopenia. Otherwise internal monitoring is safe.

COMPUTERIZED FHR MONITORING

Measured by interobserver agreement, the reliability of electronic FHR monitoring is not very good. **There is insufficient evidence to assess if computerized evaluation of electronic FHR monitoring improves perinatal outcomes**, as there is no trial available (25).

MANAGEMENT OF ABNORMAL FHR (FIG. 10.7)

The best time to evaluate the FHR tracing is after a contraction. The frequency with which the FHR should be evaluated depends on the risk status of pregnancy (see above). To correctly interpret the FHR pattern, the clinician must be cognizant of the gestational age, medications (Table 10.3) (26), prior fetal assessment, and obstetric and medical conditions. There is no evidence to support the prophylactic use of betamimetics during the second stage of labor. Compared with placebo, prophylactic betamimetic therapy is associated with an increase in forceps deliveries in one trial (27).

Digital Scalp or Vibroacoustic Stimulation

The presence of acceleration usually assures that the fetus is not acidotic (pH < 7.20). If spontaneous acceleration is not present, and/or NRFHR is present, **digital scalp or vibroacoustic stimulation** should be done to elicit an acceleration (see definition in Table 10.1). Allis clamp and scalp puncture have been used to elicit an acceleration but are less safe. Digital scalp stimulation (gentle stroking of the fetal scalp for 15 seconds) is the test with the best predictive accuracy among these four (28). There are currently no RCTs that address the safety and efficacy of digital scalp or vibroacoustic stimulation used to assess fetal well-being in labor in the presence of NRFHR. If the FHR increases, then labor should continue since an acceleration following fetal stimulation indicates that the likelihood of low scalp pH is 2% (28). In the absence of an acceleration, the likelihood is 38%.

Scalp pH

With persistent NRFHR tracing, a **scalp pH** should be attempted, if available. There are no statistically significant differences for any fetal/neonatal/infant outcomes when

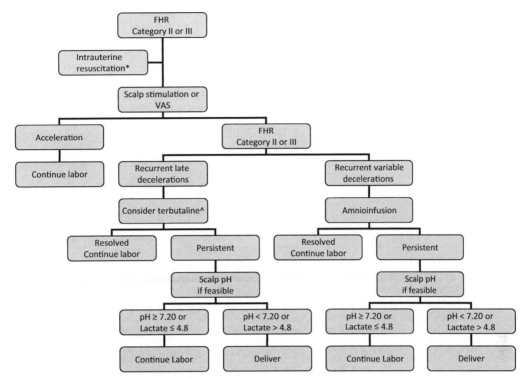

*Discontinue labor stimulant, change maternal position, hydration, and oxygenation
^Use with caution among women with diabetes or thyroid storm

Figure 10.7 Algorithm for the management of abnormal FHR in labor. *Abbreviation*: VAS, vibroacoustic stimulation.

Table 10.3 Effect of Medications and FHR Patterns

Medications	Study design	Effect on FHR
Butorphanol	Case:control	Transient sinusoidal FHR pattern
Cocaine	Case:control	No characteristic changes in FHR pattern
Corticosteroid	RCT	Decrease in FHR variability with betamethasone but not dexamethasone
Magnesium sulfate	RCT and retrospective	A significant decrease in the FHR baseline and variability; inhibits the increase in accelerations with advancing gestational age
Meperidine	RCT	No characteristic changes in FHR pattern
Morphine	Case:control	Decreased number of accelerations
Nalbuphine	RCT	Decreased the number of accelerations, long- and short-term variations
Terbutaline	Retrospective	Abolishment or decrease in frequency of late and variable decelerations
Zidovudine	Case:control	No difference in the FHR baseline, variability, number of accelerations or decelerations

Abbreviations: FHR, fetal heart rate; bpm, beats per minute; RCT, randomized clinical trial.
Source: Adapted from Ref. 26.

lactate is compared with pH estimation of fetal blood samples in labor, with a 10% higher success rate for obtaining lactate compared with pH values (29). If the results are scalp pH < 7.20 or lactate >4.8 mm/L, then delivery should be accomplished expeditiously, usually by CD (30) (Fig. 10.7). The sensitivities of abnormal scalp pH or lactate to predict moderate to severe hypoxic-ischemic encephalopathy are 50% and 66%, respectively, while the corresponding specificities are 73% and 76% (30). If the results are scalp pH ≥7.20 or lactate ≤4.8 mm/L, continuous careful FHR monitoring should continue, with repeat scalp stimulation and/or pH if NRFHR persists. Several RCTs of continuous versus intermittent FHR monitoring in labor used scalp pH in concomitance with continuous FHR monitoring (6). Scalp pH may not be feasible in cases with cervical dilatation <3 cm. To be beneficial, the scalp pH machine needs to be reliable and readily available with prompt results. If neither acceleration nor a scalp pH can be obtained, then the management of NRFHR tracing depends on the abnormality.

Amnioinfusion

When the FHR abnormality is **recurrent variable decelerations** (usually with preceding oligohydramnios), then **amnioinfusion** to relieve cord compression can be utilized (Fig. 10.7) (31). Prophylactic (for oligohydramnios, and therefore suspicion of later variable decelerations) or therapeutic (for variable decelerations) **transcervical** amnioinfusion significantly **reduces the rate of persistent variable decelerations,** Apgar score <7 at 5 minutes, low cord arterial pH (usually <7.20), neonatal hospital stay >3 days, **CD for suspected NRFHR, and overall CD**, compared with no amnioinfusion (31). Postpartum endometritis is decreased, too. There is a nonsignificant 49% decrease in perinatal mortality (31). Transabdominal amnioinfusion may be considered if amniotomy cannot be done and an intrauterine pressure catheter placed, because it has similar effects, relieving persistent recurrent variable decelerations and lowering the incidence of umbilical arterial pH <7.20 in two small trials (32,33). The limited evidence available suggests that there is no advantage to using amnioinfusion prophylactically as opposed to therapeutically (see chap. 18).

Because the trials involving amnioinfusion are small, it is not feasible to address the possibility of rare but serious maternal adverse effects of amnioinfusion.

The mechanism of effectiveness of amnioinfusion is relief of the umbilical cord compression thought to be causing the variable decelerations.

Amnioinfusion can be done by bolus or continuous infusion technique, with similar ability to relieve recurrent variable decelerations. Neither pumps nor warmers are necessary with amnioinfusion. In fact, the use of infusion pump during amnioinfusion significantly increases the risk of NRFHR. Either lactated Ringer's solution or normal saline can be used to place a crystalloid solution into the uterus without altering the neonatal electrolyte balance (20).

Tocolysis

For **bradycardia, or recurrent late or variable decelerations**, tocolytics can be used to abolish uterine contractions, especially if hyperstimulation is present. During suspected NRFHR, compared with no treatment, betamimetics (terbutaline 0.25 mg subcutaneously or hexoprenaline 10 µg intravenously) are associated with fewer failed improvements in FHR abnormalities (34). There is insufficient evidence to evaluate the effect on important neonatal outcomes such as umbilical artery pH, given small numbers. When terbutaline is compared with magnesium sulfate (4 g over 10 minutes), the betamimetic is faster acting and more effective, with similar maternal cardiovascular side effects (35). Thus betamimetics may be a useful treatment in selected cases of NRFHR diagnosed during labor. The time gained with this intervention may be useful for preparing for cesarean section or operative delivery, setting up regional analgesia, transferring a woman at home or in a unit without the necessary surgical or neonatal facilities to an appropriate hospital, or reviewing the need for urgent delivery.

Intrauterine Resuscitation

In the presence of NRFHR, concomitantly with performing scalp stimulation and/or scalp pH, intrauterine resuscitation can be attempted with the following (Fig. 10.7):

- **Maternal position** change to left or right lateral
  - There is insufficient evidence (no trial) to assess by itself the effect of intrapartum maternal position change on fetal status.
- **Hydration**
  - There is insufficient evidence (no trial) to assess by itself the effect of intrapartum maternal hydration on fetal status.
- **Oxygenation**
  - There is insufficient evidence (no trial) to assess by itself the effect of intrapartum maternal oxygen on fetal status.

- **Labor stimulant** should be discontinued.
  - There is insufficient evidence (no trial) to assess by itself the effect of labor stimulant discontinuation on fetal status.

Intravenous fluid bolus of 1000 mL, lateral positioning, and oxygen administration at 10 L/min via nonbreather face mask are effective resuscitative measures to improve fetal oxygen saturation (FSpO$_2$) during labor (36). The evidence is from patients with normal FHR, and at present it is a reasonable assumption that the findings are applicable to NRFHR pattern.

Other Interventions

Additional steps with the management of NRFHR tracing might include (no trials available) the following:

- **Tocomonitoring** assessment for hyperstimulation.
- **Cervical examination** to assess rapid dilation or descent, and to ensure that the umbilical cord has not prolapsed.
- **Maternal blood pressure** monitoring, especially among those who have received regional anesthesia. If hypotension is present in conjunction with NRFHR pattern, ephedrine or phenylephrine may be utilized (5).

Piracetam for NRFHR in Labor

Piracetam, a derivative of γ-aminobenzoic acid, is thought to promote the metabolism of the brain cells when they are hypoxic. There is not enough evidence to evaluate the use of piracetam for NRFHR in labor. Compared with placebo, piracetam is associated with a nonsignificant trend to reduced need for cesarean section, and similar incidences of low Apgar scores, or neonatal respiratory problems and signs of hypoxia (37).

Operative Delivery for NRFHR in Labor

There are no contemporary trials of operative delivery versus conservative management of suspected NRFHR. In the only old (1959) trial, there is no difference in perinatal mortality (38).

Fetal Electrocardiogram for Fetal Monitoring in Labor

The use of the fetal electrocardiogram (ECG) has been evaluated **as an adjunct to continuous electronic FHR monitoring during labor** (39–46). The use of internal monitoring with a scalp lead is mandatory to obtain ECG. In most labors, technically satisfactory cardiotocographic traces can be obtained by external ultrasound monitors, which are less invasive than internal scalp electrodes. One study assessed PR intervals and is insufficient to make recommendations (46). Five RCTs assessed the ST segment (41–46).

Compared with cardiotocography (CTG) alone, ST segment analysis (STAN) with CTG in fetuses at ≥36 weeks' gestation is associated with similar incidences of metabolic acidosis (0.81% vs. 1.12%, RR 0.80, 95% CI 0.44–1.47), perinatal death, neonatal encephalopathy, Apgar score <7 at 5 minutes, admission to neonatal intensive care unit (NICU), and CD. Operative vaginal delivery is lower in the STAN with CTG compared with CTG alone (13.56% vs. 15.20%, RR 0.89, 95% CI 0.83–0.97), as is the use of fetal scalp samples (40). **As there is no difference in perinatal outcomes between STAN with CTG compared with CTG alone, this modality cannot be yet recommended for routine clinical care.**

If STAN is considered for clinical use, the protocols used in trials (40) recommended no action if CTG is normal, regardless of ST waveform analyses. A better approach might be to restrict fetal ST waveform analysis to those fetuses demonstrating NRFHR on FHR monitor.

Fetal Pulse Oximetry

A normal $FSpO_2$ in labor is 35% to 65%. Fetal pulse oximetry (FPO) showing $FSpO_2$ <30% for at least >2 minutes is associated with a higher risk for declining fetal arterial pH and metabolic acidosis. The fetal oxygen sensor lies against the fetal cheek. The use of the FPO has been evaluated **as an adjunct to continuous electronic FHR monitoring during labor** (47–52).

FPO with continuous FHR tracing is associated with **similar overall cesarean section rate, as well as similar CDs for NRFHR** compared with continuous FHR only (47). No differences are seen for endometritis, intrapartum or postpartum hemorrhage, uterine rupture, low Apgar scores, umbilical arterial pH or base excess, admission to the NICU, or fetal/neonatal death (47,48). Given the above evidence, **routine use of FPO in labor is not recommended.**

REFERENCES

1. Chen HY, Chauhan SP, Ananth CV, et al. Electronic fetal heart rate monitoring and infant mortality: a population-based study in the United States. Am J Obstet Gynecol 2011; 204:491.e1–491.10. [II-3]
2. Macones GA, Hankins GDV, Spong CY, et al. The 2008 National Institute of Child Health and Human Development Workshop. Electronic fetal heart rate monitoring: update on definitions, interpretation, and research guidelines. Obstet Gynecol 2008; 112:661–666. [Review]
3. American College of Obstetricians and Gynecologists. ACOG Committee Opinion No. 197:. Inappropriate use of the terms fetal distress and birth asphyxia. Washington, D.C.: ACOG, 1998. [Review]
4. Chauhan SP, Magann EF, Scott JR, et al. Cesarean delivery for fetal distress: rate and risk factors. Obstet Gynecol Surv 2003; 58:337–350. [Review of 392 articles published in English from 1990 to 2000]
5. American College of Obstetricians and Gynecologists. ACOG Practice Bulletin No. 106: Intrapartum fetal heart rate monitoring: nomenclature, interpretation, and general management principles. Washington, D.C.: ACOG, 2009. [Review]
6. Alfirevic Z, Devane D, Gyte GM. Continuous cardiotocography (CTG) as a form of electronic fetal monitoring (EFM) for fetal assessment during labour. Cochrane Database Syst Rev 2006; (3): CD006066. [Meta-analysis]
7. Renou P, Chang A, Anderson I, et al. Controlled trial of fetal intensive care. Am J Obstet Gynecol 1976; 126:470–476. [Level I]
8. Macdonald D, Grant A, Sheridan-Pereira M, et al. The Dublin randomized controlled trial of intrapartum fetal heart rate monitoring. Am J Obstet Gynecol 1985; 152:524–539. [Level I]
9. Leveno KJ, Cunningham FG, Nelson S, et al. A prospective comparison of selective and universal electronic fetal monitoring in 34,995 pregnancies. N Engl J Med 1986; 315:615–619. [Level I, $n = 34,995$]
10. Luthy DA, Shy KK, van Belle G, et al. A randomized trial of electronic fetal monitoring in preterm labor. Obstet Gynecol 1987; 69:687–695. [Level I]
11. Vintzileos AM, Antsaklis A, Varvarigos I, et al. A randomized trial of intrapartum electronic fetal heart rate monitoring versus intermittent auscultation. Obstet Gynecol 1993; 81:899–907. [Level I]
12. Begg C, Cho M, Eastwood S, et al. Improving the quality of reporting of randomized controlled trials. The CONSORT statement. JAMA 1996; 276:637–639. [Level III]
13. Vintzileos AM. Evidence-based compared with reality-based medicine in obstetrics. Obstet Gynecol 2009; 113:1335–1340. [Level III]
14. Hundley V, Ryan M, Graham W. Assessing women's preferences for antepartum care. Birth 2001; 28:254–263. [Level II-3]
15. Vandenbussche FPHA, De Jong-Potjer LC, Stiggelbout AM, et al. Difference in the valuation of birth outcomes among pregnant women, mothers, and obstetricians. Birth 1999; 28:178–183. [Level II-3]
16. Vintzileos AM, Nochimson DJ, Antsaklis A, et al. Comparison of continuous electronic fetal heart rate monitoring versus intermittent auscultation in detecting fetal acidemia at birth. Am J Obstet Gynecol 1995; 173:1021–1024. [Level I-1]
17. Morrison JC, Chez BF, Davis ID, et al. Intrapartum fetal heart rate assessment: monitoring by auscultation or electronic means. Am J Obstet Gynecol 1993; 168:63–66. [Level II-1]
18. Phelan JP, Ahn MO. Perinatal observations in forty-eight neurologically impaired term infants. Am J Obstet Gynecol 1994; 171:424–431. [Level II-3]
19. Society of Obstetricians and Gynaecologists of Canada Policy Statement. Fetal health surveillance in labour. J Soc Obstet Gynaecol Can 1995; 17:865–901. [Review]
20. Royal College of Obstetricians and Gynaecologists. The use of electronic fetal monitoring. The use and interpretation of cardiotocography in intrapartum surveillance. Evidence-Based Clinical Guidelines No. 8. London: RCOG Press, 2001:136. [Review]
21. Chauhan SP, Klauser CK, Woodring TC, et al. Intrapartum nonreassuring fetal heart rate tracing and prediction of adverse outcomes: interobserver variability. Am J Obstet Gynecol 2008; 199:623.e1–623.e5. [II-3]
22. Nielsen PV, Stigsby B, Nickelsen C, et al. Intra-and inter-observer variability in the assessment of intrapartum cardiotocograms. Acta Obstet Gynecol Scand 1987; 66:421–424. [Level II-3]
23. Zain HA, Wright JW, Parrish GE, et al. Interpreting the fetal heart rate tracing: effect of knowledge of neonatal outcome. J Repro Med 1998; 43:367–370. [Level II-3]
24. Nelson KB, Dambrosia JM, Ting TY, et al. Uncertain value of electronic fetal monitoring in predicting cerebral palsy. NEJM 1996; 324:613–618. [II-2]
25. Devoe LD, McDaniel T. Visual vs. computerized analysis of FHR tracings. Cont Obstet Gynecol 2002; May:65–80. [Review]
26. Chauhan SP, Macones GA. ACOG Practice Bulletin No. 62: Intrapartum fetal heart rate monitoring. Obstet Gynecol 2005; 105(5 pt 1):1161–1169. [Review]
27. Hofmeyr GJ, Kulier R. Tocolysis for preventing fetal distress in second stage of labour. Cochrane Database Syst Rev 1996; (1): CD000037. [Meta-analysis: 2 RCTs, $n = 164$]
28. Skupski DW, Rosenberg CR, Eglinton GS. Intrapartum fetal stimulation tests: a meta-analysis. Obstet Gynecol 2002; 99:129–134. [Meta-analysis: 11 studies (not RCTs)].
29. East CE, Leader LR, Sheehan P, et al. Intrapartum fetal scalp lactate sampling for fetal assessment in the presence of a nonreassuring fetal heart rate trace. Cochrane Database Syst Rev 2010; (3):CD006174. [Meta-analysis: 2 RCTs, $n = 3348$]
30. Kruger K, Hallberg B, Blennow M, et al. Predictive value of fetal scalp blood lactate concentration and pH markers of neurologic disability. Am J Obstet Gynecol 1999; 181:1072–1078. [Level II-3]
31. Hofmeyr GJ. Amnioinfusion for potential or suspected umbilical cord compression in labour. Cochrane Database Syst Rev 1998; (1):CD000013. Updated 2010; (8). [Meta-analysis: 14 RCTs, most with <200 women each]
32. Busowski J, Pendergraft JS, Parsons M, et al. Transabdominal amnioinfusion prior to induction of labor. Am J Obstet Gynecol 1995; 172:287. [RCT, $n = 31$. *Decreased amniotic fluid prior to induction of labour.* Transabdominal amnioinfusion with 250 mL normal saline over 20 minutes under ultrasound guidance using a 22-gauge needle ($n = 16$), compared with no amnioinfusion ($n = 15$)]
33. Vergani P, Ceruti P, Strobelt N, et al. Transabdominal amnioinfusion in oligohydramnios at term before induction of labor with intact membranes: a randomized clinical trial. Am J Obstet

Gynecol 1996; 175:465–470. [RCT, $n = 79$. Oligohydramnios (largest amniotic fluid pocket $<2 \times 2$ cm on perpendicular planes); no FHR abnormality. Transabdominal amnioinfusion under ultrasonographic guidance: normal saline 500 mL at 37°C infused through a 20-gauge spinal needle at 30 mL/min. Sulbactam-ampicillin 3 g given intravenously ($n = 39$), compared with no amnioinfusion ($n = 40$)]

34. Kulier R, Hofmeyr GJ. Tocolytics for suspected intrapartum fetal distress. Cochrane Database Syst Rev 1996; (1):CD000037. Updated 2010; (8). [Meta-analysis: 3 RCTs, $n = 103$]

35. Magann EF, Cleveland RS, Dockery JR, et al. Acute tocolysis for fetal distress: terbutaline versus magnesium sulphate. Aust NZ J Obstet Gynaecol 1993; 33:362–364. [RCT, $n = 46$]

36. Simpson KR, James DC. Efficacy of intrauterine resuscitation techniques in improving fetal oxygen status during labor. Obstet Gynecol 2005; 105:1362–1368. [RCT, $n = 56$]

37. Huaman EJ, Hassoun R, Itahashi CM, et al. Results obtained with piracetam in foetal distress during labour. J Int Med Res 1983; 11:129–136. [RCT, $n = 96$. Peru L. Fetal distress: meconium-stained amniotic fluid and/or pathological fetal heart rate pattern. Piracetam ($n = 48$) vs. placebo ($n = 48$), intravenously 6 ampoules at once and 2 ampoules hourly]

38. Walker N. A case for conservatism in management of foetal distress. BMJ 1959; 2:1221–1226. [RCT, $n = 350$. Fetal distress: meconium-stained liquor; fetal heart rate below 110/minute, above 160/minute, or irregular. Drawn envelop from drum for either operative delivery or expectant management]

39. Neilson JP. Fetal electrocardiogram (ECG) for fetal monitoring during labour. Cochrane Database Syst Rev 2006; (3):CD000116. Updated 2009; (3). [Meta-analysis; 5 RCTs, $n = 10,628$]

40. Potti S, Berghella V. ST waveform analysis (STAN) vs cardiotocography alone for intrapartum monitoring: a meta-analysis. Am J Obstet Gynecol 2011; 204:s262. [Meta-analysis]

41. Amer-Wahlin I, Hellsten C, Noren H, et al. Cardiotocography only versus cardiotocography plus ST analysis of fetal electrocardiogram for intrapartum fetal monitoring: a Swedish randomised controlled trial. Lancet 2001; 358:534–538. [RCT, $n = 4966$. CTG plus ST analysis of fetal ECG (2519 women) versus CTG alone (2477). The monitoring device was the STAN S21 (Neoventa Medical, Gothenburg) that incorporates an "expert system" to provide advice to clinical staff. In this, it constitutes a technically more advanced system than used in the Westgate 1993 trial.]

42. Westgate J, Harris M, Curnow JSH, et al. Plymouth randomized trial of cardiotocogram only vs ST waveform plus cardiotoco-

gram for intrapartum monitoring in 2400 cases. Am J Obstet Gynecol 1993; 169:1151–1160. [RCT, $n = 2434$]

43. Ojala K, Vaarasmaki M, Makikallio K, et al. A comparison of intrapartum automated fetal electrocardiography and conventional cardiography—a randomized controlled study. Br J Obstet Gynecol 2006; 113:419–423. [RCT, $n = 1483$]

44. Vayssiere C, David E, Meyer N, et al. A French randomized controlled trial of ST-segment analysis in a population with abnormal cardiotocograms during labor. Am J Obstet Gynecol 2007; 197(3):299.e1–299.e6. [RCT, $n = 799$]

45. Westerhuis ME, Visser GH, Moons KG, et al. Cardiotocography plus ST analysis of fetal electrocardiogram compared with cardiotocography only for intrapartum monitoring: a randomized controlled trial. Obstet Gynecol 2010; 115(6):1173–1180. [RCT, $n = 5681$]

46. Strachan BK, van Wijngaarden WJ, Sahota D, et al, for the FECG Study Group. Cardiotocography only versus cardiotocography plus PR-interval analysis in intrapartum surveillance: a randomised, multicentre trial. Lancet 2000; 355:456–459. [RCT, $n = 957$]

47. East CE, Begg L, Colditz PB. Fetal pulse oximetry for fetal assessment in labour. Cochrane Database Syst Rev 2007; (2): CD004075. [Meta-analysis: 6 RCTs, $n = 7654$]

48. Garite TJ, Dildy GA, McNamara H, et al. A multicenter controlled trial of fetal pulse oximetry in the intrapartum management of nonreassuring fetal heart rate patterns. Am J Obst Gynecol 2000; 183(5):1049–1058. [RCT, $n = 1010$. Control group: fetal heart rate monitoring (CTG) (Doppler/fetal scalp electrode). Study group: CTG plus fetal pulse oximetry. Protocol for action with reassuring and nonreassuring fetal oximetry values]

49. Kuhnert M, Schmidt S. Intrapartum management of nonreassuring fetal heart rate patterns: a randomized controlled trial of fetal pulse oximetry. Am J Obstet Gynecol 2004; 191:1989–1995. [RCT, $n = 146$]

50. Klauser CK, Christensen EE, Chauhan SP, et al. Use of fetal pulse oximetry among high-risk women in labor: a randomized clinical trial. Am J Obstet Gynecol 2005; 192:1810–1819. [RCT, $n = 360$]

51. East CE, Brennecke SP, King JK, et al. The effect of intrapartum fetal pulse oximetry, in the presence of nonreassuring fetal heart pattern, on operative delivery rates: a multicenter, randomized, controlled trial (the FOREMOST trial). Am J Obstet Gynecol 2006; 194:606–616. [RCT, $n = 600$]

52. Bloom SL, Spong CY, Thom E, et al.; National Institute of Child Health and Human Development Maternal-Fetal Medicine Units Network. Fetal pulse oximetry and cesarean delivery. N Engl J Med 2006; 355(21):2195–2120. [RCT, $n = 5341$].

11

Analgesia and anesthesia

Rolf Alexander Schlichter and Valerie Arkoosh

KEY POINTS

- **In every hospital providing labor and delivery services, anesthesia personnel has to be available on a 24-hour basis,** with the ability to perform a cesarean delivery (CD) within 30 minutes from decision.
- **Intravenous pain relief is inferior to neuraxial analgesia,** minimally effective, and associated with several maternal and fetal/neonatal side effects.
- **Neuraxial analgesia provides the best pain relief in labor,** and should be **available to all laboring women upon request.**
- In the absence of a medical condition associated with coagulopathy, it is not necessary to obtain a platelet count before neuraxial analgesia/anesthesia. In general, women with platelet counts of $\geq$75,000/μL can safely receive neuraxial analgesia. Women with platelet counts of 50,000 to 75,000/μL, or less, are potential candidates for neuraxial analgesia.
- As there is no benefit to obstetric outcome from delaying neuraxial analgesia until an arbitrary cervical dilation has been reached, **the decision of when to initiate neuraxial analgesia should be made individually with each woman.**
- **The patient should be counseled regarding the effects of neuroaxial analgesia in labor. These include the following:**
  - **Neuroaxial anesthesia is associated with much better pain relief** compared with any other intervention for pain relief, and with lower risk of umbilical cord pH < 7.20 compared with systemic opioids.
  - **Neuraxial analgesia is associated with an increased incidence of hypotension, pruritus, urinary retention, and modest maternal fever; increased need for oxytocin administration; increased duration of the second stage (by about 15 minutes); and increased risk of instrumental vaginal birth.**
  - **Rare complications of neuraxial analgesia include postdural puncture headache (PDPH), respiratory depression from opioid use, epidural or spinal hematoma or abscess.**
- Discontinuation of neuraxial analgesia in the second stage does not impact obstetric outcome.
- Use of **low doses of anesthetic medications, prophylactic prehydration,** and **phenylephrine or ephedrine** can **decrease** the incidence of **maternal hypotension and associated** nonreassuring fetal heart rate **(NRFHR).**
- Compared with the standard epidural approach, combined spinal epidural **(CSE)** has been shown to **produce a quicker** (by about 6 minutes) **onset of analgesia,** result in a **lower total dose of local anesthetic** over the course of the labor, achieve a **lower median visual analog pain score earlier in labor, increase** the incidence of **maternal satisfaction,** have a **lower incidence of incomplete block,** and

possibly lower incidence of instrument-assisted deliveries, **but is associated with an increased likelihood of maternal pruritus.**
- **For CD, neuraxial anesthesia is the anesthetic technique of choice. Spinal (intrathecal) anesthesia has advantages over epidural anesthesia including quicker onset of surgical anesthesia, simplicity, lower total drug dose, and superior abdominal muscle relaxation.** Compared with epidural anesthesia, the spinal technique is associated with a similar failure rate, need for supplemental intraoperative analgesia, need for conversion to general anesthesia intraoperatively, maternal satisfaction, need for postoperative pain relief and neonatal intervention.
- **Hypotension** following spinal analgesia for CD can **be decreased by crystalloid or colloid administration, phenylephrine (bolus or infusion), ephedrine, and lower limb compression.**
- **General anesthesia for CD should be avoided if at all possible** as it is associated with a threefold risk of maternal death compared with neuraxial analgesia. Risks include inability to intubate or ventilate the patient at the induction of general anesthesia as well as airway complications at emergence from anesthesia. There are no evident advantages to general anesthesia in the absence of a contraindication to a neuraxial approach.

HISTORIC NOTES

In 1847, Dr James Young Simpson first administered chloroform to a woman during childbirth. The practice of obstetric anesthesia has changed markedly since. In 2006, about 60% (2.4 millions) of laboring U.S. women chose and received epidural or CSE analgesia. Women in labor now receive analgesia, rather than anesthesia, with the goal of enabling maternal mobility during labor. Refined anesthetic techniques for women requiring CD have decreased substantially the number of maternal deaths directly related to anesthesia.

DEFINITIONS

Analgesia: From the Greek, "no pain"—partial or complete relief of pain sensation (absence of sensitivity to pain) without loss of consciousness

Anesthesia: From the Greek, "no sensation"—historically defined as loss of sensation and total/partial consciousness

GENERAL COMMENTS

Labor is associated with two sources of pain: visceral pain at T10 through L1 from uterine contractions and cervical dilation, and somatic pain transmitted by the pudendal nerve at S2 through S4 from descent and consequent pressure of the fetal head on the pelvic floor, vagina, and perineum (1). This pain is amenable to safe intervention. **While not all laboring women desire the services of an anesthesiologist, maternal request is a sufficient medical indication for pain relief in labor** (2).

Pregnant women have a **unique physiology** compared with the general population. After the first trimester, they are at increased risk for aspiration of gastric contents, have decreased oxygen reserve, and are much more likely to be difficult to intubate than a nonpregnant woman. Maternal mortality associated with general anesthesia is estimated at approximately 32/1,000,000 live births, versus 1.9/1,000,000 live births for neuraxial analgesia (1).

Pregnant patients should be positioned with **left uterine displacement** when supine after about 22 to 24 weeks of gestational age. Left uterine displacement prevents aortocaval compression, which can result in a marked decrease in venous return to the heart and a subsequent drop in cardiac output. The ability to compensate for aortocaval compression is compromised in the presence of neuraxial analgesia or anesthesia.

When considering anesthesia or analgesia, one must take into account that pregnant women are **more sensitive to sedative hypnotics, local anesthetics, and the inhaled anesthetic agents** than nonpregnant women. Also, the pregnant patient is, in reality, *two patients* and occasionally the needs of one must be prioritized over the other. An informed consent should be attempted in case of an emergency, and the patient's wishes for an unmedicated birth always respected.

Hospitals providing labor and delivery services must have **anesthesia personnel available on a 24-hour basis**, with the ability to perform a CD within 30 minutes from decision (3). Availability of licensed practitioners to administer anesthetics and support vital functions in emergencies is recommended (2,3). Successful initiation of breastfeeding is not affected by neuraxial analgesia.

NONNEURAXIAL LABOR ANALGESIA
Acupuncture and Acupressure
Compared with no intervention or placebo, **acupuncture** for pain in labor is associated with less intense pain, increased satisfaction with pain relief, and reduced use of pharmacological analgesia, in small trials. Compared with no intervention or placebo, **acupressure** has been associated with less pain intensity, in small trials (4). Therefore, acupuncture and acupressure may have a role with reducing pain, increasing satisfaction with pain management and reduced use of pharmacological management. However, there is a need for further research before a recommendation for their routine use.

Biofeeback
Despite some positive results shown in some very small trials, there is insufficient evidence that biofeedback is effective for the management of pain during labor (5).

Aromatherapy
The limited evidence available does not show benefit, or harm, from aromatherapy for labor pain relief compared to no aromatherapy (6).

Hypnosis
Women taught self-hypnosis have decreased requirements for pharmacological analgesia, including epidural analgesia, and are more satisfied with their pain management in labor compared with controls (7).

Massage
There is insufficient evidence to assess the effect of massage therapy on labor pain (8).

Relaxation
There is insufficient evidence to assess the effect of relaxation techniques on labor pain (9).

Transcutaneous Nerve Stimulation
There is only limited evidence that transcutaneous nerve stimulation (TENS) reduces pain in labor and it does not seem to have any impact (either positive or negative) on other outcomes for mothers or neonates (10). The use of TENS at home in early labor has not been evaluated. Where TENS was used as an adjunct to epidural analgesia, there was no evidence that it reduced pain.

Systemic Analgesia
Opioids (IV/IM). Numerous choices exist for systemic analgesia during the first stage of labor, including intravenous opioid agonist-antagonists such as buprenorphine (Buprenex), butorphanol (Stadol), or nalbuphine (Nubain), or pure opioid agonists such as meperidine, fentanyl (Duragesic), morphine, hydromorphone, or their derivatives. Characteristics of some of these drugs are shown in Table 11.1.

Efficacy. These drugs are similarly efficacious, or better stated, similarly minimally efficacious in relief of maternal labor pain. In one small study, **compared with placebo, meperidine (Demerol, pethidine) 100 mg IM in early labor**

Table 11.1 Intravenous or Intramuscular Opioid Agents for Maternal Pain Relief in Labor

Agent	Usual dose (mg)	Frequency (every hour)	Onset (min)	Neonatal half-life (hours)
Tramadol	50–100 mg	4		
Pentazocine	30 mg IV or IM	3–4		
Meperidine	25–50 IV	1–2	5	13–22
	50–100 IM	2–4	30–45	>60
Fentanyl	50–100 µg IV	1	1	5
Nalbuphine	10 IV or IM	3	2–3 (IV)	4
			15 (IM)	
Butorphanol	1–2 IV or IM	4	1–2 (IV)	4
			10–30 (IM)	
Morphine	2–5 IV	4	5 (IV)	7
	10 IM		30–40 (IM)	

Source: Adapted from Ref. 1.

is associated with a very modest (17 mm) reduction in the visual analogue scale (VAS) pain score at 30 minutes (11,12). Request for epidural analgesia is delayed to 232 minutes compared with 75 minutes for parturients receiving placebo, with no further requests for analgesia in 32% versus 4% of women receiving meperidine or placebo, respectively (12).

There is not enough evidence to definitively evaluate the comparative efficacy of the various systemic opioids used to provide labor analgesia. There are problems with the methodological quality of some trials, and lack of consistency in the way various outcomes are reported. Nonetheless, using a variety of measures, including pain relief, maternal satisfaction with analgesia, interval to delivery, and obstetric outcome, there is no evidence of significant differences between meperidine, and tramadol (Ultram, meptazinol), or pentazocine (Talwin) (11).

Safety. Maternal: There is not enough evidence to definitively evaluate the comparative safety of the various systemic opioids used to provide labor analgesia. Common side effects include maternal sedation, nausea, hypotension, respiratory depression, and potential for neonatal respiratory depression. There is weak evidence of more frequent adverse effects such as maternal nausea, vomiting, and drowsiness with meptazinol compared to meperidine. However, both tramadol and pentazocine have fewer maternal side effects when compared with meperidine (11), making these two agents the ones with the best evidence of both moderate efficacy and lowest incidence of side effects among the opioid analgesic agents.

Fetal: Intravenous opioids cross the placenta and can affect the fetus/neonate. When compared with neuraxial analgesia, intravenous opioids are associated with increased incidence of NRFHR, lower fetal base excess, and decreased fetal respirations and tone at birth. Drugs with active metabolites, such as meperidine (active metabolite normeperidine), are associated with more prolonged neonatal sedation. Agonist/antagonists such as nalbuphine can result in both cardiac and respiratory depression in the baby although there is no data that demonstrates adverse outcomes. Naloxone is a pure opioid antagonist and is the drug of choice in treatment of maternal or neonatal respiratory and neurobehavioral depression secondary to opioid agonist agents. Repeated doses might be necessary, but excess use can be associated with neonatal withdrawal seizures.

Compared with neuraxial analgesic techniques, systemic medications are much less effective at decreasing visual analog pain scores (see below).

Nonneuraxial Blocks

First stage. Pain from cervical dilation (but not uterine contractions) can be blocked by a paracervical block. There are no trials to assess the effectiveness of paracervical block in labor. Risks include maternal local anesthetic toxicity from intravenous injection, fetal local anesthetic toxicity from inadvertent fetal injection, and a strong association with fetal bradycardia.

In women with severe lower back pain, four injections of sterile water, either 0.1 mL intracutaneously or 0.5 mL subcutaneously in the lumbar-sacral region, has been shown to be effective in reducing severe back pain (13).

Second stage. During the second stage of labor, perineal pain (e.g., from episiotomy) can be blocked with a pudendal block. There are no trials to assess the effectiveness of pudendal block in labor. There is a small risk of maternal local anesthetic toxicity due to accidental intravenous injection.

NEURAXIAL (REGIONAL) LABOR ANALGESIA (EPIDURAL, SPINAL, OR CSE)
Overview of Techniques
Neuraxial labor analgesia is also commonly called regional analgesia. It can be provided via the epidural space, the intrathecal (spinal) space, or both.

Medications injected into the epidural space have a relatively slow analgesic onset of 8 to 15 minutes. Block height is determined by the volume of medication injected into the epidural space. For example, to achieve a dermatome level of T10 to L2 for early labor analgesia, a volume of 8 to 10 mL is usually sufficient, contrasted with 20 to 25 mL to achieve a block height of T4 for CD. In the epidural space, injecting low-concentration local anesthetic produces analgesia and injecting high-concentration local anesthetic produces anesthesia.

By contrast, medication injected into the intrathecal space has a quick onset of 2 to 5 minutes. Block height is determined primarily by the baricity [density relative to cerebrospinal fluid (CSF)] of the injectate and, to some extent the total volume of drug. Intrathecal analgesia is produced when small doses of local anesthetic are injected (i.e., bupivacaine 2.5 mg for labor analgesia), whereas anesthesia is produced with higher doses (i.e., bupivacaine 15 mg for CD anesthesia).

Epidural Analgesia
Technique. The epidural space is located using a special needle and a loss of resistance (to air or saline) technique (Figure 11.1) (14). A onetime injection is rarely used; instead, a small catheter is placed into the epidural space through which local anesthetics and opioids can be either intermittently injected (bolus) or given as a continuous infusion.

Local anesthetic choices include low-concentration bupivacaine, ropivacaine, or lidocaine. Opioids can be used alone early in labor, but are more often combined with local anesthetics. The semisynthetic opioids fentanyl and sufentanil are used most commonly. Their addition to local anesthetics produces an additive effect that results in a lower concentration of local anesthetic being required to produce adequate labor analgesia. A lower concentration of local anesthetic increases maternal mobility and decreases the potential for maternal systemic toxicity. There is insufficient evidence comparing concentrations, type of anesthetic used, and several other technical aspects of epidural anesthesia in labor to recommend one specific drug "cocktail" (15).

The epidural infusion rate can be either controlled by the anesthesiologist or the patient. Patient-controlled epidural analgesia (PCEA) typically employs a background infusion of local anesthetic and opioid together with enabling the parturient to augment the infusion with a bolus dose every 10 to 15 minutes. This technique can also be used with a spinal catheter with appropriately reduced doses.

Indications. The primary indication for neuraxial analgesia is maternal request during labor (1). Other indications may include anticipated difficulty in intubation, history of malignant hyperthermia, high risk for CD, the presence of a comorbidity that would benefit from the reduced catecholamine levels produced by adequate labor analgesia (e.g., selected respiratory or cardiac disease) or prophylaxis against autonomic hyperreflexia in the woman with a high spinal cord lesion. Functioning epidural catheters can also be used to provide anesthesia for instrumented delivery and extraction of a retained placenta. PCEA is very useful for patients laboring for an extended period of time. Additionally, it can be used as a manpower extender for a busy obstetric anesthesia service.

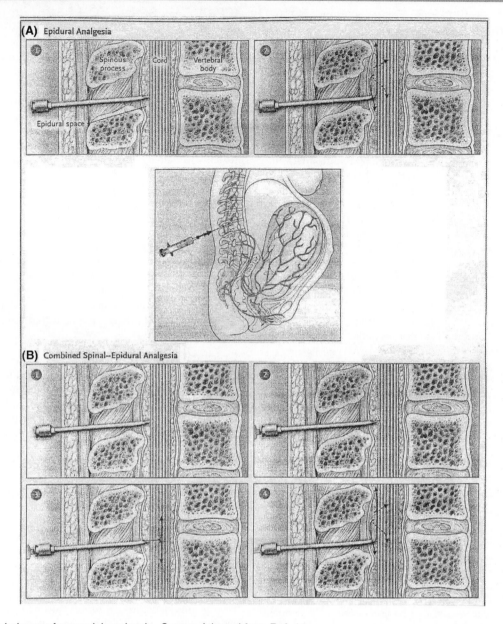

Figure 11.1   Techniques of neuraxial analgesia. *Source*: Adapted from Ref. 14.

In some cases, an epidural catheter can be intentionally inserted into the intrathecal space to provide continuous spinal analgesia. However, the resulting PDPH incidence may be high. Nonetheless, this risk is acceptable in certain situations such as the presence of certain maternal comorbidities (typically cardiac), the severely morbidly obese parturient with an airway that appears extremely difficult or impossible to intubate, or following an inadvertent dural puncture during a difficult epidural placement.

Efficacy and advantages.   Compared with nonpharmacologic techniques or to intravenous opioids, epidural analgesia provides **significantly better pain relief** (15). In >85% of cases, the pain relief is optimal. **As labor results in severe pain for many women, and neuraxial analgesia is the most effective intervention to decrease or eliminate this pain, neuraxial analgesia should be offered, when available, to all women in labor (assuming no medical contraindication)** (15).

Compared with systemic opioids, **epidural anesthesia is associated with much better pain relief, lower risk of umbilical cord pH <7.20**; and no significant effect on the incidence of CD (RR 1.07, 95% CI 0.93–1.23), long-term backache, low neonatal Apgar scores at 5 minutes, and other maternal and neonatal outcomes. No studies reported on rare but potentially serious adverse effects of epidural analgesia (15). Neuraxial analgesia is the least depressant method of analgesia for the fetus/neonate.

There is no reason to delay epidural placement until an arbitrary cervical dilation has been reached. Data suggest that neuraxial analgesia can be offered as early as 2 cm without adversely affecting labor outcome or incidence of CD. Epidural placement at ≤2 to 5 cm is associated with similar maternal (instrumental delivery, CD, etc.) and neonatal outcomes compared with epidural placement at ≥3 to 5 cm in women in spontaneous labor or receiving oxytocin (16–20). Therefore, **the** decision of when to place epidural analgesia should be made individually with each woman (1).

PCEA gives the patient control over her analgesia. Patients receive less local anesthetic overall (and therefore have less motor blockade) and receive fewer "top offs" (manual boluses from the anesthesiologist) (15,21). As patient satisfaction is high with epidural analgesia, PCEA is not associated with additional improvement in maternal satisfaction.

There is insufficient evidence to support the hypothesis that discontinuing epidural analgesia late in labor (e.g., at the beginning of the second stage) reduces the rate of instrumental delivery. There is evidence that it increases the rate of inadequate pain relief in the second stage of labor (22).

Safety, disadvantages, and complications. Compared with nonneuraxial analgesia, epidural analgesia is associated with an increased risk of mild maternal **fever, hypotension,** and **urinary retention; increase need for oxytocin administration; increase duration of the second stage (by about 15 minutes); increased risk of instrumental vaginal birth** (RR 1.38, 95% CI 1.24–1.53) (15).

The etiology of the occasional **increase in maternal temperature** associated with epidural use is uncertain. This effect can lead to increased maternal and neonatal antibiotic treatments, as well as neonatal sepsis evaluations, but with no difference in the corresponding rate of neonatal infection or sepsis (23). In centers with structured protocols for neonatal sepsis workups, there are no increases in the incidence of neonatal sepsis workups in babies born to mothers with epidural analgesia.

Maternal **hypotension** following neuraxial analgesia can occur and can affect both mothers and their babies. Hypotension is associated with an increased incidence of NRFHT that **rarely (1–2%) necessitates** CD. Left uterine displacement should be maintained whenever possible as it will increase maternal preload and increase uterine perfusion. Measures such as fluid preloading and concurrent administration of phenylephrine or ephedrine can mitigate or prevent maternal hypotension.

Although the risk of long-term **backache** in women who utilize epidural analgesia is similar to controls (IM meperidine), it is quite common for a woman to experience soreness or tenderness at the site of epidural insertion for 2 to 3 days (24).

Disadvantages of epidural analgesia include a slower onset compared with intrathecal (spinal) injection, incomplete blockade of pain (in about 10–15% of patients), and inadvertent intrathecal or intravascular catheter placement. While the PCEA gives the patient more control and entails less intervention from anesthesiologists, this can lead to underdosing and therefore inadequate analgesia: for example, if the patient does not self-administer a bolus (if she is asleep), or if there is a pump malfunction.

Other complications include a 1% to 2% chance of **PDPH** following accidental lumbar puncture, and rarely, epidural **hematoma, respiratory arrest** due to the unrecognized injection of an epidural dose of opioid into the intrathecal space, systemic local anesthetic toxicity due to unrecognized intravenous injection, or total spinal anesthesia from an unrecognized intrathecal injection of a dose of local anesthetic meant for the epidural space. See under spinal analgesia and anesthesia emergencies for further details on these complications and strategies for their prevention and treatment.

Women should be counseled about these risks before labor (23).

Interventions to avoid some disadvantages and complications of epidural analgesia. **Preloading with IV fluids to prevent hypotension:** Preloading with IV fluids (500–1000 mL, or weight-based formula 10–20 mL/kg) prior to traditional high-dose local anesthetic blocks may have some beneficial fetal and maternal effects in healthy women (25). Using the now recommended **low-dose** analgesic solutions for epidural techniques, preloading with IV fluids is associated with **no significant difference in maternal hypotension,** although only a very large effect was excluded. There is, however, a **trend toward less frequent fetal heart rate** abnormalities (25), thus some fluid preloading is still recommended.

Prophylactic ephedrine to prevent NRFHR: Compared with no ephedrine, ephedrine 10 mg IV bolus, followed by a 20 mg continuous infusion over 60 minutes, started in the first minutes after the epidural test dose, significantly **decreases the incidence of NRFHT** from 15% to 3% (26).

Spinal Analgesia

Technique. Using a small-bore spinal needle (typically a pencil point–type needle that minimizes trauma to the dura and thus reduces the incidence of PDPH), a dural puncture is made and proper location confirmed by CSF aspiration (Fig. 11.1). A single injection of an analgesic dose (much less than for epidural analgesia) of an opioid such as fentanyl, or sufentanil, with or without a local anesthetic such as bupivacaine or ropivacaine, is administered.

Indications. Indications for single injection spinals include advanced labor where delivery is imminent, forceps deliveries in women without epidurals and for patients with retained placentas.

Advantages. Advantages for single injection spinals include ease and speed of onset, completeness of block, and lower incidence of PDPH compared with epidural analgesia.

Disadvantages and complications. Disadvantages for single injection spinals are inability to re-dose (which can be solved with a spinal catheter or CSE).

Postdural puncture headache: PDPH occurs with a frequency of approximately 1% to 2% after either spinal or CSE analgesia when administered using a small-gauge pencil-point needle. PDPH is believed to be caused by leak of CSF through the punctured dura. The leak of CSF and subsequent decreased spinal fluid pressure leads to downward traction or stretch on the meninges with resulting symptoms. PDPH is characterized by a frontal-occipital headache that is exacerbated by being upright (gravity worsening stretch on the meninges), improving when the patient is supine. Diploplia, tinnitus, nausea, and vomiting (from stretch on the cranial nerves) are also common. **Although pencil-point design spinal needles have significantly reduced the incidence of PDPH following spinal analgesia,** there are no proven interventions to prevent PDPH following inadvertent dural puncture with an epidural needle. Usual early interventions include analgesics, supine positioning, caffeine, and hydration. In about 1/3 of cases, the headache persists and is severe enough to require an epidural blood patch procedure. An epidural blood patch is performed by drawing 15 to 20 mL of the patient's blood and sterilely injecting it into the patient's epidural space at the level of the dural puncture. Resolution of symptoms with blood patch occurs in 70% to 85% of women. Expected side effects following epidural blood patch include backache and leg pain (27).

Respiratory depression or arrest: Respiratory depression or arrest due to intrathecal opioids occurs rarely, 1 in 5000 to 10,000 patients. Naloxone reverses this complication and should be readily available, along with airway management equipment when administering labor analgesia.

Hematoma: Hematoma after epidural or spinal analgesia is extremely rare (1/168,000), and if suspected the patient should undergo prompt definitive imaging (MRI) of her neuraxis, followed by surgical decompression after diagnosis. Surgical decompression within approximately 6 hours following the onset of symptoms often prevents permanent neurologic injury. The risk of persistent neurologic injury from epidural is about 1/240,000 (14).

Combined Spinal Epidural

Technique (Fig. 11.1). The anesthesiologist first identifies the epidural space. Then a small-bore spinal needle, 1 cm longer than the epidural needle, is placed through the epidural needle into the cerebral spinal fluid. An intrathecal dose of local anesthetic and opioids is injected through the spinal needle, which is then removed, leaving the epidural needle in place. An epidural catheter is inserted and an epidural local anesthetic and opioid infusion is started. The intrathecal dose generally lasts about 2 hours, at which point, the epidural infusion should be providing adequate analgesia.

Indications. A CSE technique provides the benefit of immediate onset of spinal analgesia coupled with the indefinite duration of an epidural catheter technique. The CSE technique is particularly useful for women in advanced labor requesting pain relief. There are data that associate CSE with an increased rate of cervical dilatation and shorter length of labor compared with both intravenous opioid and epidural analgesia (28–30). Indications for a CSE are the same as those for both epidural and spinal techniques.

Advantages. Both CSE and epidural techniques provide effective pain relief in labor. The type (opioids with or without local anesthetics) and concentration of local anesthetic used in the CSE or epidural technique impact maternal mobilization and other outcomes more than the technique itself (31). **There appears to be little basis for offering CSE over epidurals in labor, with no difference in overall maternal satisfaction despite a slightly faster onset (about 6 minutes) with CSE, and less pruritus with epidurals.** There is some evidence that CSE compared with an epidural is associated with a faster rate of cervical dilatation in nulliparous women less than 5 cm (29), and women close to imminent birth may benefit from the speed of onset a CSE offers. There is no difference in ability to mobilize, obstetric outcome, or neonatal outcome (31).

Disadvantages. Disadvantages of CSE are similar to epidural and spinal techniques. Although data is limited, no differences are reported between intravenous preloading and no preloading to prevent hypotension (25). Women who receive intrathecal opioids experience **more pruritus** than with a standard epidural (31). However, pruritus is very common after both spinal and epidural opioids. Pruritus from neuraxial opioid injection results from μ-opioid receptor stimulation in the brainstem. Thus, either naloxone or nalbuphine are effective interventions. Diphenhydramine and other antihistamines are not effective in treating opioid-induced pruritus because opioids administered via the intrathecal or epidural route do not cause histamine release. **The significantly higher incidence of urinary retention and rescue interventions with traditional techniques would favor the use of low-dose epidurals** (31). It is not possible to draw any meaningful conclusions as to possible differences between CSE and epidural in producing rare complications such as nerve injury and meningitis.

Contraindications to Regional Anesthesia

Coagulopathy. A routine platelet count is not necessary before administering neuraxial analgesia in the healthy parturient. Indications for platelet count may include severe preeclampsia, hemolysis, elevated liver enzymes, and low platelets (HELLP) syndrome, idiopathic thrombocytopenia purpura (ITP), abruption, or other risks for disseminated intravascular coagulation (DIC). Assuming the patient is not in DIC, a platelet count of $\geq 100,000/\mu L$ is considered safe, but several studies have also confirmed that platelets levels of 50,000 to 99,000/μL are not associated with higher risk of complications (2). Women on prophylactic unfractionated heparin or low-dose aspirin are not at increased risk for complications from neuraxial blocks. Women on therapeutic unfractionated heparin can receive regional analgesia if the activated partial thromboplastin time (PTT) is normal. If the PTT is elevated, protamine may be used to reverse the heparin effect. Women on low–molecular weight heparin should not receive regional analgesia until 12 to 24 hours from last dose, given a higher rate of epidural hematoma with placement during this period. Therefore, consideration should be given to converting women who require anticoagulation from low-molecular to unfractionated heparin as they approach term.

The coagulation status of parturients with medical conditions associated with coagulopathy such as the HELLP syndrome should be thoroughly evaluated before initiating a neuraxial block. Patients with platelets less than 75,000/μL should be examined for stigmata of coagulopathy (easy bruising, bleeding from the IV site, etc.) before instrumentation. A prothrombin time, a partial thrombin time, and a platelet count should all be reviewed before proceeding. A fibrinogen level and a d-dimer level are useful to assess the presence of DIC if any of the aforementioned tests are abnormal. A bleeding time is not indicated. Patients with known platelet dysfunction including those on antiplatelet medication (e.g., clopidogrel) should not receive regional analgesia. Aspirin therapy is considered an acceptable risk (32).

Infection. **Systemic:** Patients with suspected meningitis (bacterial or viral), sepsis, or viremia should not receive neuraxial blockade. Patients with suspected chorioamnionitis can receive neuraxial analgesia/anesthesia following the administration of appropriate intravenous antibiotics. Chronic herpes simplex virus (HSV) outbreak is not a contraindication to neuraxial techniques, however a primary outbreak places the parturient at risk for herpetic viremia and meningitis. HIV/AIDS is not a contraindication to spinal or epidural anesthesia, or epidural blood patch.

Localized: Patients with localized skin or soft tissue infections should not be instrumented at those sites.

ANESTHESIA AND MATERNAL COMORBIDITIES
Hypertensive Disorders

Advantages of analgesia. Patients with gestational hypertension may benefit from neuraxial analgesia, as it may improve uterine perfusion through several pathways (localized neuraxial vasodilatory effect, reduced catecholamine release). **Neuraxial analgesia is the analgesia of choice in hypertensive pregnant women.**

Disadvantages. Patients with gestational hypertension, preeclampsia, and eclampsia are at increased risk for hemodynamic instability during both labor and surgical anesthesia. Neuraxial techniques can be used safely with increased vigilance for maternal hypotension. Methods to prevent hypotension as described above should be employed.

Cautions. Caution must be taken in fluid management in this population as there is altered vascular leaking, decreased oncotic pressure, and a higher incidence of pulmonary edema. Also, there can be an exaggerated hypertensive response to ephedrine and phenylephrine. The prevention, rather than treatment, of hypotension has been associated with better outcomes for the fetus. Women with severe preeclampsia who must undergo general anesthesia are at risk for an extremely exaggerated hypertensive response to intubation and often benefit from pretreatment with an antihypertensive such as labetalol immediately prior to induction. Treatment with magnesium sulfate for preeclampsia/eclampsia can potentiate neuromuscular blockade in patients receiving general anesthesia, so care must be taken when using intermediate- to long-acting nondepolarizing muscle relaxants.

Maternal Cardiac Disease

Heart disease in the parturient is the leading cause of maternal mortality outside of obstetric complications. Understandably, the risk increases with severity of maternal disease. The normal changes in maternal cardiac physiology resulting from pregnancy can either unmask subclinical or worsen clinical cardiac disease. Every effort should be made to care for these patients in facilities equipped to provide the multidisciplinary approach that is required to ensure the best possible outcome for mother and neonate.

Valvular heart disease. Patients with acquired valvular disease (rheumatic fever, mitral valve prolapse, artificial valves, and endocarditis) are at increased risk for arrhythmias, pulmonary edema, and cardiac ischemia from the increased heart rate, cardiac output, metabolic demand, and decreased oxygen reserve associated with pregnancy and the pain of labor. Patients with arrhythmias or artificial valves may also be on heparin or low–molecular weight heparin.

Advantages of neuraxial analgesia: Epidurals (and CSE) block the pain and stress of contractions therefore reducing tachycardia and increased cardiac output. Ablation of the bearing down reflex can be advantageous in patients with aortic or mitral regurgitation.

Disadvantages: Hypotension is the largest disadvantage with neuraxial analgesia; even transient hypotension can lead to coronary hypoperfusion, ischemia, arrhythmias, or arrest. This is especially dangerous in patients with moderate to severe aortic stenosis. However, parturients with aortic stenosis have safely undergone both neuraxial labor analgesia and anesthesia for CD. Meticulous anesthetic technique and allowing adequate time to slowly administer the requisite medication is the key to safe provision of neuraxial anesthesia in these patients. Inadvertent intravenous injection of local anesthetics is also a significant risk in patients with underlying arrhythmias due to impairment of cardiac automaticity and conduction (especially with bupivacaine).

Congenital heart disease. Women with congenital heart disease (e.g., tetralogy of Fallot, hypoplastic left ventricle, transposition of the great vessels, and septal defects) are now surviving to childbearing years. Depending on the adequacy of their surgical repair, pregnancy may or may not severely impact these patients with underlying cyanotic heart disease. The increased cardiac output, oxygen consumption, changes in systemic and pulmonary resistance, and aortocaval compression can exacerbate preexisting right to left shunts increasing the risk of maternal cyanosis and death.

Advantages of epidural analgesia: Although the hypotension of large-dose spinal anesthesia can be associated with risk of shunting and cyanosis, slowly administered epidural, low-dose spinal, or continuous spinal analgesia are advantageous to these patients by reducing catecholamine levels and preventing maternal expulsive reflexes. Additionally, if an instrumented delivery or CD is required, a surgical anesthetic level can be slowly produced, avoiding the risks of general anesthesia in these patients.

Disadvantages: The largest disadvantage of neuraxial analgesia is the risk of hypotension. Hemodynamic management of these patients should be aggressive and tailored to the underlying cardiac defect.

Previous Lumbar Surgery

Previous lumbar surgery (e.g., discectomy, placement of Harrington Rods) is not a contraindication for lumbar epidural or spinal analgesia or anesthesia. One case series found that successful block can be achieved, although at a lower rate (55%) than in the control population. There were no cases of spine infection, low back pain, or headaches (33).

Maternal Obesity

The incidence of maternal obesity has been rapidly increasing worldwide. Obese parturients have higher rates of miscarriages, stillbirths, hypertension, diabetes, preeclampsia, and chorioamnionitis compared with normal weight women (see chap. 3 in *Maternal-Fetal Evidence Based Guidelines*). Also, the risks of low Apgar scores, neonatal intensive care unit admission, cesarean section, fetal death, and perinatal death are increased (34). Respiratory, gastrointestinal, and anatomical changes of pregnancy significantly increase the **risk of a failed intubation and aspiration, which is as high as 15% to 33% in obese pregnant women**. Venous access can be difficult increasing the need for central venous access. Bony landmarks and increased adipose and soft tissue can complicate placement of neuraxial analgesia and anesthesia with initial **epidural failure as high as 42%**. Obese patients are also more at risk for hypoventilation and apnea after administration of opioids, complicating postpartum and postoperative pain control. Relative immobility also increases the risk of thromboembolic events (35).

CESAREAN DELIVERY ANESTHESIA

Current guidelines recommend a fasting period of 6 to 8 hours prior to scheduled CD.

Epidural

Indications
Epidural anesthesia can be used for planned (scheduled) CD and, if a functioning catheter is in place, for most urgent or emergent deliveries. Patients with existing labor epidurals usually can have their block extended to an adequate level for surgery using a large volume of high-concentration local anesthetic, opioids, and epinephrine (which is thought to produce analgesia via α2 receptors in the spinal cord).

Advantages
The benefit of an epidural is the ability to re-dose the epidural in the event of a delayed or prolonged surgery. Also, long-acting epidural opioids can be given to augment postoperative pain control.

Disadvantages

Disadvantages include longer onset time for surgical block compared with spinal anesthesia and the possibility of incomplete or patchy block, making epidural anesthesia a less attractive option than spinal anesthesia in the case of an emergency (when an epidural catheter is not already in place). The higher doses of local anesthetics used in epidural blocks (compared with spinal) increase the risk of systemic local anesthetic toxicity. Occasionally, an epidural catheter that functioned adequately for labor analgesia is inadequate for CD anesthesia.

Spinal

Indications

Spinal anesthesia can be used for both planned cesarean sections and in most emergencies. Intrathecal morphine can be given to augment postoperative pain control.

Advantages

Intrathecal anesthesia produces adequate anesthesia significantly faster than epidural anesthesia (36). Other advantages are its simplicity, lower drug doses, and superior abdominal muscle relaxation. **Compared with epidural, spinal technique is associated with similar failure rate, need for additional intraoperative analgesia, need for conversion to general anesthesia intraoperatively, maternal satisfaction, need for postoperative pain relief, and neonatal intervention** (36). Compared with epidural, spinal anesthesia for cesarean section is associated with reduced time, by about 8 minutes, from start of the anesthetic to start of the operation.

Although regional anesthesia is preferred in a large majority of CD, general anesthesia can be done with relative safety. Compared with general anesthesia, women who had either epidural or spinal anesthesia have a significantly lower difference between pre- and postoperative hematocrit, and a lower estimated maternal blood loss (~127 mL). Compared with general anesthesia, women who had either epidural or spinal anesthesia have significantly more nausea, and a lower incidence of preferring to have the same anesthesia again. No significant difference is seen in terms of neonatal Apgar scores of <7 at 5 minutes and need for neonatal resuscitation with oxygen. Many of the studies involved in this meta-analysis are from the early 1980s and from many different countries, and may not reflect modern anesthetic practice (37).

Disadvantages

Hypotension, possibly profound, is increased in incidence 23% with spinal versus epidural anesthesia (36). No intervention reliably prevents hypotension due to spinal anesthesia for cesarean delivery, but five interventions have been found to reduce the incidence of hypotension: (*i*) **crystalloid** preload versus no crystalloid (25), (*ii*) **preemptive colloid administration** versus crystalloid; (*iii*) **ephedrine** versus no ephedrine or crystalloids; (*iv*) phenylephrine versus controls (38), and (*v*) **lower limb compression** versus no intervention (39). No differences were detected for different doses, rates or methods of administering colloids or crystalloids. No significant differences in hypotension were seen between ephedrine and phenylephrine. High rates or doses of ephedrine may increase the incidences of hypertension and tachycardia. Ephedrine is associated with dose-related maternal hypertension and tachycardia, and fetal acidosis of uncertain clinical significance. Alternatively, newer studies have shown that **phenylephrine** is as safe as ephedrine; in fact, fetal pH is higher and the incidence of maternal nausea

lower with phenylephrine (40). Different methods of compression appeared to vary in their effectiveness. No other comparisons between different physical methods such as position were shown to be effective. In summary, **interventions such as crystalloids, colloids, ephedrine, phenylephrine, or lower-leg compression can reduce the incidence of hypotension**, but none have been shown to eliminate the need to treat maternal hypotension during spinal anesthesia for cesarean section. No conclusions can be drawn regarding rare adverse effects due to the relatively small numbers of women studied.

Patients who receive intrathecal bupivacaine with prophylactic intravenous phenylephrine infusion have less hypotension than those without phenylephrine (38).

Limited duration is another disadvantage of spinal anesthesia. CSEs and spinal catheters combine the advantages of the rapid onset of spinal anesthesia with the ability to redose in the case of prolonged surgical time.

High/total **spinal** is discussed under anesthetic emergencies.

In summary, both spinal and epidural techniques are shown to provide effective anesthesia for cesarean section. Both techniques are associated with moderate degrees of maternal satisfaction. Spinal anesthesia has a shorter onset time, but treatment for hypotension is more likely if spinal anesthesia is used. No conclusions can be drawn about intraoperative side effects and postoperative complications because they were of low incidence and/or not reported. Because of its safety and effectiveness, **spinal anesthesia has developed in most L&Ds as the regional technique of choice for cesarean delivery** due in particular to rapidity of anesthetic onset, quality of anesthesia, and ease of performance of block.

General Anesthesia

Indications

In the case of failed regional anesthesia, an obstetric emergency preventing extension of an epidural or placement of a spinal, a contraindication for regional anesthesia, or objection by the patient to regional anesthesia, general anesthesia is used for CD. Additionally, halogenated anesthetic agents, in high concentrations, produce potent uterine muscle relaxation. This property can be useful in the management of uterine inversion, fetal entrapment, or retained placenta. Intravenous nitroglycerine and terbutaline are other options in these situations.

If a general anesthetic is chosen, patients must receive acid aspiration prophylaxis that may include a nonparticulate oral antacid and/or metoclopramide. Time permitting, an H2 blocker, which takes 45 minutes to be effective, can confer additional protection. Airway protection with an endotracheal tube is mandatory.

Precautions

There is insufficient evidence to assess prevention of aspiration at general anesthesia. To decrease the risk of harm from aspiration of gastric contents, the stomach should be empty with a high pH. When compared with no treatment or placebo, there is a significant reduction in the risk of intragastric pH < 2.5 with antacids, H_2 antagonists, and proton pump antagonists (41). H_2 antagonists are associated with a reduced risk of intragastric pH < 2.5 at intubation when compared with proton pump antagonists, but compared with antacids the findings were unclear. The combined use of "antacids plus H_2 antagonists" is associated with a significant reduction in the risk of intragastric pH < 2.5 at intubation when compared with placebo or compared with antacids alone (RR 0.12, 95% CI 0.02

to 0.92, 1 trial, 119 women). In general, the quality of the evidence is insufficient to make a recommendation. None of the studies assessed potential adverse effects or substantive clinical outcomes (41).

Advantages
There are *no evident advantages* to general anesthesia in the absence of a contraindication to a neuraxial approach.

Disadvantages
Compared with neuraxial anesthesia, general anesthesia is associated with a threefold risk of maternal death. The **biggest risk is from the inability to intubate or ventilate the patient**. Parturients have increased upper airway edema, lower pulmonary functional residual capacity, increased metabolic oxygen consumption, decreased lower esophageal sphincter tone, and delayed gastric emptying. These conditions increase the risk of both hypoxemia and aspiration. Airway edema can also make anesthetizing the airway for awake, fiberoptic intubation more difficult. The incidence of failed intubation in obstetric population is approximately 1 in 200 patients, versus 1 in 800 patients in the general surgical population.

    Compared with nonobstetric surgery, the risk of maternal awareness under general anesthesia is increased (0.4% vs. 0.2% for nonobstetric surgery) (42). This stems from the effort to minimize fetal exposure to medications that reduce the risk of maternal awareness. Typically, the use of sedative hypnotic medications such as benzodiazepines and opioids is limited or omitted prior to delivery of the fetus. Although benzodiazepines and opioids can depress the fetus, they are pharmacologically reversible and maternal administration should be considered if their use would benefit the mother. For instance, the judicious use of preintubation opioids can be considered in the hypertensive parturient. Opioids effectively attenuate the hypertensive response elicited by direct laryngoscopy and may be necessary to safely intubate the already hypertensive patient. The ultra-short-acting synthetic opioid remifentanil can provide this benefit with minimal effect on the neonate.

    General anesthesia is also associated with higher incidence of postoperative nausea and vomiting, maternal sedation, and increased time to breastfeeding.

    General anesthesia's effect on the fetus depends on the length of time from induction to umbilical cord clamp; length of time from hysterotomy to cord clamp is also important. Fetal exposure to inhaled anesthetics of >5 to 8 minutes is associated with neonatal depression. General anesthesia compared with neuraxial anesthesia has been shown to increase the incidence of fetal acidosis, drug exposure, and lower Apgar scores. Intravenous induction agents, opioids, and hypnotics readily cross the placenta while neuromuscular blocking agents do not (43).

Post-CD Analgesia
First 24 Hours
There are several safe and effective options for providing postcesarean analgesia. Preservative-free **morphine** hydrochloride administered **at the time of spinal** anesthesia **or** following cord clamp when using **epidural** anesthesia provides effective pain relief in the first 12 to 24 hours (1). An alternative is **patient-controlled epidural analgesia**, which can be associated with increased maternal motor weakness. However, following major surgery, such as cesarean hysterectomy, the effectiveness of continuous epidural analgesia may justify the potential for increased maternal motor weakness.

Keep in mind that opioids administered via a spinal or epidural are associated with a 35% to 55% incidence of maternal pruritus severe enough to require treatment (44). The epidural catheter should be removed after 24 hours to reduce urinary retention, pruritus, and infection risks.

    Intravenous patient-controlled opioids are another reasonable alternative, using morphine, hydromorphone hydrochloride, or fentanyl.

    Oral analgesia with oxycodone-acetaminophen 5/325 mg two tablets every 3 hours for 12 hours and then one/two tablets every 4 hours as needed is associated with superior pain control and fewer side effects compared with morphine patient-controlled intravenous analgesia in one trial (45).

    The transversus abdominis plane (TAP) block is performed by injection of local anesthetic between the internal oblique and transversus abdominis muscles. The goal is to provide anesthesia to the T7–11 intercostal nerves, the subcostal nerve (T12), and the iliohypogastric and ilioinguinal nerves (L1). TAP blocks do not block peritoneal visceral pain. The block has traditionally been done blindly; however, ultrasound guidance has improved the efficacy of the block while reducing complications such as liver, bowel, or intraperitoneal injection. Under ultrasound guidance, a catheter can be placed for prolonged analgesia. The TAP block is a reasonable alternative in a patient with a contraindication to a neuraxial block (46).

After 24 Hours
Nonsteroidal anti-inflammatory drugs reduce maternal opioid consumption after CD, even in the first 24 hours, and should be the main intervention for pain control after the first 24 hours. Use of oral narcotics should be quickly weaned.

ANESTHETIC EMERGENCIES
An anesthetic emergency in the obstetric patient necessitates clear and precise communication and cooperation between the anesthesia and obstetric teams. The goal is to stabilize the mother while, if necessary, safely and quickly delivering the neonate.

Total Spinal
A total spinal occurs with cephalad spread of local anesthetic to the breathing centers of the brainstem. This can occur with normal doses of spinally administered drug or be the result of an overdose of spinally administered medication. This can occur with accidental intrathecal placement of an epidural dose of medication or from subdural catheter placement with subsequent migration of the catheter. Control of the airway with endotracheal intubation, and blood pressure control with uterine displacement, sympathomimetic medications, and fluid should be achieved quickly. Once the airway has been secured, assessment of the fetus should be facilitated. If the fetus is stable, delivery can await maternal recovery, usually about 20 to 30 minutes.

Local Anesthetic Toxicity
Intravenous injection of local anesthetics can lead to systemic toxicity including seizures and cardiovascular collapse. The mother's airway should be controlled as rapidly as possible and delivery of the fetus is often indicated because of maternal instability. Seizures can usually be stopped quickly with small doses of most sedative-hypnotic drugs. In the case of cardiovascular collapse, sympathomimetic therapy, IV fluids, and in

some cases cardiopulmonary bypass should be initiated. In the case of bupivacaine toxicity, intravenous Intralipid, a 20% fat emulsion, has been shown to increase the survival rate of patients who experience cardiac arrest (47).

Failed Intubation

The risk of failed intubation is increased in the parturient (about 1 in 200 for the pregnant patient vs. about 1 in 800 for the general population). Increased edema in the upper airway, increased breast size, and increased friability of the mucosa increase chance of failure. In addition, parturients have decreased functional residual capacity that decreases their apneic oxygen reserve and are at higher risk for aspiration secondary to decreased gastric emptying and increased abdominal pressure. In the case of a failed intubation, the obstetric team can assist the anesthesia team by calling for help, helping to set up emergency equipment (fiberoptic bronchoscope, laryngeal mask airway, cricothyrotomy with jet ventilation) and maintaining communication. Delivery of the fetus is indicated if the mother cannot be ventilated at all and is becoming hypoxic as evidenced by a falling pulse oximetry reading.

Maternal Hemorrhage, Resuscitation, and Massive Transfusion

Maternal hemorrhage can lead to exsanguination and the need for massive transfusion, defined as the need for 10 or more units of packed red blood cells (PRBC) in 24 hours. Volume resuscitation with crystalloid, nonbiologically active colloid, and PRBCs can lead to a dilutional coagulopathy necessitating the transfusion of clotting factors and platelets. Recent retrospective studies from both military and civilian trauma have shown improved outcomes using an empirical ratio of FFP: RBC (fresh frozen plasma:red blood cells) 1:1 in settings that require massive transfusion. Keep in mind that FFP has relatively low amounts of fibrinogen so in patients with low fibrinogen levels cryoprecipitate may also be needed. Parturients may already have dilutional thrombocytopenia, thus transfusion of platelets may also be warranted; however, the optimal ratio of platelet units to other factors is not known. Risks of massive transfusion include transfusion reactions, viral infection, fluid overload, pulmonary edema, and transfusion related acute lung injury (TRALI) (48).

Cardiopulmonary Resuscitation in the Pregnant Patient

In the rare and unfortunate case that a pregnant patient experiences cardiac arrest, cardiopulmonary resuscitation (CPR) is not as effective due to aortocaval compression by the gravid uterus. Control of the airway with subsequent immediate delivery of the fetus is the priority (with delivery of the fetus being as or more important than control of the airway). Resuscitation of a pregnant woman should never be abandoned until some period of time after the fetus is delivered.

REFERENCES

1. American College of Obstetricians and Gynecologists. ACOG Practice Bulletin, number 36: Obstetric analgesia and anesthesia. Washington, D.C.: American College of Obstetricians and Gynecologists, 2002. [Review]
2. Practice Guidelines for Obstetric Anesthesia: An updated report by the American Society of Anesthesiologists Task Force on Obstetric Anesthesia. Anesthesiology 2007; 106:843–863. [Review]
3. American College of Obstetricians and Gynecologists. Optimal goals for anesthesia care in obstetrics. ACOG Committee Opinion. Washington, D.C.: American College of Obstetricians and Gynecologists, 2008. [Review]
4. Smith CA, Collins CT, Crowther CA, et al. Acupuncture or acupressure for pain management in labor. Cochrane Database Syst Rev 2011; (7):CD009232. [Meta-analysis: 13 RCTs, n = 1986]
5. Barragán Loayza IM, Solà I, Juandó Prats C. Biofeedback for pain management during labour. Cochrane Database Syst Rev 2011; (6):CD006168. [Meta-analysis: 4 RCTs, n = 186]
6. Smith CA, Collins CT, Crowther CA. Aromatherapy for pain management in labour. Cochrane Database Syst Rev 2011; (7): CD009215. [Meta-analysis: 2 RCTs, n = 535]
7. Smith CA, Collins CT, Cyna AM, et al. Complementary and alternative therapies for pain management in labour. Cochrane Database Syst Rev 2006; (4):CD003521. [Meta-analysis: Hypnosis: 5 RCTs, n = 729]
8. Smith CA, Collins CT, Cyna AM, et al. Complementary and alternative therapies for pain management in labour. Cochrane Database Syst Rev 2006; (4):CD003521. [Meta-analysis: Massage: 1 RCTs, n = 60]
9. Smith CA, Collins CT, Cyna AM, et al. Complementary and alternative therapies for pain management in labour. Cochrane Database Syst Rev 2006; (4):CD003521. [Meta-analysis: Relaxation: 1 RCTs, n = 30]
10. Dowswell T, Bedwell C, Lavender T, et al. Transcutaneous electrical nerve stimulation (TENS) for pain relief in labour. Cochrane Database Syst Rev 2009; (2):CD007214. [Meta-analysis: 19 RCTs; 1671]
11. Elbourne D, Wiseman RA. Types of intra-muscular opioids for maternal pain relief in labour. Cochrane Database Syst Rev 2005; (3). [16 RCTs; n = >5000]
12. Tsui MHY, Ngan Kee WD, Ng FF, et al. A double blinded randomized placebo-controlled study of intramuscular pethidine for pain relief in the first stage of labour. Br J Obstet Gynecol 2004; 111:648–655. [RCT, n = 112]
13. Martensson L, Wallin G. Labour pain treated with cutaneous injections of sterile water: a randomized controlled trial. Br J Obstet Gynecol 1999; 106:633–637. [RCT, n = 99]
14. Hawkins JL. Epidural analgesia for labor and delivery. N Engl J Med 2010; 362:1503–1510. [Review]
15. Anim-Somuah M, Smyth R, Howell C. Epidural versus nonepidural or no analgesia in labour. Cochrane Database Syst Rev 2005; (4). [Meta-analysis: 21 RCTs, n = 6664; 20/21 compared epidural analgesia with opiates]
16. Chestnut DH, McGrath JM, Vincent RD, et al. Does early administration of epidural analgesia affect obstetric outcome in nulliparous women who are spontaneous labor? Anesthesiology 1994; 80:1201–1208. [RCT, n = 344]
17. Chestnut DH, Vincent RD, McGrath JM, et al. Does early administration of epidural analgesia affect obstetric outcome in nulliparous women who are receiving intravenous oxytocin? Anesthesiology 1994; 80:1193–1200. [RCT, n = 150]
18. Luxman D, Wolman I, Groutz A, et al. The effect of early epidural block administration on the progression and outcome of labor. Int J Obstet Anesth 1998; 7:161–164. [RCT, n = 60]
19. Ohel G, Gonen R, Vaida S, et al. Early versus late initiation of epidural analgesia in labor: does it increase the risk of cesarean section? A randomized trial. Am J Obstet Gynecol 2006; 194:600–605. [RCT, n = 449]
20. Wassen MMLH, Zuijlen J, Roumen LJM, et al. Early versus late epidural analgesia and risk on instrumental delivery in nulliparous women: a systematic review. Br J Obstet Gynecol 2011; 118 (6):655–661. [Meta-analysis: 6 RCTs, 1 cohort, n = 15,399]
21. Usha Kiran TS, Thakur MB, Bethel JA, et al. Comparison of continuous infusion versus midwife administered top-ups of epidural bupivicaine for labour analgesia: effect on second stage of labour mode of delivery. Int J Obstet Anesth 2003; 12:9–11. [RCT]
22. Torvaldsen S, Roberts CL, Bell JC, et al. Discontinuation of epidural analgesia late in labour for reducing the adverse delivery outcomes associated with epidural analgesia. Cochrane Database Syst Rev 2005; (3). [5 RCTs, n = 462]

23. Segal S. Labor epidural analagesia and maternal fever. Anesth Analg 2010; 111:1467–1475. [Review]

24. Koughnan F, Crli M, Romney M, et al. Epidural analgesia and backache: a randomized controlled comparison with intramuscular meperidine for analgesia during labor. Br J Anaesth 2002; 89(3):466–472. [RCT]

25. Hofmeyr GJ, Cyna AM, Middleton P. Prophylactic intravenous preloading for regional analgesia in labour. Cochrane Database Syst Rev 2005; (3). [6 RCTs, $n = 473$]

26. Kreiser D, Katorza E, Seidmen DS, et al. The effect of ephedrine on Intrapartum fetal heart rate after epidural analgesia. Obstet Gynecol 2004; 104:1277–1281. [RCT, $n = 145$]

27. Harrington BE. Postdural puncture headache and the development of the epidural blood patch. Reg Anesth Pain Med 2004; 29:136–163. [II-2]

28. Rawal N, Van Zundert A, Holmstrom B, et al. Combined-spinal technique. Reg Anesth 1997; 22:406–423. [Review]

29. Tsen LC, Brad T, Datta S, et al. Is combined spinal-epidural analagesia associated with more rapid cervical dilatation in nulliparous patients when compared with conventional epidural analgesia. Anesthesiology 1999; 91:920–925. [RCT; $n = 100$]

30. Wong CA, Scavone BM, Peaceman AM, et al. The risk of cesarean delivery with neuraxial analgesia given early versus late in labor. N Engl J Med 2005; 352:655–665. [RCT, $n = 750$]

31. Simmons SW, Cyna AM, Dennis AT, et al. Combined spinal-epidural versus epidural analgesia in labour. Cochrane Database Syst Rev 2007; (3)CD003401. [Meta-analysis: 19 RCTs, $n = 2658$]

32. American Society of Regional Anesthesia and Pain Medicine Consensus Conference. Regional Anesthesia in the Anticoagulated Patient-Defining the Risks. American Society of Regional Anesthesia and Pain Medicine, 2002. [Review]

33. Ho AM, Kee WD, Chung DC. Should laboring parturients with Harrington rods receive lumbar epidural analgesia? Int J Gynaecol Obstet 1999; 67(1): 41–43. [II-3]

34. Raatikainen K, Heiskanen N, Heinon S. Transition from overweight to obesity worsens pregnancy outcome in a BMI-dependent manner. Obesity 2006; 14:165–171. [II-3]

35. Saravanakumar K, Rao SG, Cooper GM. Obesity and obstetric anaesthesia. Anaesthesia 2006; 61:36–48. [II-3]

36. Ng K, Parsons J, Cyna AM, et al. Spinal versus epidural anaesthesia for caesarean section. Cochrane Database Syst Rev 2005; (4). [Meta-analysis: 10 RCTs, $n = 751$]

37. Afolabi BB, Lesi AFE, Merah NA. Regional versus general anaesthesia for caesarean section. Cochrane Database Syst Rev 2006; (4):CD004350. [Meta-analysis: 16 RCTs, $n = 1586$]

38. Langesaeter E, Rosseland LA, Stubhaug A. Continuous invasive blood pressure and cardiac output monitoring during cesarean delivery: a randomized, double-blind comparison of low-dose versus high-dose spinal anesthesia with intravenous phenylephrine or placebo infusion a randomized, double-blind comparison of low-dose vs. high-dose spinal anesthesia with intravenous phenylephrine or placebo infusion. Anesthesiology 2008; 109:856–863. [RCT]

39. Emmett RS, Cyna AM, Andrew M, et al. Techniques for preventing hypotension during spinal anaesthesia for caesarean section. Cochrane Database Syst Rev 2005; (4). [Meta-analysis: 25 RCTs, $n = 1477$]

40. Lee A, Ngan Kee WD, Gin T. A quantitative, systematic review of randomized controlled trials of ephedrine versus phenylephrine for the management of hypotension during spinal anesthesia for cesarean delivery. Anesth Anal 2002; 94:920–926. [Meta-analysis]

41. Paranjothy S, Griffiths JD, Broughton HK, et al. Interventions at caesarean section for reducing the risk of aspiration pneumonitis. Cochrane Database Syst Rev 2010; (1):CD004943. [Meta-analysis: 22 RCTs, 2658]

42. Lyons G. MacDonald: Awareness during cesarean section. Anesthesia 1991; 46:62–64. [II-2]

43. Littleford J. Effects on the fetus and newborn of maternal analgesia and anesthesia: a review. Can J Anesth 2004; 51:585–609. [Review]

44. Dahl JB, Jeppesen IS, Jorgensen H, et al. Intraoperative and postoperative analgesic efficacy and adverse effects of intrathecal opioids in patients undergoing cesarean section with spinal anesthesia: a qualitative and quantitative systematic review of randomized controlled trials. Anesthesiology 1999; 91:1919–1927. [Meta-analysis: 11 RCTs]

45. Davis KM, Esposito MA, Meyer BA. Oral analgesia compared to intravenous patient-controlled analgesia for pain after cesarean delivery: a randomized controlled trial. Am J Obstet Gynecol 2006; 194:967–971. [RCT, $n = 93$]

46. Mukhtar K. Transversus abdominis plane (TAP) block. J N Y School Reg Anesth 2009; 12:28–33. [II-3]

47. Rosenblatt MA, Abel M, Fischer GW, et al. Successful use of a 20% lipid emulsion to resuscitate a patient after a presumed bupivicaine-related cardiac arrest. Anesthesiology 2006; 105:217–218. [III, case report]

48. Bolliger D, Gorlinger K, Tanaka KA. Pathophysiology and treatment of coagulopathy in massive hemorrhage and hemodilution. Anesthesiology 2010; 113:1205–1219. [Review]

Operative vaginal delivery

Jay Goldberg and Ariella B. Glazer

KEY POINTS

- **Vacuum- and forceps-assisted deliveries** have the **same indications**. There are **no circumstances where operative vaginal delivery is definitely indicated**. Alternatives, including allowing the patient to labor longer, oxytocin augmentation, and cesarean delivery, should always be considered.
- **When used by experienced operators, operative vaginal delivery is safe for both mother and baby** and **effective in obtaining vaginal delivery**, with **forceps having slightly higher success rates**.
- **Forceps achieve a vaginal delivery more often than vacuum, 91% versus 86%, respectively. Complication rates differ between vacuum and forceps**, with the predominant differences being that **maternal third- and fourth-degree perineal (14% vs. 7.5%) and vaginal wall (26% vs. 8%) injuries are more common with forceps-assisted delivery. Neonatal facial injury is uncommon with operative delivery, 1.7% with forceps, and 0.2% with vacuum.** The choice of instrument is decided after appropriate counseling and depends also on operator experience.
- There is insufficient evidence to compare different types of forceps.
- **Soft vacuum cups fail at attaining vaginal delivery more often than by rigid cups** but have a lower rate of significant fetal scalp trauma. Rigid cups may be better for occiput posterior and other more difficult deliveries, while soft cups may be better suited for less complicated, routine deliveries.
- If attempted, **vacuum application should not last more than 5 minutes** and, in general, should be **discontinued if the vacuum cup pops off the fetal head three times**.
- **Attempting to use a different extraction instrument after failing with one should be avoided due to increased incidence of fetal injury.**

HISTORICAL PERSPECTIVES

Operative vaginal delivery has been practiced for centuries. Its initial function was fetal extraction during prolonged dysfunctional labor in an attempt to preserve the life of the laboring women. The invention of modern forceps can be traced back to the Chamberlain family in Europe during the 16th century. Vacuum extraction was first described by Dr James Yonge in 1705. The modern evolution of **vacuum delivery (also called ventouse)** can be attributed to Malmström's metal cup vacuum system developed in 1954. Operative vaginal delivery has evolved significantly and today implies a mechanism for facilitating vaginal delivery of a healthy infant while minimizing maternal risk.

INCIDENCE

Rates of operative vaginal deliveries have been declining in the United States since about 1996. The 2007 rate for birth by forceps or vacuum delivery was 4.3% compared with the 1995 rate of 9.4% (1). In 2007, forceps-assisted deliveries accounted for only 0.8% of live births.

INDICATIONS

Both **forceps and vacuum have the same indications**. Use should depend mostly on proper evaluation of the patient's labor, risk factors, clinical pelvimetry, estimated fetal weight, and operator experience. There are **no circumstances where operative vaginal delivery is definitely indicated. Alternatives, including allowing the patient to labor longer, oxytocin augmentation, and cesarean delivery, should always be considered.** Operative vaginal delivery is usually considered for the following:

- **Maternal: inefficient maternal effort** (e.g., exhaustion or underlying medical condition precluding pushing)
- **Fetal: nonreassuring fetal heart rate tracing**
- **Other: prolonged second stage:** nulliparas ≥ 2 hours without regional anesthesia or ≥ 3 hours with regional anesthesia; multiparas ≥ 1 hour without regional anesthesia or ≥ 2 hours with regional anesthesia (2).

"Elective" forceps delivery, that is, without an indication, is associated with increased maternal perineal trauma and, given the other potential maternal and neonatal complications, should not be preferred to spontaneous vaginal delivery (3).

CONTRAINDICATIONS TO OPERATIVE VAGINAL DELIVERY

Contraindications to operative vaginal delivery are listed in Table 12.1. Severe scalp trauma and unexplained active bleeding may be relative contraindications in individual cases. Operative vaginal delivery should be used with extreme caution in women with maternal diabetes, prolonged labor, and fetal macrosomia, with appropriate preparations due to an increased risk of shoulder dystocia.

RISKS FOR FAILED OPERATIVE VAGINAL DELIVERY

Risks for failed vacuum or forceps vaginal delivery include increased maternal age, increased body mass index, diabetes, polyhydramnios, African-American race, induction of labor, occiput posterior (also increases rates of third- and fourth-degree perineal lacerations), dysfunctional labor, and prolonged labor (4).

Table 12.1 Contraindication to Operative Vaginal Delivery

- Nonvertex presentation
- Unengaged fetal head
- Unknown fetal head position
- Fetal prematurity such as <34 wk
- Known fetal coagulation disorders (e.g., hemophilia and NAIT)
- Known fetal bone demineralization conditions (e.g., osteogenesis imperfecta)

Abbreviation: NAIT, neonatal alloimmune thrombocytopenia.

CLASSIFICATION OF OPERATIVE VAGINAL DELIVERY (2)

- **Outlet:** Scalp is visible at introitus without separating the labia, fetal skull has reached pelvic floor, sagittal suture is anteroposterior (AP) diameter or right or left occiput anterior or posterior position, fetal head is at or on perineum, and rotation ≤45°.
- **Low:** Leading point of the fetal skull is at station ≥ +2 cm and not on the pelvis floor, rotation is ≤45° (left or right occiput anterior to occiput anterior or left or right occiput posterior to occiput posterior), or rotation is >45°.
- **Mid:** Station is above +2 cm but head is engaged.

Originally devised for forceps, this classification is valid for any operative delivery, including vacuum (5).

TYPES OF FORCEPS

There are many different designs for forceps, but all consist of two separate halves that each have the same four basic components: blade, shank, lock, and handle. **There is insufficient evidence to compare different types of forceps.** In the only small trial performed, severe facial abrasion was decreased from 4.1% to 1.9% from the regular forceps compared with soft forceps, as were minimal markings (from 61% to 34%, respectively) (6). Unfortunately successful delivery rates for the two different forceps were not reported, and the soft forceps were self-made. Given the paucity of data, choice of forceps type is somewhat operator dependent.

- **Classical forceps:** These have cephalic and pelvic curvatures. Usually indicated when no rotation of the fetal head is necessary before delivery. Common types include the following: Simpson forceps (fenestrated blades and nonoverlapping shanks), Tucker–McLane forceps (nonfenestrated blades and overlapping shanks), and Elliot forceps (fenestrated blades, overlapping shanks, and largest cephalic curvature). Many of these forceps have been modified with a Luikart pseudofenestration of the blade.
- **Rotational forceps:** These have cephalic curvature but lack a pelvic curvature. Also have a sliding lock to allow forceps to slide to correct asynclitism of the fetal head if present. After rotation of the fetal head is accomplished classical forceps should be used to complete the delivery. Types include Kielland, Luikart, Barton, and Salinas forceps.
- **Forceps for breech delivery:** These are indicated to help with the aftercoming head in a breech delivery. These forceps lack a pelvic curvature and have blades that are beneath the plane of the shank. Types include Piper and Laufe forceps.

TYPES OF VACUUM EXTRACTORS

Vacuum extractors were originally designed with a rigid metal cup. Subsequently, soft cups have been developed. **Several types of rigid (metal or plastic) and soft (silicone plastic or rubber) vacuums are in clinical use** (7–9). Among different types of vacuums, **the metal cup is more likely to result in a successful vaginal birth** than the soft cup (9% vs. 17%), with **more cases of scalp injury** (41% vs. 30%) **and cephalohematoma** (14% vs. 8%). The handheld ventouse is associated with more failures than the metal ventouse, and a trend to fewer than the soft ventouse (7–11).

Rigid cups may be better for occiput posterior and other more difficult deliveries, while **soft cups are better suited for less complicated, routine deliveries** (7). Maternal injury, low Apgar scores at 1 or 5 minutes, umbilical artery pH < 7.20, hyperbilirubinemia/phototherapy, retinal/intracranial hemorrhage, and perinatal death do not differ between soft and rigid vacuum cups (7,10,11). Soft vacuum cups have largely replaced the rigid cup in routine clinical practice. For a comprehensive review of vacuum delivery, see Ref. 12.

COMPARISON OF FORCEPS- VS. VACUUM-ASSISTED DELIVERY (11)
Safety/Complications
Maternal

- **There is a trend for less regional (37% vs. 40%), and significantly less general anesthesia (1% vs. 10%) with vacuum** compared to forceps-assisted deliveries. We do not use general anesthesia for operative delivery.
- **Third- and fourth-degree perineal (14% vs. 7.5%; RR 1.89, 95% CI 1.51–2.37) and vaginal wall lacerations (26% vs. 8%; RR 2.48, 95% CI 1.59–3.87) (maternal trauma) are significantly increased with forceps** compared with vacuum.
- **Severe perineal pain at 24 hours is decreased (9% vs. 15%) with vacuum** compared to forceps-assisted deliveries (11).
- Flatus incontinence or altered continence is more common with forceps compared to vacuum in a small trial (59% vs. 33%; RR 1.77, 95% CI 1.19–2.62).
- Rates of moderate/severe pain at delivery, endoanal ultrasound abnormalities (13), and other maternal outcomes are similar.

Fetal/Neonatal

- **Facial injury** is more likely with forceps (1.7% vs. 0.2%; RR 5.10, 95% CI 1.12–23.25).
- Using a random effects model because of heterogeneity between studies, there was a trend toward **fewer cases of cephalohematoma with forceps** (5% vs. 9%; RR 0.64, 95% CI 0.37–1.11). Rates of cephalohematomas occur in about 10% versus 4% in vacuum and forceps, respectively (11). Cephalohematomas have an overall rate of 2.5% in the general population (14). However, the diagnosis of cephalohematoma can be falsely positive in up to 75% of cases (15).
- **Retinal hemorrhages** trended to be less common in forceps than vacuum deliveries (5% vs. 8%; RR 0.68, 95% 0.43–1.06) (11). One study found retinal hemorrhages occurred in 18% in spontaneous vaginal deliveries (16). The clinical significance of retinal hemorrhages remains unclear (14).
- Rates of scalp/face injury other than cephalohematoma, use of phototherapy, perinatal death, readmission to

hospital, and hearing or vision disability are similar between forceps and vacuum-assisted vaginal deliveries (11,17).

- Other possible uncommon fetal complications associated with operative vaginal delivery include facial nerve injury, corneal abrasions, facial bruising, and lacerations. Very rare findings include facial nerve palsy, skull fractures, cervical spine injury, and intracranial hemorrhage. **With vacuum-assisted delivery**, life-threatening neonatal injuries include **subgaleal (subaponeurotic) hematoma** (0–4%). **Intracranial hemorrhage** is a rare complication of operative vaginal delivery (0–2.5%).
- Most neonatal complications, in particular intracranial hemorrhage, associated with operative vaginal delivery have been found in some studies to be similar to those of similar pregnancies who instead elect cesarean delivery (18). Therefore abnormal labor may be the common risk factor for neonatal intracranial hemorrhage, and not the procedure itself.
- **Long-term infant outcome:** There are no **neurologic or cognitive differences** in infants and children who underwent operative vaginal delivery with forceps or vacuum compared with each other or to infants delivered by spontaneous vaginal delivery (19,20).

Efficacy

Both vacuum- and forceps-assisted delivery have high delivery success rates (with vacuum from 83% to 94% and with forceps 78% to 92%) (11,15). **Forceps are less likely than the vacuum to fail to achieve a vaginal birth with the allocated instrument** (9% vs. 14%; RR 0.65, 95% CI 0.45–0.94) (11).

Cesarean delivery occurred in 4.5% of forceps, and 2.6% of vacuum deliveries, as in these studies unfortunately failed vacuum would at times be followed by forceps, which, in general, should not be done (11).

Summary

There is a recognized place for forceps and all types of vacuum in clinical practice (11). The role of operator training with any choice of instrument must be emphasized. The **increasing risks of failed delivery with the chosen instrument from forceps to metal cup to handheld to soft cup vacuum**, and **trade-offs between risks of maternal and neonatal trauma** (see Table 12.2) need to be considered when choosing an instrument. **Overall forceps or the metal cup appears to be most effective at achieving a vaginal birth, but with increased risk of maternal trauma with forceps and neonatal trauma with the metal cup** (11).

MANAGEMENT
Preoperative Assessment
Counseling

Review with the patient the indication, risks (possible complications) and benefits, and type of instrument to be used for operative vaginal delivery. The option of cesarean delivery, including its risks and benefits, should also be reviewed. Obtain verbal or written informed consent prior to operative vaginal delivery.

Preparation/Documentation (Table 12.3)

Maternal: Sufficient analgesia, clinical assessment of pelvis, lithotomy position, ± empty bladder.

Table 12.2   Comparison of Forceps Vs. Vacuum for Operative Vaginal Delivery

Fetal		Maternal	
Favors forceps	Favors vacuum	Favors forceps	Favors vacuum
		Less likely to fail to deliver vaginally the baby (9% vs. 14%)	Less third- and fourth-degree perineal tears (7.5% vs. 14%) and vaginal wall (8% vs. 26%) lacerations
	Less facial injury (0.2% vs. 1.7%)		Less severe perineal pain postpartum (9% vs. 15%)

Source: From Ref. 11.

Table 12.3   Preoperative Checklist Before Operative Delivery

Maternal criteria	Fetal criteria	Uteroplacental criteria	Other criteria
Sufficient analgesia[a]	Vertex presentation	Cervix fully dilated	Alert nursing, anesthesia, and neonatology
Patient in the lithotomy position	The fetal head must be engaged in the pelvis	Membranes ruptured	An experienced operator who is fully acquainted with the use of the instrument
Consider emptying the bladder	The position of the fetal head must be known with certainty[a]	No placenta previa	Ability to monitor fetal well-being continuously
Clinical pelvimetry must be adequate in dimension and size to facilitate an atraumatic delivery	The station of the fetal head must be + 2 or more		The capability to perform an emergency cesarean delivery if required
Verbal or written consent obtained	The estimated fetal weight must be documented (ideally 2500–4500 g)		Be prepared for shoulder dystocia
	The attitude of the fetal head and the presence of caput succedaneum, molding, or asynclitism should be evaluated		

[a]Especially for forceps delivery.

Fetal: Vertex presentation, head engaged (lower part of bony vertex—not caput—at or lower than level of ischial spines), knowledge of the position of the head (consider ultrasound for confirmation), asynclitism, and estimated fetal weight.

Uteroplacental: Cervix completely dilated, ruptured membranes, absence of placenta previa, or other contraindications.

Other: Alert nursing, anesthesia, and neonatology of plan for operative vaginal delivery. Be prepared for possible shoulder dystocia. Willingness to discontinue the procedure if it does not proceed as planned (2).

Episiotomy

There is insufficient evidence (no trials) to assess the benefits and risks of episiotomy in operative deliveries. In a large observational study, mediolateral episiotomy protected significantly for anal sphincter damage in both vacuum extraction (OR 0.11, 95% CI 0.09–0.13) and forceps delivery (OR 0.08, 95% CI 0.07–0.11), compared with no episiotomy. The number of mediolateral episiotomies needed to prevent one sphincter injury in vacuum extractions was 12, whereas 5 mediolateral episiotomies could prevent one sphincter injury in forceps deliveries (21). Episiotomy should not be routinely performed, as it is associated with perineal lacerations in nonoperative vaginal deliveries (see chap. 8).

Antibiotic Prophylaxis

Antibiotic prophylaxis cannot be recommended solely for the indication "operative vaginal delivery." Two grams cefotetan IV at the time of vacuum or forceps delivery are associated with a nonsignificant decrease (0% vs. 3.5%) in endometritis (22).

Vacuum Application

Vacuum application, if performed, should begin with low suction and be slowly increased to vacuum of about 0.7 to 0.8 kg/cc^2 (500–600 mmHg). Compared with stepwise negative pressure for vacuum delivery, rapid negative pressure application is associated with reduced duration (by 6 minutes) of vacuum procedure, but no other maternal or perinatal effects, in a small trial (23). No torque or rocking motions should be applied to the vacuum. Traction should only be in the direct line of the vaginal canal. The risk of cephalohematoma increases as the time of vacuum application increases. Vacuum application **should not last more than 5 minutes** and should be **discontinued if the vacuum cup pops off the fetal head three times** (2).

Failed Operative Delivery

Attempting to use a different extraction instrument after failing with one should be avoided, as cephalopelvic disproportion may be present, and the highest incidence of neonatal intracranial hemorrhage, as well as other neonatal injuries, is highest among infants delivered using forceps and vacuum sequentially (17,24,25). At that point, cesarean is usually offered and performed.

Postpartum

It is essential to examine carefully both the fetus and the maternal perineum after operative vaginal delivery.

REFERENCES

1. Martin JA, Hamilton BE, Sutton PD, et al. Births: final data for 2007. Natl Vital Stat Rep 2007; 58:1–125. [Data report]
2. American College of Obstetricians and Gynecologists. Practice Bulletin No. 17: Operative vaginal delivery. Washington, DC: ACOG, 2000 (reaffirmed 2009). [Review]
3. Yancey MK, Herpolsheimer A, Jordan GD, et al. Maternal and neonatal effects of outlet forceps delivery compared with spontaneous vaginal delivery in term pregnancies. Obstet Gynecol 1991; 78:646–650. [II-2, $n = 333$]
4. Gopalani S, Bennett K, Critchlow C. Factors predictive of failed operative vaginal delivery. Am J Obstet Gynecol 2004; 191:896–902. [II-3]
5. Weinstein L, Calvin S, Trofatter KR. Operative vaginal delivery: risks and benefits. ACOG Update 2001; 27:5. [Review]
6. Roshan DF, Petrikovski B, Sichinava L, et al. Soft forceps. Int J Obstet Gynecol 2005; 88:249–252. [RCT, $n = 96$]
7. O'Mahony F, Hofmeyr GJ, Menon V. Choice of instruments for assisted vaginal delivery. Cochrane Database Syst Rev 2010; (11). [DOI: 10.1002/14651858.CD005455.pub2]
8. Attilakos G, Sibanda T, Winter C, et al. A randomized controlled trial of a new handheld vacuum extraction device. Br J Obstet Gynecol 2005; 112:1510–1515. [RCT, $n = 194$]
9. Groom KM, Jones BA, Miller N, et al. A prospective randomized controlled trial of the Kiwi Omnicup versus conventional ventouse cups for vacuum-assisted vaginal delivery. Br J Obstet Gynecol 2006; 113:183–189. [RCT, $n = 404$]
10. Ismail NAM, Saharan WSL, Zaleha MA, et al. Kiwi Omnicup versus Malmstrom metal cup in vacuum assisted delivery: a randomized comparative trial. J Obstet Gynaecol Res 2008; 34:350–353. [RCT]
11. O'Mahony F, Hofmeyr GJ, Menon V. Choice of instruments for assisted vaginal delivery. Cochrane Database Syst Rev 2010; (11): CD005455. [Meta-analysis: 32 RCTs, $n = 6597$]
12. Vacca A. Handbook of Vacuum Delivery in Obstetric Practice. Brisbane, Australia: Vacca Research, 2009. [Review]
13. Fitzpatrick M, Behan M, O'Connel PR, et al. Randomized clinical trial to assess anal sphincter function following forceps or vacuum assisted vaginal delivery. Br J Obstet Gynecol 2003; 110:424–429. [RCT, $n = 130$]
14. Uhing M. Management of birth injuries. Clin Perinatol 2005; 32 (1):19–38. [II-3]
15. Williams M, Knuppel R, O'Brien W, et al. A randomized comparison of assisted vaginal delivery by obstetric forceps and polyethylene vacuum cup. Obstet Gynecol 1991; 78:789–794. [RCT, $n = 99$]
16. Williams M, Knuppel R, O'Brien W, et al. Obstetric correlates of neonatal retinal hemorrhage. Obstet Gynecol 1993; 81:688–694. [II-2, $n = 278$]
17. Bofill JA, Rust OA, Schorr SJ, et al. A randomized prospective trial of the obstetric forceps versus the M-cup vacuum extractor. Am J Obstet Gynecol 1996; 175:1325–1330. [RCT, $n = 637$]
18. Towner D, Castro MA, Eby-Wilkens E, et al. Effect of mode of delivery in nulliparous women on neonatal intracranial injury. N Engl J Med 1999; 341:1709–1714. [II-2]
19. Wesley BD, van den Berg BJ, Reece EA. The effects of forceps delivery on cognitive development. Am J Obstet Gynecol 1993; 169:1091–1095. [II-2]
20. Ngan HY, Miu P, Ko L, et al. Long-term neurological sequelae following vacuum extractor delivery. Aust N Z J Obstet Gynaecol 1990; 30:111–114. [II-2]
21. De Leeuw J, De Wit C, Kuijken J, et al. Mediolateral episiotomy reduces the risk for anal sphincter injury during operative vaginal delivery. Br J Obstet Gynecol 2008; 115:104–108. [II-2]
22. Heitmann JA, Benrubi GI. Efficacy of prophylactic antibiotics for the prevention of endomyometritis after forceps delivery. South Med J 1989; 82:960–962. [RCT, $n = 393$]
23. Suwannachat B, Lumbiganon P, Laopaiboon M. Rapid versus stepwise negative pressure application for vacuum extraction assisted vaginal delivery. Cochrane Database Syst Rev 2008; (3): CD006636. [Meta-analysis: 1 RCT, $n = 94$]
24. Edozien LC, Williams JL, Chattopadhyay I, et al. Failed instrumental delivery: how safe is the use of a second instrument? J Obstet Gynaecol 1999; 19:460–462. [III]
25. Demissie K, Rhoads GG, Smulian JC, et al. Operative vaginal delivery and neonatal and infant adverse outcomes: population based retrospective analysis. BMJ 2004; 329(7456):24–29. [II-2]

13

Cesarean delivery

Vincenzo Berghella

See also specific chapters on anesthesia (chap. 11), TOLAC (chap. 14), and postpartum care (chap. 27).

KEY POINTS

- A cesarean delivery on maternal request (CDMR) or a planned repeat CD without other indication should not be performed before 39 weeks.
- Prophylactic antibiotics should be administered before every CD. The evidence suggests the use of a single dose of ampicillin or cefazolin IV given within 1 hour prior to skin incision.
- All women undergoing CD should receive mechanical venous thromboembolism (VTE) prophylaxis with either pneumatic compression devices or compression stockings. These should be inserted preoperatively and continued until full ambulation.
- Left lateral tilt is associated with a lower incidence of hypotension.
- Compared with no scrub, vaginal irrigation with povidone-iodine immediately before CD significantly reduces the incidence of postcesarean endometritis.
- Adhesive drapes for CD are associated with a higher incidence of wound infection.
- A transverse skin incision with either the Joel–Cohen or Pfannenstiel technique is the preferred one for CD.
- Developing a bladder flap at CD may be detrimental and can be avoided.
- The uterine incision should be performed with the scalpel in a transverse fashion and expanded cephalad-caudad with fingers.
- Oxytocin IV or IM is effective at preventing postpartum hemorrhage.
- Uterine massage, associated with cord traction, is associated with less blood loss.
- Spontaneous placental removal should be preferred to manual removal given the significant decrease in blood loss and endometritis.
- The uterus should be repaired with sutures with full-thickness bites, in a continuous fashion, probably without locking.
- Compared with two (double) layers, one (single) layer of suture for uterine incision repair is associated with a statistically significant reduction in mean blood loss; duration of the operative procedure; and presence of postoperative pain. It might be reasonable to omit the second layer if the woman is planning no more pregnancies (e.g., receives tubal ligation). For women planning future pregnancies, the uterus can be closed in two layers.
- There is no evidence to justify the time taken and the cost of peritoneal closure, so avoid it.
- The evidence supports routine subcutaneous suture closure in women with a subcutaneous tissue depth ≥2 cm.
- There is no conclusive evidence about how the skin should be closed after CD.
- Gum chewing three times/day for at least 30 minutes each time after CD is associated with a earlier return of bowel sounds (by 5 hours), earlier passage of flatus (by about 5 hours), and less (12% vs. 21%) symptoms of mild ileus.
- There is insufficient evidence for a strong recommendation, but early oral fluids and even food after CD seem to be safe and possibly beneficial.
- Reclosure of the disrupted laparotomy wound of CD is associated with success in >80% of women, faster healing times, and fewer office visits.

HISTORIC NOTES

The word cesarean is probably derived either from the "Lex Regia," later called "Cesarea," which allowed in ancient Rome the postmortem abdominal delivery of the child, or from the Latin "caesare," which means "to cut." Until the late 1800s, most CDs were done after maternal death, for attempt at fetal salvage. In 1882, the era of modern CD began when Saenger advocated closing all uterine incisions immediately after surgery. The lower uterine segment incision was introduced by Kronig in 1912 and popularized in the United States by DeLee in 1922. The transverse uterine incision was described by Munro-Kerr in 1926 (1). CD has been associated with relatively low maternal mortality for about 100 years. Safety has improved in the last 50 years, as the above techniques have become more widely used, and antibiotics have been introduced.

DIAGNOSIS/DEFINITION

Birth via abdominal route by laparotomy.

EPIDEMIOLOGY/INCIDENCE

CD is now the most common surgical procedure in the United States with over 1 million performed each year. Its incidence has increased to 32% of deliveries in the United States in 2008 (2). This increase has been fueled at least in part by increased incidence of multiple gestations and decreased incidences of vaginal births after CD and vaginal breech deliveries. Women's demand for scheduled CD (CDMR) has increased as complications from the procedure diminish, women have fewer children, and fear and concerns about vaginal delivery do not abate.

INDICATIONS

Common accepted indications for CD are failure to progress (aka failure to dilate, failure to descend, cephalopelvic disproportion, dystocia, etc.), nonreassuring fetal heart rate tracing

(NRFHT), nonvertex presentation, etc. See specific chapters for details.

There is insufficient evidence (lack of any trial) to assess the benefits and risks of a policy of CDMR (only indication: woman's desire; also called elective CD) compared with trial of labor in term women with singleton gestations in cephalic presentation. The most common reason for a request for CDMR is fear of labor pain. CDMR should not be motivated by the unavailability of effective pain medication. There is also no randomized controlled trial (RCT) to evaluate the obstetrician recommendation for CD not based on an accepted indication. As there are no such trials, there is insufficient evidence to assess the long-term maternal and neonatal morbidity and mortality of CD or labor. There is insufficient evidence on the impact of counseling during pregnancy with the aim of reducing the incidence of CDMR (3). The incidence of women (without prior CD) preferring CDMR in a systematic review of studies is about 10%, and even less in developed countries (4). A practitioner is not obligated to perform a CDMR but should appropriately refer the woman as necessary.

A CDMR or a planned repeat CD without other indication should not be performed before 39 weeks.

OPTIMAL CD RATE
The optimal CD rate is unknown. Maternal and neonatal morbidity and mortality are the important outcomes, not CD rate per se. Increasing CD rate, if CD is performed for appropriate indications, has several times been associated with a lower mortality rate in normally formed term babies (5). As the CD rate increases, an increasing number of CDs have to be performed to achieve smaller benefits in perinatal mortality.

There are **limited data of nonclinical interventions aimed at decreasing the unnecessary CD rate** (6). Implementation of guidelines with **mandatory second opinion** can lead to a small reduction in CD rates, predominately in **intrapartum CDs** (7). **Peer review, including precesarean consultation, mandatory secondary opinion, and postcesarean surveillance,** can lead to a reduction in repeat cesarean section rates. **Guidelines** disseminated with endorsement and support from local opinion leaders may increase the proportion of women with previous CD being offered a trial of labor in

certain settings (see also chap. 14). **Nurse-led relaxation classes and birth preparation classes** may reduce CD rates in low-risk pregnancies (6). There is insufficient evidence that prenatal education and support programs, computer-based patient decision aids, decision-aid booklets, and intensive group therapy are effective. There is insufficient evidence that audit and feedback, training of public health nurses, insurance reform, external peer review, and legislative changes are effective.

PREOPERATIVE CONSIDERATIONS
See Tables 13.1 and 13.2 for summary of recommendations on how to perform a CD (8).

Consent should always be obtained after counseling. Counseling should include at least indication, and possible complications.

A checklist, including possibly pre-, intra-, and postoperative steps aimed at preventing complications, has been associated with benefits in general surgery (9) and should probably be implemented at CD (Table 13.2).

Prophylactic Antibiotics
Who to Give it to
Prophylactic antibiotics should be administered before every CD. They are associated with decrease in incidence of endometritis of 62%, in wound infection of 61%, in fever of 55%, and in serious maternal infectious complications by 69% (10,11). Urinary tract infections (UTI) are also markedly decreased. These results are similar for planned or not-planned (e.g., in labor) CDs.

Which Antibiotics to Use and How
Comparing which antibiotic to give, the **efficacy of ampicillin is equivalent to that of first-generation cephalosporins such as cefazolin** (Ancef) (12). These are the recommended agents to use, unless there are drug allergies to them. Later-generation (e.g., second or third), or more expensive broad-spectrum agents, do not improve efficacy further (11). A multiple-dose regimen for prophylaxis appears to offer no added benefit over a single-dose regimen (10,11). Systemic (after cord clamping)

Table 13.1 Standard Recommendation Language and Quality of Evidence According to the Method Outlined by the U.S. Preventive Services Task Force (USPSTF)

Recommendation:
A.—The USPSTF strongly recommends that clinicians provide [the service] to eligible patients. The USPSTF found good evidence that [the service] improves important health outcomes and concludes that benefits substantially outweigh harms.
B.—The USPSTF recommends that clinicians provide [this service] to eligible patients. The USPSTF found at least fair evidence that [the service] improves important health outcomes and concludes that benefits outweigh harms.
C.—The USPSTF makes no recommendation for or against routine provision of [the service]. The USPSTF found at least fair evidence that [the service] can improve health outcomes but concludes that the balance of benefits and harms is too close to justify a general recommendation.
D.—The USPSTF recommends against routinely providing [the service] to asymptomatic patients. The USPSTF found at least fair evidence that [the service] is ineffective or that harms outweigh benefits.
I.—The USPSTF concludes that the evidence is insufficient to recommend for or against routinely providing [the service]. Evidence that the [service] is effective is lacking, of poor quality, or conflicting and the balance of benefits and harms cannot be determined.

Quality of evidence:
Good: Evidence includes consistent results from well-designed, well-conducted studies in representative populations that directly assess effects on health outcomes.
Fair: Evidence is sufficient to determine effects on health outcomes, but the strength of the evidence is limited by the number, quality, or consistency of the individual studies, generalizability to routine practice, or indirect nature of the evidence on health outcomes.
Poor: Evidence is insufficient to assess the effects on health outcomes because of limited number or power of studies, important flaws in their design or conduct, gaps in the chain of evidence, or lack of information on important health outcomes.

Source: From Ref. 8.

Table 13.2 Evidence-Based Recommendations for Cesarean Delivery

CD technical aspect	Recommendation[a]	Quality[a]	Comment
Prophylactic antibiotics			
Yes or no	A	Good	All CD
Antibiotic type	A	Good	Amp. or first gen. cephalo.[b]
Route of administration	A	Good	IV
Single dose	B	Good	[c]
Timing	A	Good	Within 60 min before skin incision
Prophylaxis for VTE	C	Poor	Pneumatic compression devices, or compression stockings, for all CDs
Lateral tilt	B	Fair	15° to left
No indwelling bladder catheterization	C	Poor	No complications with its avoidance
No hair removal	C	Poor	Avoid if possible, do not use razor
Skin cleaning	B	Poor	Povidone-iodine[c]
Vaginal irrigation	C	Poor	Povidone-iodine[c]
No adhesive drapes	B	Fair	Avoid
Skin incision			
Type	C	Fair	Transverse, Pfannenstiel or Joel–Cohen
Length	I	Poor	15 cm
No need to changing to a second knife	C	Fair	[c]
Subcutaneous dissection	I	Poor	[c](we prefer bluntly)
Fascial incision	I	Poor	[c]
No rectus muscle cutting	B	Fair	Avoid
Dissection of fascia off rectus	I	Poor	[c]
Opening of peritoneum	I	Poor	[c]
Bladder flap			
No development	B	Fair	Avoid development of the bladder flap
Use of bladder blade	I	Poor	Operator preference
Uterine incision			
Type	B	Fair	Transverse
No stapling device	B	Fair	Not recommended
Expansion of uterine incision	A	Good	Bluntly
No instrumental delivery	B	Poor	[c]
Prevention of uterine atony			
Oxytocin[d]	I	Poor	IV or IM[c]
Oxytocin infusion rate	C	Poor	Optimal rate unclear[c]
Carbetocin	B	Fair	Carbetocin is superior to oxytocin, should be used if available[c]
Uterine massage	B	Fair	Perform with cord traction
Placental removal			
Spontaneous	A	Good	Avoid manual removal
No glove change	B	Fair	Not recommended
Uterine exteriorization	C	Fair	Operator preference
Cleaning of uterus	I	Poor	[c]
No cervical dilation	I	Poor	Avoid[c]
Closure of uterine incision			
Two vs. one layers	B	Fair	[c]
Incorporation of decidua/serosa	B	Fair	[c]
Continuous	B	Fair	Not interrupted
Sharp needles	I	Poor	[c]
No intra-abdominal irrigation	B	Fair	Not recommended
No peritoneal closure	A	Good	Not recommended (for both parietal and visceral)
No reapproximation of rectus muscles	C	Poor	[c]
Fascial closure	I	Poor	[c]
Subcutaneous tissue closure			
≥2 cm thickness	A	Good	Closure recommended
No subcutaneous tissue drain	A	Good	Not recommended
Closure of skin			
Staples vs. subcuticular	I	Fair	[c]

[a]Level of evidence was based on the U.S. Preventive Services Task Force recommendations (Table 13.1).
[b]Ampicillin or first-generation cephalosporin.
[c]See text for more details.
[d]Based on trials of women with vaginal delivery, not CD.
Abbreviations: CD, cesarean delivery; RCTs, randomized controlled trials.

versus lavage routes of antibiotic administration seem to have similar efficacy (10,11). If ampicillin or a first-generation cephalosporin has already been given in labor (e.g., for chorioamnionitis), there may be no need for additional prophylactic antibiotics at CD. If preoperative antibiotics were not given, prophylaxis should include an extended-spectrum regimen, involving azithromycin or metronidazole (13).

When to Give the Antibiotics
Compared with after cord clamp, **administration of antibiotics within 1 hour before skin incision is associated with a lower incidence of endometritis and wound infection** (14–19).

Summary
This evidence suggests the use of a **single dose of ampicillin or cefazolin IV given within 1 hour prior to skin incision.**

Prophylactic Agents to Prevent Venous Thromboembolism

There is insufficient evidence on which to base recommendations for thromboprophylaxis during pregnancy and the early postnatal period. The three most commonly used interventions are pneumatic compression devices, compression stockings, and anticoagulants such as unfractionated (UH) or low–molecular weight heparin (LMWH).

Pneumatic compression devices have been recommended based on retrospective data (20). They appear to be safe and effective.

While there are two RCTs on UH versus placebo, two RCTs of LMWH versus placebo, and three RCTs on LMWH versus UH, the RCTs are, in general, small and the data are insufficient to make any recommendation (21). It is not possible to assess the effects of any of these interventions on most outcomes, and especially on rare outcomes such as VTE, death, and osteoporosis, because of small sample sizes and the small number of RCTs making the same comparisons. There was some evidence of side effects associated with thromboprophylaxis.

In summary, given the higher risk of VTE at CD compared with vaginal delivery, **all women undergoing CD should receive mechanical VTE prophylaxis with either pneumatic compression devices or compression stockings** (21). These should be **inserted preoperatively and continued until full ambulation.**

In women undergoing CD with BMI > 50 kg/m², previous VTE, or two or more additional risk factors for VTE (such as smoking, multiple gestation, BMI > 30 kg/m², prolonged immobility, and infection), one can consider adding to mechanical prophylaxis pharmacological VTE prophylaxis, with either enoxaparin 40 mg daily or UH 5000 every 12 hours. This pharmacological prophylaxis can start postoperatively, at 6 to 12 hours, after concerns for hemorrhage have decreased, and can continue until full ambulation (21).

Fetal Heart Monitoring

1. *If external monitoring* has been employed, it should be continued up until the abdominal prep has begun. This includes the time when regional anesthesia is administered. If continuous fetal monitoring is not possible, reapply the external monitor for 2 to 3 minutes if feasible after completion of the regional anesthesia to determine the postanesthesia fetal status.

2. *If internal monitoring* has been employed, the scalp electrode can be kept on until delivery of the fetal head, at which point the lead can be cut and the fetus delivered or the fetus delivered with the electrode attached. The OR team will be responsible to document on the count sheet the location of the scalp electrode after delivery.

3. If the cesarean section is done for **nonreassuring fetal status**, all attempts should be made to perform continuous fetal monitoring until the delivery occurs. This may not apply when the cesarean section is done in an emergent manner.

There is no trial regarding optimal **time of "decision to incision"** for CD. Thirty minutes for CD for NRFHR and 60 minutes for CD for dystocia and most other indications have been proposed but are not based on trials (22).

Steroids for Fetal Maturity

Betamethasone 12 mg × 2 doses 24 hours apart at 37 weeks or beyond before planned CD has been shown to reduce the incidence of respiratory distress syndrome (RDS) to 0.2% from 1.1%. The incidence of admission to special care nursery for RDS is decreased to 0.24% from 0.51% (23). Given there is only one RCT on this subject, and that it was not placebo controlled, not blinded, and with very low incidences of disease in the control group, these data are insufficient for a definite recommendation. Steroids for fetal maturity should not be given at ≥39 weeks since the incidence of RDS is extremely small.

Music

Playing music during planned cesarean section under regional anesthesia may improve pulse rate and birth satisfaction score. However, the magnitude of these benefits is small and the methodological quality of the one included trial is questionable. Therefore, the clinical significance of music is unclear (24).

PREPARATIONS ON THE OPERATIVE TABLE
Maternal Position

There is **insufficient evidence to support or clearly disprove the value of the use of tilting or flexing the table, the use of wedges and cushions, or the use of mechanical displacers at CD** (25). Most of the results below are from small single RCTs. The incidence of air embolism is not affected by head up versus horizontal position. **Lateral tilt** involves tilting the woman toward her left side 10° to 15° to avoid vena caval compression by the gravid uterus. There is no change in hypotensive episodes when comparing left lateral tilt (RR 0.11, 95% CI 0.01–1.94), right lateral tilt (RR 1.25, 95% CI 0.39–3.99), and head down tilt [mean difference (MD) −3.00; 95% CI −8.38 to 2.38] with horizontal positions or full lateral tilt with 15° tilt (RR 1.20, 95% CI 0.80–1.79). **Hypotensive episodes are decreased with** manual displacers (RR 0.11, 95% CI 0.03–0.45), a right lumbar wedge compared to a right pelvic wedge (RR 1.64, 95% CI 1.07–2.53), and increased in right lateral tilt (RR 3.30, 95% CI 1.20–9.08) versus **left lateral tilt**. Position does not affect systolic blood pressure when comparing left lateral tilt or head down tilt to horizontal positions, or full lateral tilt with 15° tilt. Manual displacers showed decreased fall in mean systolic blood pressure compared with left lateral tilt. Position does not affect diastolic blood pressures when comparing left lateral tilt versus horizontal positions. The mean diastolic pressure is a bit lower in head down tilt when compared with horizontal positions. There are no statistically significant changes in maternal pulse rate, 5-minute Apgars, maternal blood pH, or cord blood pH when comparing different positions (25).

Indwelling Bladder Catheterization

Compared with use of indwelling urinary catheters inserted pre-CD and removed ≥12 hours after CD, nonuse is associated with lower incidence of UTI (RR 0.08, 95% CI 0.01–0.64), lower rate of discomfort at first voiding (RR 0.06, 95% CI 0.03–0.12), less time to first voiding (by 16 minutes), and less time (by about 6 minutes) until ambulation. No differences in intraoperative difficulties, complications, or time are seen (26). Given that these studies were both performed in developing countries, that the quality of the RCTs was poor, and the use of prophylactic antibiotics and other important confounders was not reported, there is still insufficient evidence to justify the routine use of bladder catheterization, but **its avoidance does not seem to be associated with complications**.

Hair Removal

There is insufficient evidence to assess any effect of pubic hair removal before CD. We avoid it as much as possible, and perform it only by electric shaver or clipping, not by razor, based on data presented in chapter 7.

Skin Cleansing

Skin cleansing techniques for CD have been studied insufficiently for an evidence-based recommendation. Compared with 7.5% povidone-iodine (p-i) scrub and then p-i 10% solution, the addition of preceding parachlorometaxylenol scrub for 5 minutes, in the women who had received prophylactic antibiotics for CD, is not associated with differences in incidences of endometritis or wound infection in a small, possibly underpowered trial (27). Skin is impossible to sterilize. In nonpregnant adults, there are no differences in wound infection with different types and times of scrubs. Therefore, the use of an iodine solution alone (better than saline) is considered reasonable. Some insist on the importance of letting the iodine dry for best infection prophylaxis.

Vaginal Irrigation

Compared with no scrub, **vaginal irrigation with p-i immediately before CD** significantly reduces the incidence of postcesarean endometritis from 9.4% in control groups to 5.2% in vaginal cleansing groups (RR 0.57, 95% CI 0.38–0.87) (28). The risk reduction was particularly strong for women with ruptured membranes (1.4% in the vaginal cleansing group vs. 15.4% in the control group; RR 0.13, 95% CI 0.02–0.66). No other outcomes realized statistically significant differences between the vaginal cleansing and control groups. No adverse effects were reported with the p-i vaginal cleansing (28). Most of these studies used also p-i skin cleansing, and prophylactic antibiotics, but not all studies. As a simple, generally inexpensive intervention, providers should consider implementing preoperative vaginal cleansing with p-i.

Compared with matching placebo, metronidazole gel 5 g intravaginally before CD is associated with a decrease from 17% to 7% in the incidence of endometritis, but no other significant changes in important outcomes (29).

Adhesive Drapes

Adhesive drapes for CD are associated with a **higher incidence of wound infection** (13.8%) compared with the control group (10.4%) (30,31). Therefore, adhesive drapes should be avoided.

SURGICAL TECHNIQUE
Skin Incision

Skin incision techniques for CD have been evaluated separately from other aspects of CD in limited studies (32,33). In general, a **transverse skin incision** is recommended, since this is associated with less postoperative pain and improved cosmetic effect compared with a vertical incision. The **Pfannenstiel** (slightly curved, 2–3 cm or 2 fingers above the symphysis pubis, with the midportion of the incision lying within the shaved area of the pubic hair) and **Joel–Cohen** (straight, 3 cm below the line joining the anterior superior iliac spines, and therefore slightly more cephalad than the Pfannenstiel) are the preferred transverse incisions. Most RCTs do not only evaluate type of skin incision but also other technical aspects of CD, making it often impossible to evaluate the effect of only the type of skin incision (34). The best larger trial reveals no differences in total operative time (32 vs. 33 minutes), intra- and postoperative complications, and neonatal outcomes, with the extraction time 50 seconds shorter for the Joel–Cohen group (32). Considering the absence of clinical benefits to the mother and fetus, **there is no clear indication for preferring either a Pfannenstiel or a Joel–Cohen incision for CD**. In contrast, a smaller, less well-designed trial (33) shows significantly shorter operating times, reduced blood loss and postoperative discomfort associated with the Joel–Cohen compared with the Pfannenstiel incision (35).

There are probably **no absolute indications for performing a vertical skin incision**. Compared with transverse skin incision, vertical skin incision is associated with slightly shortened incision-to-delivery intervals of about 1 minute for primary and about 3 minutes for repeat CD (36).

Skin incision length has not been studied in a trial. Abdominal surgical incision size should provide probably about 15 cm (size of a standard Allis clamp) of exposure to assure optimal outcome of both mother and term fetus (1).

Changing to a second scalpel after the first scalpel has been used for skin incision versus no such change has never been evaluated in a trial, or in any obstetrical literature. From general surgery data, one scalpel is probably adequate to use throughout the whole surgical procedure.

Subcutaneous Tissue Opening

Subcutaneous tissue possible incision and general opening have not been studied separately in a trial. We use the scalpel as little as possible, opening layers bluntly from medial to lateral to avoid injury to tissue and the inferior epigastric vessels. Blunt dissection has been associated with shorter operating times. **There are no trials to evaluate the safety or efficacy of electrosurgery, electrocautery, or diathermy (Bovie) during CD.**

Fascial Incision

Fascial incision has **not been studied separately in a trial**. A transverse incision is usually performed with the scalpel, and then extended with scissors. Digital extension can alternatively be accomplished by separating the forefingers in a cephalad-caudad direction after inserting the fingers into a small, midline transverse fascial incision.

Rectus Muscle Cutting

Rectus muscle cutting with Maylard technique is not associated with any difference in operative morbidity, difficult deliveries, postoperative complications or pain scores compared with Pfannenstiel (no muscle cutting) technique (37–39), but abdominal muscle strength at 3 months tends to be better in the Pfannenstiel group (39). Therefore, **rectus muscle cutting is probably not necessary** (35).

Dissection of Fascia

Dissection of the fascia off the recti muscles has not been studied separately in a trial. There seems to be no necessity of this commonly used technical step of CD (1).

Opening of the Peritoneum

Opening of the peritoneum has not been studied separately in a trial. The peritoneum is usually carefully opened with blunt or sharp dissection, and blunt expansion, high above the bladder, avoiding injury to organs below.

Retractors

There is insufficient evidence for comparing different types of retractors in CD.

Bladder Flap

Development (incision and opening) of a bladder flap is associated with longer (7 vs. 5 minutes) incision-to-delivery interval, longer (40 vs. 35 minutes) total operating time, and greater (1 vs. 0.5 g/dL) change in hemoglobin compared to just direct incision 1 cm above the bladder fold (40). Forming a bladder flap is also associated with more (47% vs. 21%) postoperative microhematuria and greater (55% vs. 26%) need for analgesia at 2 days after CD. No long-term effects (e.g., adhesions, bladder function, and fertility) have been evaluated. As bladder injury at CD is an uncommon event (1–3/1000), a sample size over 40,000 women would be required to show a difference in this outcome (40). **Developing a bladder flap at CD may be detrimental and can be avoided.**

The use of a bladder blade to protect the bladder has not been studied separately in a trial.

Uterine Incision

Uterine incision type has not been studied separately in a trial. The **transverse incision in the lower uterine segment** is usually recommended (1). Some experts advocate the classical vertical or at least low vertical incision if the lower uterine segment is not large enough to allow a transverse incision, for example, for the very preterm (<28 weeks) uterus, and fibroids, but this has been associated with increased blood loss compared with low transverse incision (41).

Uterine Stapling

Use of uterine stapling (autosuture) device for opening and closing of the uterus is associated with no difference in the amount of blood loss during the procedure, but a statistically significant increase in the duration of the procedure (by about 3 minutes) and no differences in other perinatal morbidity outcomes compared with traditional opening and closure of the uterine scar (42,43). **There is no enough evidence to justify the routine use of stapling devices** to extend the uterine incision at lower segment cesarean section, especially since there is a possibility that stapling **could cause harm** by prolonging the time to deliver the baby.

Expansion of Uterine Incision

Expansion of the uterine incision with fingers (blunt) is associated with significantly decreased estimated blood loss (by about 43 mL), change in hematocrit, incidence of postpartum hemorrhage (9% vs. 13%), need for transfusion (0.4% vs. 2%), and total number of extensions compared with expansion with scissors (sharp) (44,45). As it is also quicker, and associated with less risk of inadvertently cutting the neonate or cord, **blunt should be preferred to sharp expansion of the uterine incision** (42).

Compared with transversal expansion, **cephalad-caudad expansion** of the low transverse uterine incision is associated with significant less incidence of blood loss >1500 mL (0.2% vs. 2%) and less unintended uterine extensions (3.7% vs. 7.4%) (46).

Instrumental Delivery

Instrumental delivery of the fetal head by either vacuum or forceps compared with manual means has been insufficiently evaluated for a firm recommendation in women with cephalic (47) or breech presentation undergoing CD. As instrumentation has been associated with maternal (especially for forceps) or fetal (especially for vacuum) harm in vaginal deliveries, the principle of "primum non nocere" ("first do no harm") should be applied in this setting, therefore **favoring manual delivery of the fetal head whenever possible** until further data are available.

Tocolysis for assisting in delivery of the fetal head at CD has been insufficiently studied (48).

Prevention of Uterine Atony and Postpartum Hemorrhage

Prevention of uterine atony and postpartum hemorrhage has not been comprehensively studied for CD but has been studied extensively for the third stage of labor after vaginal delivery (see chap. 9).

Oxytocin

In the setting of vaginal delivery, **both IV and IM oxytocin effectively reduce postpartum hemorrhage** and the need for therapeutic uterotonics by at least 40% compared with placebo or no routine prophylactic agent. **Oxytocin is as effective and has fewer side effects than ergot alkaloids.**

For CD, regarding oxytocin infusion rates, 10 units of oxytocin in 500 cc (infusion rate 333 mU/min) lactated ringer over 30 minutes after cord clamping are associated with an increased need for another uterotonic medication (39% vs. 19%) and similar change in hematocrit compared with 80 units of oxytocin in 500 cc (infusion rate 2667 mU/min) (49). Given this is the only trial on this subject, and many obstetricians use different infusion rates, **the optimal infusion rate for oxytocin at CD is still unclear.**

For CD, **carbetocin as a single 100-g dose is associated with more effective prevention of uterine atony and lower need for additional uterotonics compared with oxytocin 8- or 16-hour infusion** (50,51). Carbetocin (where available) may be recommended over oxytocin for prevention of uterine atony.

For CD, oxytocin 20 IU IV is as effective as ergometrine plus oxytocin, with less vomiting, in a small RCT (52).

Uterine Massage

Uterine massage, associated with cord traction, is associated with less blood loss compared with no such interventions (53).

Collection and Drainage of Cord Blood

At CD, drainage of fetal blood from the umbilical cord is associated with less incidence of feto-maternal transfusion (measured by Kleihauer–Betke test) compared with no drainage (54). The clinical significance of this finding is unknown.

Placental Removal

Placental removal options are either spontaneous (with gentle cord traction) or manual (55). Manual removal of the placenta is associated with more endometritis (RR 1.64, 95% CI 1.42–1.90); more blood loss (by 94 mL); more blood loss >1000 mL (RR 1.81, 95% CI 1.44–2.28); lower hematocrit after delivery (by about 1.6%); greater hematocrit fall after delivery (by about 0.4%); and longer duration of hospital stay (by about 0.4 days). The duration of surgery was shorter in one trial but not overall.

There were no significant differences in feto-maternal hemorrhage, blood transfusion, and puerperal fever (numbers studied for these outcomes were small) (55).

Blood loss may be increased in manual removal because dilated sinuses in the uterine wall are not closed yet. Bacterial contamination of the lower uterine segment and incision may contaminate the surgeon's dominant hand, and therefore the upper segment in manual removal, or the glove may be itself contaminated. **Spontaneous placental removal should be preferred to manual removal** given the **significant decrease in blood loss and endometritis**.

Change of Gloves

Changing the operator's glove before manual removal of the placenta does not alter the incidence of endometritis (56).

Uterine Exteriorization

Uterine exteriorization (extra-abdominal uterine incision repair) is associated with no significant effects in incidences of fever; endometritis; wound infection; blood loss; blood transfusion; intraoperative nausea and vomiting, pain, or hypotension; and operative time compared with leaving the uterus intra-abdominally for uterine incision repair (57,58). So the balance of the benefits and harms is too close to justify a general recommendation, but many obstetricians subjectively prefer to exteriorize the uterus for easier uterine incision repair.

Cleaning the Uterus

Cleaning any placental remnants or blood clots from the uterus with a sponge or other means is a technique frequently used after placental removal, but not studied in any trial.

Cervical Dilation

Routine cervical dilation at CD before uterine incision repair has been insufficiently studied, but it is not associated with an effect on maternal fever, wound infection, or change in hemoglobin (59).

Closure of Uterine Incision

At least one-layer uterine closure is always done, as the uterus should not be left open. Closure of uterine incision involves several decisions. These include use of blunt versus sharp needles; type of suture; full- versus split-thickness repair; continuous versus interrupted sutures; locking versus non-locking of sutures; and if to perform a second layer or not.

Blunt needles for closure of the uterus, peritoneum, and rectus sheath are associated with similar outcome compared with sharp needles in one RCT (60). In another RCT, glove perforation was significantly less with use of blunt compared to sharp needles, especially for the assistant surgeon. However, physicians reported decreased satisfaction performing CD with blunt needles (61). In summary, **there is still limited evidence to recommend blunt versus sharp needles at CD.**

There is insufficient evidence to compare different sutures at closure at CD.

Compared with split-thickness repair (avoiding the endometrium), **full-thickness uterine incision repair** is associated with a lower incidence of incomplete healing (documented by split in uterine muscle seen on transvaginal ultrasound about 40 days after the CD) of the uterine incision after CD (62). Experts usually advocate incorporating all of the muscle up to the serosa in a one-layer closure also to avoid bleeding from edges.

There is insufficient evidence to compare continuous versus interrupted sutures for single-layer closure of the uterine incision at CD. **Continuous single-layer closure** may save operating time and reduce blood loss compared with interrupted single-layer closure (63).

Locking of sutures in the first layer has been insufficiently studied, but associated with poorer healing.

Compared with two (double) layers, one (single) layer of suture for uterine incision repair is associated with a statistically significant reduction in the following: mean blood loss (by 70 mL); duration of the operative procedure (by 7.4 minutes); presence of postoperative pain (RR 0.69, 95% CI 0.52–0.91); and similar need for transfusion and endometritis rates (64).

Based on short-term outcomes, one would select one-layer repair. But long-term outcomes, especially the chance of uterine rupture with a future pregnancy, are probably much more important (65). Unfortunately, the women followed-up are too few to detect a significant difference in rare but extremely important long-term outcomes such as rates of rupture in the next pregnancy (63–65), with contradictory results of retrospective studies. Since there is as of yet no trial demonstrating benefit from two- versus one-layer uterine closure, **it might be reasonable to omit the second layer if the woman is planning no more pregnancies (e.g., receives tubal ligation). For women planning future pregnancies, the uterus can be closed in two layers** (66).

Intra-abdominal Irrigation

Intra-abdominal irrigation with 500 to 1000 mL of normal saline before abdominal wall closure **should not be routinely performed** since it provides no significant differences in blood loss, intrapartum complications, hospital stay, return of gastrointestinal function, or incidence of infectious complications versus no irrigation (67).

Adhesion Formation Prevention

There is insufficient evidence to assess if any intervention is effective at adhesion prevention at CD.

Appendectomy

Performing a planned appendectomy without indications at CD is not associated with inpatient morbidity in a small RCT (68). No clear benefits were shown, either. The evidence is insufficient to make a recommendation regarding this non-indicated procedure.

Intra-abdominal Drain

There is insufficient evidence to evaluate the effect of placing a drain in the abdominal cavity at CD. In one RCT, liberal use of a subrectus sheath drain was not associated with any effect compared with the restricted use of such intervention (69).

Peritoneal Nonclosure

Compared with closure, **peritoneal nonclosure** is associated with a reduction in operating time whether both or either visceral or parietal peritoneal layer was not sutured. For both layers, the operating time was reduced by about 6 minutes (70). Peritoneal nonclosure is also associated with significantly less postoperative fever and reduced postoperative stay in hospital for visceral peritoneum and for both layer nonclosure. The number of postoperative analgesic doses is reduced in the peritoneal nonclosure group. There are no other statistically significant differences. The trend for wound infection tended to favor nonclosure, while endometritis results were variable.

Long-term follow-up in one trial showed no significant differences. Long-term follow-up (71) after 7 years showed no differences in pain, fertility, urinary symptoms, and adhesions. Long-term studies following cesarean section are limited; there is therefore no definite evidence for nonclosure until long-term data become available (72). A review of general surgery and gynecological data concluded that "we encourage clinicians not to close both parietal and visceral peritoneum" (73). Observational studies have shown that the peritoneum regenerates in 5 to 6 days. The hypothetical benefits of closing these layers for anatomic barrier, reduction of wound dehiscence, and minimization of adhesion have not been proven, and in fact have been invalided by trials. **There is no evidence to justify the time taken and the cost of peritoneal closure.**

Reapproximation of Rectus Muscles

Reapproximation of rectus muscles has not been studied in any trial. Most clinicians agree that they do find the right anatomic place, and suturing them together can cause unnecessary pain when the woman starts to move postoperatively.

Fascial Closure

Techniques of fascial closure have not been studied in any trial of CD. Most experts suggest continuous nonlocking closure with delayed absorbable suture.

Subcutaneous Tissue

Irrigation
Irrigation of the subcutaneous tissue to minimize wound infections and other complications has not been studied versus no irrigation in a trial of CD. The type of irrigation, with saline or antibiotic solution, has also not been studied in a trial.

Suture Closure
Subcutaneous tissue closure versus nonclosure by suture should be analyzed by the thickness of the subcutaneous tissue, as results differ according to <2 cm versus ≥2 cm of subcutaneous tissue thickness (74). Most studies used 3-0 Vicryl for suture closure.

Any subcutaneous thickness: *Suture closure* of subcutaneous fat in women with *any subcutaneous thickness* is overall associated with less wound disruption *versus nonclosure*, but the presence of women with both <2 cm and ≥2 cm thickness, which can have differing outcomes, and inability to blind represent a possible source of confounding and bias (74).

Less than 2 cm subcutaneous thickness: Routine subcutaneous tissue closure in women with a depth <2 cm has been insufficiently studied. It is not associated with any effects on outcome, and therefore cannot be recommended (74).

Greater than or equal to 2 cm subcutaneous thickness: *Suture closure* of subcutaneous fat in women with ≥2 *cm thickness* is associated with a significant decrease in wound disruptions, defined as any wound complication that required intervention, and seromas, compared with nonclosure. **The evidence supports routine subcutaneous suture closure in women with a subcutaneous tissue depth ≥2 cm** (74).

Drainage
Some RCTs have evaluated drainage of subcutaneous tissue, compared with no drainage, or compared with tissue closure.

In meta-analyses of all RCTs, there is no evidence of a difference in the risk of wound infection, other wound complications, febrile morbidity, or endometritis in women who had wound drains compared with those who did not (75). Drainage of subcutaneous tissue (i.e., wound drainage) in women with any thickness and who did not receive prophylactic antibiotics with a 2-cm corrugated rubber drain, left to drain open, coming out of one end of incision, and removed the following day is associated with a trend toward increased wound infection (75). Drainage is also not as effective as tissue closure for women with ≥2 cm of subcutaneous fat. Drainage was usually performed with a 7-mm Jackson–Pratt drain (75). Therefore, **routine subcutaneous tissue drainage in women undergoing CD cannot be recommended.** These trials do not answer the question of whether wound drainage is of benefit when hemostasis is not felt to be adequate.

Closure of Skin

Closure of skin at CD has been most commonly performed with either sutures or metal staples. Compared with sutures, staple closure is associated with higher wound infection or separation (13% vs. 7%), and a shorter duration of surgery, with no other significant differences in pain, cosmesis, or patient satisfaction (76). In these studies there is no blinding possible, and no long-term outcome reported. Additionally, often the staples were removed <4 days after CD, which might not allow sufficient healing. The types of sutures or method of suturing have never been compared. The general surgery literature seems to support the evidence that subcuticular suture is associated with less pain and better cosmesis. CD is considered a clean-contaminated procedure, with a relatively high risk of wound infection. In clean-contaminated procedures, the general surgical literature would suggest avoiding a continuous method of wound closure. In contrast with interrupted closure (with staples or sutures), continuous wound closure does not allow selective, minimal wound opening in cases of infection or collections. Therefore, **there is no conclusive evidence about how the skin should be closed after CD.**

POSTOPERATIVE CARE
Gum Chewing

Compared with no gum chewing, **gum chewing three times/ day for at least 30 minutes each time after CD is associated with a earlier return of bowel sounds (by 5 hours), earlier passage of flatus (by about 5 hours), and less (12% vs. 21%) symptoms of mild ileus** (77).

Oral Fluids and Feeding

Compared with delayed (usually ≥24 hours) oral fluids or food, **early oral fluids or food** are associated with reduced time (by about 7 hours) to first food intake; reduced time (by about 4 hours) to return of bowel sounds; reduced postoperative hospital stay (by about 0.75 days) following surgery under regional analgesia; and a trend to reduced abdominal distension (RR 0.78, 95% CI 0.55–1.11). No significant differences were identified with respect to nausea, vomiting, time to bowel action/passing flatus, paralytic ileus, and number of analgesic doses, based on a few small RCTs (78). In summary, **there is insufficient evidence for a strong recommendation, but early oral fluids and even food after CD seem to be safe and possibly beneficial.**

Pain Relief after CD

See also chapter 11. **Nonsteroidal anti-inflammatory drugs** (NSAIDs; e.g., ibuprofen) and/or **narcotics** (e.g., oxycodone) are commonly used in the United States for post-CD pain relief. There is no RCT evaluating oral narcotic use or oral NSAIDs use. **Local analgesia wound infiltration** and **abdominal nerve blocks** as adjuncts to regional analgesia and general anesthesia seem to be of benefit in CD by reducing opioid consumption in small RCTs. NSAIDs (even as a wound infiltration) as an adjuvant may confer additional pain relief (79).

In detail, in women who had CD performed under regional analgesia, wound infiltration is associated with a decrease in morphine consumption at 24 hours compared with placebo. In women with regional analgesia and also a local anesthetic, NSAID cocktail wound infiltration is associated with less morphine use compared with local anesthetic control. Women who have regional analgesia with abdominal nerves blocked have decreased opioid consumption. In women under general anesthesia, with CD wound infiltration and peritoneal spraying with local anesthetic, the need for opioid rescue is reduced (79).

MANAGEMENT OF COMPLICATIONS
Disrupted (Open) Laparotomy Wound

Compared with healing by secondary intention, **reclosure of the disrupted laparotomy wound is associated with success in >80% of women, faster healing times** (16–23 vs. 61–72 days), **and fewer office visits** (80). No serious morbidity or mortality is associated with either method. There is insufficient evidence to assess optimal timing (probably 4–6 days after disruption if noninfected) and technique (superficial vertical mattress or "en bloc" reclosure of entire wound thickness with absorbable sutures, or adhesive tape) of reclosure, as well as utility of antibiotics. **Compared with reclosure using sutures, reclosure using permeable, adhesive tape** (Cover-Roll; Biersdorf, Inc., Norwalk, Connecticut, U.S.) is associated with faster procedure, less pain scores, and similar healing times in a small RCT (81).

Postoperative Counseling

Interval until next pregnancy after a CD should be 12 to 24 months, as shorter intervals have been associated with increased risk of uterine rupture. See also chapter 14.

REFERENCES

1. Berghella V, Baxter JK, Chauhan SP. Evidence-based surgery for cesarean delivery. Am J Obstet Gynecol 2005; 193:1607–1617. [Systematic review]
2. CDC National Vital Statistics Report. Births: preliminary data for 2008. December, 2010. Available at: http://www.cdc.gov/nchs/data/nvsr/nvsr58/nvsr58_16.pdf. [Data review]
3. Saisto T, Salmela-Aro K, Nurmi JE, et al. A randomized controlled trial of intervention in fear of childbirth. Obstet Gynecol 2001; 98(5):820–826. [RCT, n = 176]
4. Mazzoni A, Althabe F, Liu NH, et al. Women's preference for caesarean section: a systematic review and meta-analysis of observational studies. Br J Obstet Gynecol 2011; 118:391–399. [Meta-analysis of 23 observational studies, n = 13,922]
5. Matthews TG, Crowley P, Chong A, et al. Rising cesarean section rates: a cause for concern? Br J Obstet Gynecol 2003; 110:346–349. [Review]
6. Khunpradit S, Tavender E, Lumbiganon P, et al. Non-clinical interventions for reducing unnecessary caesarean section. Cochrane Database Syst Rev 2011; (6):CD005528. [Meta-analysis: 16 RCTs]
7. Althabe F, Belizan JM, Villar J, et al. Mandatory second opinion to reduce rates of unnecessary caesarean sections in Latin America: a cluster randomized controlled trial. Lancet 2004; 363:1934–1940. [RCT]
8. U.S. Preventive Services Task Force. Agency for health care research and quality. Available at: www.ahcpr.gov. [Guideline]
9. Haynes AB, Weiser TG, Berry WR, et al. A surgical safety checklist to reduce morbidity and mortality in a global population. N Engl J Med 2009; 360:491–499. [II-2]
10. Hopkins L, Smaill FM. Antibiotic prophylaxis regimens and drugs for cesarean section. Cochrane Database Syst Rev 1999; (2):CD001136. [51 RCTs, n = >10,000]
11. Smaill FM, Gyte GML. Antibiotic prophylaxis versus no prophylaxis for preventing infection after cesarean section. Cochrane Database Syst Rev 2010; (1): CD007482. [Meta-analysis: 86 RCTs, n = 13,000]
12. Alfirevic Z, Gyte GML, Dou L. Different classes of antibiotics given to women routinely for preventing infection at caesarean section. Cochrane Database Syst Rev 2010; (10):CD008726. [Meta-analysis: 25 RCTs, n = 2627]
13. Tita ATN, Rouse DJ, Blackwell S, et al. Emerging concepts in antibiotic prophylaxis fro cesarean delivery. Obstet Gynecol 2009; 113:675–682. [Meta-analysis of RCTs]
14. Gordon HR, Phelps D, Blanchard K. Prophylactic cesarean section antibiotics: maternal and neonatal morbidity before or after cord clamping. Obstet Gynecol 1979; 53:151–156. [RCT, n = 114]
15. Cunningham FG, Leveno KJ, DePalma RT, et al. Perioperative antimicrobials for cesarean delivery: before or after cord clamping? Obstet Gynecol 1983; 62:151–154. [RCT, n = 305]
16. Wax JR, Hersey K, Philput C, et al. Single dose cefazolin prophylaxis for postcesarean infections: before vs. after cord clamping. J Matern Fetal Med 1997; 6:61–65. [RCT, n = 90]
17. Thigpen BD, Hood WA, Chauhan S, et al. Timing of prophylactic antibiotic administration in the uninfected laboring gravida: a randomized clinical trial. Am J Obstet Gynecol 2005; 192:1864–1871. [RCT, n = 303]
18. Ohly NT, Baxter JK, Mackeen AD, Berghella V. Timing of antibiotic prophylaxis for preventing postpartum infectious morbidity in women undergoing cesarean delivery. Cochrane Database Syst Rev 2012 (in press).
19. Clark SL, Belfort MA, Dildy GA, et al. Maternal death in the 21st century: causes, prevention, and relationship to cesarean delivery. Am J Obstet Gynecol 2008; 199(1):36.e1–36.e5. [II-1]
20. Tooher R, Gates S, Dowswell T, et al. Prophylaxis for venous thromboembolic disease in pregnancy and the early postnatal period. Cochrane Database Syst Rev 2010; (5):CD001689. [Meta-analysis: 13 RCTs, n = 1774]
21. SMFM, Publication Committee, with Varner MW. Thromboprophylaxis for cesarean delivery. Cont Obstet Gynecol 2011; 6:30–33. [Review]
22. Chauhan SP, Macones GA. ACOG Practice Bulletin No. 62: intrapartum fetal heart rate monitoring. Obstet Gynecol 2005; 105(5 pt 1):1161–1169. [Review]
23. Stuchfield P, Whitaker R, Russell I, et al. Antenatal betamethasone and incidence of neonatal respiratory distress after elective caesarean section: pragmatic randomized trial. BMJ 2005; 331:662–668. [RCT; n = 942]

24. Laopaiboon M, Lumbiganon P, Martis R, et al. Music during caesarean section under regional anaesthesia for improving maternal and infant outcomes. Cochrane Database Syst Rev 2009; (2):CD006914. [Meta-analysis: 1 RCT, $n = 76$]

25. Cluver C, Novikova N, Hofmeyr GJ, et al. Maternal position during caesarean section for preventing maternal and neonatal complications. Cochrane Database Syst Rev 2010; (6):CD007623. [Meta-analysis: 9 RCTs, $n = 683$]

26. Li L, Wen J, Wang L, et al. Is routine indwelling catheterization of the bladder for caesarean section necessary? A systematic review. Br J Obstet Gynecol 2011; 118:400–409. [Meta-analysis: 2 RCTs, $n = 690$]

27. Magann EF, Dodson MK, Ray MA, et al. Preoperative skin preparation and intraoperative pelvic irrigation: impact on post cesarean endometritis and wound infection. Obstet Gynecol 1993; 81:922–925. [RCT, $n = 50$]

28. Haas DM, Morgan Al Darei S, Contreras K, Vaginal preparation with antiseptic solution before cesarean section for preventing postoperative infections. Cochrane Database Syst Rev 2010; (3): CD007892. [Meta-analysis: 4 RCTs, $n = 1198$]

29. Pitt C, Sanchez-ramos L, Kaunitz AM. Adjunctive intravaginal metronidazole for the prevention of postcesarean endometritis: a randomized controlled trial. Obstet Gynecol 2001; 98:745–750. [RCT, $n = 224$]

30. Cordtz T, Schouenborg L, Lauren K, et al. The effect of incision plastic drapes and redisinfection of operation site on wound infection following caesarean section. J Hosp Infect 1989; 13:267–272. [RCT, $n = 1340$]

31. Ward HRG, Jennings OGN, Potgieter P, et al. Do plastic adhesive drapes prevent post caesarean wound infection? J Hosp Infect 2001; 47:230–234. [RCT, $n = 605$]

32. Franchi M, Ghezzi F, Raio L, et al. Joel-Cohen or Pfannenstiel incision at cesarean delivery: does it make a difference? Acta Obstet Gynecol Scand 2002; 81:1040–1046. [RCT, $n = 366$]

33. Mathai M, Ambersheth S, George A. Comparison of two transverse abdominal incisions for cesarean delivery. Int J Gynecol Obstet 2002; 78:47–49. [RCT, $n = 101$ (411 total)]

34. Hofmeyr GJ, Mathai M, Shah AN, et al. Techniques for caesarean section. Cochrane Database Sys Rev 2008; (1):CD004662. [Meta-analysis: 8 RCTs, $n = 412$]

35. Mathai M, Hofmeyr GJ. Abdominal surgical incisions for caesarean section. Cochrane Database Sys Rev 2007; (1):CD004453. [Meta-analysis: 4 RCTs]

36. Wylie BJ, Gilbert S, Landon MB, et al. Comparison of transverse and vertical skin incision for emergency cesarean delivery. Obstet Gynecol 2010; 115:1134–1140. [II-1]

37. Ayers JWT, Morley GW. Surgical incision for cesarean section. Obstet Gynecol 1987; 70:706–708. [RCT, $n = 97$]

38. Berthet J, Peresse JF, Rosier P, et al. Comparative study of Pfannesteil's incision and transverse abdominal incision in gynecologic and obstetric surgery. Presse Med 1989; 18:1431–1433. [RCT]

39. Giacalone PL, Daures JP, Vignal J, et al. Pfannesteil versus Maylard incision for cesarean delivery: a randomized controlled trial. Obstet Gynecol 2002; 99:745–750. [RCT, $n = 97$]

40. Hohlagschwandtner M, Ruecklinger E, Husslein P, et al. Is the formation of a bladder flap at cesarean necessary? A randomized trial. Obstet Gynecol 2001; 98:1089–1092. [RCT, $n = 102$]

41. Lao TT, Halpern SH, Crosby ET, et al. Uterine incision and maternal blood loss in preterm caesarean section. Arch Gynecol Obstet 1993; 252:113–117. [II-2]

42. Dodd JM, Anderson ER, Gates S. Surgical techniques for uterine incision and uterine closure at the time of caesarean section. Cochrane Database Sys Rev 2008; (3):CD004732. [Meta-analysis: 2 RCTs, $n = 397$]

43. Wilkinson C, Enkin MW. Absorbable staples for uterine incision at caesarean section. Cochrane Database Sys Rev 2005; (1): CD004549. [Meta-analysis: 4 RCTs, $n = 526$]

44. Rodriguez AI, Porter KB, O'Brien WF. Blunt versus sharp expansion of the uterine incision in low-segment transverse cesarean section. Am J Obstet Gynecol 1994; 171:1022–1025. [RCT, $n = 286$]

45. Magann EF, Chauhan SP, Bufkin L, et al. Intra-operative haemorrhage by blunt versus sharp expansion of the uterine incision at caesarean delivery: a randomised clinical trial. Br J Obstet Gynaecol 2002; 109:448–452. [RCT, $n = 945$]

46. Cromi A, Ghezzi F, Dinaro E, et al. Blunt expansion of the low transverse uterine incision at cesarean delivery: a randomized comparison of 2 techniques. Am J Obstet Gynecol 2008; 199:292. e1–292.e6. [RCT, $n = 811$]

47. Bofill JA, Lencki SG, Barhan S, et al. Instrumental delivery of the fetal head at the time of elective repeat cesarean: a randomized pilot study. Am J Perinatol 2000; 17(5):265–269. [RCT, $n = 44$]

48. David M, Halle H, Lichtenegger W, et al. Nitroglycerin to facilitate fetal extraction during cesarean delivery. Obstet Gynecol 1998; 91:119–124. [RCT, $n = 97$]

49. Munn MB, Owen J, Vincent R, et al. Comparison of two oxytocin regimens to prevent uterine atony at cesarean delivery: a randomized controlled trial. Obstet Gynecol 2001; 98:386–390. [RCT, $n = 321$]

50. Boucher M, Horbay GLA, Griffin P, et al. Double-blind, randomized comparison of the effect of carbetocin and oxytocin on intraoperative blood loss and uterine tone of patients undergoing cesarean section. J Perinat 1998; 18:202–207. [RCT, $n = 57$]

51. Dansereau J, Joshi AK, Helewa ME, et al. Double-blind comparison of carbetocin versus oxytocin in prevention of uterine atony after cesarean section. Am J Obstet Gynecol 1999; 180:670–676. [RCT, $n = 694$]

52. Balki M, Dhumme S, Kasodekar S, et al. Oxytocin-ergometrine co-administration does not reduce blood loss at caesarean delivery for labour arrest. Br J Obstet Gynecol 2008; 115:579–584. [RCT, $n = 48$]

53. Anorlu RI, Maholwana B, Hofmeyr GJ. Methods of delivering the placenta at caesarean section. Cochrane Database Sys Rev 2008; (3):CD004737. [Meta-analysis: 15 RCTs, $n = 4694$]

54. Leavitt BG, Huff DL, Bell LA, et al. Placental drainage of fetal blood at cesarean delivery and feto-maternal transfusion. Obstet Gynecol 2007; 110:608–611. [RCT, $n = 86$]

55. Wilkinson C, Enkin MW. Manual removal of placenta at cesarean section. Cochrane Database Sys Rev 2004; (4):CD000085. [Meta-analysis: not yet updated, should include 12 RCTs, $n = >3000$]

56. Atkinson MW, Owen J, Wren A, et al. The effect of manual removal of the placenta on post-cesarean endometritis. Obstet Gynecol 1996; 87:99–102. [RCT, $n = 643$]

57. Jacobs-Jokhan D, Hofmeyr GJ. Extra-abdominal versus intra-abdominal repair of the uterine incision at caesarean section. Cochrane Database Sys Rev 2005; (1). [Meta-analysis: 6 RCTs, $n = 1221$]

58. Walsh CA, Walsh SR. Extraabdominal vs intraabdominal uterine repair at cesarean delivery: a metaanalysis. Am J Obstet Gynecol 2009; 200:625. [Meta-analysis: 11 RCTs, $n = 3183$]

59. Ahmed B, Abu Nahia F, Abushama M. Routine cervical dilatation during elective cesarean section and its influence on maternal morbidity: a randomized controlled study. J Perinat Med 2005; 33 (6):510–513. [RCT, $n = 131$]

60. Stafford MK, Pitman MC, Nanthakumaran N, et al. Blunt-tipped versus sharp-tipped needles: wound morbidity. J Obstet Gynecol 1998; 18:18–19. [RCT, $n = 203$]

61. Sullivan S, Williamson B, Wilson LK, et al. Blunt needles for the reduction of needlestick injuries during cesarean delivery. Obstet Gynecol 2009; 114:211–216. [RCT, $n = 194$]

62. Yazicioglu F, Gokdogan A, Kelekci S, et al. Incomplete healing of the uterine incision after caesarean section: is it preventable? Eur J Obstet Gynecol Reprod Biol 2006; 124:32–36. [RCT, $n = 78$]

63. Hohlagschwandtner M, Chalubinski K, Nather A, et al. Continuous vs interrupted sutures for single-layer closure of uterine incision at cesarean section. Arch Gynecol Obstet 2003; 268:26–28. [II-2, $n = 81$]

64. Enkin MW, Wilkinson C. Single versus two layer suturing for closing the uterine incision at caesarean section. Cochrane Database Sys Rev 2005; (1). [Meta-analysis: 2 RCTs, $n = 1006$]

65. Chapman SJ, Owen J, Hauth JC. One-versus two-layer closure of a low transverse cesarean: the next pregnancy. Obstet Gynecol 1997; 89:16–18. [Follow-up of RCT]

66. Bujold E, Goyet M, Marcoux S, et al. The role of uterine closure in the risk of uterine rupture. Obstet Gynecol 2010; 116:43–50. [II-2, n = 98 cases of uterine rupture]
67. Harrigill KM, Miller HS, Haynes DE. The effect of intraabdominal irrigation at cesarean delivery on maternal morbidity: a randomized trial. Obstet Gynecol 2003; 101:80–85. [RCT, n = 196]
68. Pearce C, Torres C, Stallings S, et al. Elective appendectomy at the time of cesarean delivery: a randomized controlled trial. Am J Obstet Gynecol 2008; 199:491. [RCT, n = 93]
69. The CAESAR Study Collaborative Group. Caesarean section surgical techniques: a randomized factorial trial. Br J Obstet Gynecol 2010; 117:1366–1376. [RCT, n = 3033]
70. Bamigboye AA, Hofmeyr GJ. Closure versus non-closure of the peritoneum at caesarean section. Cochrane Database Sys Rev 2003; (4):CD000163. [Meta-analysis: 14 RCTs, n = 2908]
71. Roset E, Boulvain M, Irion O. Nonclosure of the peritoneum during cesarean section: long term follow-up of a randomized controlled trial. Eur J Obstet Gynecol Reprod Biol 2003; 108:40–44. [Follow-up of RCT]
72. Bamigboye AA, Hofmeyr GJ. Closure versus non-closure of the peritoneum at caesarean section. Cochrane Database Sys Rev 2005; (1):CD004549. [Meta-analysis: 9 RCTs, n = 1811]
73. Tulandi T, Al-Jaroudi D. Nonclosure of peritoneum: a reappraisal. Am J Obstet Gynecol 2003; 189:609–612. [Review]
74. Hellums EK, Lin MG, Ramsey PS. Prophylactic subcutaneous drainage for prevention of wound complications at cesarean delivery—a meta-analysis. Am J Obstet Gynecol 2007; 229–235. [Meta-analysis: 6 RCTs]
75. Gates S, Anderson ER. Wound drainage for caesarean section. Cochrane Database Sys Rev 2005; (1):CD004549. [Meta-analysis: 9 RCTs, n = 2421]
76. Tuuli MG, Rampersad RM, Carbone JF, et al. Staples compared to subcuticular suture for skin closure after cesarean delivery. Obstet Gynecol 2011; 117:682–690. [Meta-analysis: 5 RCTs]
77. Shang H, Yang Y, Tong X, et al. Gum chewing slightly enhances early recovery from postoperative ileus after cesarean section: results of a prospective, randomized, controlled trial. Am J Perinatol 2010; 27:387–391. [RCT, n = 288]
78. Mangesi L, Hofmeyr GJ. Early compared with delayed oral fluids and food after caesarean section. Cochrane Database Sys Rev 2002; (3):CD003516. [Meta-analysis: 6 RCTs, n = about 500]
79. Bamigboye AA, Hofmeyr GJ. Local anaesthetic wound infiltration and abdominal nerves block during caesarean section for postoperative pain relief. Cochrane Database Sys Rev 2009; (3): CD006954. [Meta-analysis: 20 RCTs, n = 1150]
80. Wechter ME, Pearlman MD, Hartmann KE. Reclosure of the disrupted laparotomy wound. Obstet Gynecol 2005; 106:376–383. [Meta-analysis: 8 RCTs, n = 324. Includes both CDs, gyn and GI laparotomies]
81. Harris RL, Magann EF, Sullivan DL, et al. Extrafascial wound dehiscence: secondary closure with suture versus noninvasive adhesive bandage. J Pelvic Surg 1995; 1:88–91. [RCT, n = 27]

14

Trial of labor after cesarean

Amen Ness

KEY POINTS

- A woman with a prior cesarean delivery (CD) has two options for mode of delivery in the subsequent pregnancy: a planned repeat cesarean delivery (PRCD) or a trial of labor after cesarean (TOLAC) to try to achieve a vaginal birth after cesarean (VBAC).
- There is insufficient evidence to compare the safety, complications, maternal and fetal/neonatal morbidity and mortality between these two options, as only a small randomized trial focused on psychological outcomes has been reported to date.
- TOLAC is a "reasonable option" for most women with a single prior low transverse CD with no other contraindications to a vaginal birth.
- Absolute contraindications to TOLAC are as follows:
  - Medical or obstetrical complications that preclude vaginal delivery
  - Inability to perform emergency CD
  - Vertical (classical) uterine scar or fundal or perifundal complete (from endometrium to serosa) uterine scar from other surgery (e.g., myomectomy)
  - Prior uterine rupture
- Successful VBAC rates in the general population of women with previous low transverse uterine incisions vary from 60% to 80%. Women with prior CD and without prior VBAC may have success rates of ≤50% if they have >2 prior CD, weight >300 lb or BMI >30, macrosomia >4000 g, etc. (Table 14.2). No screening tool is sensitive enough to be clinically useful in predicting an unsuccessful trial of labor. One available for clinical use is at www.bsc.gwu.edu/mfmu/vagbirth.html.
- Rates of maternal and perinatal complications are in general similar and low with both TOLAC and PRCD, except for the risk of uterine rupture, which confers both maternal and perinatal risks. Uterine rupture is the main complication associated with TOLAC. Most maternal and perinatal morbidity results from repeat CD after TOLAC.
- The overall risk of uterine rupture during a TOLAC at term is 0.7% after one prior low transverse CD, versus 0.26% after PRCD. The lowest risk (0.4%) of rupture is with spontaneous labor TOLAC. With prior VBAC, TOLAC has also a very low (about 0.5%) risk of rupture. The risk is increased with >1 prior CD, prior vertical scar, prior rupture, induction of labor with no prior vaginal deliveries (especially when using prostaglandin ripening agents), augmentation with higher doses of oxytocin, interval between deliveries <18 months, maternal age >30-year-old, fetal macrosomia, single-layer closure, fever at time of prior CD, etc. (Table 14.2).
- With term uterine rupture, the risks of fetal/neonatal morbidity/mortality are about 33% risk of pH < 7.00, 40% admission to neonatal intensive care unit (NICU), 6%

risk of hypoxic-ischemic encephalopathy (HIE), and 1.8% risk of neonatal death (rupture-related risk of neonatal death: 1/10,000 TOLAC) in equipped academic centers. In other centers, these risks are higher, including risk of neonatal death from rupture up to 10% to 25%.
- Compared with PRCD, TOLAC is associated with slightly higher rates of adverse perinatal outcome: cord pH < 7.00 (1.5/1000 TOLAC), HIE (5–8/10,000), and perinatal death (13/10,000 with TOLAC vs. 1/10,000 for PRCD) (Table 14.3). The overall risk of adverse perinatal outcome is 1/2000 with TOLAC, slightly higher than with PRCD.
- When compared with women without a previous CD (instead of with those having a planned primary CD), the perinatal mortality for TOLAC is higher than PRCD (10/10,000 vs. 0.4/10,000 births), but this rate is twice as high as that of a non-VBAC multipara in labor and the same as that of a nullipara in labor.
- Appropriate counseling including risks as described should be provided to the woman with a prior CD deciding on subsequent mode of delivery. The ultimate decision regarding TOLAC or PRCD is up to the patient.
- To minimize risks, an experienced obstetrician, anesthesia, nursing, and OR personnel, and ability to perform emergency CD must be immediately available throughout the TOLAC.

HISTORICAL PERSPECTIVE

Each year almost 1.5 million childbearing U.S. women have cesarean deliveries, and this population continues to increase. Most of these are primary CDs but, the largest single indication for CD is prior CD, accounting for over half a million CDs each year (1). In order to reduce this trend, there is a need to both reduce the frequency of a first CD and increase the use of a TOLAC in appropriate candidates.

Until the late 1970s, "Once a cesarean always a cesarean" was the general rule among most obstetricians. This phrase did not derive from formal studies and was clearly not evidence based. A classical uterine incision was used until the1920s when the low transverse incision was first introduced. The low transverse incision was associated with a tenfold decreased rate of uterine rupture in labor than the classical incision. On the basis of studies in the 1970s, when the VBAC rate was very low, the National Institutes of Health (NIH) in 1980 and then the American College of Obstetricians and Gynecologists (ACOG) in 1988 and in 1994, in an attempt to lower CD rates, suggested that a trial of labor (TOL) after a previous low transverse CD is a reasonable option (2). ACOG encouraged all women with a single prior low transverse cesarean section to consider a TOLAC. In response to these recommendations, the VBAC rate in the United States increased from 3.5% in 1980 to 28.3% in 1996 (Figure 14.1).

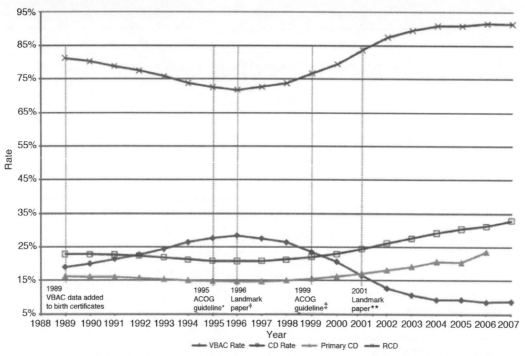

*1995 ACOG guidelines states "In the absence of contraindications, a woman with one previous cesarean delivery with a lower transverse uterine incision is a candidate for VBAC and should be counseled and encouraged to undergo a trial of labor."

† 1996 Landmark paper by McMahon (6).

‡1999 ACOG states "VBAC should be attempted in institutions equipped to respond to emergencies with physicians immediately available to provide emergency care."

**2001 Landmark paper by Lydon-Rochelle (60).

Figure 14.1   Rates of vaginal birth after cesarean (VBAC rate), total cesarean deliveries (CD rate), primary cesarean deliveries (Primary CD), and repeat cesarean delivery (RCD). *Source*: From Refs. 1,3.

As more VBACs were attempted, more ruptures were seen and litigation for complications of a TOL also increased. As a result, in 1999, ACOG addressed these risks and added the requirements of a "readily available" physician "throughout labor" and "availability of anesthesia and personnel for emergency CD." Since that time, after declining until about 1997, CDs have increased globally, 33% in the United States in 2009 and 24% in England in 2010 (3,4). At the same time, **VBAC rates have decreased rapidly to just 8.5% in the United States in 2007** (Fig. 14.1), although they have remained relatively high in the United Kingdom at 33% (range 6–64%) (5). The ACOG requirement for "immediately available" personnel for women undergoing a TOLAC, but not for other laboring women, eliminated the option of TOLAC/VBAC in many community hospitals. Since 1996, about one-third of hospitals and one-half of physicians have stopped offering TOLAC/ VBAC in the United States (5).

DEFINITIONS

TOLAC: Trial of labor after cesarean.
  VBAC: Vaginal delivery after cesarean delivery.
  PRCD: Planned repeat cesarean delivery (before labor).
  VBAC rate: Number of vaginal births after previous CD per 100 live births to all women with a previous CD. (Same denominator as the CD rate)

TOLAC rate: If the average success rate of a TOLAC is about 70%, then the TOLAC rate is the VBAC rate/0.7.
  Adjusted VBAC rate: Number of women with prior CD **and no contraindications to TOL** who had a VBAC per 100 live births to all women with a previous CD.
  Successful VBAC rate: Percentage of women with prior CD who attempted a TOLAC achieving VBAC.
  Successful adjusted VBAC rate: Percentage of women with prior CD **and no contraindications to TOLAC** achieving a VBAC.
  Failed TOLAC (failed VBAC): TOLAC that results in a repeat CD.
  Uterine dehiscence: Disruption of the uterine muscle **with intact serosa** (4). It can include asymptomatic opening if the uterine scar is from prior surgery, without protrusion of fetus/fetal organs outside the uterus.
  Uterine rupture: Disruption or tear of the uterine muscle and visceral peritoneum, or separation of the uterine muscle with **extension to the bladder or broad ligament** (4). It includes symptomatic gross rupture of the uterine scar from prior surgery, with or without protrusion of fetus/fetal organs outside the uterus.

GENERAL CONSIDERATIONS

A woman with a prior CD has two options for mode of delivery in the subsequent pregnancy: a **PRCD or a TOLAC** to try to achieve a VBAC. There is only one small RCT to compare these two options, and it focuses on psychological outcomes, not maternal and fetal safety and complications (6). Virtually all studies on VBAC, except for a few exceptions (7), are retrospective and often use differing criteria for patient selection and differ in their ability to correctly ascertain (make sure all cases are included) and define uterine rupture. Most studies also include women at various gestational ages and may therefore not specifically apply to women at term considering their options of delivery after a prior CD. Studies with <1000 TOLAC cannot adequately assess maternal and fetal/neonatal morbidity and mortality, as these complications are rare, and meta-analyses (8–10) might compound errors from different retrospective studies. Many studies do not differentiate between asymptomatic uterine dehiscence and true acute symptomatic uterine rupture.

The **main issues** regarding TOL after CD (attempt at VBAC) are the following: (*i*) Which women are **candidates** for TOLAC, and which should instead be recommended a PRCD? (*ii*) Among women who attempt a TOLAC, what is the **VBAC rate** (successful TOLAC) and the factors that influence it? (*iii*) What are the short- and long-term **maternal and perinatal benefits and harms** of attempting TOLAC versus PRCD, and what factors influence benefits and harms? Complications and safety are especially related to the risk of **uterine rupture**.

These issues are important in order to **properly counsel** women who are considering a TOLAC (5). This information should be shared with the woman in a way best suited to her understanding. When a TOLAC and a PRCD are medically equivalent options, the woman's preference should be honored if possible (1).

CANDIDATES FOR TOLAC

The choice of candidates for TOLAC should be based on an acceptable balance between the chance of achieving a VBAC and fetal and maternal risks. The ACOG and the 2010 NIH consensus statement acknowledged that **TOLAC is a reasonable option for most women with a single prior low transverse CD with no other contraindications to a vaginal birth** (2,5). Criteria to be a candidate, and absolute and relative contraindications for TOLAC are shown in Table 14.1.

Table 14.1 Candidates, and Absolute and Relative Contraindications for Trial of Labor After Cesarean

- Singleton gestation
- Clinically adequate pelvis
- One prior low transverse cesarean delivery
- No other uterine scars or previous rupture

Limited evidence
- A twin pregnancy who is a candidate for VBAC
- Unknown uterine scar (low clinical suspicion of prior classical uterine incision)

Absolute contraindications
- Medical or obstetrical complications that preclude vaginal delivery
- Inability to perform emergency CD
- Vertical (classical) uterine scar
- Fundal or perifundal complete (from endometrium to serosa) uterine scar from other surgery (e.g., myomectomy)
- Prior uterine rupture

Relative contraindications
- Multiple uterine scars (e.g., ≥2 prior CDs)
- Any other factor associated with a risk of rupture of >1% (see text)

FACTORS FOR SUCCESSFUL TOLAC

Vaginal delivery rates for TOLAC in the general population of women with previous low transverse uterine incisions vary from 60% to 80% (7,8,11). In tertiary care centers the rates may be higher, about 73% to 76% (7,12). The rate is highly dependent on demographic and obstetric factors (Table 14.2). Based on these factors, **women with a probability for VBAC of at least 60% to 70% have similar or less maternal and perinatal morbidity with a TOLAC than a PRCD** (13,14). Conversely, women with less than a 60% probability of VBAC have a greater likelihood of morbidity with TOLAC than if they had a PRCD. One study demonstrated that composite neonatal morbidity is similar between TOLAC and PRCD for the women with the greatest probability of achieving VBAC (13,15). Factors that influence the likelihood of VBAC after TOLAC, and their effect of success rates, are shown in Table 14.2, and described below.

Maternal Demographics

Age

There is inconsistent evidence regarding the effect of age on VBAC after a TOLAC. Recent prospective studies did not show any relationship although overall there appears to be a small inverse association between maternal age and the likelihood of vaginal delivery (1).

Race/Ethnicity

Race and ethnicity are the strongest demographic predictors of VBAC. **Hispanic and African-American women have lower rates of VBAC** than non-Hispanic white women.

Obesity

Obese women attempting a VBAC have **lower vaginal delivery rates**. This appears to be true whether measured at first prenatal visit (per BMI unit) or at delivery (BMI > 30) [adjusted ORs (aORs) 0.94, 95% CI 0.93–0.95 and 0.55, 95% CI 0.51–0.60, respectively] (16,17). **Obese women, weighing ≥300 lb, had rates of VBAC of only 15%,** while women weighing 200 to 300 lb had rates of 56% (18). Women ≥300 lb also have a >50% chance of infectious morbidity (vs. 17.8% in women weighing 200–300 lb) (19). PRCD in the obese group significantly reduced the infectious morbidity by almost 50% compared with those with a TOLAC (20). **Greater maternal height and body mass index below 30 kg/m² are associated with an increased likelihood of VBAC.**

Others

Single marital status and less than 12 years of education also have been associated with lower rates of VBAC.

Obstetric History

Prior Vaginal Delivery

A prior vaginal delivery, either before or after a prior CD, is the strongest predictor of a VBAC after a TOLAC. A previous successful VBAC is the most predictive (21). **The VBAC rate is >85%, even 90% in some reports, for women with a prior VBAC,** compared with 65% for women without a prior vaginal delivery (22,23). Based on data from the Maternal-Fetal Medicine Units (MFMU) cohort, the rate of VBAC increases with each prior VBAC (24). Women with zero, one, two, three, and four or more prior VBACs had likelihoods of VBAC of 63%, 88%, 91%, 91%, and 91% (*p* < 0.001), respectively (24).

Prior Indication for Cesarean

Breech presentation or other **nonrecurring indication** (e.g., nonreassuring fetal monitoring) for the prior CD significantly increase the chances for a vaginal delivery (85%) compared

Table 14.2 Factors Associated with Success and Risk of Uterine Rupture Associated with TOLAC

Factor	Effect on success rates[a]	Effect on risk of uterine rupture with TOLAC (% risk)	Comment (references)
Maternal demographics			
Older age	↓	↑	
Obesity	↓↓	NA	
Obstetric history			
Prior vaginal delivery	↑↑	↓↓ (0.2%)	Especially prior VBAC. **Recommend TOLAC** (4,16,37)
No prior uterine scars	NA	NA (<0.01%)	
Prior nonrecurring indication for CD	↑		For example, prior CD for malpresentation
Labor before primary CD		↓	(45)
More than 1 prior CDs	↓	↑ (see below)	10–15% lower success rate per CD
1 Prior LT CD (no prior VBAC)		(0.7%, range 0.5–1.0)[b]	(4,5)
1 Prior LT CD (prior VBAC)		↓ (<0.5%)	(13,39,40)
2 Prior LT CD (no prior VBAC)		↑ (1.8%, 1–3.7%)	(8,39,40)
2 Prior LT CD (prior VBAC)		↓ (0.5%)	(39)
Prior vertical (classical) CD		↑↑ (4–10%)	**Avoid TOLAC** (1)
Prior low-vertical CD		↑ (1–2%)	(4,6)
Prior "unknown uterine scar" CD		(0.5–2%)	(4)
1-Layer uterine closure		↑ (1–2%)	(6,41,42)[c]
Fever at prior CD		↑	If both intra- and postpartum fever
Prior preterm CD		↑ (1%)	
Prior uterine rupture		↑↑ (6% if lower segment rupture; 32% if upper segment rupture)	**Avoid TOLAC** (1)
Short interpregnancy interval		↑↑ (2–5%)	<18 months; avoid TOLAC (49–52)
Current labor factors			
PRCD	NA	(0–0.15% in labor) (0.5 risk of dehiscence)	(4,60)
Favorable cervical status	↑↑	↓↓	Bishop score >8, or CL < 15 mm
Postdates	↓	–	Uterine rupture rate increased if induced/augmented
Fetal macrosomia (e.g., BW ≥4000–4500 g)	↓	↑	Uterine rupture rate increased by relative risk 2.3 (21)
Induction/augmentation of labor	↓	↑ (mostly 1–2%)	Avoid misoprostol; avoid PGE2 followed by oxytocin; avoid oxytocin >20 mU/min. See below (4,44–48)
Misoprostol induction		↑↑ (>5%)	**Avoid**
PGE2 only induction		↑ (1%)	Cannot predict if PGE2 will be sufficient
PGE2 then oxytocin induction		↑ (1–3%)	Probably avoid
Foley induction		–	Probably safe
Oxytocin only induction		↑ (1.1%)	
Oxytocin augmentation		↑ (0.9%)	

[a]Chance of achieving vaginal birth after CD.
[b]Used as reference.
[c]See chapter 13.
Abbreviations: CD, cesarean delivery; PRCD, planned repeat CD; TOLAC, trial of labor after CD; NA, not applicable; BW, birth weight.

with CD done for dystocia or failure to progress. These rates are similar to vaginal delivery rates in nulliparous women. Nevertheless, about 60% to 70% of women undergoing a TOLAC for **dystocia** (failure to progress) deliver vaginally (1). In addition, most studies show no reduction in the rates for a successful TOLAC after a **prior CD done for failure to progress in the second stage of labor** (75–80%), with no increased risk of operative vaginal delivery (1,25,26).

Uterine Scar Type
Vaginal delivery rates appear to be **similar** for low transverse, low vertical, and for unknown incision types (9,17). Most women with unknown scar types have had low transverse incisions.

Number of Prior Cesarean Deliveries
Previous studies had reported that 75% to 80% of women attempting a VBAC with a single prior cesarean will deliver vaginally versus about **60% to 70% (decreased) with more than one prior cesarean**. Recent studies have shown that **the greater the number of prior CDs, the lower the chances for a vaginal delivery (about 10–15% lower per CD)** (9). But a large retrospective multicenter study found similar rates of vaginal delivery after TOL in women with two versus one prior CD (75%) (27), while a recent meta-analysis of six studies that compared outcomes between women having a TOL after one or two CD found similar vaginal delivery rates of 77% and 72%, respectively (28).

Interdelivery Interval
Interdelivery interval of < 19 months may be associated with similar success rates of TOL after CD compared to longer intervals (9), but in one study, rates were lower with induction (29).

Current Labor Factors
Cervical Status
Labor factors associated with a higher VBAC rate include greater cervical dilation at admission or at rupture of membranes (1). The more **favorable** the **cervix**, the greater the odds for a vaginal delivery. Fetal head engagement and a lower station also increase the likelihood of VBAC.

Gestational Age
Preterm patients with prior CD have a slightly higher VBAC success rate than term patients (82 vs. 74%) (30).

Gestational age greater than 40 weeks is associated with a decreased rate of VBAC. Lower gestational age at delivery is associated with increased VBAC rates when compared with term gestational age at delivery. There is conflicting data regarding the chance of VBAC after TOLAC in **postterm** pregnancy. Successful VBAC rates of 65% to 82% have been reported for women past 40 weeks, with the higher rates in women with prior vaginal deliveries (1). In the MFMU cohort, women >41 weeks had a lower chance for vaginal delivery than women less than 41 weeks (aOR 0.61, 95% CI 0.55–0.68) (17). **If VBAC is still desired after 40 weeks, awaiting the onset of spontaneous labor may be a better option than induction before 40 weeks for women planning a VBAC.** On the other hand, since the rate of uterine rupture is significantly increased for women who are induced regardless of the gestational age, and because women induced before or at 40 weeks or those who enter spontaneous labor after 40 weeks have similar (30–35%) CD rates, it may be reasonable to offer an AROM/oxytocin induction around the estimated date of conception (EDC) to women with a prior vaginal delivery and a favorable cervix.

Induction/Augmentation of Labor
The overall estimated rate of vaginal birth with a TOLAC after any method of labor induction is 63% (1). **Women who receive oxytocin for induction or augmentation have rates of vaginal delivery about 10% lower than those that are allowed or able to labor spontaneously** (9,10). Studies demonstrate that the rate of VBAC ranges from 54% for induction of labor with mechanical (transcervical balloon catheter) to 69% for induction with pharmacologic methods. There are no high-quality studies comparing VBAC rates with different induction methods (1).

Fetal Macrosomia
The most consistent infant factor associated with an increased likelihood of VBAC is birth weight less than 4000 g. As expected, large for gestational age/macrosomia, especially birth weight >4000 g, decreases the odds of a VBAC after TOLAC (31). The success rates for VBAC in women with a previous CD and no other births is about **60% in the >4000 g group** and **71% in the ≤4000 g group** (32). There is a progressive reduction in VBAC success rates as birth weight increases. **With a prior VBAC or a vaginal delivery,** there is **no success rate below 63% for any of the birth weight strata.** But **with no previous vaginal delivery, VBAC** success rates can drop **below 50% as neonatal weight exceeds 4000 g** (22,31). This

success rate can decrease further if the indication for the previous CD is cephalopelvic disproportion or failure to progress. **There is limited data regarding prenatal estimated fetal birth weight and VBAC success.** Even so, VBAC rates after TOL were noted to be 60% to 70% in fetuses suspected to be macrosomic (22). This is likely due to the limitations of estimating birth weight by ultrasound. Thus, suspected macrosomia alone should not rule out a TOLAC (15).

Multiple Gestations
Vaginal delivery rates of both twins after prior CD generally range from 65% to 84% (9,33,34). In most series, rates do not seem to differ from success rates in singletons, without increased risk for maternal morbidity or uterine rupture (33,34).

Prediction Tools for Vaginal Delivery
Given the associations above, several different scoring systems have been proposed to predict the likelihood of vaginal delivery or cesarean in women undergoing a TOLAC (16,22,35,36). The best studies used scoring systems that were validated in separate data sets and in external studies (1). These scoring systems performed as well in the validation testing as they did in the original dataset. Unfortunately, although these models are accurate at predicting which women will have a VBAC, they are limited in their ability to predict who will have a repeat cesarean following a TOLAC. Half of women with unfavorable risk factors had a vaginal delivery.

The authors of the NIH-sponsored review of prediction tools recommend clinicians use a sequential approach to screening (37) (Table 14.2). Initially, prenatal predictors such as previous vaginal delivery and previous indication for CD and possibly patient demographics and fetal estimated weight should be considered. This can then be modified by intrapartum predictors such as onset of spontaneous labor or the need for induction, and cervical status can be used to reevaluate the likelihood of vaginal delivery (16). One available tool can be found at http://www.bsc.gwu.edu/mfmu/vagbirth.html.

Nevertheless, **none of these screening tools is sensitive enough to be clinically helpful in predicting an unsuccessful trial of labor, and none have been validated prospectively to improve outcomes.**

UTERINE RUPTURE
Complications and safety of TOLAC are especially related to the risk of **uterine rupture**. Uterine rupture is the most serious complication associated with TOLAC. It is defined as a complete separation through the entire thickness of the uterine wall (including serosa). At all gestational ages, pooled data from one review indicate that uterine rupture occurs in approximately 470/100,000 (0.47%, 95% CI 0.28–0.47) of women undergoing TOLAC and in 26/100,000 (0.026%, 95% CI 0.009–0.082) of women undergoing a PRCD (RR 20.74, 95% CI 9.77–44.02; $p < 0.0010$) (1). At term, the overall risk for rupture is 778/100,000 (0.78%, 95% CI 0.62–0.96). This means that overall there are about 5 to 6 additional ruptures per 1000 in women undergoing a TOLAC (1).

No maternal deaths due to uterine rupture have been reported (1,38). **Perinatal death occurs in about 6% of women with uterine rupture, which translates to an overall risk of intrapartum fetal death rate of about 20/100,000,** and a risk of perinatal death at term of about 0% to 2.8% in women undergoing a TOLAC (1).

The risk for rupture is modified by a number of important factors (39) listed in Table 14.2 and described below. Prior vaginal delivery and prior VBAC reduce the risk of uterine rupture, while number of prior CDs, vertical scars, single-layer closure, induction or augmentation, greater maternal age, fever, prior preterm CD, and TOLAC at ≥40 weeks are associated with higher rupture rates.

Maternal Age
Maternal age (>30 years old) is associated with an increased risk (1.4%) of uterine rupture (40).

Prior Vaginal Delivery
Prior vaginal delivery significantly reduces the risk for rupture during TOLAC from 1.1%, in women with no prior vaginal deliveries, to **0.2%.** After controlling for maternal demographics and labor characteristics, prior vaginal delivery reduced the risk for rupture fivefold (OR 0.2, 95% CI 0.04–0.08) (41). This protective effect was also confirmed by recent large retrospective (OR 0.30, 95% CI 0.23–0.62) (42) and prospective (OR 0.66, 95% CI 0.45–0.95) (7) studies.

Number of Prior Cesareans
Women with ≥2 prior low transverse CD may be at increased risk of uterine rupture compared with women with one prior CD, but the absolute risk is small. **Current ACOG recommendations now allow this option regardless of whether there is a prior vaginal delivery** (15). **Most ruptures occur in women undergoing induction or augmentation and in those without a prior vaginal delivery** (43). Earlier data had indicated an overall relative increased risk of rupture (about 2- to 3-fold) in women having a TOL after two low transverse CD compared with one (38,43,44). A recent meta-analysis that included the more recent data of Macones et al. (43) and the MFMU cohort confirmed these findings **(0.9% 1 prior CD vs. 1.8% 2 prior CD)**. A follow-up case-control analysis of the study by Macones et al. (42) showed no increased risk (OR 1.46, 95% CI 0.87–2.44), and in the MFMU cohort (39) there was no difference in the incidence of rupture after two CDs compared with one (0.9% vs. 0.7%). Furthermore, the rupture rate in women with a prior vaginal delivery and two prior CD is only 0.5%, no greater than a VBAC with only one prior CD (43).

Prior CD Characteristics
Labor Before Primary CD
Labor before the primary CD has been associated with a lower risk of uterine rupture in a future TOLAC compared with no labor before the primary CD (45).

Direction of Scar
Classical and low vertical uterine scars have higher rates of rupture compared with low transverse uterine incisions (4–10%, and 1–2%, respectively) (2). **Records regarding the prior CD(s) should be obtained, with special care in documentation of direction of scar. If a woman has had a prior vertical (classical) CD, PRCD at 36 to 37 weeks is recommended** (15,46).

Layers of Closure
There is insufficient evidence to assess if the numbers of layers performed at prior uterine closure affects the outcomes for future pregnancies. Randomized trials have insufficient follow-up numbers (see chap. 13). Compared with women who had double-layer closure, women with a single-

layer closure have been reported to have either similar or up to a fourfold increased risk of uterine rupture compared with those with a double-layer closure (9,47). A recent large multicenter case-controlled study by the same authors that examined operative reports again confirmed an increased rate of rupture with single versus two layer closure (3.1% vs. 0.5%; aOR 2.69, 95% CI 1.37–5.28) (48).

Fever
The presence of both intrapartum and postpartum fever at CD, but not either alone, may increase the risk of uterine rupture in a subsequent pregnancy (49).

Previous Preterm CD
The MFMU Network data showed a **higher risk of rupture** in women with a prior preterm CD compared with in those with a prior term CD (1% vs. 0.68%; aOR 1.6, 95% CI 1.01–2.50) (50). No difference in rupture rates were found in a secondary analysis of the recent retrospective, multicenter cohort study comparing prior CD before and after 34 weeks (aOR 1.5, 95% CI 0.7–3.5) (51).

Prior CD for Twins
Compared with women with prior CD for singletons, women with prior CD for twins have similar risk of uterine rupture and TOLAC success (52).

Prior Uterine Rupture
As prior uterine rupture is associated with **high rates (6–32%) of recurrent rupture** with TOLAC, these pregnancies should have an **PRCD before labor**, possibly around 36 to 37 weeks (46).

Interval Between Deliveries
Interval between deliveries **of <24 months** are associated with an **increased risk of rupture** (2.3–4.8%) compared with longer intervals (0.9–1.1%) in a number of studies (53,54). Interdelivery intervals less than 18 months are at the highest risk for rupture (2.7–4.8%) (55,56).

Post Dates
The risk of uterine rupture does not increase substantially after 40 weeks, but is increased with induction of labor regardless of gestational age (57).

Preterm
In one study there was a trend toward a lower uterine rupture rate in preterm patients who attempted a VBAC (30).

Induction/Augmentation
The rate of uterine rupture in women with one prior low transverse CD undergoing TOLAC with spontaneous labor is about 0.4%. Almost all studies of sufficient size report **higher rates of uterine rupture (up to 1–2%) with induction** at any gestational age and of any kind (7,58). At term, the risk of rupture is not statistically significantly greater than women with spontaneous labor (OR 1.42, 95% CI 0.57–3.52). But women induced at >40 weeks have higher risk of rupture than those induced between 37 and 40 weeks (3.2% vs. 1.5%) (1). In the MFMU cohort, induction increased the risk of rupture **only in women without a prior vaginal delivery** (induced 1.5%, vs. spontaneous 0.8%). In women with a prior vaginal delivery, the incidence of rupture was similar (0.6% vs. 0.4%) (59).

The risks of uterine rupture with induction in women who had one prior cesarean section may also depend on the

type of induction. Risk of rupture may be as high as **1.4% to 2.5% with induction with prostaglandin** (with or without oxytocin) (7,60), and about **1.1% with oxytocin alone** (74). The MFMU data, which included all prostaglandins, and Grobman et al., which excluded misoprostol, did not find an increased risk for rupture when prostaglandins were used alone, but they did note a **threefold increased risk with sequential use of prostaglandins and oxytocin versus spontaneous labor** (7,59).

ACOG therefore advises that induction with **sequential use of prostaglandins and oxytocin be avoided.** It also states use of **misoprostol in women at ≥ about 30 weeks with a prior CD should be discouraged** (15). There is insufficient evidence to assess the safety of mifepristone induction in women with a prior CD. Women with prior CD should be made aware of these higher risks of rupture associated with induction.

Augmentation may be associated with an increased risk of rupture, up to about 1%, but the risk is mainly related to higher doses of oxytocin (7,61). A secondary analysis of a large retrospective cohort and a follow-up nested case-control study reported a dose-response relationship between the maximum oxytocin dose and increased risk for uterine rupture (fourfold increased risk with 21–30 mU/min vs. no oxytocin; attributable risk of 2.9–3.6%) (61,62). **Oxytocin should be used judiciously in women undergoing TOLAC, with a possible maximum dose of 20 mU/min.**

Second Trimester Induction of Labor
Induction of labor in the second trimester with misoprostol is associated with **0.4% risk of uterine rupture** (with 0% risk of hysterectomy and 0.2% risk of transfusion) **after one prior low transverse CD**, and about 50% risk with a prior classical CD (63).

Macrosomia >4000 g
Macrosomia >4000 is associated with a slightly increased risk of rupture (31).

A recent multicenter case-control study showed that birth weight >3500 g had twice the risk for rupture (OR 2.03, 95% CI 1.21–3.38) (31).

Twins
The risk of rupture or maternal mortality is not increased with prior CD and subsequent TOL with twins, with uncommon perinatal morbidity at ≥34 weeks (33).

BENEFITS AND HARMS ASSOCIATED WITH TOLAC
The majority of benefits and the least morbidity of a TOLAC are dependent on having a VBAC, while the potential harms of a TOLAC are associated with an unsuccessful TOLAC resulting in CD. Studies comparing TOLAC to PRCD usually include both VBAC and TOLAC ending in CD. Thus, the outcomes for women who have a TOLAC reflect both of these possibilities. These data is therefore appropriate for women with a previous CD who are deciding on the mode of delivery for the current pregnancy. Rates of all maternal and perinatal complications except rupture are infrequent and similar with both TOL and PRCD (4,11,12).

Maternal (Table 14.3)
Surgical Complications
Overall rates of surgical injury are low, but may be **slightly higher with TOLAC** compared with PRCD. This is primarily due to those women who have a TOLAC but deliver with a repeat CD in labor (6,7,13,64,65). There are no studies that specifically evaluated the risks of complications due to subsequent surgery after a TOLAC or PRCD. Nevertheless, increasing number of abdominal surgeries is commonly associated with increased risks of adhesions, injury to bowel and bladder, and other complications at the time of subsequent CD or non-pregnancy-related hysterectomy.

Table 14.3 Maternal and Perinatal Risks of TOLAC Vs. PRCD

			TOLAC	
	Favors	PRCD	1 prior CD	≥2 prior CDs
Maternal complications				
Uterine rupture	PRCD	1/200–250	1/111–140	1/55–140
Operative injury	PRCD	1/166–200	1/250	1/250
Hysterectomy	–	0–1/250	1/200–500	1/166
Transfusion	–	1/71–100	1/58–140	1/31
VTE	–	1/1,000	4/10,000	NA
Endometritis	–	1/47–66	1/34	1/32
Hospitalization	TOLAC			
Death	–	1/2,500–5,000	1/5,000	NA
Satisfaction	–			
Long-term risks	*			
Perinatal complications				
Stillbirth	PRCD	1/1,000	2–4/1,000	NA
Low cord pH	NA	NA	1.5/1,000	NA
Neonatal death	–	5/10,000	8/10,000	NA
Perinatal death	PRCD	1/10,000	13/10,000	NA
Respiratory	TOLAC	1–5/100	0.1–1.8/100	NA
Hyperbilirubinemia	TOLAC	5.8/100	2.2/100	NA
HIE	PRCD	1/10,000	5–8/10,000	NA

Please notice that some numbers may contradict each other as they are from different sources.
*See text.
Abbreviations: CD, cesarean delivery; TOLAC, trial of labor after CD; PRCD, planned repeat CD; NA, not available; HIE, hypoxic-ischemic encephalopathy.
Source: From Refs. 7, 15, 27, 39.

Hysterectomy
The risk of hysterectomy is about 1 to 2/1000 TOLAC (6–8,12,60,66), and similar to PRCD (7).

Transfusion
The risk of transfusion is very low, and not significantly different for TOLAC or PRCD (0.9% vs. 1.2%) (1,7). It has been estimated at about 2 units pRBC/1000 TOLAC (8). The risk is higher when labor is induced with no prior vaginal deliveries, and it is related to the need for CD following a TOLAC (7).

Venous Thromboembolism
The risk is about 4/10,000 with TOLAC, similar to PRCD (1/1,000) (7).

Endometritis
The risk is very similar for TOLAC or PRCD [6% vs. 7–8%, fever (10); or 3% vs. 2% in academic centers (7)]. The overall absolute risk for any fever with TOLAC is 6.5 % (1). Morbid obesity, cesarean after TOLAC, and increased number of cesarean deliveries increase infection rates.

Hospitalization
Overall, because most women deliver vaginally, a TOLAC results in a shorter **hospitalization** compared with PRCD. This benefit does not apply to morbidly obese women.

Maternal Mortality
The risk of **maternal mortality is lower overall for women having a TOLAC** (3–4/100,000) compared with PRCD (13.4/100,000). This compares to the overall U.S. maternal mortality rate of 11–15/100,000. At term, maternal mortality is lower: 1.9 for TOLAC versus 9.6 PRCD per 100,000 live births (1). Based on limited evidence, mortality is lower for TOLAC in high-volume hospitals (more than 500 deliveries per year) (67).

Short-Term Satisfaction
Anxiety, depression, psychological well-being, and satisfaction scores are similar between women who choose TOLAC versus those who elect for PRCD (6).

Long-Term Maternal Risks
There is a clear association between the number of CDs and abnormal placentation as well as other surgical complications. This complication is an important consideration for the 28% of women who have more than two births. For each CD, the risk for placenta previa significantly increases, occurring in 900, 1700, and 3000 per 100,000 women who have one, two, and three or more prior CDs. The overall risk for placenta accreta also increases (0.2% in the first CD to 0.3%, 0.6%, 2.1%, 2.3%, and 6.7% for 2nd, 3rd, 4th, 5th, and ≥6th CD). In the presence of placenta previa, the risk for abnormal placentation is markedly increased for each additional CD (3.3%, 11%, 40%, and >60% for the 1st, 2nd, 3rd, and ≥4th CDs, respectively) (68). Even without a placenta previa, the incidence of abnormal placentation, although much lower, increases with the number of CDs (see chap. 25). **The major benefit of TOLAC is the about >70% chance of a VBAC and avoidance of multiple CDs.**

In addition, as noted above, women who undergo multiple CDs are at increased risk for many complications unrelated to placentation, including hysterectomy, adhesions, injury to bowel and bladder, transfusions >4U, need for postoperative ventilation, ICU admission, and increased operative time and hospital stay (68). There is insufficient evidence regarding long-term pelvic floor function comparing TOLAC with PRCD. PRCD should not be used as a way to prevent pelvic floor disorders (1).

A decision analysis evaluating both the immediate and subsequent risks of the delivery decision for women with a prior CD suggested that **for women planning only one additional pregnancy, PRCD results in fewer hysterectomies than TOLAC**, while for women planning two or more additional pregnancy, a TOL provides the lowest risk (69).

Therefore, when counseling women about risks and benefits of a TOLAC compared with PRCD, the discussion should address her plans for future pregnancies.

Perinatal
The most serious fetal risk in women with prior CD is from uterine rupture during TOLAC. Risks of fetal/neonatal morbidity/mortality with term uterine rupture are **33% risk of pH < 7.00, 40% admission to NICU, 6% risk of hypoxic-ischemic encephalopathy (HIE), and 1.8% risk of neonatal death. The rupture-related risk of neonatal death is 1/10,000 in equipped academic centers (7). In other centers, these risks are higher, including risk of neonatal death from rupture up to 10% to 25%.**

Stillbirth
The rates of stillbirths are **2 to 6/1000 for TOLAC versus 1 to 2/1000 for PRCD**. At 39 weeks or more, the rate of antepartum stillbirth in the MFMU cohort was 1/1000 with TOLAC and 3/10,000 with PRCD (7). This difference might be due to stillbirths occurring at ≥39 weeks with TOLAC, and/or to encouragement for TOLAC with diagnosis of stillbirth (7).

Low cord pH
The risk of cord pH < 7.00 is about 1.5/1000 TOLAC (8).

Neonatal Death
Neonatal death rates are similar between the TOLAC versus PRCD (0.08% vs. 0.05%, respectively) in academic centers, with the neonatal death rate associated with a rupture at term of about 1.8% (7).

Perinatal Death
Perinatal death rates at term (excluding malformations) are **1.3/1000 with TOLAC versus 0.5/1000 for PRCD** (9). **Overall risk of adverse perinatal outcome is 1/2000 with TOLAC, slightly higher than with PRCD** (7). In one study of women at term with vertex presentations, the risk of delivery-related perinatal mortality with a TOLAC was 11 times that of PRCD (OR 11.6, 95% CI 1.6–86.7). When compared with women **without a previous CD** (instead of to those having a PRCD), the **perinatal mortality for TOLAC was the same as that of a nullipara in labor,** but about twice as high as that of a non-TOLAC multipara in labor (12).

Respiratory Complications
Rates of **respiratory complications**, transient tachypnea of the newborn, and need for oxygen and ventilator support may be **slightly higher in infants delivered by PRCD** versus those delivered by VBAC (1,70). It is unclear if there is a difference in respiratory outcomes in infants born by PRCD versus those born by repeat CD after a TOLAC.

Hypoxic-Ischemic Encephalopathy

Aside from perinatal death, HIE is the most serious adverse outcome of uterine rupture and is one of the primary concerns regarding the decision to have a TOLAC. The incidence is **46/100,000 live births for TOLAC**, versus none in the PRCD (7). The overall risk of rupture-related HIE is 1 in 2500 TOLAC. In term infants, the overall incidence for HIE is 100/100,000 live births.

MANAGEMENT

Patients with contraindications (Table 14.1) **to TOLAC should receive a PRCD at 39 weeks, or earlier if labor starts or in certain cases (e.g., prior early uterine rupture). TOLAC can be offered if the risk of uterine rupture is estimated to be <2%, possibly <1% (Table 14.2), and if spontaneous labor starts by 40 weeks. If the patient reaches her EDC with no labor and an unfavorable cervix, a PRCD should be recommended.**

Counseling

TOLAC can be offered to most women with a prior CD, but several safety and success factors should be considered and discussed with the woman (Tables 14.1–14.3).

The composite of **maternal complications** is slightly **higher with TOLAC** compared with PRCD group **primarily due to the risk of rupture, and the increased risks of a CD in labor.** These estimates do not take into account the long-term increased risks of repetitive CD and the associated risks of placenta previa and accreta. This is why **counseling should take into account how many future pregnancies are planned**.

The overall risk of serious **perinatal complications** is about 1 in 2000 **TOLAC**, which is **slightly greater** than that of PRCD (7). Combining all poor perinatal outcomes, **more than 600 PRCD would need to be performed to prevent one poor perinatal outcome.** Although a woman with a TOLAC is at higher risk of uterine rupture than any other group, the risk of perinatal death is similar to that of any nulliparous woman in labor (12).

For the approximately 60% to 80% of women having TOLAC **who will deliver vaginally,** the maternal and perinatal morbidity and mortality are lower than PRCD.

About 50% of women with prior CD have a 70% or higher chance of successful VBAC (http://www.bsc.gwu.edu/mfmu/vagbirth.html), **and they have no higher risk of maternal or perinatal morbidity and mortality compared** with those who have PRCD. PRCD is safer than a TOLAC that results in a CD (11).

Although the risks of TOLAC are higher than PRCD, the absolute risks are small and comparable to other potential complications of labor.

Efforts to reduce the frequency of the first CD reduce the need for a TOLAC or repeat CD.

Women at lowest risk for adverse outcomes and highest chance for a vaginal delivery include those with a prior vaginal delivery (especially a prior VBAC), in spontaneous labor, with a favorable cervix (Table 14.2).

TOLAC should be approached with caution in those with the lowest chance of vaginal delivery and highest risk of rupture: for example, induction of labor in obese women over age 40 with an unfavorable cervix and no prior vaginal deliveries.

All women with a single prior low transverse CD without other indications for a CD are candidates for a TOLAC.

Women with two prior CD can also be considered for TOLAC, but induction should be avoided.

The ultimate decision regarding whether to have a TOLAC or PRCD should be based on the patient choice, after appropriate counseling and the availability of adequate resources and personnel to respond to obstetric emergencies. Most women should decide before term, and their decision should be documented in the medical record. The decision may be deferred until term in women who want to assess if spontaneous labor and/or favorable cervix make their chances of complications lower and of success higher. There is no evidence that examining the adequacy of the pelvis benefits outcomes.

Prenatal Education

Individualized prenatal education directed toward avoidance of a PRCD does not increase the rate of VBAC (71).

Consent

Specific consent for TOL after CD or PRCD should be signed by the woman after appropriate counseling.

Nonvertex Presentation

External cephalic version (ECV) can safely be performed in women with a prior CD. The success rate for ECV is similar or higher in women with a prior CD compared to controls without a prior CD (82% vs. 61%) (72). Women with a successful version have successful VBAC rates of 65% to 76% (72,73).

Ultrasound of Lower Uterine Segment

Due to the uncommon nature of rupture, several thousand women need to be studied to assess if measuring the thickness of the lower uterine segment predicts complications in women with a prior CD who elect TOLAC, and therefore there is insufficient evidence to assess the clinical utility of this screening test. No women with a lower uterine segment thickness of ≥4.5 mm in the late third trimester seem to have dehiscence or rupture, while the proportion of these complications rises as this thickness decreases, with **women with large defects, or lower uterine thickness <3.5 mm (especially <2.0 mm), or myometrial layer <2.0 mm (especially <1.4 mm) in the third trimester, possibly benefiting from PRCD** (44,74).

Requirements to Minimize Risks (1)

To minimize risks, the following must be immediately available throughout TOLAC:

- **Experienced obstetrician**
- **Anesthesia**
- **Nursing and OR personnel**
- **Ability to perform emergency CD**

Labor and delivery units with >500/1000 births per year have lower risks of uterine rupture and complications compared with units with less volume (6). If centers cannot provide the above resources, this does not mean TOLAC should not be offered. Referral should be made to adequate facilities early during prenatal care so that TOLAC is safely available.

Detecting Rupture Intrapartum

Fetal heart rate (FHR) disturbances are the most common (but not universal) sign of uterine rupture (55–85%) (75). The most commonly reported FHR disturbance is repetitive progressively severe variable decelerations and prolonged bradycardia, although in most cases they are not caused by rupture.

Nevertheless, **in women with a prior CD, in the presence of such FHR disturbances, uterine rupture must be considered.**

Abdominal pain over the area of the prior uterine scar is a poor predictor of uterine rupture. Epidural usually does not mask rupture. Epidural should not be withheld in women attempting TOL after prior CD.

Intrauterine pressure catheter (IUPC) monitoring has not been shown to be helpful (76). Significant loss of fetal station especially in the second stage may occur with rupture, but is of limited predictive value. There is insufficient data to assess the utility of uterine exploration after a successful VBAC.

Cost-Effectiveness

Cost savings with TOLAC may occur only if success rate is ≥70%.

REFERENCES

1. Agency for Healthcare Research and Quality. Evidence Report/Technology Assessment Number 191. Vaginal Birth After Cesarean: New Insights. Rockville, MD: Agency for Healthcare Research and Quality, 2010. [Review]
2. American College of Obstetricians and Gynecologists. ACOG Practice Bulletin No. 54: Vaginal birth after previous cesarean delivery. Washington, D.C.: American College of Obstetricians and Gynecologists, 2004. [Review]
3. National Vital Statistics System. 2009. Available at: www.cdc.gov/nchs/pressroom/states/CESAREAN_STATE_2009.pdf. Accessed August 28, 2011. [Epidemiologic data]
4. The Information Centre for Health and Social Care, Maternity Statistics, England: 2009–2010. Statistical Bulletin 2010. Available at: www.ic.nhs.uk. [Epidemiologic data]
5. National Institute of Health. Consensus Development Conference Statement: Vaginal Birth After Cesarean: New Insights. Bethesda: NIH, 2010. [Review]
6. McMahon MJ, Luther ER, Bowes WA, et al. Comparison of a trial of labor with an elective second cesarean section. N Engl J Med 1996; 335(10):689–695. [II-2, $n = 6138$]
7. Landon MB, Hauth JC, Leveno KJ, et al. Maternal and perinatal outcomes associated with a trial of labor after prior cesarean delivery. N Engl J Med 2004; 351(25):2581. [II-2; prospective; $n = 33,699$]
8. Chauhan SP, Martin JN, Henrichs CE, et al. Maternal and perinatal complications with uterine rupture in 142,075 patients who attempted vaginal birth after cesarean delivery: a review of the literature. Am J Obstet Gynecol 2003; 189(2):408–417. [Meta-analysis: 72 studies, $n = 142,075$]
9. Guise J, Hashima J, Osterweil P. Evidence-based vaginal birth after caesarean section. Best Pract Res Clin Obstet Gynaecol 2005; 19(1 spec. iss.):117–130. [Meta-analysis: 61 studies, $n = >10,000$]
10. Guise JM, Berlin M, McDonagh M, et al. Safety of vaginal birth after cesarean: a systematic review. Obstet Gynecol 2004; 103(3):420. [Meta-analysis: $n = 20$ studies]
11. Miller D, Diaz FG, Paul RH. Vaginal birth after cesarean: a 10 year experience. Obstet Gynecol 1994; 84:255–258. [II-2, $n = 17,322$]
12. Smith G, Pell JP, Cameron AD, et al. Risk of perinatal death associated with labor after previous cesarean delivery in uncomplicated term pregnancies. JAMA 2002; 287(20):2684. [II-2; $n = 15,515$]
13. Cahill AG, Stamilio DM, Odibo AO, et al. Is vaginal birth after cesarean (VBAC) or elective repeat cesarean safer in women with a prior vaginal delivery? Am J Obstet Gynecol 2006; 195(4):1143–1147. [II-2, $n = 6619$]
14. Grobman WA, Lai Y, Landon MB, et al. Can a prediction model for vaginal birth after cesarean also predict the probability of morbidity related to a trial of labor? Am J Obstet Gynecol 2009; 200(1):56.e1–56.e6. [Review: prediction]
15. American College of Obstetricians and Gynecologists. ACOG Practice Bulletin No. 115: Vaginal birth after previous cesarean

delivery. Washington, D.C.: American College of Obstetricians and Gynecologists, 2010. [Review]
16. Grobman WA, Lai Y, Landon MB, et al. Development of a nomogram for prediction of vaginal birth after cesarean delivery. Obstet Gynecol 2007; 109(4):806. [II-2; prospective; $n = 7660$]
17. Landon MB, Leindecker S, Spong C, et al. The MFMU Cesarean Registry: factors affecting the success of trial of labor after previous cesarean delivery. Am J Obstet Gynecol 2005; 193:1016–1023. [II-2; prospective; $n = 14,529$]
18. Durnwald CP, Ehrenberg HM, Mercer BM, The impact of maternal obesity and weight gain on vaginal birth after cesarean section success. Am J Obstet Gynecol 2004; 191:954–957. [II-2, $n = 510$]
19. Chauhan SP, Magann EF, Carroll CS, et al. Mode of delivery for the morbidly obese women with prior cesarean delivery: vaginal versus repeat cesarean section. Am J Obstet Gynecol 2001; 185:349–354. [II-2, $n = 30$ women >300 lb with TOL after CD vs. 39 with PRCD]
20. Edwards R, Harnsberger S, Johnson I, et al. Deciding on route of delivery for obese women with a prior cesarean delivery. Am J Obstet Gynecol 2003; 189:385–390. [II-2]
21. Hendler I, Bujold E. Effect of prior vaginal delivery or prior vaginal birth after cesarean delivery on obstetric outcomes in women undergoing trial of labor. Obstet Gynecol 2004; 104 (2):273. [II-2, $n = 2204$]
22. Flamm BL, Geiger AM. Vaginal birth after cesarean delivery: an admission scoring system. Obstet Gynecol 1997; 90:907–910. [II-2]
23. Caughey AB, Shipp TD, Repke JT, et al. Trial of labor after cesarean delivery: the effect of previous vaginal delivery. Am J Obstet Gynecol 1998; 179(4):938–941. [II-2, $n = 800$]
24. Mercer BM, Gilbert S, Landon MB, et al. Labor outcomes with increasing number of prior vaginal births after cesarean delivery. Obstet Gynecol 2008; 111(2 pt 1):285. [II-2; prospective; $n = 13,532$]
25. Jongen WM, Halfwerk MGC, Bouwer WK. Vaginal delivery after previous caesarean section for failure of second stage of labour. Br J Obstet Gynecol 1998; 105:1079–1081. [II-2]
26. Kwon JY, Jo YS, Lee GS, et al. Cervical dilatation at the time of cesarean section may affect the success of a subsequent vaginal delivery. J Matern Fetal Neonatal Med 2009; 22(11):1057–1062. [II-2]
27. Macones GA, Peipert J, Nelson DB, et al. Maternal complications with vaginal birth after cesarean delivery: a multicenter study. Am J Obstet Gynecol 2005; 193(5):1656–1662. [II-2, multicenter $n = 25,005$]
28. Tahseen S, Griffiths M. Vaginal birth after two caesarean sections (VBAC-2)-a systematic review with meta-analysis of success rate and adverse outcomes of VBAC-2 versus VBAC-1 and repeat (third) caesarean sections. Br J Obstet Gynecol 2009; 117(1):5–19. [Meta-analysis: 20 studies]
29. Huang WH, Nakashima DK, Rumney PJ, et al. Interdelivery interval and the success of vaginal birth after cesarean delivery. Obstet Gynecol 2002; 99(1):41–44. [II-2]
30. Quinones JN, Stamilio DM, Paré E, et al. The effect of prematurity on vaginal birth after cesarean delivery: success and maternal morbidity. Obstet Gynecol 2005; 105(3):519–524.
31. Elkousy MA, Sammel M, Stevens E, et al. The effect of birth weight on vaginal birth after cesarean delivery success rates. Am J Obstet Gynecol 2003; 188:824–830. [II-2, $n = 9960$]
32. Zelop C, Shipp T, Repke J, et al. Outcomes of trial of labor following previous cesarean delivery among women with fetuses weighing >4000 g. Am J Obstet Gynecol 2001; 185:903–905. [II-2]
33. Varner MW, Leindecker S, Spong CY, et al. The Maternal-Fetal Medicine Unit cesarean registry: trial of labor with a twin gestation. Am J Obstet Gynecol 2005; 193(1):135–140. [II-2, $n = 186$ women with prior CD and subsequent TOL]
34. Cahill A, Stamilio DM, Pare E, et al. Vaginal birth after cesarean (VBAC) attempt in twin pregnancies: Is it safe? Am J Obstet Gynecol 2005; 193:1050–1055. [II-2, $n = 535$ twins with prior CD].
35. Hashima JN, Eden KB, Osterweil P, et al. Predicting vaginal birth after cesarean delivery: a review of prognostic factors and screening tools. Am J Obstet Gynecol 2004; 190(2):547–555. [Review: prediction]

36. Dinsmoor MJ, Brock EL. Predicting failed trial of labor after primary cesarean delivery. Obstet Gynecol 2004; 103(2):282–286. [Review: prediction]

37. Eden KB, McDonagh M, Denman MA, et al. New insights on vaginal birth after cesarean: can it be predicted? Obstet Gynecol 2010; 116 (4):967–981. [Meta-analysis: 203 total, 16 using scored models]

38. Guise JM, McDonagh MS, Osterweil P, et al. Systematic review of the incidence and consequences of uterine rupture in women with previous caesarean section. Br Med J 2004; 329(7456):1–7. [Meta-analysis: 21 studies]

39. Landon MB, Spong CY, Thom E, et al. Risk of uterine rupture with a trial of labor in women with multiple and single prior cesarean delivery. Obstet Gynecol 2006; 108(1):12–20. [II-2; prospective; $n = 17,898$]

40. Shipp TD, Zelop C, Repke JT, et al. The association of maternal age and symptomatic uterine rupture during a trial of labor after prior cesarean delivery. Obstet Gynecol 2002; 99(4):585–588. [II-2]

41. Zelop C, Shipp T, Repke J, et al. Effect of previous vaginal delivery on the risk of uterine rupture during a subsequent trial of labor. Am J Obstet Gynecol 2000; 183:1184–1186. [II-2]

42. Macones GA, Cahill AG, Stamilio DM, et al. Can uterine rupture in patients attempting vaginal birth after cesarean delivery be predicted? Am J Obstet Gynecol 2006; 195(4):1148–1152. [II-2]

43. Macones GA, Cahill A, Pare E, et al. Obstetric outcomes in women with two prior cesarean deliveries: is vaginal birth after cesarean delivery a viable option? Am J Obstet Gynecol 2005; 192(4):1223–1228. [II-2; $n = 20,175$ with 1 prior CD and 3970 with 2 prior CD].

44. Caughey AB, Shipp TD, Repke JT, et al. Rate of uterine rupture during a trial of labor in women with one or two prior cesarean deliveries. Am J Obstet Gynecol 1999; 181(4):872–876. [II-2, $n = 3891$ TOL with 1 or 2 prior CD]

45. Algert CS, Morris JM, Simpson JM, et al. Labor before a primary cesarean delivery reduced risk of uterine rupture in a subequent trial of labor for vaginal birth after ceasrean. Obstet Gynecol 2008; 112:1061–1066. [II-1]

46. Spong CY, Mercer BM, D'Alton M, et al. Timing of indicated late-preterm and early-term birth. Obstet Gynecol 2011; 118:323–333. [Review]

47. Bujold E, Bujold C, Hamilton EF, et al. The impact of a single-layer or double-layer closure on uterine rupture. Am J Obstet Gynecol 2002; 186(6):1326–1330. [II-2, $n = 1980$ with 1 or 2 layers]

48. Bujold E, Goyet M, Marcoux S, et al. The role of uterine closure in the risk of uterine rupture. Obstet Gynecol 2010; 116(1):43–50. [II-2]

49. Shipp TD, Zelop C, Cohen A, et al. Post-cesarean delivery fever and uterine rupture in a subsequent trial of labor. Obstet Gynecol 2003; 101(1):136–139. [II-2]

50. Sciscione AC, Landon MB, Leveno KJ, et al. Previous preterm cesarean delivery and risk of subsequent uterine rupture. Obstet Gynecol 2008; 111(3):648–653. [II-2, prospective; $n = 41,367$]

51. Harper LM, Cahill AG, Stamilio DM, et al. Effect of gestational age at the prior cesarean delivery on maternal morbidity in subsequent VBAC attempt. Am J Obstet Gynecol 2009; 200(3): 276.e1–276.e6. [II-2]

52. Varner, Thom E, Spong CY, et al. Trial of labor after one previous cesarean delivery for multifetal gestation. Obstet Gynecol 2007; 110:814–819. [II-1]

53. Shipp TD, Zelop CM, Repke JT, et al. Interdelivery interval and risk of symptomatic uterine rupture. Obstet Gynecol 2001; 97(2): 175. [II-2, $n = 2409$]

54. Bujold E, Mehta S, Bujold C, et al. Interdelivery interval and uterine rupture. Am J Obstet Gynecol 2002; 187:1199–1202. [II-2, $n = 1527$]

55. Bujold E, Gauthier RJ. Risk of uterine rupture associated with an interdelivery interval between 18 and 24 months. Obstet Gynecol 2010; 115(5):1003–1006. [II-2, $n = 1768$]

56. Stamilio DM, DeFranco E, Paré E, et al. Short interpregnancy interval: risk of uterine rupture and complications of vaginal birth after cesarean delivery. Obstet Gynecol 2007; 110(5):1075–1082. [II-2, $n = 13,331$]

57. Zelop CM, Shipp TD, Cohen A, et al. Trial of labor after 40 weeks' gestation in women with prior cesarean. Obstet Gynecol 2001; 97(3):391–393. [II-2]

58. McDonagh MS, Osterweil P, Guise JM. The benefits and risks of inducing labour in patients with prior caesarean delivery: a systematic review. Br J Obstet Gynecol 2005; 112(8):1007–1015. [Meta-analysis: 14 studies (only 2 RCTs)]

59. Grobman W, Gilbert S, Landon MB, et al. Outcomes of induction of labor after one prior cesarean. Am J Obstet Gynecol 2007; 109:262–269. [II-2; prospective; $n = 11,778$]

60. Lydon-Rochelle MT, Cahill AG, Spong CY. Birth after previous cesarean delivery: short-term maternal outcomes. Semin Perinatol 2010; 34:249–257. [Review]

61. Cahill A, Stamilio D, Odibo A, et al. Does a maximum dose of oxytocin affect risk for uterine rupture in candidates for vaginal birth after cesarean delivery? Am J Obstet Gynecol 2007; 197(5):495.e1–495.e5. [II-2, $n = 13,523$]

62. Cahill A, Waterman B, Stamilio D, et al. Higher maximum doses of oxytocin are associated with an unacceptably high risk for uterine rupture in patients attempting vaginal birth after cesarean delivery. Am J Obstet Gynecol 2008; 199(1):32.e1–32.e5. [II-2]

63. Berghella V, Airoldi J, O'Neill A, et al. Misoprostol for second trimester pregnancy termination in women with prior caesarean: a systematic review. BJOG 2009; 116(9):1151–1157. [II-2 and review of the literature]

64. Silver RM, Landon MB, Rouse DJ, et al. Maternal morbidity associated with multiple repeat cesarean deliveries. Obstet Gynecol 2006; 107(6):1226–1232. [II-2, prospective; $n = 30,132$]

65. Spong CY, Landon MB, Gilbert S, et al. Risk of uterine rupture and adverse perinatal outcome at term after cesarean delivery. Obstet Gynecol 2007; 110(4):801. [II-2, prospective; $n = 39,117$]

66. Wen SW, Rusen ID, Walker M, et al. Comparison of maternal mortality and morbidity between trial of labor and elective cesarean section among women with previous cesarean delivery. Am J Obstet Gynecol 2004; 191(4):1263–1269. [II-2; $n = 308,755$ with 5839 prior preterm CD]

67. Law LW, Pang MW, Chung TK, et al. Randomized trial of assigned mode of delivery after a previous cesarean section—impact on maternal psychological outcomes. J Matern Fetal Neonatal Med 2010; 23:1106–1113. [RCT, $n = 298$]

68. Silver RM. Delivery after previous cesarean: long-term maternal outcomes. Semin Perinatol 2010; 34:258–266. [Review]

69. Paré E, Quiñones JN, Macones GA. General obstetrics: vaginal birth after caesarean section versus elective repeat caesarean section: assessment of maternal downstream health outcomes. Br J Obstet Gynecol 2005; 113(1):75–85. [II-2]

70. Kamath BD, Todd JK, Glazner JE, et al. Neonatal outcomes after elective cesarean delivery. Obstet Gynecol 2009; 113:1231–1238. [II-1]

71. Fraser W, Maunsell E, Hodnett E, et al. Randomized controlled trial of a prenatal vaginal birth after cesarean section education and support program. Am J Obstet Gynecol 1997; 176:419–425. [RCT; $n = 1275$]

72. Flamm BL, Fried MW, Lonky NM, et al. External cephalic version after previous cesarean section. Am J Obstet Gynecol 1991; 165:370–372. [II-2]

73. De Meeus JB, Ellia F, Magnin G. External cephalic version after previous cesarean section: a series of 38 cases. Eur J Obstet Gynecol Reprod Bio 1998; 81(1):65–68. [II-2]

74. Bujold E, Jastrow N, Simoneau J, et al. Prediction of complete uterine rupture by sonographic evaluation of the lower uterine segment. Am J Obstet Gynecol 2009; 201(3):320.e1–320.e6. [II-2, prospective; $n = 236$]

75. Ridgeway JJ, Weyrich DL, Benedetti TJ. Fetal heart rate changes associated with uterine rupture. Obstet Gynecol 2004; 103(3):506–512. [II-2]

76. Devoe L, Croom C, Youssef A, et al. The prediction of controlled uterine rupture by the use of intrauterine pressure catheters. Obstet Gynecol 1992; 80:626–629. [II-2]

15

Early pregnancy loss

Michele Berghella and Alexi E. Achenbach

KEY POINTS

- Threatened pregnancy loss can be defined as vaginal bleeding in pregnancy before 20 weeks of gestation. Several **interventions** have been studied, but **none has been confirmed to be beneficial.**
- **Diagnosis of recurrent early pregnancy loss (REPL)** is ≥2 **consecutive losses of pregnancy <14 weeks.**
- **Workup** includes **uterine study, antiphospholipid antibodies (APAs),** and **parental karyotypes,** as well as **karyotype of products of conception (POC)** (if available).
- Prognosis with negative workup is for a 60% to 70% subsequent successful pregnancy in women <35 years old and 40% to 50% in women ≥35 years old.
- Women with **REPL and APA** should be **treated** with **low-dose aspirin and heparin** in subsequent pregnancy (see chap. 26 in *Maternal-Fetal Evidence Based Guidelines*). Women with unexplained REPL should not receive anticoagulant therapy.
- Women with **REPL and uterine septum, synechiae, or submucous myomata** can consider **hysteroscopic resection** of these abnormalities.
- Couples with abnormal parental karyotype can be offered genetic counseling, prenatal diagnosis, and/or gamete donation.
- There is insufficient evidence for universal screening for diabetes mellitus (DM), thyroid disease, progesterone deficiency [luteal phase defect (LPD)], infections, thrombophilia, etc.
- Women should **not be tested for alloimmunization or receive any of the immune therapies,** since they are ineffective and at times detrimental.
- Women should **not receive estrogen supplementation,** as this is unsafe, as it is detrimental to the future offspring, and ineffective.
- There is very limited evidence that supportive care and progesterone are beneficial interventions.
- There is insufficient evidence to support human chorionic gonadotropin (hCG), aspirin, and vitamins as interventions.

BACKGROUND

This chapter is mostly focused on recurrent pregnancy loss, with a brief limited part on early pregnancy loss.

DIAGNOSIS/DEFINITIONS

Pregnancy loss (PL): Spontaneous loss of pregnancy from conception to <20 weeks. The term spontaneous abortion (SAB) is equivalent but should be avoided since women associate negative feeling with this term. **Miscarriage** is a lay term for PL.

Anembryonic PL: No embryo identified, as embryonic disk has failed to develop or has already been resorbed (e.g., blighted ovum).

Embryonic PL: Embryo identified, but then nonviable, as in failure of an embryo, previously identified, to grow and/or retain a heart beat over time (e.g., missed abortion) (see also chap. 29).

First-trimester PL: PL from conception to <14 weeks. This guideline concerns mostly this type of recurrent loss (REPL).

Early first-trimester PL: Loss of pregnancy between conception and 9 6/7 weeks.

Late first-trimester PL: Loss of pregnancy between 10 and 13 6/7 weeks.

Second-trimester (late or fetal) PL: Loss of pregnancy between ≥14 and 19 6/7 weeks (see end of chapter).

Recurrent PL (RPL): ≥2 consecutive losses.

INCIDENCE

Early first-trimester PL is very common and occurs up to 20% or more of pregnancies.

RPL occurs in about 1% of reproductive-age women.

ETIOLOGY/BASIC PATHOPHYSIOLOGY

Most early PLs are secondary to genetic defects.

Etiology of REPL is not established in at least 50% of cases after workup (see below).

CLASSIFICATION

Primary REPL: no intervening live births; secondary REPL: intervening live births.

RISK FACTORS/ASSOCIATIONS

Maternal age <20 years, ≥35 years; maternal medical diseases, especially poorly controlled [e.g., hypertension (HTN) and DM].

PREGNANCY CONSIDERATIONS

Human reproduction is relatively inefficient (Table 15.1). Only 30% of fertilized eggs result in a viable pregnancy. Sporadic early PL is very common in humans. At least 15% to 20% of clinically identified pregnancies (implanted) physiologically end with early PL, and **only 50% to 60% of all conception advance to ≥20 weeks** (1). Most PLs represent failure of implantation and are difficult to recognize clinically. The prognosis after one uncomplicated early PL in a healthy young woman is for >70% to 80% chance of a viable pregnancy in the successive pregnancy. Therefore **no workup or therapy is usually indicated after one PL.** Oocyte quality and normal karyotype are most important for normal implantation, a lot more than uterine factors.

Table 15.1 Natural History of Pregnancies Following Prior Pregnancy Losses

	Prior PL (n)	Probability of live born (%)
Women with prior live born	0	90
	1	80
	2	75
	3	70
	4	60–65
Women without prior live born	≥3	55–60

Abbreviation: PL, pregnancy loss.

THREATENED PREGNANCY LOSS
Threatened PL can be defined as vaginal bleeding in pregnancy before 20 weeks of gestation. Several **interventions** have been studied, but **none has been confirmed to be beneficial**.

Complications
Vaginal bleeding in the first trimester has been associated with several complications in pregnancy, including antepartum hemorrhage (OR 2.47), preterm premature rupture of membranes (PPROM) (OR 1.78), preterm birth (PTB) (OR 2.05), intrauterine growth restriction (IUGR) (OR 1.54), low birth weight (LBW) (OR 1.83), and perinatal mortality (OR 2.15) (2). The presence of a subchorionic hematoma detected on ultrasound (usually between 5 and 20 weeks) is associated with increased risks of SAB (OR 2.18), abruptio (OR 5.71), intrauterine fetal demise (IUFD) (OR 2.09), PPROM (OR 1.64), and PTB (OR 1.40) (3).

Prevention
Vitamin
In non-high-risk women, multivitamin supplementation before 20 weeks is associated with similar total fetal loss (early/late miscarriage and stillbirth), early or late miscarriage or stillbirth, and most other outcomes compared with controls (4). Multivitamin supplementation is associated with a 38% higher incidence to have a multiple pregnancy, probably associated with vitamin A as well as folic acid supplementation. Therefore, **vitamin supplementation cannot be recommended for prevention of miscarriage**.

Progesterone
There is no evidence to support the routine use of progesterone to prevent miscarriage in early to midpregnancy. The meta-analysis of all women, regardless of gravidity and number of previous miscarriages, showed no statistically significant difference in the risk of miscarriage between progesterone and placebo or no treatment groups (OR 0.98, 95% CI 0.78–1.24) and no statistically significant difference in the incidence of adverse effect in either mother or baby (5). Therefore, **progesterone supplementation cannot be recommended for prevention of miscarriage**.

Therapy
Bed Rest
There is insufficient evidence of high quality that supports a policy of bed rest in order to prevent miscarriage in women with confirmed fetal viability and vaginal bleeding in first half of pregnancy. There is no statistically significant difference in the risk of miscarriage in the bed rest group versus the no bed rest group (placebo or other treatment) (RR 1.54, 95% CI 0.92–

2.58). Neither bed rest in hospital nor bed rest at home shows a significant difference in the prevention of miscarriage. There is a higher risk of miscarriage in those women in the bed rest group than in those in the hCG therapy group with no bed rest (RR 2.50, 95% CI 1.22–5.11). The small number of participants included in these studies makes these analyses inconclusive (6). Therefore, **bed rest cannot be recommended for prevention of miscarriage**. In fact, it might be harmful, given the higher rates of venous thromboembolism (VTE), muscle atrophy, and other detriments associated with bed rest.

Progesterone
There is insufficient evidence to assess the effect of progesterone supplementation in women with threatened miscarriage. There was no evidence of effectiveness with the use of vaginal progesterone compared with placebo in reducing the risk of miscarriage (RR 0.47, 95% CI 0.17–1.30) (7).

Human Chorionic Gonadotropin
The current evidence does **not support the routine use of hCG in the treatment of threatened miscarriage**. There is no statistically significant difference in the incidence of miscarriage between hCG and "no hCG" (placebo or no treatment) groups (RR 0.66, 95% CI 0.42–1.05). There was no report of adverse effects of hCG on mother or baby (8).

Muscle Relaxant
There is **insufficient evidence** to support the use of uterine muscle relaxant drugs for women with threatened miscarriage, and **therefore they should not be used**. In one poor-quality randomized controlled trial (RCT), compared with placebo, buphenine (a β-agonist) was associated with a lower risk of intrauterine death (RR 0.25, 95% CI 0.12–0.51). PTB was the only other outcome reported (RR 1.67, 95% CI 0.63–4.38) (9).

RECURRENT PREGNANCY LOSS
Workup (Screening)
Appropriate diagnostic workup of REPL is essential for choosing the proper intervention (Table 15.2) (10). Screening tests should not only discover diagnosis (etiology) but also lead to interventions effective in increasing the incidence of subsequent live birth. **The following women should be offered evaluation:**

1. Women with ≥2 primary REPLs
2. Women with ≥3 secondary REPLs

Initial part of workup consists of **history** (smoking, alcohol and caffeine, illicit drug use, environmental exposures, working conditions, as well as detailed obstetrical and gynecological history) and **physical exam** (pelvic). Often obstetrical history is mixed, with early PL, second-trimester PL, PTB, and/or fetal death, so that workup may include other tests (see specific chapters, including chapter 54 in Maternal-Fetal Evidence Based Guidelines).

RECOMMENDED SCREENING TESTS
Mother/Father

- Maternal **uterine study** [e.g., 3D sonohysterography (recommended—day 8–10 of follicular phase), hysterosalpingogram (HSG), hysteroscopy, 2D sonohysterography, or MRI]

    Ten to fifteen percent of women with REPL have uterine anomalies. Most common associated anomaly is septate uterus, followed by didelphys and bicornuate. Arcuate uterus has not been consistently associated with REPL. Uterine synechiae (Asherman's syndrome) and

Table 15.2 Evaluation of a Woman with Recurrent Miscarriages

Assessment

Medical history	Comment
Determine pattern and gestational age of preembryonic, embryonic, or fetal death, if such information is available.	Preembryonic and embryonic losses before 10 wk of gestation are the most common type of miscarriage, although the onset of symptoms may be later.
Evaluate for features suggestive of the antiphospholipid syndrome.	Features include thrombosis, fetal death, autoimmune disease, and thrombocytopenia.
Assess whether patient has history of uterine malformations (e.g., seen on previous ultrasonographic examination or during intra-abdominal surgery).	Previous obstetrical complication such as preterm labor or breech presentation suggests possibility of uterine malformation.
Assess whether patient has had another fetus or infant with congenital anomaly.	A congenital anomaly suggests the possibility of a parental karyotype abnormality, although these abnormalities may be present in the absence of such a history.
Determine whether patient has history of symptoms suggestive of thyroid disease or diabetes.	
Physical examination	
Perform pelvic examination with particular focus on findings compatible with uterine or cervical abnormalities.	
Examine patient for other physical findings suggestive of thyroid disease or diabetes.	
Recommended tests[a]	
Lupus anticoagulant, anticardiolipin antibodies, and anti-β_2-glycoprotein 1 antibodies	Tests for lupus anticoagulant are reported as either positive or negative; levels of anticardiolipin and anti-β_2-glycoprotein 1 antibodies are clinically significant only in medium-to-high titers as defined by the laboratory; antiphospholipid syndrome is diagnosed when tests are repeatedly positive at least 12 wk apart[b]
Sonohysterography	Sonohysterography and hysterosalpingography are noninvasive screening tests used to evaluate uterine cavity and shape; MRI, hysteroscopy, or both may be more informative but are more expensive and invasive, respectively; all are useful in detecting a uterine abnormality.
Chromosome analyses of father and mother	Parental karyotyping is expensive and not always covered by third-party payers; because treatment options are limited and do not surpass results of spontaneous conception, some couples may choose to forgo this testing.
Chromosome analysis of products of conception	Karyotype testing of the conceptus is somewhat controversial, but an aneuploid conceptus indicates a more favorable outcome of a subsequent pregnancy and may avert further unnecessary evaluation and treatment.
Other laboratory tests (e.g., thyrotropin measurement or screening for diabetes), if suggested by history or physical examination.	

[a]Routine testing for thyroid disease, diabetes, the polycystic ovary syndrome, heritable thrombophilias, bacteria and viruses, and alloimmune abnormalities is not recommended.
[b]See also chapter 26 in *Maternal-Fetal Evidence Based Guidelines*.
Abbreviation: MRI, magnetic resonance imaging.
Source: Adapted from Ref. 10.

diethylstilbestrol (DES) exposure are associated with REPL. Myomata have not been consistently associated with REPL. Available intervention is hysteroscopic resection of septum, synechiae, or submucous myomata. Surgical correction of these and other uterine anomalies has not been studied in trials.

- Maternal APAs

    Three to fifteen percent of women with REPL have APAs. Tests should be positive twice, ≥12 weeks apart. See chapter 26 in *Maternal-Fetal Evidence Based Guidelines* for tests [lupus anticoagulant, anticardiolipin antibodies (ACAs), and β-2 glycoprotein 1] and effective intervention (e.g., low-dose aspirin and prophylactic heparin).

- Parental karyotype

    Two to four percent of couples with REPL have one parent with balanced translocation, or less commonly a chromosome inversion. Available intervention is donor gametes.

- If family history or clinical suspicion of DM: fasting glucose
- If clinical symptoms/suspicion of thyroid disease: thyroid-stimulating hormone (TSH) and free thyroxine (T4)

Products of Conception

- POC karyotype

    Management of women with ≥2 REPLs can be based on genetic evaluation of POCs (Fig. 15.1) (11). Fifty to sixty percent of early PL tested have aneuploidy, especially if prior PL with aneuploidy and/or advanced maternal age (AMA) (70–80%); aneuploidy is present in >50% of embryos tested preimplantation in women with REPL. More than 50% of aneuploidies are trisomies; most common single aneuploidy is 45XO. 46XX karyotype is often associated with maternal cell contamination, so that caution is necessary; microsatellite analysis decreases this confusion. This test can identify probable etiology; decrease further workup; and provide couple with explanation, shown to decrease self-blame (12).

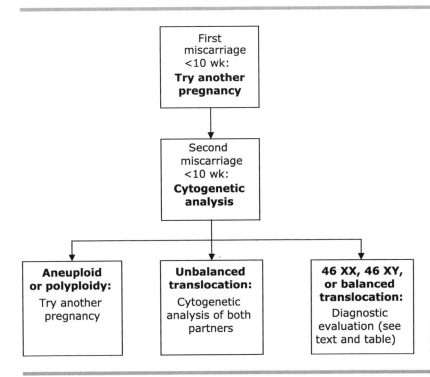

Figure 15.1 Evaluation of patients with early pregnancy loss based on cytogenetic analysis of products of conception. *Source*: Adapted from Ref. 11.

TESTS THAT CANNOT BE ROUTINELY RECOMMENDED
Mother

*   Endometrial biopsy or progesterone levels
    Hypothesis: Corpus luteum fails to make enough progesterone to sustain early decidua for placentation (LPD). It is normal to have at least two consecutive out-of-phase (≥2 days discrepancy) biopsies (diagnosis of LPD) on endometrial histology (late luteal phase—day 25 or 26—after presumed ovulation) in 50% of menstrual cycles; there is also high interobserver variation on interpretation of endometrial biopsies. There is insufficient evidence that intervention [such as progesterone supplementation—17P, micronized progesterone tablets 100 mg po bid or Crinone cream (8%) one application per vagina daily (beginning 2 days after ovulation until 10 weeks' gestation or menses)] improves outcomes specifically in women with REPL and LPD (13,14). 17P is efficacious in improving pregnancy outcomes in women with in vitro fertilization (IVF), and in decreasing PTB in women with prior PTB (see chapter 16).
*   Alloimmune tests [includes fecal occult blood (FOB)]
    No consistent association and no efficacious intervention—see below.
*   Thyroid antibodies
    No consistent association and no intervention studies.
*   Antinuclear antibody (ANA)
    No consistent association and no intervention studies.

Products of Conception

*   POC molecular genetic abnormalities (e.g., X-chromosome inactivation)
    Commercially available tests are not widely available for this testing.

Both

*   Thrombophilia
    Thrombophilic mutations [factor V Leiden, prothrombin G20210, fasting hyperhomocysteinemia (methylenetetrahydrofolate (MTHFR), antithrombin III deficiency, protein S, and protein C] have not been consistently associated with REPL. Second-trimester PL has been associated with thrombophilic mutations. There is insufficient evidence regarding any interventions in women with PL and thrombophilias (see chap. 27 in *Maternal-Fetal Evidence Based Guidelines*).
*   Infections
    No infectious agent has been proven to cause REPL. *Listeria*, *Toxoplasma gondii*, and many viruses have been associated with sporadic early PL. Chlamydia, mycoplasma/ureoplasma (proposed diagnosis with endometrial biopsy, with treatment of woman and partner with either doxycycline 100 mg po bid or ciprofloxacin 250 mg po bid), and bacterial vaginosis are associated with sporadic PL, not REPL.

MANAGEMENT
Prevention

Optimize preconception medical care of all maternal diseases.

Preconception Care

Informative and sympathetic counseling. Workup is best done preconception (Table 15.2). When workup is positive, counsel regarding specific association. If workup is negative (>50% of couples), counseling should include the fact that 60% to 70% of couples with unexplained REPL have successful pregnancies in the next gestation (Table 15.1). This percentage decreases to 40% to 50% in women ≥40 years old. Offer all women with REPL a support group (Unite, etc.).

Prenatal Care

See subsection "Preconception Care."

Therapy (Specific for Workup)

Abnormal Uterine Cavity

Septum, synechiae, and/or submucous myomata can be resected hysteroscopically, but **there are no trials regarding this intervention. There is a high likelihood of successful pregnancy in women with unrepaired septa, so that some suggest against surgical repair in nulligravid women with uterine septa** (10). **Repair of bicornuate or unicornuate uteri is also usually not suggested in these women, as outcomes are usually good without repair, whereas surgical correction is associated with higher risk of complications.** Consider referral to reproductive endocrinology specialist if necessary. **There is unfortunately insufficient evidence to give a recommendation for women with fibroids and REPL.**

Antiphospholipid Syndrome

Prophylactic unfractionated heparin (UFH) and aspirin (see chap. 26 in *Maternal-Fetal Evidence Based Guidelines*):

Therapy is usually begun once fetal viability is established. **Low-dose aspirin** is usually about **75 to 100 mg** daily. For prophylactic **UFH: 5000 to 7500 U first trimester, 7500 to 10,000 U second trimester, and 10,000 U third trimester SQ q12h.** Heparin used in positive trials was UFH, and even if low–molecular weight heparin (LMWH) is associated with less side effects in nonpregnant adults, RCTs of LMWH in pregnancy for RPL in antiphospholipid syndrome (APS) women have not shown benefit.

UFH combined with aspirin is associated with a significant reduction in PL compared with aspirin alone (RR 0.46, 95% CI 0.29–0.71; 3 trials, $n = 140$). There is no advantage in high-dose, over low-dose, UFH (1 trial, $n = 50$).

LMWH combined with aspirin compared with aspirin does not significantly reduce PL (OR 0.70, 95% CI 0.34–1.45; 5 trials, $n = 398$) (15). For prophylactic LMWH either enoxaparin (Lovenox) 30 to 40 mg SQ q12h or dalteparin (Fragmin) 5000 U SQ q12h were used in RCTs, and clinicians may adjust prophylaxis in high-risk cases to heparin (anti-Xa) level range of 0.2 to 0.3.

Three trials of **aspirin alone** ($n = 135$) show no significant reduction in PL (RR 1.05, 95% CI 0.66–1.68).

Prednisone and aspirin (3 trials, $n = 286$) result in a significant increase in prematurity when compared with placebo, aspirin, and heparin combined with aspirin, and an increase in gestational diabetes, but no significant benefit.

Intravenous immunoglobulin (IVIG) ± UFH and aspirin (2 trials, $n = 58$) is associated with an increased risk of PL or premature birth when compared with UFH or LMWH combined with aspirin (RR 2.51, 95% CI 1.27–4.95). When compared with prednisone and aspirin, IVIG (1 trial, $n = 82$) is not significantly different in outcomes (16).

In summary, **therapy with UFH and aspirin can be recommended to the woman with REPL and APS**, as it reduces the chance of PL by 54% compared with aspirin alone.

Abnormal Parental Chromosomes

Offer genetic counseling, prenatal diagnosis, and gamete donation. Preimplantation genetic screening with IVF is not supported by RCTs and should therefore not be recommended (10).

Medical Condition

If a medical condition is identified (e.g., DM, thyroid disease), treat as indicated (see specific chapters in *Maternal-Fetal*

Evidence Based Guidelines). Metformin has not been shown to reduce the risk of miscarriage in women with REPL and polycystic ovary syndrome (10).

Inherited Thrombophilia

As stated above, a workup for inherited thrombophilia is not indicated. If positive inherited **thrombophilia** is incidentally or previously identified, no intervention has been consistently shown to improve outcomes. Please also refer chapter 27 in *Maternal-Fetal Evidence Based Guidelines*, and see below if one prior second trimester PL.

Negative Workup

Progesterone. In women who had ≥3 consecutive miscarriages, progesterone treatment is associated with a statistically significant **61% decrease in miscarriage** rate compared with placebo or no treatment in three small trials (5,17–19). No statistically significant differences, probably because of small numbers, were found between the route of administration of progesterone (oral, intramuscular, and vaginal) versus placebo or no treatment (5,17–19), so the best route and dose of progesterone for prevention of REPL are still unknown. In summary, **progesterone treatment for women with REPL may be warranted given the reduced rates of miscarriage in the treatment group and the finding of no statistically significant difference between treatment and control groups in rates of adverse effects** suffered by either mother or baby (5).

Supportive care. **Consider** intensive supportive early prenatal care, focusing on antenatal counseling and psychological support. There are **no properly controlled trials to assess the effect of this intervention**. Three studies (not RCTs) showed improved outcome versus standard or no prenatal care (20–22).

Human chorionic gonadotropin. There is **not enough evidence** to evaluate the use of hCG during pregnancy in order to prevent miscarriage in women with a history of unexplained recurrent spontaneous miscarriage because the trials are small, and have significant (especially two studies) limitations (23–27). hCG is associated with a 74% reduced risk of miscarriage for women with a history of recurrent miscarriage (23–27). All studies showed at least a trend favoring benefit of hCG. This result should be interpreted cautiously because the apparent effect is greatly influenced by the two methodologically weaker studies.

Low-dose aspirin. Compared with placebo, low-dose (50 mg/day) aspirin was associated with similar live birth rates (both 81%) in 54 pregnant women with recurrent (≥3) SAB occurring before 22 weeks without detectable ACAs (28,29). In another RCT, aspirin 80 mg had effects similar to placebo in women with unexplained recurrent miscarriages (30). Therefore, low-dose aspirin should not be recommended for women with recurrent unexplained early PLs.

Unfractionated heparin. There is **insufficient evidence** to assess the effect of UFH in women with unexplained REPL.

Low–molecular weight heparin. There are several RCTs that show **no effect of LMWH on prevention of PL in women with unexplained REPL**. Compared with low-dose aspirin, enoxaparin (a LMWH) was associated with similar live birth rates, respectively 82% and 84% (RR 0.97, 95% CI 0.81–1.16), in 107 women with consecutive recurrent miscarriage (≥3 consecutive first-trimester miscarriages or ≥2 consecutive second-trimester miscarriages) without any apparent cause and no hereditary thrombophilia (31). In 340 women with ≥3 unexplained first-trimester REPLs, enoxaparin 20 mg daily from fetal viability until 34 weeks was associated with a slight nonsignificant reduction in both early (4.1% vs. 8.8%) and late (1.1% vs. 2.3%) miscarriages, but no other effects on other perinatal outcomes.

No reduction in PL was observed when LMWH and low-dose aspirin were used in combination to treat 297 women with idiopathic recurrent miscarriage (22% in pharmacologic intervention group vs. 20% in surveillance group) (32). In women with 364 unexplained REPLs, nadroparin and low-dose aspirin were associated with similar outcomes compared with either low-dose aspirin alone or to placebo (30).

Vitamin

There is no specific adequate trial on multivitamin supplementation of any kind for women with prior REPL.

Diethylstilbestrol

DES should not be used in pregnancy for any indication. Data are mostly from studies of women without risk factors, women with "threatened abortion" in the current pregnancy, or diabetics (most women with RPL). **DES use in pregnancy is significantly associated with several harmful consequences for both mother and baby.** DES given in the first trimester leads to a 37% increased rate of miscarriage and 61% increased rate of PTB (33–40). There is also a 48% increase in the numbers of babies weighing less than 2500 g. Stillbirth and neonatal death are not influenced by the intervention (DES) as compared with the control group. Preeclampsia is similar in the two groups. Exposed female offsprings have a nonsignificant trend toward more cancer of the genital tract and cancer other than of the genital tract. Primary infertility, adenosis of the vagina/cervix in female offsprings, and testicular abnormality in male offsprings are significantly higher in those exposed to DES before birth.

The vast use in the 50s to 70s of a medication with no benefit proven by evidence-based medicine is the best example of the importance of using data from trials and meta-analyses to guide effective practice.

Immunotherapy

The various forms of immunotherapy did not show significant differences between treatment and control groups in terms of subsequent live births (41):

- Paternal cell immunization (12 trials, 641 women), OR 1.38, 95% CI 0.90 to 2.12 (42–52)
- Third-party donor cell immunization (3 trials, 156 women), OR 1.39, 95% CI 0.68 to 2.82 (43,45,51)
- Trophoblast membrane infusion (1 trial, 37 women), OR 0.40, 95% CI 0.11 to 1.45 (53)
- IVIG (8 trials, $n = 303$), OR 0.98, 95% CI 0.61 to 1.58 (54–60)

Immunization using viable mononuclear cells carries the **risk of any blood transfusion** such as hepatitis B virus or human immunodeficiency virus (HIV). Reactions have been uncommon but include soreness and redness at the injection site, fever, maternal platelet alloimmunization, blood group sensitization, and one cutaneous graft-versus-host-like reaction. Women who have received lymphocyte immune therapy may have a higher incidence of subsequent miscarriage than women who did not receive such cellular products (49). The Director of the Office of Therapeutics Research and Review, U.S. Food and Drug Administration (FDA), sent a letter on January 30, 2002, to physicians believed to be using lymphocyte immune therapy to prevent miscarriages. He informed them that the injectable products used in lymphocyte immune therapy do not have the required FDA approval and are considered investigational new drugs that pose several significant safety concerns. Administration of such cells or cellular products in humans can only be performed in the United States as part of clinical investigations, and then only if there is an investigational new drug (IND) application in effect. IVIG therapy is expensive and in relatively short supply.

Immunotherapies should not be offered as treatment for unexplained RPL. Women should be spared the pain and grief associated with false expectations that an ineffective treatment might work.

ANTEPARTUM TESTING
No specific testing indicated.

DELIVERY
No specific precaution.

ANESTHESIA
No specific precaution.

POSTPARTUM/BREASTFEEDING
No specific precaution.

FUTURE
Effective treatment of an alleged alloimmune cause of recurrent miscarriage awaits more complete knowledge of the underlying pathophysiology. A specific assay to diagnose immune-mediated early PL and a reliable method to determine which patients might benefit from manipulation of the maternal immune system are urgently needed. It is not presently known exactly how many REPLs are the result of anembryonic or chromosomally abnormal conceptuses, anatomic or structural abnormalities, and how many are embryonic or fetal deaths. It is likely that some unexplained early losses are due to as yet undefined subchromosomal genetic abnormalities impairing early development of the conceptus. New molecular techniques should be directed at understanding the factors responsible for successful pregnancy as well as PL.

SECOND-TRIMESTER PREGNANCY LOSS
If loss ≥ 14 and <20 weeks, obtain any available autopsy, chromosomes, and other workup from that loss (see also chapter 54 in Maternal-Fetal Evidence Based Guidelines). Placental pathology from previous pregnancies may be reexamined by an expert.

$\geq$10 Weeks Loss
Compared with low-dose aspirin, in women who had had a previous fetal loss after the 10th week and had a thrombophilic defect (heterozygous factor V Leiden, prothrombin G20210, or protein S deficiency), enoxaparin 40 mg daily treatment is associated with a 10-fold increased live birth rate, as compared with low-dose aspirin in just one trial (61).

See also chapter 16.

For management of early PL, see chapter 29.

REFERENCES

1. American College of Obstetricians and Gynecologists. ACOG Practice Bulletin No. 24: Management of recurrent early pregnancy loss. Washington, D.C.: ACOG, 2001. [Review]
2. Saraswat L, Bhattacharya S, Maheshwari A, et al. Maternal and perinatal outcome in women with threatened miscarriage in the first trimester: a systematic review. Br J Obstet Gynecol 2010; 117:245–257. [Systematic review]
3. Tuuli MG, Norman SM, Odibo AO, et al. Perinatal outcomes in women with subchorionic hematoma—a systematic review and meta-analysis. Obstet Gynecol 2001; 117:1205–1212. [Meta-analysis, $n = 1735$]
4. Rumbold A, Middleton P, Pan N, et al. Vitamin supplementation for preventing miscarriage. Cochrane Database Syst Rev 2011; (1): CD004073. [Meta-analysis: 28 RCTs, $n = 96{,}674$]
5. Haas DM, Ramsey PS. Progestogen for preventing miscarriage. Cochrane Database Syst Rev 2008; (2):CD003511. [Meta-analysis: 15 RCTs, $n = 2118$]
6. Aleman A, Althabe F, Belizán JM, et al. Bed rest during pregnancy for preventing miscarriage. Cochrane Database Syst Rev 2005; (2):CD003576. [Meta-analysis: 2 RCTs, $n = 84$]
7. Wahabi HA, Abed Althagafi NF, Elawad M, et al. Progestogen for treating threatened miscarriage. Cochrane Database Syst Rev 2011; (3):CD005943. [Meta-analysis: 2 RCTs, $n = 84$]
8. Devaseelan P, Fogarty PP, Regan L. Human chorionic gonadotrophin for threatened miscarriage. Cochrane Database Syst Rev 2010; (5):CD007422. [Meta-analysis: 3 RCTs, $n = 312$]
9. Soltan MH. Buphenine and threatened abortion. Eur J Obstet Gynecol Reprod Biol 1986; 22:319–324. [RCT, $n = 170$]
10. Branch DW, Gibson M, Silver RM. Recurrent miscarriage. N Engl J Med 2010; 363:1740–1766. [Review]
11. Stephenson MD. Recurrent early pregnancy loss: is miscarriage evaluation the missing link? Contemp OB/GYN 2008; 10:505. [Review]
12. Nikcevic AV, Tunkel SA, Kuczmierczyk AR, et al. Investigation of the cause of miscarriage and its influence on women's psychological distress. Br J Obstet Gynecol 1999; 106:808–813. [II-2]
13. Karamardian LM, Grimes DA. Luteal phase deficiency: effect of treatment on pregnancy rates. Am J Obstet Gynecol 1992; 167:1391. [Meta-analysis: 1 RCT, $n = 44$ and 3 controlled studies]
14. Balasch J, Vanrell J, Marquez M, et al. Dehydrogesterone versus vaginal progesterone in the treatment of the endometrial luteal phase deficiency. Fertil Steril 1982; 37:751–754. [RCT, $n = 44$]
15. Ziakas PD, Pavlou M, Voulgarelis M. Heparin treatment in antiphospholipid syndrome with recurrent pregnancy loss: a systematic review and meta-analysis. Obstet Gynecol 2010; 115(6):1256–1262. [Meta-analysis: 5 RCTs, $n = 398$]
16. Empson MB, Lassere M, Craig JC, et al. Prevention of recurrent miscarriage for women with antiphospholipid antibody or lupus anticoagulant. Cochrane Database Syst Rev 2005; (2):CD002859. [Meta-analysis: 13 RCTs, $n = 840$]
17. Goldzieher JW. Double-blind trial of a progestin in habitual abortion. J Am Med Assoc 1964; 188(7):651–654. [RCT, $n = 16$. Women who had either: never had a term pregnancy and who had had two or more miscarriages or who had had one or more term pregnancy followed by a minimum number of two consecutive miscarriages. All women had to have a urinary pregnanediol of <5 mg/day before 8 weeks' gestation and/or <7 mg/day by 14 weeks' gestation. 10 mg/day of oral medroxyprogesterone. Placebo: yes. Duration: not stated.]
18. Le Vine L. Habitual abortion. A controlled clinical study of progestational therapy. West J Surg 1964; 72:30–36. [RCT, $n = 30$. Women who had had three consecutive miscarriages, were less than 16 weeks' gestation, and with no signs of threatened miscarriage in the current pregnancy. 500 mg/wk IM of hydroxyprogesterone caproate. Duration: until miscarriage or the 36th week of gestation. Placebo: yes.]
19. Swyer GIM, Daley D. Progesterone implantation in habitual abortion. BMJ 1953; 1:1073–1086. [RCT, $n = 47$ (out of 113 total). Women having had two or more consecutive miscarriages before 12 weeks' gestation. 6 × 25 mg progesterone pellets inserted within the gluteal muscle either: (i) as soon as pregnancy was confirmed or (ii) not later than 10th week of gestation, or (iii) not later than the earliest previous miscarriage. Placebo: no but had a no-treatment control group.]
20. Stray-Pedersen B, Stray-Pedersen S. Recurrent abortion: the role of psychotherapy. In: Beard RW, Sharp F, eds. Early Pregnancy Loss. London: Springer-Verlag, 1988:433–440. [II-2]
21. Liddell HS, Pattison NS, Zanderigo A. Recurrent miscarriage—outcome after supportive care in early pregnancy. Aust NZ Obstet Gynecol 1991; 31:320–322. [II-1]
22. Clifford K, Rai R, Regan L. Future pregnancy outcome in unexplained recurrent first trimester miscarriage. Hum Reprod 1997; 12:387–389. [II-2]
23. Scott JR, Pattison N. Human chorionic gonadotrophin for recurrent miscarriage. Cochrane Database Syst Rev 2005; (4). [Meta-analysis: 4 RCTs, $n = 180$. Variable quality trials]
24. Harrison RF. Treatment of habitual abortion with human chorionic gonadotrophin: results of open and placebo-controlled studies. Eur J Obstet Gynecol Reprod Biol 1985; 20:159–168. [RCT, $n = $ spontaneous miscarriage of *three previous consecutive pregnancies without evidence of a cause*, normal investigative profile included: chromosomal analysis of both partners; no systemic disease; normal bacteriological investigations of semen and cervical secretions; normal HSG, normal serum FSH, LH, estradiol, and prolactin; normal or low progesterone. Initially 10,000 IU hCG by IM injection followed by 5000 IU twice weekly up to 12 weeks, followed by 5000 IU weekly until 20 weeks.]
25. Harrison RF. Human chorionic gonadotrophin (HCG) in the management of recurrent abortion; results of a multi-centre placebo-controlled study. Eur J Obstet Gynecol Reprod Biol 1992; 47:175–179. [RCT. "Modus operandi" described as identical to Harrison 1985 study. hCG 10,000 IU IM starting before 8 weeks. hCG 5000 IU IM twice weekly until 12 weeks. hCG 5000 IU IM once weekly from 12 to 16 weeks. Identically packaged vs. placebo vials given as same regime]
26. Quenby S, Farquharson R. Human chorionic gonadotropin supplementation in recurring pregnancy loss: a controlled trial. Fertil Steril 1994; 62:708–710. [RCT, $n = 104$. Two or more consecutive first-trimester miscarriages. Profasi (Serono) 10,000 U IM initially and 5000 U twice weekly until 14 weeks' gestation. Control group: placebo of normal saline IM "in an identical fashion."]
27. Svigos J. Preliminary experience with the use of human chorionic gonadotrophin therapy in women with repeated abortion. Clin Reprod Fertil 1982; 1:131–135. [RCT. Two unexplained (normal genital tract and chromosomes) miscarriages. Treatment group managed in one of two ways according to serum progesterone. A low progesterone precipitated compliance with the intended treatment. A normal progesterone precipitated no treatment (i.e., managed as a control). Groups analyzed on an intention-to-treat basis. 9000 IU, IM × 3 per week from 6 to 7 weeks until 12 weeks vs. no treatment.]
28. Kaandorp S, Di Nisio M, Goddijn M, et al. Aspirin or anticoagulants for treating recurrent miscarriage in women without antiphospholipid syndrome. Cochrane Database Syst Rev 2009; (1):CD004734. [Meta-analysis: 2 RCTs; $n = 74$ subgroup analyses; only Tulppala is pertinent for this analysis.]
29. Tulppala M, Marttunen M, Soderstrom-Anttila V, et al. Low-dose aspirin in the prevention of miscarriage in women with unexplained or autoimmune related recurrent miscarriage: effect on prostacyclin and thromboxane A2 production. Hum Reprod 1997; 12(7):1567–1572. [RCT, $n = 54$ with negative ACA—subcategory of 82 women with a history of at least three consecutive miscarriages in whom no obvious cause for their previous pregnancy losses was found. Interventions: aspirin (50 mg/daily) vs. placebo, started as soon as a urinary pregnancy test became positive.]
30. Kaandorp SP, Goddijn M, van der Post JAM, et al. Aspirin plus heparin or aspirin alone in women with recurrent miscarriages. N Engl J Med 2010; 362:1586–1596. [RCT, $n = 364$]
31. Dolitzky M, Inbal A, Segal Y, et al. A randomized study of thromboprophylaxis in women with unexplained consecutive recurrent miscarriages. Fertil Steril 2006; 86(2):362–366. [RCT, $n = 107$]

32. Clark P, Walker ID, Langhorne P, et al. SPIN (Scottish Pregnancy Intervention) study: a multicenter, randomized trial of low-molecular-weight heparin and low-dose aspirin in women with recurrent miscarriage. Blood 2010; 115:4162–4167. [RCT, $n = 294$, multicenter, ≥ 2 recurrent pregnancy losses at 24 or fewer weeks, randomized to enoxaparin 40 mg SQ QD and aspirin 75 mg PO QD until 36 weeks, or to pregnancy surveillance only.]

33. Bamigboye AA, Morris J. Oestrogen supplementation, mainly diethylstilbestrol, for preventing miscarriages and other adverse pregnancy outcomes. Cochrane Database Syst Rev 2005; (4): CD002859. [Meta-analysis: 7 RCTs, $n = 2897$]

34. Bender S. The effect of diethylstilboestrol on recurrent miscarriage. Personal communication February 1988. [RCT, $n = 58$ women with prior SAB. DES in one clinic vs. control in another clinic]

35. Crowder RE, Bills ES, Broadbent JS. The management of threatened abortion. A study of 100 cases. Am J Obstet Gynecol 1950; 60(4):896–899. [RCT, $n = 100$. Women admitted for threatened abortion and diabetic. DES 25 mg every 30 minutes for 6 hours then 100 mg daily until asymptomatic for 24 hours, then 50 mg daily until 28 weeks of pregnancy. Both DES and control group had phenobarbitone and demerol.]

36. Dieckmann WJ, Davis ME, Rynkiewcz SM, et al. Does the administration of diethylstilbestrol during pregnancy have therapeutic value? Am J Obstet Gynecol 1953; 66(5):1062–1081. [RCT, $n = 1646$ (all women). 5 mg of DES administered from 7 to 8 weeks in graduated fashion up to 150 mg at 34–35 weeks vs. placebo. Many long-term follow-up manuscripts]

37. Ferguson JH. Effect of stilbestrol on pregnancy compared to the effect of a placebo. Am J Obstet Gynecol 1953; 65(3):592–601. [RCT, $n = 393$ (all women). DES 6.3–137.5 mg depending on gestational age vs. placebo]

38. Medical Research Council. The use of hormones in the management of pregnancy in diabetics. Lancet 1955; 2:833–836. [RCT, $n = 147$ (High-risk diabetic women). Incremental doses of 50–200 mg DES daily from about 16 weeks to term. Ethisterone, 25 mg/day from 16 weeks, incrementally to 250 mg/day at 32 weeks to term. Ethisterone was given incrementally. Graduated dosing with stilbestrol from 50 mg at 19 weeks or less to 200 mg at 32 weeks or more. Ethisterone from 25 mg/day at 19 weeks or less to 250 mg at 32 weeks or more vs. placebo]

39. Robinson D, Shettles LB. The use of diethylstilboestrol in threatened abortion. Am J Obstet Gynecol 1952; 63(6):1330–1333. [RCT, $n = 93$. Women admitted for threatened abortion. DES 5–125 mg depending on gestational age vs. placebo]

40. Swyer GIM, Law RG. An evaluation of the prophylactic antenatal use of stilboestrol. Preliminary report. Proceedings of the society for endocrinology. J Endocrinol 1954; 10:36–37. [RCT, $n = 460$ (all primigravidas). 5 mg of DES administered from 7 to 8 weeks in graduated fashion up to 150 mg at 34–35 weeks vs. placebo (as Dieckman).]

41. Porter TF, LaCoursiere Y, Scott JR. Immunotherapy for recurrent miscarriage. Cochrane Database Syst Rev 2006; (2):CD000112. [Meta-analysis: 20 RCTs—see below]

42. Cauchi MN, Lim D, Young DE, et al. Treatment of recurrent aborters by immunization with paternal cells—controlled trial. Am J Reprod Immunol 1991; 25:16–17. [RCT]

43. Christiansen OB, Mathiesen O, Husth M, et al. Placebo-controlled trial of active immunization with third party leukocytes in recurrent miscarriage. Acta Obstet Gynecol Scand 1994; 3:261–268. [RCT]

44. Gatenby PA, Cameron K, Simes RJ, et al. Treatment of recurrent spontaneous abortion by immunization with paternal lymphocytes: results of a controlled trial. Am J Reprod Immunol 1993; 29:88–94. [RCT]

45. Ho HN, Gill TJ, Hsieh HJ, et al. Immunotherapy for recurrent spontaneous abortions in a Chinese population. Am J Reprod Immunol 1991; 25:10–15. [RCT]

46. Illeni MT, Marelli G, Parazzini F, et al. Immunotherapy and recurrent abortion: a randomized clinical trial. Hum Reprod 1994; 9:1247–1249. [RCT]

47. Kilpatrick DC, Liston W. Abstracts of contributors' individual data submitted to the Worldwide Prospective Observation Study on Immunotherapy for Treatment of Recurrent Spontaneous Abortion. Am J Reprod Immunol 1994; 32:264. [RCT]

48. Mowbray JF, Gibbings C, Liddell H, et al. Controlled trial of treatment of recurrent spontaneous abortion by immunisation with paternal cells. Lancet 1985; 1:941–943. [RCT]

49. Ober C, Karrison T, Odem RB, et al. Mononuclear-cell immunisation in prevention of recurrent miscarriages: a randomised trial. Lancet 1999; 354:365–369. [RCT, $n = 183$]

50. Reznikoff-Etievant MF. Abstracts of contributors' individual data submitted to the Worldwide Prospective Observation Study on Immunotherapy for Treatment of Recurrent Spontaneous Abortion. Am J Reprod Immunol 1994; 32:266–267. [RCT]

51. Scott JR, Branch WD, Dudley DJ, et al. Immunotherapy for recurrent pregnancy loss: the University of Utah perspective. In: Dondero F, Johnson P, eds. Reproductive Immunology. Serono Symposium Publications, Raven Press, San Diego, U.S.A: 1997:255–257. [RCT]

52. Stray-Pederson S. Department of Obstetrics and Gynecology, University of Oslo, Oslo, 1 Norway. Personal communication 1994 (in Cochrane, Ref. 28 above). [RCT]

53. Johnson PM, Ramsden GH, Chia KV, et al. A combined randomised double-blind and open study of trophoblast membrane infusion (TMI) in unexplained recurrent miscarriage. In: Chaouat G, Mowbray J, eds. Cellular Molecular Biology of the Materno-Fetal Relationship. Vol. 212, Colloque INSERM/John Libbey Eurotext Ltd, Paris, France: 1991:277–284. [RCT]

54. Christiansen OB, Mathieson O, Husth M, et al. Placebo-controlled trial of treatment of unexplained secondary recurrent spontaneous abortions and recurrent late spontaneous abortions with iv immunoglobulin. Hum Reprod 1995; 10:2690–2695. [RCT, $n = 34$]

55. Christiansen OB, Pedersen B, Rosgaard A, et al. A randomized, double-blind, placebo-controlled trial of intravenous immunoglobulin in the prevention of recurrent miscarriage: evidence for a therapeutic effect in women with secondary recurrent miscarriage. Hum Reprod 2002; 17(3):809–816. [RCT, $n = 58$]

56. Coulam CB, Krysa L, Stern JJ, et al. Intravenous immunoglobulin for treatment of recurrent pregnancy loss. Am J Reprod Immunol 1995; 34:333–337. [RCT, $n = 95$]

57. German RSA/IVIG Group. Intravenous immunoglobulin for treatment of recurrent miscarriage. Br J Obstet Gynecol 1994; 101:1072–1077. [RCT]

58. Jablonowska B, Selbing A, Palfi M, et al. Prevention of recurrent spontaneous abortion by intravenous immunoglobulin: a double-blind placebo-controlled study. Hum Reprod 1999; 14:838–841. [RCT, $n = 41$]

59. Perino A, Vassiliadis A, Vuceticha R, et al. Short-term therapy for recurrent abortion using intravenous immunoglobulins: results of a double-blind placebo-controlled Italian study. Hum Reprod 1997; 12:2388–2392. [RCT, $n = 46$]

60. Stephenson MD, Dreher K, Houlihan E, et al. Prevention of unexplained recurrent spontaneous abortion using intravenous immunoglobulin: a prospective, randomized, double blinded, placebo controlled trial. Am J Reprod Immunol 1998; 39:82–88. [RCT, $n = 62$]

61. Gris J-C, Mercier E, Quere I, et al. Low-molecular-weight heparin versus low-dose aspirin in women with one fetal loss and a constitutional thrombophilic disorder. Blood 2004; 103:3695–3699. [RCT, $n = 160$. Open-label, quasi-random. Women with a history of one fetal loss after the 10th week of gestation and factor V Leiden, FII 20210A mutation, or protein S deficiency. Subcutaneous enoxaparin (40 mg/daily from the 8th week of amenorrhoea after a positive pregnancy test) vs. aspirin (100 mg/daily from the 8th week of amenorrhoea after a positive pregnancy test.]

16

Preterm birth prevention

Vincenzo Berghella

KEY POINTS

- See also chaps. 17 (Preterm Labor) and 18 (Preterm Premature Rupture of Membranes).
- **Gestational age (GA) determination is of outmost importance in prevention of preterm birth (PTB) and management of presumed threatened PTB.**
- **PTB** is defined as birth between 20 0/7 and 36 6/7 weeks. It is the **number one cause of perinatal morbidity and mortality**, and these complications are inversely proportional to GA at birth. **Over 1 million babies die of the consequences of PTB every year in the world**, 1 every 30 seconds.
- An accurate history should be taken regarding risk factors for PTB, especially obstetric-gynecological (ob-gyn) history, maternal lifestyle, and prepregnancy weight (Table 16.1).
- **Primary prevention strategies** for PTB aimed at the general population include family planning, avoidance of lifestyle risks, and proper nutrition. A reproductive-age woman should **avoid** (as feasible) **extremes of age, of interpregnancy interval (18–23 months is optimal interval between last delivery and next conception), induced termination of pregnancy (TOP) without ripening, multiple gestations, illegal drugs (e.g., cocaine), physical abuse, sexually transmitted infections (STIs),** poverty, poor education, and **a prepregnancy weight of** <50 kg (<120 lb). A normal BMI at the start of pregnancy, not dieting but instead a balanced diet during pregnancy achieving weight gain of >5 kg by 30 weeks for underweight and normal-weight women, can certainly help avoid PTB. Supplementation with docosahexaenoic acid (DHA) is associated with a reduction in PTB <34 weeks in multiple randomized controlled trials (RCTs) in low-risk women. **Screening with transvaginal ultrasound (TVU) cervical length (CL) at 19 to 23 weeks should be offered to all singleton gestations. If CL < 21 mm develops, vaginal progesterone (e.g., 200 mg daily until 36 weeks) should be recommended.**
- **Secondary prevention of PTB** is based on identification and treatment (or avoidance) of risk factors. **A screening test aimed at prediction of PTB is only beneficial if an intervention reduces the outcome once the screening test is positive.** Secondary prevention of PTB has been shown in the following groups for the following interventions:
  - In women who **smoke, smoking cessation counseling/** support programs
  - In women with ≥1 prior PTBs, now carrying **a singleton gestation,**
    - **17α-hydroxyprogesterone caproate** 250 mg IM q week starting at 16 to 20 weeks until 36 weeks
    - **cerclage if the CL is <25 mm between 14 and 23 6/7 weeks**
    - **moderate (≥3 meals/wk) fish intake**
  - In women with **≥3 prior PTBs or second-trimester losses (STLs), history-indicated cerclage**
  - In women with **cervical dilatation ≥1 cm before 24 weeks, physical exam–indicated cerclage**
  - In women with **asymptomatic bacteriuria of** >100,000 **bacteria/mL, appropriate antibiotics**
  - In women with **asymptomatic group B streptococcus (GBS) bacteriuria of any colony count,** appropriate antibiotics (usually **penicillin**)
- All other screening and treatment interventions for prevention of PTB are not supported by evidence for recommending their clinical use.

BACKGROUND

Prevention of preterm birth is the number one issue in pregnancy, as being born preterm is the number one cause of neonatal mortality in many developed countries, including the United States (1). This chapter reviews evidence-based guidelines for women without symptoms related to PTB. The following two chapters deal with women with symptoms of PTB: first preterm labor (PTL) (chap. 17), then preterm premature rupture of membranes (PPROM) (chap. 18).

DIAGNOSES/DEFINITIONS

Gestational age determination is of outmost importance in prevention of preterm birth and management of presumed threatened PTB (see chap. 4 for best GA determination criteria).

Definitions regarding prematurity vary in different publications, but the ones most commonly accepted and used in trials are the following:

Preterm birth: birth between 20 0/7 and 36 6/7 weeks (2)

- Very early preterm birth: birth between 20 0/7 and 23 6/7 weeks
- Early preterm birth: birth between 24 0/7 and 33 6/7 weeks
- Late preterm birth: birth between 34 0/7 and 36 6/7 weeks

Pregnancy loss (PL): loss of pregnancy from conception to <20 weeks. The term spontaneous abortion is equivalent but should be avoided since women associate negative feeling with this term. Miscarriage is a lay term for PL (see also chaps. 15 and 29).

Second-trimester PL (aka second-trimester loss—STL): birth between 14 0/7 and 19 6/7 weeks.

Cervical insufficiency (CI) (formerly called incompetence): recurrent painless dilatation leading to STLs (3). A better definition can be a **CL < 25 mm before 24 weeks in women with prior PTB < 37 weeks.**

Preterm labor (PTL): uterine contractions (≥4/20 min or ≥8/hr) and documented cervical change with intact membranes at 20 to 36 6/7 weeks. A better definition is **uterine contractions (≥4/20 min or ≥8/h) with TVU CL < 20mm, or**

Table 16.1 Risk Factors for Spontaneous Preterm Birth

History:

- Obstetrical-gynecological history: prior spontaneous PTB; prior STL; prior D&Es; prior cone biopsy; uterine anomalies; DES exposure; myomatas; extremes of interpregnancy interval; ART
- Maternal lifestyle (smoking, drug abuse, STIs, etc.);
- Maternal prepregnancy weight <120 lb (<50 kg) or low BMI; poor nutritional status
- Maternal age (<19; >35)
- Race (especially Afro-American)
- Education (<12 grades)
- Certain medical conditions (e.g., DM and HTN)
- Low socioeconomic status
- Limited prenatal care
- Family history of spontaneous PTB (poorly studied)
- Vaginal bleeding (especially during second trimester)
- Stress (mostly related to above risks)

Identifiable by screening:

- Anemia
- Periodontal disease
- TVU CL <25 mm (especially <24 weeks)
- fFN positive (>50 ng) (between 22 to 34 weeks)

Usually symptomatic:

- Uterine contractions

Not spontaneous (indicated/iatrogenic):

- Fetal demise/Major anomaly/Compromise/Polyhydramnios
- Placenta previa
- Placental abruption
- Major maternal disease (HTN complications, DM, etc.)

Abbreviations: PTB, preterm birth; STL, second-trimester loss; DES, diethylstilbestrol; ART, assisted reproductive technology; STI, sexually transmitted infection; BMI, body mass index; DM, diabetes mellitus; HTN, hypertension; TVU, transvaginal ultrasound; CL, cervical length; fFN, fetal fibronectin.

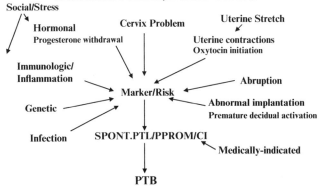

Figure 16.1 Preterm birth is the final common pathway of many associated possible etiologies. *Abbreviations*: SPONT. PTL, spontaneous preterm labor; PPROM, preterm premature rupture of membranes; CI, cervical insufficiency.

ETIOLOGY/BASIC PATHOPHYSIOLOGY

Just like cardiac disease, PTB is a final common manifestation of multifactorial, complex etiology. Several processes leading to PTB are shown in Figure 16.1.

CLASSIFICATION

PTB can be spontaneous, and follow PTL (50%; chap. 17), PPROM (30%; chap. 18), or, rarely, CI; or be iatrogenic (20%). CI may comprise about 1% of spontaneous PTB (SPTB) and/or STLs (see below). CI represents one extreme of SPTB, as PTB is continuous.

RISK FACTORS/ASSOCIATIONS

Many women who have a PTB have no identifiable risk factors. Risk factors for SPTB (presenting as PTL, PPROM, or CI) are similar (Table 16.1).

COMPLICATIONS

PTB is the **number one cause of perinatal mortality.** Seventy five percent of perinatal mortality occurs in preterm babies; more than two-third of perinatal mortality (60% of total) occurs in infants aged <32 weeks. **Mortality and morbidities are inversely associated with GA at birth.** Morbidities include respiratory distress syndrome (RDS), bronchopulmonary dysplasia (BPD), intraventricular hemorrhage (IVH), necrotizing enterocolitis (NEC), sepsis, retinopathy, etc.

PREDICTION AND PREVENTION OF PTB

A screening test aimed at prediction of PTB is only beneficial if an intervention (prevention) reduces the outcome once the screening test is positive. Several predictive strategies have poor sensitivity and specificity.

Prevention is preferable, rather than treatment once symptoms have been identified. Prevention can be divided into three categories (Table 16.2). Primary and secondary prevention are preferable, rather than tertiary prevention of symptomatic women with PTL or PPROM. This chapter refers to prevention of SPTB mostly in **singleton gestations,** unless otherwise specified. Prevention of PTB in multiple gestations

20 to 29 mm with positive fFN at 20 to 36 6/7 weeks. (see also chap. 17).

Premature preterm rupture of membranes (PPROM): vaginal pooling, nitrazine and/or ferning at 16 to 36 6/7 weeks (see PPROM guidelines).

- Early PPROM: PPROM between 24 and 33 6/7 weeks
- Very early PPROM: PPROM between 16 and 23 6/7 weeks

EPIDEMIOLOGY/INCIDENCE

Incidence of PTB < 37 weeks varies between 5% and 25% in different countries, and accounted for 12.2% of all U.S. births in 2009. PTB < 32 weeks: 2% in United States; ≤1% in most other developed countries. **Over 1 million babies die of the consequences of PTB every year in the world, 1 every 30 seconds** (1). The high incidence of PTB in many developed countries may be due to assisted reproductive technology (ART)-related multiple gestations, older and sicker mothers, earlier GA of registered births and neonatal improvements, better and earlier timing of births (related to ultrasound), worsening socioeconomic factors, and other factors.

GENETICS

While a genetic predisposition in certain ethnic groups and families has been reported, no clinical genetic studies are yet recommended for prediction/prevention of PTB due to insufficient evidence.

Table 16.2 Definition of the Different Categories of Prevention of Preterm Birth

	Definition	Examples
Primary prevention	Prevention strategies aimed at **all asymptomatic** pregnant women at risk for PTB (i.e., aimed at all pregnant women).	Give every pregnant woman a baby aspirin.
Secondary prevention	Prevention strategies aimed at **identifying asymptomatic women at high risk for PTB through screening.** Screen for predictive risk factor (prediction) in asymptomatic women and avoid/treat (preventive intervention).	Screen for infection, and treat the ones identified with infection with antibiotics.
Tertiary prevention	Prevention strategies aimed at women with active **symptoms** of PTB	Interventions for women with PTL (chap. 17) or PPROM (chap. 18)

Source: PTB, preterm birth; PTL, preterm labor; PPROM, preterm premature rupture of membranes.

is also discussed in chapter 43 in *Maternal-Fetal Evidence Based Guidelines.*

For women at risk for **iatrogenic (indicated) PTB,** one should aim to keep the pregnant woman as healthy as non-pregnant adult. Appropriate prevention and therapy of any maternal medical or fetal/congenital anomaly disorder is paramount, as is appropriate prevention and therapy for preeclampsia and fetal growth restriction (FGR) (please see specific chapters in *Maternal-Fetal Evidence Based Guidelines*) (1).

All **prepregnancy evaluations** of the cervix (e.g., hysterosalpingogram, no. 8 Hegar dilator passage, and catheter traction test) aimed at screening for CI have either been inadequately studied or been shown not to be sufficiently predictive and therefore useful in a prevention program (no trial ever reported).

An accurate history should be taken regarding risk factors for PTB, especially ob-gyn history, maternal lifestyle, and prepregnancy weight (Table 16.1).

A Creasy's score or other similar history-based systems to predict PTB have been associated with a low (10–30%) positive predictive value (PPV) for PTB, and not clinically useful given negative intervention trials (see below).

There are four main risk factors for which there are effective interventions for prevention of PTB: smoking; short TVU CL; prior PTB; and asymptomatic bacteriuria (Table 16.3). **TVU CL at 16 to 24 weeks is indicated in all women with a singleton gestation** (see below).

Evidence does not support the use of home uterine activity monitoring (HUAM) or bacterial vaginosis (BV) screening in asymptomatic low-risk women. There are insufficient data to support the use of salivary estriol or fetal fibronectin (fFN) in asymptomatic women (even if fFN is one of the best predictive screening tests). Cytokines, matrix metalloproteinases, corticotropin-releasing hormone (CRH), salivary estriol, relaxin, human chorionic gonadotropin (HCG), prothrombin, fetal DNA, and many other tests remain research tools for prediction of PTB and are not yet clinically beneficial.

Primary Prevention

Primary prevention includes prevention strategies aimed at **all asymptomatic pregnant women** at risk for PTB (i.e., aimed at all pregnant women). Unfortunately most primary prevention interventions have been so far either insufficiently studied or found not to be effective.

Preconception/Early Pregnancy

Family planning. There are no trials to assess interventions. **Avoiding extremes of age, of interpregnancy interval** (18–23 months is optimal interval between last delivery and

Table 16.3 Effective Interventions for Prevention of Preterm Birth

Avoid (as feasible)	<ul><li>Extremes of age</li><li>Interpregnancy interval <6 months</li><li>Induced termination of pregnancy without ripening</li><li>Multiple gestation</li><li>Illegal drugs (e.g., cocaine)</li><li>Physical abuse</li><li>STIs</li><li>Poverty</li><li>Poor education</li><li>Prepregnancy weight of <50 kg (<120 lb).</li></ul>

Risk	**Intervention**
Smoking	Smoking cessation programs
Short CL<21 mm (screen every singleton with TVU CL at 19–23 wk)*	Vaginal progesterone (e.g., 200 mg daily)
Prior spontaneous PTB (SPTB)*	17OH Progesterone caproate
Prior SPTB *and* CL<25 mm between 16–23 6/7 wk*	Moderate (≥3 meals/wk) fish intake Ultrasound-indicated cerclage
Prior ≥3 PTB/STL*	History-indicated cerclage
Asymptomatic bacteriuria	Appropriate antibiotics

Abbreviations: TVU, transvaginal ultrasound; CL, cervical length; PTB, preterm birth; SPTB, spontaneous PTB; STL, second-trimester loss; STIs, sexually transmitted infections.
*For singleton gestations

next conception) (4), **and multiple gestations** (through ART improvements) seem self-evident for efficacy in preventing PTB when feasible.

Induced TOP is associated with a higher risk of PTB, even if just one early TOP is performed (5). **Avoiding TOPs seems to be an effective preventive strategy to avoid PTB.** If TOP is unavoidable, the D&E should be performed with preoperative cervical ripening (e.g., misoprostol, mifepristone, or laminaria), as this is associated with no or very low risk for PTB (5).

Avoidance of lifestyle risks. There are no trials to assess interventions. **Avoiding illegal drugs** (e.g., cocaine and amphetamines), **physical abuse, and STIs** (chlamydia, gonorrhea, syphilis, HIV, etc.) seem self-evident for efficacy in preventing PTB (6). **Poverty, poor education,** lack of women's empowerment, and several other social stressors (Table 16.1) are all linked profoundly to an increased risk of PTB and should be avoided as possible, especially through political and social changes. There are no trials on modifying other potential risks, such as physically demanding job, prolonged standing, night work, or others.

Proper nutrition, weight gain. **A prepregnancy weight of <50 kg (<120 lb) should be avoided.** The available evidence is inadequate to evaluate potential effects of balanced protein/energy supplementation as provided in most trials on prevention of PTB (7). **A normal BMI at the start of pregnancy, not dieting but instead a balanced diet during pregnancy achieving weight gain of >5 kg by 30 weeks for underweight and normal-weight women, can certainly help to avoid PTB.**

Balanced protein supplementation alone (i.e., without energy supplementation) does not reduce PTB and is unlikely to be of benefit to pregnant women or their infants. This conclusion appears to apply even to undernourished women (8). High-protein diet (>25% of total energy content) cannot be recommended in pregnancy (9) (see also chap. 2).

Early Pregnancy

Fish intake. Maternal fish intake is also associated with better child cognitive test performance (10).

Omega-3 fatty acids. Low-risk women without a prior PTB have a similar incidence of PTB <37 weeks when given 12 eggs with either 133 mg DHA or with 33 mg DHA per week starting at 24 to 28 weeks (11). Supplementation has been shown to prolong pregnancy by 3 to 8 days in different populations. When all RCTs are examined, women allocated a marine oil supplement had a mean gestation that was 2.6 days longer than women allocated to placebo or no treatment. This was not reflected in a clear difference between the two groups in PTB < 37 weeks, although women allocated marine oil did have a **lower risk of PTB < 34 weeks** (RR 0.69, 95% CI 0.49–0.99). Birth weight was slightly greater (47 g) in infants born to women in the marine oil group compared with controls. However, there were no overall differences between the groups in the proportion of low birth weight (LBW) or small-for-gestational age babies. There was no clear difference in the relative risk of preeclampsia between the two groups (12). A more recent large RCT found that **DHA 800 mg supplementation before 21 weeks was associated with a decrease in PTB < 34 weeks** (RR 0.49, 95% CI 0.25–0.94) (13). Therefore, **supplementation with DHA is associated with a reduction in PTB < 34 weeks in multiple RCTs in low-risk women.**

Shark, swordfish, king mackerel, or tilefish contain high levels of mercury and should be avoided or eaten infrequently (≤1/wk) in pregnancy. Canned light tuna, salmon, pollock, grouper, mussels, scallops, shrimp, and catfish are common fishes low in mercury, and two portions (6 oz = 1 portion) of these per week can be eaten. Albacore ("white") tuna has more mercury and should be consumed up to 6 oz/wk. In general, for other fishes, smaller fishes have less mercury than larger ones. More information on fish and mercury intake in pregnancy is available at www.cfsan.fda.gov and www.epa.gov/ost/fish. PrimaCare vitamin supplement contains 150 mg of omega-3 fatty acids and has not been evaluated in a trial. The possible beneficial effects of omega-3 fatty acids to later fetal/neonatal/infant cognition remain not fully proven. For omega-3 supplementation in high-risk women, see subsection "Risk: Prior PTB."

Probiotics. Women who report habitual intake of probiotic diary foods (e.g., yogurt) have been associated with lower incidence of PTB in non-RCT (14). Currently, there are **insufficient data** from RCTs to demonstrate any impact of probiotic foods supplementation in low-risk women on PTB and its complications (15).

Other nutritional changes. There are no trials with specific aim of prevention of PTB to evaluate other nutritional changes, such as vitamin supplementation (see chap. 2), HCG, and anticytokine supplements. **Prepregnancy weight < 120 lb (< 50 kg) is a very significant risk factor for PTB and should be avoided if possible.** Suggested pregnancy weight gain in pregnancy is 25 to 35 lb for women with normal BMI, but there are no trials on proper prepregnancy weight or pregnancy weight gain.

Vitamins C and E. Maternal supplementation with vitamin C 1000 mg and vitamin E 400 mg daily from 9 to 16 weeks until delivery in nulliparous low-risk women is **not associated with a reduction in PTB** (16).

Magnesium supplementation. There is **no sufficient high-quality evidence** to show that dietary magnesium supplementation during pregnancy is beneficial. In the analysis of all trials, oral magnesium treatment from before the 25th week of gestation was associated with a lower frequency of PTB (RR 0.73, 95% CI 0.57–0.94), a lower frequency of LBW (RR 0.67, 95% CI 0.46–0.96), and fewer small-for-gestational age infants (RR 0.70, 95% CI 0.53–0.93) compared with placebo. In addition, magnesium-treated women had fewer hospitalizations during pregnancy (RR 0.66, 95% CI 0.49–0.89) and fewer cases of antepartum hemorrhage (RR 0.38, 95% CI 0.16–0.90) than placebo-treated women (17). In the analysis excluding the large cluster randomized trial, the effects of magnesium treatment on the frequencies of PTB, LBW, and small-for-gestational age were not different from placebo (17). Of the seven trials included in the review, only one was judged to be of high quality. **Poor-quality trials,** several of which did not have PTB as primary outcome, and some of which included women with risk factors for preeclampsia and/or PTB, are likely to have resulted in a bias favoring magnesium supplementation.

Progesterone. The mechanism of action of progesterone for prevention of PTB is poorly understood but probably involves an anti-inflammatory action. Safety for the fetus/neonate has not been yet proven with 100% certainty, but progesterone is known not to be a teratogen, and long-term detrimental effects have not been shown. The effect of progesterone supplementation should be **evaluated according to different patient populations, and according to type of progesterone.** Here we review progesterone for low-risk women (see below for other risk groups).

In a small RCT including women in active military duty with only a 3% rate of prior PTB and unknown CL, 17α- hydroxyprogesterone (17P) 1000 mg IM weekly starting at 16 to 20 weeks was **not associated with any effect** on incidence of PTB or perinatal outcomes compared with placebo (18). No RCT has evaluated the effect of vaginal progesterone in this population.

In summary, there is **insufficient evidence to determine the impact on PTB of progesterone in singleton gestations with no prior PTB**, with unknown or normal CL.

Secondary Prevention

Secondary prevention strategies involve screening for a predictive risk factor (prediction) in asymptomatic women, and avoiding it or treating it (preventive intervention) (Table 16.3).

Risk: Smoking

Intervention: smoking cessation programs. It is estimated that 10% to 15% of PTB may be due to smoking. In the United States, about 20% of women start pregnancy as a smoker, and 11% continue to smoke throughout pregnancy (2008 data). All interventions for promoting smoking cessation in pregnancy are associated with a 6% decrease in smoking (19). The trials with validated smoking cessation, a high-intensity intervention, and a high-quality score are associated with an absolute decrease in continued smoking in late pregnancy of 5%. Most studies had as intervention **provision of information on risks to fetus/infant, and benefits of quitting; and use of written material.** Often cognitive/behavioral strategies for quitting were included. The American College of Obstetricians and Gynecologists (ACOG) has recommended use of the five As— ask, advice, assess, assist, arrange—approach (20). The most effective intervention for smoking cessation in pregnancy is **social support and a reward component** (23% decrease) (21,22). If above approach is not successful, consider nicotine replacement therapy (NRT) (see chap. 22 in *Maternal-Fetal Evidence Based Guidelines*).

Smoking cessation counseling/support programs are associated with a 14% reduction in PTB and a 17% reduction in LBW. Other outcomes (e.g., perinatal mortality) have not been adequately evaluated (19).

Intervention: nicotine replacement therapy. NRT is associated with a trend for benefit in reduction in the incidence of smoking (23–25) (see chap. 22 in *Maternal-Fetal Evidence Based Guidelines*). One concern about its use in pregnancy is the possibility of adverse effects of nicotine on the fetus, through alterations in uterine, placental, or blood flow, or directly on the brain. As there are still too few trials to assure safe use in pregnancy, and animal studies suggest nicotine may be toxic to the developing central nervous system, registries of women using NRT should be established to gather more outcome data. **There is insufficient evidence to assess the safety NRT, or nicotine gum, and also the effect on incidence of PTB.** No trial has been done using bupropion. Interventions to increase smoking cessation among the partners of pregnant women, with the additional aim of facilitating cessation by the women themselves, have been insufficiently studied (only 1 trial) (19). Stages of change, or feedback, do not show benefit (19).

Risk: "Pregnancy High-Risk for PTB"

Intervention: bed rest. There is no evidence supporting bed rest to prevent PTB. **Bed rest (rest 1 hour tid) in (asymptomatic and symptomatic) "high-risk" singleton pregnancies is not associated with prevention of PTB over no bed rest** (26). Bed rest can be associated with an increased incidence of complications; in-hospital extended strict bed rest for PTL or PPROM is associated with an up to 1% to 2% incidence of thromboembolic disease. Moreover, muscle wasting, cardiovascular deconditioning, bone demineralization, impaired glucose tolerance, heartburn, constipation, failure of volume expansion, headaches, dizziness, fatigue, depression, anxiety, stress, as well as lost wages, lost domestic productivity, and other costs may be other detrimental consequences of bed rest.

It is true that rest decreases uterine activity, and exercise increases it, but these are small effects that do not change rates of PTB. In nonrandomized studies, **exercise in pregnancy has been associated with a decrease in PTB** (27), while physically demanding work, prolonged standing, shift and night work, and high cumulative work fatigue score have been associated with PTB. Despite its use in about 20% of pregnancies, bed rest for prevention of PTB cannot be recommended. It should be studied in trials before clinical use. If prescribed bed rest, women should be allowed to ambulate to the bathroom a few times a day to limit complications of strict bed rest. It is possible that women at real risk of PTB from the above or other

risk factors have not been studied adequately with this intervention of bed rest.

Intervention: support. Programs of additional support during at-risk pregnancy (varying definitions) usually by a professional (social worker, midwife, or nurse) **do not reduce PTB** or LBW (28). "Additional support" was defined as some form of emotional support (e.g., counseling, reassurance, and sympathetic listening) with or without additional information/ advice, occurring during home visits, clinic appointments, and/ or by telephone; most of the times these were intensive programs started in the first or second trimesters to the end of pregnancy. Other significant outcomes are as follows: anxiety is decreased; satisfaction with care is increased; TOP is increased; and cesarean delivery is decreased (28).

Intervention: weekly manual exams, education. A program of weekly manual cervical exams in addition to education for women at high-risk for PTB (≥10 on Creasy's score) **does not reduce PTB** (29–31).

Intervention: antibiotics. See subsection "Intervention: Antibiotics" under "Risk: Prior PTB."

Intervention: cerclage. Different specific clinical scenarios have been studied for possible benefit of cerclage. For efficacy of history-indicated cerclage, transabdominal (TA) cerclage, ultrasound-indicated cerclage, physical exam–indicated cerclage, as well as cerclage in twins, see below.

Risk: Prior PTB (Figs. 16.2 and 16.3) (32)

Intervention: fish intake. **Moderate fish intake, up to three meals per week, before 22 weeks is associated with a reduction in repeat PTB**, compared with women eating fish less than once per month (OR 0.60, CI 0.38–0.95) (33). **Moderate fish intake should be encouraged in women with prior PTB for prevention of recurrent PTB** (see also above for low-risk women).

Intervention: omega-3 fatty acids. In one RCT, omega-3 fatty acids [fish oil, Pikasol: 32% eicosapentaenoic acid (EPA), 23% DHA, and 2 mg tocopherol/mL; 4 capsules/day: 1.3 g EPA and 0.9 g DHA, total 2.7 g/day; started ≥16 weeks at an average of 29–30 weeks] were associated with reduction in PTB <37 weeks by 46% and PTB <34 weeks by 68% in women with a prior PTB <37 weeks and a singleton gestation. The same omega-3 fatty acid regimen does not reduce PTB in women with twins (34). In another larger RCT, in singleton gestations with prior SPTB and on 17P 250 mg IM, omega-3 supplementation (1200 mg EPA and 800 mg DHA) from 16 to 22 weeks until 36 weeks was associated with similar incidences of PTB < 37 weeks (38% vs. 41%; RR 0.91, 95% 0.77–1.07) and PTB < 35 weeks (RR 0.95, 95% CI 0.72–1.25) (35). In summary, **in singleton gestations with prior SPTB on 17P, omega-3 supplementations do not seem to be beneficial in preventing recurrent PTB** (see also above for low-risk women).

Intervention: antibiotics. Antibiotics to prevent PTB in women with prior PTB have been evaluated either as preconception (1 RCT) or as prenatal intervention.

In women with prior PTB < 34 weeks, **preconception** oral azythromycin 1 g twice (4 days apart) and metronidazole 750 mg daily for 7 days are not associated with an effect of subsequent PTB or miscarriage rates (36).

Clindamycin cream 2% for 7 days at 26 to 32 weeks does not reduce PTB <37 weeks in women with a prior PTB 24 to 36 weeks but may increase PTB < 34 weeks, especially in women without BV, so that antibiotics in this setting may actually be detrimental (37).

Cefetamet Pivoxil (not available in United States) 2 g × 1 at 28 to 32 weeks in women in Nairobi with prior PTB, fetal

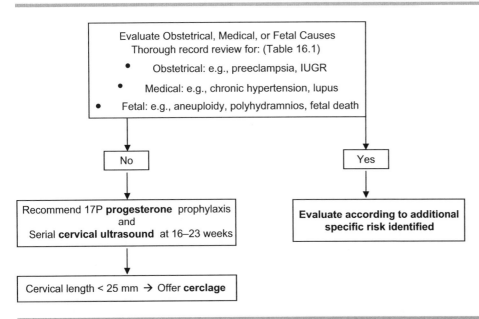

Figure 16.2 Care algorithm for women with a history of birth at 16 to 34 weeks (see exceptions in Fig. 16.3). *Source*: Adapted from Ref. 32.

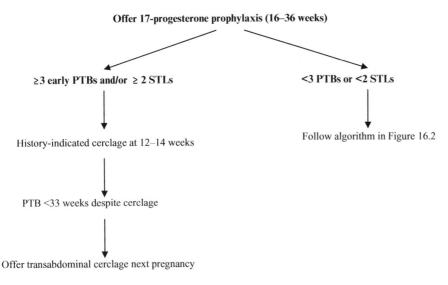

Figure 16.3 Clinical algorithm for care of asymptomatic women with multiple prior PTB or STLs (see text). *Abbreviations*: PTB, preterm birth; STL, second-trimester loss. *Source*: Adapted from Ref. 32.

death, or LBW did not affect GA at delivery (PTB was not reported) (38).

Metronidazole 250 mg tid × 7 days and erythromycin base 333 mg tid × 14 days in women with a prior PTB or prepregnancy weight <50 kg do not prevent PTB < 37 weeks but may increase PTB < 34 weeks (39,40).

In summary, **antibiotics given just because of a prior PTB do not prevent recurrent PTB.**

Intervention: progesterone. The effect of progesterone supplementation should be evaluated according to different patient populations, and according to type of progesterone. Here we review progesterone for prior PTB.

For 17P, there are at least two RCTs available in women with prior PTB. In 43 women with mostly (>90%) singleton gestation and either prior PTB or prior >1 spontaneous abortion, 17P 250 mg IM weekly started as soon as prenatal care began was associated with significant reduction in PTB < 37

weeks and perinatal mortality compared with placebo (41). In 463 women with singleton gestation and prior SPTB at 20 to 36 6/7 weeks of a singleton gestation, compounded 17P 250 mg IM weekly started at 16 to 20 6/7 weeks was associated with reduction in the incidences of PTB < 35 weeks (RR 0.66, 95% CI 0.54–0.81), PTB < 37 weeks, and <32 weeks, as well as of supplemental oxygen and IVH, compared with placebo (42). The number needed to treat to prevent one recurrent PTB was 5.4. Based mostly on this clinical trial, **17P 250 mg IM weekly started at 16 to 20 weeks is recommended for all women with prior SPTB 20 to 36 6/7 weeks** (43–45). The estimated number of prevented PTBs <37 weeks in the United States by this policy is about 9870.

For vaginal progesterone, there are at least two RCTs available in women with prior PTB. In 142 women with singleton gestations and mostly (>90%) prior PTB, vaginal progesterone 100 mg nightly from 24 to 34 weeks was associated with significant reduction in the incidences of PTB < 37 weeks (RR 0.48, 95% CI 0.25–0.96) and <34 weeks, as well as contraction frequency, compared with placebo (46). In 659 women with singleton gestation and prior SPTB 20 to 35 0/7 weeks, vaginal progesterone 90 mg every morning starting at 18 to 22 6/7 weeks until 37 0/7 weeks was not associated with significantly different rates of PTB < 37, 36, 33, 29 weeks and neonatal morbidity and mortality (47). Several women screened for this trial were excluded from inclusion because of short CL (47). Therefore, **vaginal progesterone cannot be recommended for prevention of recurrent PTB.**

For comparison of 17P versus vaginal progesterone, there is only one RCT.

In 315 women with singleton gestation and prior PTB between 20 and 34 weeks, 17P 250 mg IM weekly was associated with similar incidences of PTB and neonatal morbidities and mortality compared with vaginal progesterone 90 mg (Crinone) daily, except for significant lower incidences of PTB 28 to 31 6/7 weeks, neonatal intensive care unit (NICU) admission, and maternal side effects in the vaginal progesterone group (48). **More data are necessary** to evaluate how 17P and vaginal progesterone compare in efficacy in this as well as other populations.

For oral progesterone, there are two small RCTs. In 148 women with singleton gestation and prior SPTB 20 to 36 6/7 weeks, oral progesterone 100 mg twice a day was associated with significantly reduced incidences of PTB <37 weeks and NICU admission compared with placebo (49). In 33 women with singleton gestation and prior PTB 20 to 36 6/7 weeks, oral progesterone 400 mg daily was associated with nonsignificant reductions in the incidence of PTB <37 weeks (26% vs. 57%) and ventilator use (0% vs. 21%) compared with placebo (50). In summary, there is **insufficient evidence** to assess the efficacy of oral progesterone for prevention of PTB in women with prior PTB.

In summary, in women with prior SPTB and singleton gestation, progesterone administration is beneficial in preventing PTB. Although we have limited data comparing the different preparations of progesterone, there is at present **stronger evidence of effectiveness for 17P than for vaginal progesterone,** based on the two largest trials (42,47). **17P 250 mg IM weekly starting at 16 to 20 weeks until 36 weeks should be recommended to women with singleton gestations and prior SPTB 20 to 36 6/7 weeks.** In cases in which 17P is unavailable, other progesterone preparations may be considered (46).

Intervention: cerclage. **A history-indicated cerclage** is placed based solely on prior ob-gyn history (previously called a prophylactic or elective cerclage). Trials on women with only one or two prior PTBs have not shown benefit from history-indicated cerclage (51,52). **A history-indicated cerclage prevents PTB in women with three or more STLs or PTBs (53).** Cerclage decreases the incidence of PTB < 37 weeks from 53% (with no cerclage) to 32%, and the incidence of PTB < 32 weeks from 32% (with no cerclage) to 15% in women with three or more prior PTBs or STLs (53) (Fig. 16.3).

The other clinical indication for history-indicated cerclage might include CI, defined by some as prior painless cervical dilatation leading to recurrent STLs. Unfortunately **no trial has been done to confirm the efficacy of history-indicated cerclage in reducing PTB in women with a diagnosis of CI.** Other indications such as prior cone biopsy, Mullerian anomaly, diethylstilbestrol (DES) exposure, prior PTB not associated with CI, and Ehler-Danlos have occasionally been used clinically but have not been confirmed by any trial as indications that benefit from history-indicated cerclage. History-indicated

cerclage is usually performed at 12 to 15 weeks' gestation, and its techniques have been well described (54).

TA cerclage has been associated with less recurrent PTB compared with controls receiving transvaginal cerclage in women with a **history of a failed (SPTB <33 weeks despite cerclage) transvaginal history-indicated cerclage** in a case-control study (55). There is no trial on TA cerclage. It should be noted that in this study antibiotics and progesterone were uniformly given to the TA cerclage women. The efficacy of TA cerclage for other clinical scenarios such as a cervix with no intravaginal portion has not been adequately studied. TA cerclage is usually performed prophylactically at around 10 to 12 weeks, and its technique has been well described (54,55). Recently, TA cerclage has been successfully performed also laparoscopically and robotically, both prepregnancy and in early first trimester.

In summary, **the vast majority of women with prior PTB (e.g., those with only 1–2 prior PTBs) do not benefit from universal history-indicated cerclage,** and can **instead be followed with TVU CL starting usually at 16 weeks.** A policy of TVU CL screening with cerclage for short CL is associated with similar incidences of PTB < 37 weeks (31% vs. 32%; RR 0.97, 95% CI 0.73–1.29), PTB < 34 weeks (17% vs. 23%; RR 0.76, 95% CI 0.48–1.20), and perinatal mortality (5% vs. 3%; RR 1.77, 95% CI 0.58–5.35) compared with universal history-indicated cerclage, and saves cerclage in about 58% of these women (56). **If the CL < 25 mm is detected before 24 weeks, singleton gestations with prior PTB should undergo ultrasound-indicated cerclage** (75) (see also subsection "Risk: Short Cervix on Ultrasound").

If cerclage is performed, it should be performed according to best technique. McDonald cerclage, with suture (usually mersilene tape) placed as close to the internal os as possible (as high as possible), is recommended. There is usually no need for preoperative antibiotics or tocolytics.

Intervention: oral tocolytics. There is insufficient evidence (only 1 small old RCT) to support the use of prophylactic oral betamimetics for preventing PTB in women with prior PTB with a singleton pregnancy (57).

For a summary of care of pregnant women with prior PTB, see also Ref. 32.

Risk: Cervical Insufficiency

Intervention: cerclage. **No intervention has been specifically studied in this population** (see above under prior PTB). There is insufficient evidence to recommend a history-indicated cerclage in women with <3 prior PTBs or STLs. **A policy of TVU CL screening with ultrasound-indicated cerclage if CL shortens to < 25 mm at <24 weeks has shown to be equivalent to a policy of universal history-indicated cerclage in women with a prior loss or PTB** (54,56,58).

Risk: IVF ART

Intervention: progesterone. 17α-hydroxyprogesterone caproate or HCG supplementation in the first trimester **increase the incidences of fetal heart activity on ultrasound by 238%, and of pregnancy ≥24 weeks' rate by 380%** compared with placebo (59).

Risk: Amniocentesis

Intervention: progesterone. Natural progesterone 200 mg IM q day for 3 days postamniocentesis followed by 17α-hydroxyprogesterone caproate 340 mg IM 2×/wk until the second week after the amniocentesis **did not reduce PTB < 25 weeks** in women undergoing amniocentesis (60).

Risk: Uterine contractions detected by home uterine activity monitoring (HUAM)

Intervention: varied, per obstetrician. Uterine contractions have been associated with PTB, but their predictive value is poor. HUAM usually consists of 1 hour of tocomonitoring twice daily at 24 to 36 weeks. **HUAM with or without nursing contact and education is associated with no prevention of PTB.** Some studies show earlier (at lower cervical dilatation) detection of PTL. The lack of benefit in prevention of PTB might have been secondary to lack of effective intervention (usually tocolysis) once PTL was diagnosed. Three different populations of women at high risk for PTB have been studied: singleton gestations with risk factors for PTB (e.g., prior PTB), twin gestations, and women status-post an episode of PTL. Unfortunately there is no published meta-analysis of all trials, and most trials do not report results for each population specifically, and also report differing outcomes. My meta-analysis of published data shows no decrease in PTB < 37 weeks in any of these three subgroups: mostly singletons at high risk (9 trials; $n = 3613$) (61–70): RR 1.01, 95% CI 0.91–1.11; twins (5 trials; $n = 998$) (64,67,69–71): RR 0.91, 95% CI 0.80–1.04; or women s/p PTL episode (4 trials; $n = 218$) (67,72–74): RR 1.21, 95% CI 0.92–1.60. The largest study (70) showed more unscheduled visits and prophylactic tocolytic use in the HUAM group compared to controls. Therefore HUAM should not be routinely provided for prevention of PTB.

Risk: Short Cervix on Ultrasound

Intervention: cerclage (ultrasound-indicated cerclage). **An ultrasound-indicated cerclage** involves first screening of high-risk pregnancies with TVU of the cervix to determine during pregnancy the risk of PTB, since the majority of women at high risk by obstetrical risk factors for PTB do not develop a short CL and deliver at term even without intervention. A short CL (<25 mm) on TVU in the second trimester (between 14 and 23 6/7 weeks) significantly increases the risk of PTB in all populations studied (54). Ultrasound-indicated cerclage is defined as a cerclage performed because a short CL has been detected on TVU during pregnancy, usually in the second trimester. This cerclage has also been called in the past therapeutic, salvage, or rescue cerclage, but these terms are confusing and should be avoided. Ultrasound-indicated cerclage has differing effects in different populations.

In women with **singleton gestations, no prior PTB or other risk factors for PTB**, and **CL < 25 mm** before 24 weeks, cerclage is associated with no effect of PTB <35 weeks (RR 0.76, 95% CI 0.52–1.15) (75). Therefore, cerclage cannot be recommended in this population, but more research is needed.

In women with a **singleton gestation, prior SPTB, and CL < 25 mm** before 24 weeks, **cerclage is associated with a significant 30% reduction in PTB < 35 weeks** (28.4% vs. 41.3%; RR 0.70, 95% CI 0.55–0.89), **significant reductions also in PTB <37, <32, <28, and <24 weeks**, as well as a **significant 36% decrease in composite perinatal mortality and morbidity** (15.6% vs. 24.8%; RR 0.64, 95% CI 0.45–0.91), compared to no cerclage (75).

In twins, ultrasound-indicated cerclage for CL < 25 mm before 24 weeks is associated with an increase in PTB and should not be offered (76). There is insufficient evidence to recommend ultrasound-indicated cerclage in other populations, or after 23 weeks.

Intervention: progesterone. **Regarding 17P,** there is currently no published RCT specifically designed to address evaluating the effect of 17P in women with singleton gesta-tions, no prior PTB, and short CL compared with placebo. One such study, evaluating nulliparous women with CL < 30 mm, has recently stopped recruitment. It is particularly important to assess the effectiveness of progesterone in women without prior PTB, as most PTBs occur in these women.

In 79 women with singleton pregnancies (66% of which had no prior PTB) with CL<25 mm between 16 to 24 weeks, 17P was associated with similar incidences of PTB and neonatal morbidity and mortality compared to cerclage (77). Cerclage was significantly more effective than 17P at reducing the incidences of PTB <35 and <37 weeks in the subgroup with CL ≤15 mm (77). This RCT was stopped before planned recruitment was completed as the authors stated that "it had become impractical, unethical, and unreasonable to withhold progesterone from one study group."

Regarding vaginal progesterone, there are two large RCTs available. In 250 women with mostly (90%) singleton gestations and CL ≤15 mm at 20 to 25 weeks, of whom about 85% had no prior PTB, vaginal progesterone 200 mg nightly started at 24 weeks until 34 weeks was associated with a 44% significant decrease in SPTB < 34 weeks (19% vs. 34%, RR 0.56, 95% CI 0.36–0.86), but no significant effects on neonatal morbidities (composite neonatal adverse outcomes: RR 0.57, 95% CI 0.23–1.31) (78). A subgroup analysis of only women without prior PTB confirmed significant benefit of progesterone in preventing PTB < 34 weeks (RR 0.54, 95% CI 0.34–0.88) (78). The incidence of CL ≤15 mm was 1.7%. Based on the frequency of short CL and effectiveness for prevention of SPTB < 34 weeks from the work of Fonseca et al., the number of women needed to be screened with CL in order to prevent one SPTB <34 weeks is approximately 387, if all women with a CL ≤15 mm receive vaginal progesterone. Once the short CL ≤15 mm is identified, the number needed to treat to prevent one PTB < 34 weeks is 7.

In 458 women with singleton gestations and CL 10 to 20 mm at 19 to 23 6/7 weeks, of whom about 84% had no prior PTB, vaginal progesterone 90 mg daily started at 20 to 23 6/7 weeks until 36 6/7 weeks was associated with a 45% significant decrease in PTB < 33 weeks (9% vs. 16%, RR 0.55, 95% CI 0.33–0.92) and 43% significant decrease in composite neonatal morbidity and mortality (8% vs. 14%, RR 0.57, 95% CI 0.33–0.99) (79). The incidences of PTB <28 and <35 weeks, and RDS, were also significantly decreased. Analysis of only women without prior PTB confirmed significant benefit of progesterone in preventing PTB <33 weeks (8% vs. 15%, RR 0.50, 95% CI 0.27–0.90) (79). The incidence of CL 10 to 20 mm was 2.3%. Based on the frequency of short CL and effectiveness for prevention of PTB < 33 weeks from this study (79), the number of women needed to be screened with CL in order to prevent one PTB < 33 weeks is approximately 604, if all women with a CL 10 to 20 mm receive vaginal progesterone. Once the short CL 10 to 20 mm is identified, the number needed to treat to prevent one PTB < 33 weeks is 14.

In summary, in women with singleton gestations, no prior SPTB, and short CL, vaginal progesterone is associated with reduction in PTB and composite perinatal morbidity and mortality. Based on these results (78,79), **if a TVU CL ≤ 20 mm is identified at ≤ 24 weeks, vaginal progesterone should be offered for prevention of PTB.** There is insufficient evidence that any of the vaginal preparations or doses are superior, as they have not been compared. Vaginal progesterone 200 mg suppository has been used in the trial for CL ≤15 mm (78), and 90 mg gel for the trial for CL 10 to 20 mm (79). Therefore CL, but also cost, availability, and other factors may influence preferred dosing (80,81).

These results also support **universal screening with a single TVU assessment of CL at around 19 to 24 weeks in singleton gestations without prior SPTB.** TVU CL screening of singleton gestations fulfills all criteria for an effective screening program. Specifically, two cost-effectiveness analyses evaluating universal CL screening in singleton gestations, to identify those with short CL eligible for vaginal progesterone, have been published so far (80,81). Both reported that such a strategy would be cost-effective, and in fact cost-saving.

In one study, compared with other managements, including no screening, "universal" sonographic screening of CL in singletons was associated with a reduction of 95,920 PTBs < 37 weeks annually in the United States, and was actually cost-saving (almost $13 billion saved) (80). Even varying the variables (e.g., the cost of vaginal progesterone or of TVU screening), universal screening was the preferred strategy 99% of the time (80).

The other cost-effectiveness analysis, when analyzing universal screening of singleton gestations without prior PTB with TVU CL at 18 to 24 weeks, calculated over $12 million saved, 424 quality-adjusted life-years (QALY) gained, and 22 neonatal deaths or long-term neurologic deficits prevented for every 100,000 women screened, compared to no screening. Even varying the variables (e.g., the cost of vaginal progesterone or of TVU screening), universal screening was cost-effective over 99% of the time (81).

It should be noted that only 1.7% to 2.3% of women were identified to have short CL in the two large trials published (78,79), but that the incidence of CL ≤20 mm at 22 to 24 weeks in the largest blinded U.S. study was 5% (82). There are insufficient data to evaluate the effectiveness of vaginal progesterone for CL > 20 mm.

Screening with TVU CL at 19 to 23 weeks should be offered to all singleton gestations. If CL < 21 mm, vaginal progesterone (e.g., 200 mg daily until 36 weeks) should be recommended (78,79).

Indomethacin. There is **insufficient evidence** to evaluate the effect of indomethacin on incidence of PTB in women with a short CL on TVU (83), as no RCTs have been performed.

Antibiotics. There is **insufficient evidence** to evaluate the effect of antibiotics on incidence of PTB in women with a short CL on TVU, as no RCTs have been performed.

Risk: Prior PTB and Short Cervix on Ultrasound

Intervention: progesterone. In a secondary analysis of an RCT (47) evaluating just the 46 singleton gestations with prior SPTB < 35 weeks and short CL < 28 mm at 18 to 22 6/7 weeks, vaginal progesterone 90 mg daily started at 18 to 23 6/7 weeks until 37 weeks was associated with significant decreases in incidences of both PTB < 32 weeks and NICU admission compared wit placebo (84).

In a randomized trial that did not recruit the planned sample size, 17P and cerclage had similar effect in women for CL < 25 mm for prevention of PTB, but cerclage was more effective in women with CL < 15 mm (77). So while cerclage seems to be more efficacious (lower RRs) as the CL is shorter (85,86) progesterone seems to be most efficacious in cases of "moderate" short CL (78,79).

In summary, 17P should be recommended to women with prior SPTB starting at 16 weeks, as described above. If the cervix shortens, there is insufficient evidence to assess efficacy of a different progesterone therapy, and therefore it is reasonable to continue 17P until 36 weeks.

Intervention: Cerclage. See above under '*Risk: Short Cervix on Ultrasound*' and '*Intervention: Cerclage*' (Ultrasound Indicated Cerclage).

Risk: Cervical Dilatation

Intervention: cerclage (physical exam–indicated cerclage). Physical exam–indicated cerclage (aka emergency, or urgent) is the cerclage placed because of changes in the cervix (dilatation, effacement, etc.) detected by physical (manual) examination. Since about 50% of women with asymptomatic cervical dilatation ≥2 cm in the second trimester have microbial invasion of the amniotic cavity, **an amniocentesis should be considered before offering cerclage.**

There are insufficient data to assess efficacy of physical exam–indicated cerclage in women with cervical dilatation in the second trimester, as only one small trial has been reported. In women with membranes at or beyond the external os at around 20 to 24 weeks, **physical exam–indicated cerclage (and indomethacin) is associated with a delay in delivery of about 4 weeks** compared with controls (30 vs. 26 weeks) (87). The major limitations of this study are the small sample size and the inclusion of twins. Over 25 retrospective observational series, mostly with no controls, have claimed benefit of physical exam–indicated cerclage. The largest cohort study reported a significant decrease of 92% in prevention of PTB < 28 weeks with physical exam–indicated cerclage, compared with no cerclage, in singletons with ≥1 cm of cervical dilatation before 26 weeks (88). In summary, **physical exam–indicated cerclage in singleton gestations with a cervix dilated to ≥1 cm in the second trimester is associated with prevention in PTB.** Clearly a large, well-designed prospective randomized trial is needed to confirm benefit.

Intervention: indomethacin. There is **insufficient evidence** to evaluate the effect of indomethacin on incidence of PTB in women with a short CL on TVU (89), as no RCT has been performed.

Risk: Positive fFN

Intervention: antibiotics. fFN is a basement membrane protein present between the decidua/uterus and fetal membranes/placenta and produced by the trophoblast. Its presence (>50 ng/mL) at ≥22 weeks in the cervicovaginal canal has been associated with an increased risk for PTB. In fact fFN is one of the best predictors of PTB in all populations, including asymptomatic low- and high-risk women, twins, and women in PTL. Even at 13 to 22 weeks, higher (using 90th percentile) fFN levels are associated with two- to threefold increase risk in subsequent SPTB. In women found to be fFN positive at 21 to 25 weeks, treatment with metronidazole 250 mg tid and erythromycin 250 mg qid × 10 days is associated with similar incidences of PTB < 37 weeks to placebo. Among women with a prior PTB, this antibiotic regimen is associated with a higher incidence of PTB < 37 weeks than the placebo group (90). In women with at least one other risk factor for PTB (e.g., prior PTB), and positive fFN at 24 to 27 weeks, metronidazole 400 mg orally tid for 7 days was associated with no effect on PTB and maternal and perinatal outcomes compared with placebo (91). In summary, **screening low-risk or high-risk asymptomatic pregnant women for fFN is not effective**, as there is no intervention (the one tried has been antibiotics) shown to alter outcomes.

Risk: Prior IUGR or Preeclampsia

Intervention: low-dose aspirin. Compared to no aspirin or placebo, **low-dose aspirin (usually 50–150 mg) is associated with decreased incidence of PTB** (RR 0.22, 95% CI 0.10–0.49) in women at high risk for pregnancy complications, such as those with prior preeclampsia or prior IUGR (92) (see chaps. 1 and 44 in *Maternal-Fetal Evidence Based Guidelines*).

Risk: Periodontal Disease

    Intervention: periodontal therapy. Periodontal disease has been associated with increased risk of PTB in several observational studies. Periodontal treatment such as scaling, root planning, plaque control, and daily rinsing have been evaluated as an intervention to decrease PTB in women with periodontal disease.

    Peridontal treatment has not been associated with decrease in PTB in women with periodontal disease (RR 0.63, 95% CI 0.32–1.22), even when controlling for probing depth and attachment loss for periodontitis criteria, multiparity, prior PTB, or genitourinary infections (93–95).

Infections

Risk: Asymptomatic Bacteriuria

    Intervention: antibiotics. Asymptomatic bacteriuria occurs in 2% to 10% of pregnancies, can lead to pyelonephritis, and is associated with an increased risk of PTB. **Screening for asymptomatic bacteriuria and treating for urine colony count of >100,000 bacteria/mL reduce the incidence of PTB** by 40% (96). The optimal time to perform the urine culture is unknown; it seems reasonable to perform the urine culture and treat, as done in most studies, at the first prenatal visit. Quantitative urine culture of a midstream or clean catch urine is the gold standard for detecting asymptomatic bacteriuria in pregnancy. The choices of a sulfonamide or sulfonamide-containing combination, a penicillin, or nitrofurantoin, based on the results of susceptibility testing, are appropriate regimens for the management of asymptomatic bacteriuria. A short (3 to 7 days) course therapy of asymptomatic bacteriuria has become accepted practice, as is as effective as longer therapy. Single-day therapy has not been studied sufficiently (97). Although it is recommended that a urine culture be done following treatment, with retreatment as necessary, the evidence is insufficient to specifically evaluate the effectiveness of this strategy. Treatment of asymptomatic pregnant women with lower colony counts is not currently recommended, but further study of appropriate strategies to manage these women is warranted. **Asymptomatic women with even low (100+) colony-forming units (CFU) of GBS in the urine culture at 27 to 31 weeks have decreased PTB <37 weeks when treated with penicillin 1 million IU three times per day for 6 days** compared with placebo (98).

    Antibiotic treatment compared with placebo or no treatment is effective in clearing asymptomatic bacteriuria. The incidence of pyelonephritis is reduced. Antibiotic treatment of asymptomatic bacteriuria is then clinically indicated to reduce the risk of pyelonephritis in pregnancy. If untreated, the overall incidence of pyelonephritis is about 19%. Overall, the number of women needed to treat to prevent one episode of pyelonephritis is seven, and treatment of asymptomatic bacteriuria will lead to approximately a 75% reduction in the incidence of pyelonephritis. The apparent reduction in PTB is consistent with current theories about the role of infection as a cause of PTB. Prevention of pyelonephritis, which in early studies prior to the availability of effective antimicrobial therapy was associated with PTB, may be a factor, but treatment of bacteriuria with antibiotics may also eradicate organisms colonizing the cervix and vagina that are associated with adverse pregnancy outcomes. The use of tetracycline is contraindicated in pregnancy. Insufficient data are available to determine the effectiveness of treatment to prevent recurrent bacteriuria during pregnancy. There is a need to define the appropriate frequency of follow-up cultures and retreatment strategies (96).

Risk: Bacterial Vaginosis

    Intervention: antibiotics. BV is a massive overgrowth of organisms such as anaerobics, *Gardnerella*, *Mycoplasma*, and others in the vagina. Most of these organisms are normally present in the vagina, but are at higher concentrations in BV, while predominant normal flora such as lactobacilli is decreased.

    The diagnosis of BV is usually made clinically with at least three out of four of these (Ansel's) criteria: pH > 4.5 (most important), clue cells, thin homogenous discharge, and "amine" test, while in many studies Nugent's criteria (≥7 on Gram stain) are used for diagnosis. All these screening tests are not very accurate in predicting PTB (PPV 6% to 49% depending on PTB prevalence and patient population) in both asymptomatic and symptomatic women.

    Antibiotic therapy is effective at decreasing the presence of BV during pregnancy. In nonselected women, antibiotic treatment is not effective in reducing the incidence of **PTB < 37 weeks, PTB < 34 weeks, PTB < 32 weeks, or PPROM** (99). However, **treatment before 20 weeks** may reduce the risk of PTB < 37 weeks (OR 0.72, 95% CI 0.55–0.95).

    In women with a previous PTB, treatment did not affect the risk of subsequent PTB <37 weeks, with a 17% to 25% nonsignificant trend for benefit (99,100). It may decrease the risk of PPROM and LBW. Subgroup analysis of treatment with metronidazole or clindamycin does not alter incidence of PTB <37 weeks (100).

Risk: Trichomonas vaginalis

    Intervention: antibiotics. Antibiotics (metronidazole only one tested) **do not prevent PTB** in women with *T. vaginalis* (TV) infection (100–104). In fact, metronidazole is associated with 78% higher incidence of PTB <37 weeks (103), and similar incidences of PTB <32 weeks and perinatal mortality (100). Even in women with a prior PTB, metronidazole is associated with an 84% higher risk of PTB (100). Metronidazole does eradicate TV in >90% of pregnant women with TV. Therefore, at least for the purpose of decreasing PTB, asymptomatic women should not be screened for TV and treated with metronidazole if positive for TV. Symptomatic women with TV should still be adequately treated (see chap. 36 in *Maternal-Fetal Evidence Based Guidelines*).

Risk: BV, Candida, and Trichomonas

    Intervention: antibiotics. In one large RCT, **screening for BV** (treatment clindamycin 2% vaginal cream for 6 days), **Candida** (treatment local clotrimazole 100 mg for 6 days), and *Trichomonas* (treatment local metronidazole 500 mg for 7 days) was **associated with lower risks of PTB < 37 weeks** (3% vs. 5%; RR 0.55, 95% CI 0.41–0.75). The incidence of PTB for BW < 2500 g and <1500 g were significantly lower in the intervention group (RR 0.48, 95% CI 0.34–0.66 and RR 0.34; 95% CI 0.15–0.75, respectively) compared to screening with results unavailable to the managing physician (105). Very few women were positive for *Trichomonas*, while about 21% of women had either BV or candida, or both.

Risk: GBS Vaginal-Cervical Colonization

    Intervention: antibiotics. GBS colonization of the cervicovaginal tract is common in pregnancy (10–20%), and has been associated with a slight (OR 1.5–3, usually) increased risk of PTB. Antibiotic therapy (with erythromycin) does not prevent PTB in women with GBS colonization, or affect stillbirths. Subanalysis by heavy colonization did not change results (106).

Risk: Ureoplasma Vagino-Cervical Colonization

Intervention: antibiotics. Ureoplasma urealiticum and/or mycoplasma hominis colonization of the cervicovaginal tract is common in pregnancy and has been associated with a possible increased risk of PTB. **There is insufficient evidence to show whether giving antibiotics to women with ureaplasma in the vagina prevents PTB.** The only trial did not report data on PTB (107). Compared to placebo, erythromycin is associated with a nonsignificant 30% decrease in incidence of LBW < 2500 g (RR 0.70, 95% CI 0.46–1.07). Although some studies appeared to meet the inclusion criteria for this review, in most studies ureaplasma was not an essential entry criterion or studies reported just a post hoc subgroup analysis of ureaplasma.

There is insufficient information at this time to evaluate other interventions such as pessary. These therefore cannot be recommended for clinical use, unless in a research trial.

Multiple Gestations (See Chap. 42 in *Maternal-Fetal Evidence Based Guidelines*)

Bed Rest

In uncomplicated twin pregnancies, **prophylactic bed rest in the hospital does not reduce PTB**, perinatal mortality, LBW, and other complications of pregnancy (108). **In fact, the incidence of PTB <34 weeks is significantly increased by 84%** (109–113).

In twin pregnancies with cervical dilatation, bed rest in the hospital does not decrease PTB in women in Zimbabwe (114). In the trial in which it was recorded, only 6% of women appreciated in-hospital bed rest. For complications, see above under subsection "Intervention: Bed Rest" (singleton pregnancies).

Reduction

There is no trial to assess the effect of multifetal reduction to prevent PTB. Compared to triplets/higher order multiples, triplets/higher order multiples reduced to twins have a higher incidence of loss <24 weeks, but lower incidences of PTB <32 weeks and better neonatal outcome of the remaining twins after reduction in case-control studies. See chapter 42 in *Maternal-Fetal Evidence Based Guidelines*.

Cerclage

History-indicated cerclage does not prevent PTB in twin gestations (115). Ultrasound-indicated cerclage for pregnancies with twin gestations and TVU CL < 25 mm does not prevent PTB (76).

Progesterone

For **17P**, there are at least six RCTs available in **twins**, with **none reporting an effect in PTB or neonatal outcomes** (116–120).

Even in **twins with short CL**, there was no effect of 17P, but numbers are limited (119).

Even in women with **twins and prior PTB**, 17P did not affect incidence of PTB (120).

In triplet gestations, 17P is not associated with an effect on incidence of PTB (121,122).

Vaginal progesterone 90 mg daily starting at 24 weeks for 10 weeks, in 500 women with **twin** gestation, was not associated with significant effects in incidences of PTB or perinatal morbidity and mortality (123). No RCT has yet been reported on the effect of vaginal progesterone on triplet gestations.

In summary, **the evidence does not support the use of any type of progesterone for prevention of PTB in multiple gestations**. There is insufficient evidence to assess the effect of progesterone in women with both multiple gestation and short CL. In women with prior SPTB, and a current multiple gestation, some experts have suggested the use of 17P starting at 16 weeks based on the historic risk factor (32), but there is insufficient evidence to make this a recommendation.

For **preconception counseling, prenatal care, antepartum testing, mode of delivery, anesthesia, and postpartum/breastfeeding**, see chapter 17.

REFERENCES

1. Berghella V, ed. Preterm Birth: Prevention and Management. Wiley-Blackwell, Oxford, U.K. 2010. [Review book]
2. American College of Obstetricians and Gynecologists. ACOG Practice Bulletin No. 31: Assessment of risk factors for preterm birth. Washington, DC: ACOG, 2001. [Review]
3. American College of Obstetricians and Gynecologists. ACOG Practice Bulletin No. 48: Cervical insufficiency. Washington, DC: ACOG, 2003. [Review]
4. Zhu B-P, Rolfs RT, Nangle BE, et al. Effect of the interval between pregnancies on perinatal outcome. N Engl J Med 1999; 340:589–594. [II-2]
5. Shah PS, Zao J. Knowledge synthesis group of determinants of preterm? LBW births. Induced termination of pregnancy and low birth weight and preterm birth: a systematic review and meta-analysis. Br J Obstet Gynecol 2009; 116:1425–1442. [Meta-analysis; II-1]
6. Rodrigues T, Rocha L, Barros H. Physical abuse during pregnancy and preterm delivery. Am J Obstet Gynecol 2008; 198:171. [II-2]
7. Kramer MS, Kakuma R. Energy and protein intake in pregnancy. Cochrane Database Syst Rev 2005; (2):CD004696. [Meta-analysis: 13 RCTS, *n* = 4665]
8. Kramer MS. Isocaloric balanced protein supplementation in pregnancy. Cochrane Database Syst Rev 2005; (1). [Meta-analysis: 3 RCTs, *n* = 996]
9. Kramer MS. High protein supplementation in pregnancy. Cochrane Database Syst Rev 2005; (1). [Meta-analysis: 2 RCTs, *n* = 1076]
10. Oken E, Radesky JS, Wright RO, et al. Maternal fish intake during pregnancy, blood mercury levels, and child cognition at age 3 years in a US cohort. Am J Epidemiol 2008; 167:1171–1181. [II-1]
11. Smuts CM, Huang M, Mundy D, et al. A randomized trial of docosahexaenoic acid supplementation during the third trimester of pregnancy. Obstet Gynecol 2003; 101:469–479. [RCT, *n* = 291]
12. Makrides M, Duley L, Olsen SF. Marine oil, and other prostaglandin precursor, supplementation for pregnancy uncomplicated by pre-eclampsia or intrauterine growth restriction. Cochrane Database Syst Rev 2006; (3). [Meta-analysis: 6 RCTs, *n* = 2783]
13. Makrides M, Gibson RA, McPhee AJ, et al. Effect of DHA supplementation during pregnancy on maternal depression and neurodevelopment of young children. JAMA 2010; 304:1675–1683. [RCT, *n* = 2399]
14. Myhre R, Brantsater AL, Myking S, et al. Intake of probiotic food and risk of spontaneous preterm delivery. Am J Clin Nutr 2011; 93:151–157. [II-2]
15. Othman M, Alfirevic Z, Neilson JP. Probiotics for preventing preterm labour. Cochrane Database Syst Rev 2007; (1). [Meta-analysis: 3 RCTs]
16. Hauth JC, Clifton RG, Robert JM, et al. Vitamin C and E supplementation to prevent spontaneous preterm bith—a randomized controlled trial. Obstet Gynecol 2010; 116:653–658. [RCT, *n* = 9968]
17. Makrides M, Crowther CA. Magnesium supplementation in pregnancy. Cochrane Database Syst Rev 2006 (1). [Meta-analysis: 7 RCTs, *n* = 2689]

18. Hauth JC, Gilstrap LC, Brekken AL, et al. The effect of 17P on pregnancy outcome in an active duty military population. Am J Obstet Gynecol 1984; 146:18790. [RCT, *n* = 168]

19. Lumley J, Chamberlain C, Dowswell T, et al. Interventions for promoting smoking cessation during pregnancy. Cochrane Database Syst Rev 2009. [72 trials, *n* ≥ 25,000]

20. American College of Obstetricians and Gynecologists. ACOG Educational Bulletin No. 260: Smoking cessation during pregnancy. Washington, DC: ACOG, 2000. Available at: www.acog.org. [Review]

21. Sexton M, Hebel JR. A clinical trial of change in maternal smoking and its effect on birth weight. JAMA 1984; 251:911–915. [RCT, *n* = 935]

22. Donatelle RJ, Prows SL, Champeau D, et al. Randomised controlled trial using social support and financial incentives for high risk pregnant smokers: Significant Other Supporter (SOS) program. Tob Control 2000; 9(suppl 3):iii67–iii69. [RCT, *n* = 120]

23. Wisborg K, Henriksen TB, Secher NJ. A prospective intervention study of stopping smoking in pregnancy in a routine antenatal care setting. Br J Obstet Gynaecol 1998; 105:1171–1176. [RCT, *n* = 5156]

24. Kapur B, Hackman R, Selby P, et al. Randomized, double blind, placebo-controlled trial of nicotine replacement therapy in pregnancy. Curr Therapeut Res 2001; 62(4):274–278. [RCT, *n* = 20]

25. Hegaard H, Hjaergaard H, Moller L, et al. Multimodel intervention raises smoking cessation rate during pregnancy. Acta Obstet Gynecol Scand 2003; 82:813–819. [RCT, *n* = 647]

26. Hobel CJ, Ross MG, Bemis RL, et al. The West Los Angeles preterm birth prevention project. I. Program impact on high-risk women. Am J Obstet Gynecol 1994; 170:54–62. [RCT, *n* => 1500]

27. Hegaard HK, Hedegaard M, Damm, et al. Leisure time physical activity is associated with a reduced risk of preterm delivery. Am J Obstet Gynecol 2008; 198:180. [II-2]

28. Hodnett ED, Fredericks S. Support during pregnancy for women at increased risk of low birthweight babies. Cochrane Database Syst Rev 2005; (1). [Meta-analysis: 16 RCTs, *n* > 16,000 women]

29. Mueller-Heubach E, Rddick D, Barnett B, et al. Preterm birth prevention: evaluation of a prospective controlled trial. Am J Obstet Gynecol 1989; 160:1172–1178. [RCT, *n* = <800]

30. Main DM, Richardson DK, Hadley CB, et al. Controlled trial of a preterm labor detection program: efficacy and costs. Obstet Gynecol 1989; 74:873–877. [RCT, *n* = 376]

31. Collaborative group on preterm birth prevention. Multicenter randomized controlled trial of a preterm birth prevention program. Am J Obstet Gynecol 1993; 169:352–366. [RCT; *n* = 2395—includes Goldenberg RL, Davis RO, Copper RL, et al. The Alabama preterm birth prevention trial. Obstet Gynecol 1990; 75:933–939. [RCT, *n* = about 1000]]

32. Iams JD, Berghella V. Care for women with prior preterm birth. Am J Obstet Gynecol 2010; 203(2):89–100. [Review]

33. Klebanoff MA, Harper M, Lai Y, et al. Fish consumption, erythrocyte fatty acids, and preterm birth. Obstet Gynecol 2011; 117:1071–7. [II–1]

34. Olsen SF, Secher NJ, Tabor A, et al. Randomised clinical trials of fish oil supplementation in high risk pregnancies. Br J Obstet Gynecol 2000; 107:382–395. [RCT; *n* = 232 for singletons; *n* = 569 for twins]

35. Harper M, Thom E, Klebanoff MA, et al. Omega-3 fatty acid supplementation to prevent recurrent PTB. A controlled trial. Obstet Gynecol 2010; 115:234–242. [RCT, *n* = 852]

36. Andrews WW, Goldenberg RL, Hauth JC, et al. Interconceptional antibiotics to prevent spontaneous preterm birth: a randomized clinical trial. Am J Obstet Gynecol 2006; 194:617–623. [RCT, *n* = 124]

37. Vermeulen GM, Bruinse HW. Prophylactic administration of clindamycin 2% vaginal cream to reduce the incidence of spontaneous preterm birth in women with an increased recurrence risk: a randomized placebo-controlled double-blind trial. Br J Obstet Gynecol 1999; 106:652–657. [RCT, *n* = 168]

38. Gighangi PB, Ndinya-Achola JO, Ombete J, et al. Antimicrobial prophylaxis in pregnancy: a randomized, placebo-controlled trial with cefetamet-pivoxil in pregnant women with poor obstetrical history. Am J Obstet Gynecol 1997; 177:680–684. [RCT, *n* = 253]

39. Hauth JC, Goldenberg RL, Andrews WW, et al. Reduced incidence of preterm delivery with metronidazole and erythromycin in women with bacterial vaginosis. N Engl J Med 1995; 333:1732–1736. [RCT, *n* = 358 women with prior PTB or prepregnancy weight <50 kg, and *without BV*; rx metro AND erythromycin]

40. Thinkhamrop J, Hofmeyr GJ, Adetoro O, et al. Prophylactic antibiotic administration in pregnancy to prevent infectious morbidity and mortality. Cochrane Database Syst Rev 2005; (4). [Meta-analysis: 6 RCTs, *n* = 2189, both low- (see PNC guideline) and high-risk women]

41. Johnson JW, Austin KL, Jones GS, et al. Efficacy of 17alpha-hydroxyprogesterone caproate in the prevention of premature labor. N Engl J Med 1975; 293(14):675–680. [RCT]

42. Meis PJ, Klebanoff M, Thom E, et al. Prevention of recurrent preterm delivery by 17 alphahydroxyprogesterone caproate. N Engl J Med 2003; 348:2379–2386. [RCT, *n* = about 460]

43. American College of Obstetricians and Gynecologists. ACOG Committee Opinion No.419: use of progesterone to reduce preterm birth. Obstet Gynecol 2008; 112:963–965. [Review]

44. Kilpatrick S, SMFM Publication committee. Progesterone for prevention of prematurity. Contemp OB/GYN 2009; 54:32–33. [Review]

45. Petrini JR, Callaghan WM, Klebanoff M, et al. Estimated effect of 17 alpha-hydroxyprogesterone caproate on preterm birth in the United States. Obstet Gynecol 2005; 105(2):267–272. [II-3]

46. da Fonseca EB, Bittar RE, Carvalho MH, et al. Prophylactic administration of progesterone by vaginal suppository to reduce the incidence of spontaneous preterm birth in women at increased risk: a randomized placebo-controlled double-blind study. Am J Obstet Gynecol 2003; 188:419–424. [RCT]

47. O'Brien JM, Adair CD, Lewis DF, et al. Progesterone vaginal gel for the reduction of recurrent preterm birth: primary results from a randomized, double-blind, placebo-controlled trial. Ultrasound Obstet Gynecol 2007; 30:687–696. [RCT, *n* = 142]

48. Maher M, et al. Prevention or preterm birth in at risk pregnant women: a randomized trial of vaginal versus intramuscular progesterone J Obstet Gynecol Research 2011. [RCT] (in press).

49. Rai P, Rajaram S, Goel N, et al. Oral micronized progesterone for prevention of preterm birth. Int J Gynaecol Obstet 2009; 104 (1):40–43. [RCT]

50. Glover MM, McKenna DS, Downing CM, et al. A randomized trial of micronized progesterone for the prevention of recurrent preterm birth. Am J Perinat 2011; 28:377–381. [RCT]

51. Rush RW, Issacs S, McPherson K, et al. A randomized controlled trial of cervical cerclage in women at high risk of preterm delivery. Br J Obstet Gynecol 1984;91:724–730. [RCT]

52. Lazar P, Gueguen S, Dreyfus J, et al. Multicentre controlled trial of cervical cerclage in women at moderate risk of preterm delivery. Br J Obstet Gynecol 1984; 91:731–735. [RCT]

53. MRC/RCOG Working Party on Cervical Cerclage. Final report of the Medical Research Council/Royal College of Obstetricians and Gynaecologists multicentre randomized trial of cervical cerclage. Br J Obstet Gynecol 1993; 100:516–523. [RCT]

54. Berghella V, Baxter J, Berghella M. Cervical insufficiency. In: Apuzzio JJ, Vintzileos AM, Iffy L, eds. Operative Obstetrics. 3rd ed. United Kingdom: Taylor and Francis, 2006:157–172. [Review]

55. Davis G, Berghella V, Talucci M, et al. Patients with a prior failed transvaginal cerclage: a comparison of obstetric outcomes with either transabdominal or transvaginal cerclage. Am J Obstet Gynecol 2000; 183:836–839. [II-2]

56. Berghella V, Mackeen AD. Cervical length screening with ultrasound-indicated cerclage compared with history-indicated cerclage for prevention of preterm birth: a meta-analysis. Obstet Gynecol 2011; 118(1):148–155. [Meta-analysis: 4 RCTs, *n* = 467]

57. Mathews DD, Friend JB, Michael CA. A double-blind trial of oral isoxuprine in the prevention of premature labour. J Obstet Gynaecol Br Commonw 1967; 74:68–70. [RCT, *n* = 64]

58. Althuisius SM, Dekker GA, van Geijn HP, et al. Cervical incompetence prevention randomized cerclage trial (CIPRACT): study design and preliminary results. Am J Obstet Gynecol 2000; 183:823–829. [RCT, $n = 67$]

59. Pritts EA, Atwood AK. Luteal phase support in infertility treatment: a meta-analysis of the randomized trials. Hum Reprod 2002; 17:2287–2299. [Meta-analysis, $n =$ about 200]

60. Corrado F, Dugo C, Cannata ML, et al. A randomized trial of progesterone prophylaxis after midtrimester amniocentesis. Eur J Obstet Gynecol Reprod Biol 2002; 188:196–198. [RCT, $n = 584$]

61. Morrison JC, Martin JN, Martin RW, et al. Prevention of preterm birth by ambulatory assessment of uterine activity: a randomized study. Am J Obstet Gynecol 1987; 156:536–543. [RCT; $n = 67$ (18 twins); cannot differentiate populations]

62. Iams JD, Johnson FF, O'Shaunessy RW. A prospective random trial of home uterine activity monitoring in pregnancies at increased risk of preterm labor. Am J Obstet Gynecol 1987; 157:638–643. [RCT; $n = 142$ (40 twins); cannot differentiate]; Iams JD, Johnson FF, O'Shaunessy RW. A prospective random trial of home uterine activity monitoring in pregnancies at increased risk of preterm labor. Part II. Am J Obstet Gynecol 1988; 159:595–603. [RCT]

63. Hill WC, Fleming WC, Martin RW, et al. Home uterine activity monitoring is associated with a reduction in preterm birth. Obstet Gynecol 1990; 76:13–18. [RCT, $n = 245$; ?twins]

64. Dyson DC, Crites YM, Ray DA, et al. Prevention of preterm birth in high-risk patients: a role of education and provider contact versus home uterine monitoring. Am J Obstet Gynecol 1991; 164:756–762. [RCT; $n = 247$ (109 twins); CAN differentiate populations]

65. Mou SM, Sunderji SG, Gall S, et al. Multicenter randomized clinical trial of home uterine activity monitoring for detection of preterm labor. Am J Obstet Gynecol 1991; 165:858–866. [RCT; first report—see Corwin et al.]

66. Corwin MJ, Mou SM, Sunderji SG, et al. Multicenter randomized clinical trial of home uterine activity monitoring: pregnancy outcomes for all women randomized. Am J Obstet Gynecol 1996; 175:1281–1285. [RCT; reports PTB outcomes of Mou et al. 1991 RCT—same RCT; $n = 339$; no twins]

67. Blondel B, Breart G, Berthoux Y, et al. Home uterine activity monitoring in France; a randomized, controlled trial. Am J Obstet Gynecol 1992; 167:424–429. [RCT; $n = 52$; cannot distinguish populations of high-risk singletons vs. twins vs. PTL pts]

68. Wapner RJ, Cotton DB, Artal R, et al. A randomized multicenter trial assessing a home uterine activity monitoring devise used in the absence of daily nursing contact. Am J Obstet Gynecol 1995; 172:1026–1034. [RCT; $n = 187$; ?twins—PTB outcomes not reported]

69. The collaborative home uterine monitoring study group. A multicenter randomized trial of home uterine monitoring: active versus sham device. Am J Obstet Gynecol 1995; 173:1120–1127. [RCT (Devoe PI); $n =$ about 1125; about 215 twins. Cannot differentiate populations]

70. Dyson DC, Danbe KH, Bamner JA, et al. Monitoring women at risk for preterm labor. N Engl J Med 1998; 338:15–19. [RCT; $n = 2422$ (844 twins) can differentiate populations; data reported in %, not actual #]

71. Knuppel RA, Lake MF, Watson DL, et al. Preventing preterm birth in twin gestation: home uterine activity monitoring and perinatal nursing support. Obstet Gynecol 1990; 76(suppl): 24s–27s; 1990; 76(suppl):13s–18s. [RCT, $n = 45$]

72. Watson DL, Welch RA, Mariona FG, et al. Management of preterm labor patients at home: does daily uterine activity monitoring and nursing support make a difference? Obstet Gynecol 1990; 76(suppl):32s–35s. [RCT, $n = 67$]

73. Nagey DA, Bailey-Jones C, Herman AA. Randomized comparison of home uterine activity monitoring and routine care in patients discharged after treatment for preterm labor. Obstet Gynecol 1993; 82:319–323. [RCT, $n = 56$]

74. Brown HL, Britton KA, Brizendine EJ, et al. A randomized comparison of home uterine activity monitoring in the outpatient management of women treated for preterm labor. Am J Obstet Gynecol 1999; 180:798–805. [RCT, $n = 162$]

75. Berghella V, Rafael TJ, Szychowski JM, et al. Cerclage for short cervix on ultrasonography in women with singleton gestations and previous preterm birth: a meta-analysis. Obstet Gynecol 2011; 117(3):663–671. [Meta-analysis: 5 RCTs, $n = 504$]

76. Berghella V, Obido AO, To MS, et al. Cerclage for short cervix on ultrasound: meta-analysis of trials using individual patient-level data. Obstet Gynecol 2005; 106:181–189. [Meta-analysis: 4 RCTs, $n = 607$]

77. Keeler SM, Kiefer D, Rochon M, et al. A randomized trial of cerclage vs. 17 α-hydroxyprogesterone caproate for treatment of short cervix. J Perinal Med 2009; 37:473–479. [RCT]

78. Fonseca EB, Celik E, Parra M, et al. Progesterone and the risk of preterm birth among women with a short cervix. N Eng J Med 2007; 357:462–469. [RCT, $n = 250$]

79. Hassan SS, Romero R, Vidyadhari D, et al.; for the PREGNANT Trial. Vaginal progesterone reduces the rate of preterm birth in women with sonographic short cervix: a multicenter, randomized, double-blind, placebo-controlled trial. Ultrasound Obstet Gynecol 2011; 38:18–31. [RCT, $n = 458$]

80. Cahill AG, Odibo AO, Caughey AB, et al. Universal cervical length screening and treatment with vaginal progesterone to prevent preterm birth: a decision and economic analysis. Am J Obstet Gynecol 2010; 202(6):548.e1–548.e8. [Decision analysis]

81. Werner EF, Han CS, Pettker CM, et al. Universal cervical-length screening to prevent preterm birth: a cost-effectiveness analysis. Ultrasound Obstet Gynecol 2011; 38(1):32–37. [Decision analysis]

82. Iams JD, Goldenberg RL, Meis PJ, et al. The length of the cervix and the risk of spontaneous premature delivery. N Engl J Med 1996; 334(9):567–572. [II-1]

83. Berghella V, Rust OA, Althuisius SM. Short cervix on ultrasound: does indomethacin prevent preterm birth? Am J Obstet Gynecol 2006; 195:809–813. [II-1]

84. DeFranco EA, O'Brien JM, Adair CD, et al. Vaginal progesterone is associated with a decrease in risk for early preterm birth and improved neonatal outcome in women with a short cervix: a secondary analysis from a randomized, double-blind, placebo-controlled trial. Obstet Gynecol 2007; 30:697–705.

85. Owen J, Szychowski J. Can the optimal cervical length for placing ultrasound-indicated cerclage be identified? Am J Obstet Gynecol 2011; 204:s198– s199. [II-1]

86. Berghella V, Keeler SM, To MS, et al. Effectiveness of cerclage according to severity of cervical length shortening: a meta-analysis. Ultrasound Obstet Gynecol 2010; 35:468–473. [II-1]

87. Althuisius SM, Dekker GA, Hummel P, et al. Cervical incompetence prevention randomized cerclage trial: emergency cerclage with bed rest versus bed rest alone. Am J Obstet Gynecol 2003; 189:907. [RCT, $n = 23$]

88. Pereira L, Cotter A, Gomez R, et al. Expectant management compared with physical-examination indicated cerclage (EM-PEC) in selected women with a dilated cervix at 14–25 weeks: results from the EM-PEC international cohort study. Am J Obstet Gynecol 2007; 197:483. [II-1]

89. Berghella V, Prasertcharoensuk W, Cotter A, et al. Does indomethacin preterm preterm birth in women with cervical dilatation in the second trimester? Am J Perinatol 2009; 26:13–19. [II-1]

90. Andrews WW, Sibai BM, Thom EA, et al. Randomized clinical trial of metronidazole plus erythromycin to prevent spontaneous preterm delivery in fetal-fibronectin-positive women. Obstet Gynecol 2003; 101:847–855. [RCT, $n = 703$]

91. Shennan A, Crawshaw S, Briley A, et al. A randomized controlled trial of metronidazole for the prevention of preterm birth in women positive for cervicovaginal fetal fibronectin: the PREMET study. Br J Obstet Gynecol 2006; 113:64–74. [RCT, $n = 100$]

92. Bujold E, Roberge S, Tapp S, et al. Could early aspirin prophylaxis prevent against preterm birth? J Mat Fet Neo Med 2011; 24:966–967. [Meta-analysis]

93. Fampa Fogacci M, Vettore MV, Thome Leao AT. The effect of periodontal therapy on preterm low birth weight—a

meta-analysis. Obstet Gynecol 2011; 117:153–165. [Meta-analysis, 10 RCTs]

94. Jeffcoat MK, Hauth JC, Geurs NC, et al. Periodontal disease and preterm birth: results of a pilot intervention study. J Periodontol 2003; 74:1214–1218. [RCT, $n = 366$. Screened and rx at 21–25 weeks 3 rx groups: dental prophylaxis; SRP; SRP and metronidazole (placebo controlled)]

95. Lopez NJ, Da Silva I, Ipinza J, et al. Periodontal therapy reduces the rate of preterm low birth weight in women with pregnancy-associated gingivitis. J Perodontol 2005; 76:2144–2153. [RCT, $n = 834$]

96. Smaill F. Antibiotics for asymptomatic bacteriuria in pregnancy. Cochrane Database Syst Rev 2005; (3). [Meta-analysis: 14 RCTs, $n => 2000$]

97. Villar J, Widmer M, Lydon-Rochelle MT, et al. Duration of treatment for asymptomatic bacteriuria during pregnancy. Cochrane Database Syst Rev 2005; (3). [Meta-analysis:10 RCTs, $n = 568$]

98. Thompsen AC, Morup L, Hansen KB. Antibiotic elimination of group-B streptococci in urine in prevention of preterm labour. Lancet 1987; 1(8533):591–593. [RCT, $n = 69$]

99. McDonald HM, Brocklehurst P, Gordon A. Antibiotics for treating bacterial vaginosis in pregnancy. Cochrane Database Syst Rev 2007; (1). [Meta-analysis: 15 RCTs, $n = 5888$]

100. Okun N, Gronau KA, Hannah ME. Antibiotics for bacterial vaginosis or Trichomonas vaginalis in pregnancy: a systematic review. Obstet Gynecol 2005; 105:857–868. [Meta-analysis: 14 RCTs on BV; $n => 5500$. 2 RCTs on TV; $n = 842$]

101. Gulmezoglu AM. Interventions for trichomoniasis in pregnancy. Cochrane Database Syst Rev 2005; (3). [Meta-analysis: 2 RCTs, $n = 842$]

102. Ross SM, Van Middelkoop A. Trichomonas infection in pregnancy: does it affect outcome? S Afr Med J 1983; 63:566–567. [RCT, $n = 225$. 2 g metronidazole × 1 to women and their partners]

103. Klebanoff MA, Carey JC, Hauth JC, et al. Failure of metronidazole to prevent preterm delivery among pregnant women with asymptomatic trichomonas vaginalis infection. N Engl J Med 2001; 345:487–493. [RCT, $n = 617$. 2 g metronidazole q48 hours × 2 doses]

104. Kigozi GG, Brahmbhatt H, Wabwire-Mangen F, et al. Treatment of Trichomonas in pregnancy and adverse outcomes of pregnancy: a subanalysis of a randomized trial in Rakai, Uganda. Am J Obstet Gynecol 2003; 189:1398–1400. [RCT, $n = 206$ with TV (PTB < 37 weeks: RR 1.28, 95% CI 0.81–2.02)—subanalysis of larger trial]

105. Kiss H, Petricevic L, Husslein P. Prospective randomised controlled trial of an infection screening programme to reduce the rate of preterm delivery. BMJ 2004; 329:371. [RCT, $n = 4166$]

106. Klebanoff MA, Regan JA, Rao AV, et al. Outcome of the vaginal infections and prematurity study: results of a clinical trial of erythromycin among pregnant women colonized with group B streptococci. Am J Obstet Gynecol 1995; 172:1540–1545. [RCT, $n = 938$; vaginal-cervical GBS at 23–26 weeks: Erythromycin 333 mg tid or placebo for 10 weeks or up to 35 6/7 weeks, whichever came first]

107. McCormack WM, Rosner B, Lee Y-H, et al. Effect of birth weight of erythromycin treatment of pregnant women. Obstet Gynecol 1987; 69:202–207. [RCT, $n = 1071$]

108. Crowther CA. Hospitalization and bed rest for multiple pregnancies. Cochrane Database Syst Rev 2005; (1). [Meta-analysis: 4 RCTs, >1000 women. Mostly in Harare, Zimbabwe]

109. Crowther CA, Verkuyl DAA, Neilson JP, et al. The effects of hospitalization for rest on fetal growth, neonatal morbidity and length of gestation in twin pregnancy. Br J Obstet Gynecol 1990; 97:872–877. [RCT, $n = 118$]

110. Crowther CA, Verkuyl D, Ashworth M, et al. The effects of hospitalisation for bed rest on duration of gestation, fetal growth and neonatal morbidity in triplet pregnancy. Acta Genet Med Gemellol 1991; 40:63–68. [RCT, $n = 19$]

111. Hartikainen-Sorri AL, Jouppila P. Is routine hospitalization needed in antenatal care of twin pregnancy? J Perinat Med 1984; 12:31–34. [RCT, $n = 73$]

112. MacLennan AH, Green RC, O'Shea R, et al. Routine hospital admission in twin pregnancy between 26 and 30 weeks' gestation. Lancet 1990; 335:267–269. [RCT, $n = 141$]

113. Saunders MC, Dick JS, Brown I McL, et al. The effects of hospital admission for bed rest on the duration of twin pregnancy: a randomised trial. Lancet 1985; 2:793–795. [RCT, $n = 212$]

114. Crowther CA, Neilson JP, Verkuyl DAA, et al. Preterm labour in twin pregnancies: can it be prevented by hospital admission? Br J Obstet Gynecol 1989; 96:850–853. [RCT, $n = 139$]

115. Dor J, Shalev J, Mashiach S, et al. Elective cervical suture of twin pregnancies diagnosed ultrasonically in the first trimester following induced ovulation. Gynecol Obstet Invest 1982; 13:55–60. [RCT, $n = 100$]

116. Hartikainen-Sorri AL, Kauppila A, Tuimala R. Inefficacy of 17 a-hydroxyprogestrone caproate in the prevention of prematurity in twin pregnancy. Obstet Gynecol 1980; 56(6):692–695. [RCT]

117. Rouse DJ, Caritis SN, Peaceman AM, et al. A trial of 17 alpha-hydroxyprogesterone caproate to prevent prematurity in twins. N Engl J Med 2007; 357:454–461. [RCT]

118. Combs CA, Garite T, Maurel K, et al.; for the Obstetrix Collaborative Research Network. 17-hydroxyprogesterone caproate for twin pregnancy: a double-blind, randomized clinical trial. Am J Obstet Gynecol 2011; 204:221.e1–221.e8. [RCT]

119. Durnwald CP, Momirova V, Rouse DJ, et al. For the Eunice Kennedy Shriver National Institute of Child Health and Human Development (NICHD), Maternal-Fetal Medicine Units Network (MFMU). Second trimester cervical length and risk of preterm birth in women with twin gestations treated with 17-α hydroxyprogesterone caproate. J Matern Fetal Neonatal Med 2010; e1–e5. [RCT]

120. Briery CM, Veillon EW, Klauser CK, et al. Progesterone does not prevent preterm births in women with twins. Southern Med J 2009; 102:900–904. [RCT]

121. Caritis SN, Rouse DJ, Peaceman AM, et al.; for the Eunice Kennedy Shriver National Institute of Child Health and Human Development (NICHD), Maternal-Fetal Medicine Units Network (MFMU). Prevention of preterm birth in triplets using 17 alpha-hydroxyprogesterone caproate: a randomized controlled trial. Obstet Gynecol 2009; 113(2):285–292. [RCT]

122. Combs CA, Garite T, Maurel K, et al.; for the Obstetrix Collaborative Research Network. Failure of 17-hydroxyprogesterone to reduce neonatal morbidity or prolong triplet pregnancy: a double-blind, randomized clinical trial. Am J Obstet Gynecol 2010; 203(3):248.e1–248e9. [RCT]

123. Norman JE, Mackenzie F, Owen P, et al. Progesterone for the prevention of preterm birth in twin pregnancy (STOPPIT): a randomized, double-blind, placebo-controlled study and meta-analysis. Lancet 2009; 373:2034–2040. [RCT]

17

Preterm labor

Vincenzo Berghella

KEY POINTS

- See chapter 16 for primary and secondary prevention of preterm birth (PTB) in asymptomatic women, and for risk factors and complications.
- Preterm labor (PTL) can be defined as **uterine contractions (≥4/20 min or ≥8/hr) with transvaginal ultrasound (TVU) cervical length (CL) <20 mm, or 20 to 29 mm with positive fetal fibronectin (FFN),** at 20 to 36 6/7 weeks.
- PTL should be managed with knowledge of **TVU CL, and FFN results** (Fig. 17.1).
- Women with PTL but negative FFN and TVU CL ≥30 mm have a ≤2% chance of delivering within 1 week, and a >95% chance of delivering ≥35 weeks without therapy, and should therefore not receive any treatment.
- **Corticosteroids** (e.g., **betamethasone 12 mg IM q24h × 2 doses)** given to mother between 24 33 6/7 weeks prior to PTB (either spontaneous or indicated) are **effective in preventing respiratory distress syndrome (RDS), intraventricular hemorrhage (IVH), necrotizing enterocolitis (NEC), and neonatal mortality.**
- **Rescue (one extra course) steroid therapy should only be considered if multiple weeks have elapsed since the initial course of corticosteroids and a new episode of PTL or preterm premature rupture of membranes (PPROM) or impeding risk of PTB presents again at an early gestational age (GA). A single rescue course of betamethasone, two 12-mg doses 24 hours apart, received before 33 weeks at least 14 or more days after the first course, which was administered before 30 weeks, is associated with decreased RDS, ventilatory support, surfactant use, and composite neonatal morbidity. More than two courses of corticosteroids for fetal maturity should be avoided.**
- **Intravenous magnesium sulfate** (loading dose of 6 g infused for 20 to 30 minutes, followed by a maintenance infusion of 2 g/hr) given at 24 to 31 6/7 weeks immediately (within 12 hours) before PTB is **associated with a significant decrease in the incidence of cerebral palsy.**
- Tocolytics should not be used without concomitant use of corticosteroids for fetal maturity.
- **No tocolytic** has been shown to **improve perinatal mortality.**
- There is **no tocolytic** agent that is **more safe and efficacious. Cyclooxygenase (COX) inhibitors** are the only class of primary tocolytics shown to **decrease PTB < 37 weeks** compared with placebo. **COX inhibitors and oxytocin receptor antagonists (ORA)** have been shown to significantly **prolong pregnancy at 48 hours and 7 days compared with placebo. COX inhibitors, calcium channel blocker (CCB), and ORA** have significantly **less side effects than betamimetics. These three classes of tocolytics (CCB, COX, and ORA) are the ones best supported by evidence for safety and effectiveness.**
- There is **no maintenance tocolytic** that **prevents PTB or perinatal morbidity/mortality, and therefore maintenance tocolysis should not be used.**
- There is insufficient evidence to evaluate multiple tocolytic agents for primary tocolysis, refractory (primary agent is failing, so another is started) tocolysis, or repeated (after successful primary tocolysis) tocolysis.
- All other interventions studied to prevent PTB in women with PTL, including bed rest, hydration, sedation, and others, have not been shown to be beneficial in the management of PTL.
- **In preterm neonates, delayed cord clamping by about 30 to 60 seconds** (120 maximum) is associated with **fewer transfusions for anemia, less hypotension, and less intraventricular hemorrhage** than early clamping at less than 30 seconds.

DIAGNOSIS/DEFINITION

Preterm labor is often defined as uterine contractions (≥4/20 min or ≥8/hr) and documented cervical change with intact membranes at 20 to 36 6/7 weeks. A better definition is probably **uterine contractions (≥4/20 min or ≥8/hr) with TVU CL < 20 mm, or 20 to 29 mm with positive FFN,** at 20 to 36 6/7 weeks.

SYMPTOMS

Symptoms of PTL are often nonspecific and include cramps, abdominal "tightenings," low backache, pelvic pressure, increased vaginal discharge, spotting.

For **epidemiology/incidence, genetics, etiology/basic pathophysiology, classification, risk factors/associations,** and **complications,** see chapter 16.

WORKUP (AND DOCUMENT)

- History: assess risk factors (see Table 16.1); ensure correctness of GA estimation
- Physical exam: vital signs; frequency of uterine contractions; perform speculum exam: test for PPROM (nitrazine, pooling, ferning), FFN; then do TVU to assess CL (do after FFN has been collected); if PPROM: assess cervical exam visually (1); if no PPROM: manual cervical exam (dilatation, CL and/or effacement, station, presentation)
- Laboratory tests: rectovaginal group B streptococcus (GBS) culture; gonorrhea and chlamydia; urinalysis and urine culture (Fig. 17.1)

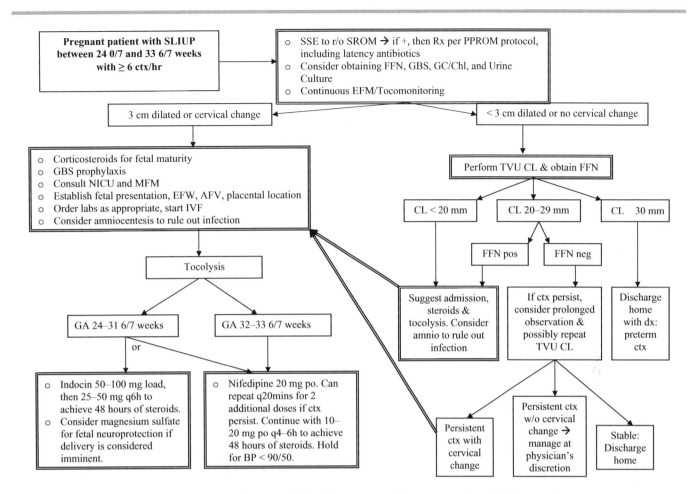

Figure 17.1 Suggested protocol for the management of PTL. *Abbreviations*: PTL, preterm labor; SLIUP, single live intrauterine pregnancy; R/O, rule out; CTX, contractions; SSE, sterile speculum exam; SROM, spontaneous rupture of membranes; Rx, treat; PPROM, preterm premature rupture of membranes; FFN, fetal fibronectin; Amnio, amniocentesis; GBS, group B streptococcus; GC, gonorrhea; Chl, chlamydia; EFM, external fetal monitoring; TVU CL, transvaginal ultrasound cervical length; dx, diagnosis; NICU, neonatal intensive care unit; MFM, maternal-fetal medicine specialist; EFW, estimated fetal weight; GA, gestational age; AFV, amniotic fluid volume; IVF, intravenous fluids; BP, blood pressure.

TVU CL

Compared to no knowledge, **knowledge of TVU CL results** is associated with a nonsignificant **decrease in PTB < 37 weeks** (22.3% vs. 34.7%, respectively; RR 0.59, 95% CI 0.26–1.32). Delivery occurred at a later GA (by about 4–5 days) in the knowledge versus no knowledge groups (2). Given the fact that management based on knowledge of TVU CL prevents PTB, **TVU CL should be used in the management of women with threatened PTL** (Fig. 17.1).

Fetal Fibronectin

Compared to no knowledge, knowledge of FFN results is associated with a decrease in the incidence of PTB < 37 weeks (15.6% vs. 28.6%; RR 0.54, 95% CI 0.34–0.87). All other outcomes for which there were available data (PTB < 34, 32, or 28 weeks; GA at delivery; birth weight less than 2500 g; perinatal death; maternal hospitalization; tocolysis; steroids for fetal lung maturity; and time to evaluate) were similar in the two groups (3). **The benefit in knowledge of FFN was seen in particular in 1 RCT, in which TVU CL was the main screening test, with FFN used only for "indeterminate" results** (4) (Fig. 17.1).

MANAGEMENT

- **Consider referral** to tertiary care center if neonatal ICU is not adequate for GA of potential neonate.
- **Counseling** regarding morbidity and mortality for preterm infant, using latest, possibly internal data (5) (Table 17.1). Current (2012) survival at our institution goes from 0% at 21 weeks to 75% at 25 weeks to >95% at 29 weeks, whereas intact survival at 18 months is about 50% after 25 weeks. Disabilities in mental and psychomotor development, neuromotor function (including cerebral palsy), or sensory and communication function are present in at least 50% of fetuses born ≤25 weeks' gestation (6). Neonatal consult at 22 to 34 weeks is indicated for counseling regarding prognosis and neonatal management.
- Pregnancies at risk for **periviable** PTB are particularly challenging to counsel and manage. The periviability period varies according to several factors, including by level of care provided in hospital and in country where the care is being provided. In many developed country, this period, in 2012, is about 22 to 25 weeks. Table 17.2

Table 17.1   Survival and Selected Major Morbidities by Gestational Age at Birth

	Survival (%)	Chronic lung disease (%)	Severe IVH (%)	Necrotizing enterocolitis (%)	Severe ROP (%)
GA Week					
<22 wk	3.3	33.3	33.3	33.3	66.7
22	6.0	77.8	52.0	11.1	57.9
23	34.3	79.2	33.8	15.9	46.9
24	59.2	74.7	29.5	12.4	34.7
25	75.3	65.9	20.1	11.6	26.2
26	80.0	51.7	17.2	10.2	14.2
27	89.4	35.9	9.7	6.8	7.0
28	91.2	25.8	6.3	7.2	3.0
29	94.3	16.2	4.3	4.9	1.0
30	96.8	11.0	1.9	3.4	0.7
31	96.7	7.3	1.9	2.4	0.6
32	97.5	4.1	1.3	1.7	0.2
33	98.1	3.1	1.4	1.0	0.9
34	98.4	4.4	1.5	0.9	0.0
35	98.2		1.8	0.6	1.1
36	97.5		1.4	0.4	0.0
37	97.9		1.8	0.5	1.5
>37 wk	98.0		1.5	0.3	0.2
All	95.4	17.3	5.3	1.5	7.2

Chronic lung disease is defined as need for oxygen therapy at 36 weeks of postmenstrual age (see Table 17.2); severe IVH: grades III and IV (see Table 17.3); necrotizing enterocolitis includes medical and surgical; severe ROP is defined as >grade 2.
Abbreviations: GA, gestational age; ROP, retinopathy of prematurity.
Source: Data from Ref. 5. Courtesy of Kevin Dysart.

Table 17.2   Suggested Management of Threatened Periviable Preterm Birth

Weeks	Obstetrical care	Neonatal care
22–22 6/7	Counseling • Corticosteroids, magnesium sulfate not recommended • Fetal monitoring not recommended • Cesarean section for fetal indications not recommended • NICU/OB joint consult, as feasible	• NICU care not offered • Comfort care provided
23 0/7–23/6/7	Counseling If mother/family choosing NICU care, consider: • Corticosteroids • Tocolysis as indicated to allow administration of corticosteroids • Magnesium sulfate for neuroprotection if imminent delivery • Fetal monitoring: discuss with family (depends mostly on willingness for cesarean) • Cesarean section for fetal indications: discuss with family • NICU/OB joint consult, as feasible	NICU consultation, decide if • Comfort care • Full invasive care to include intubation • Attempt bag/mask ventilation to determine infant's ability to respond. If no response, interventions should cease
24 0/7–24 6/7	Counseling Suggest: • Corticosteroids • Tocolysis as indicated to allow administration of corticosteroids • Magnesium sulfate for neuroprotection if imminent delivery • Fetal monitoring • Cesarean section for fetal indications	NICU consultation • Full resuscitation provided in the majority of cases • The options of comfort care and attempting bag/mask ventilation to determine infant's ability to respond and cease interventions; if no response, interventions can be considered
25 0/7–25 6/7	Counseling Recommend: • Corticosteroids • Tocolysis as indicated to allow administration of corticosteroids • Magnesium sulfate for neuroprotection if imminent delivery • Fetal monitoring • Cesarean section for fetal indications	NICU consultation • Full resuscitation provided in the majority of cases

Abbreviations: NICU, neonatal intensive care unit; OB, obstetrics.

provides some guidance for care, but should be adjusted according to local capabilities. Patients with an intrauterine demise or undergoing pregnancy termination are not to be included in this group. For patients in whom the GA has not been clearly established at prenatal care, plans for intervention and information provided to the patient should possibly lie on the greatest GA. An online calculator can be used to provide patient-specific mortality and morbidity information, if applicable (http://www.nichd.nih.gov/about/org/cdbpm/pp/prog_epbo/epbo_case.cfm). Status can be reevaluated with each new gestational week.

Principles of Management

Before treatment is ever considered, the diagnosis (see above) must be established.

Women with preterm contractions but negative FFN and TVU CL $\geq$30 mm have a $\leq$2% chance of delivering within 1 week, and a >95% chance of delivering $\geq$35 weeks without therapy, and should therefore not receive any treatment (7) (Fig. 17.1); 70% to 80% of women diagnosed with PTL (if diagnosed without using TVU CL) do not deliver preterm. Women without cervical change do not have PTL and should not receive tocolysis. Women with multiple gestations should not be treated differently than those with singletons, except that their risk of pulmonary edema is greater when exposed to betamimetics or magnesium sulfate (8). There is insufficient evidence to justify the use of steroids for fetal lung maturity and tocolysis before 23 weeks and after 33 6/7 weeks. **Amniocentesis** may be considered to assess intra-amniotic infection (IAI) (incidence about 5–15%) and fetal lung maturity (especially between 33 and 35 weeks). IAI (documented by amniotic fluid culture) rates can be estimated by pregnancy status (Table 17.3). IAI rates can also be estimated by TVU CL (9). Patients between 34 and 36 weeks should also be evaluated for etiology of PTL, though neither tocolyzed nor given steroids.

Prophylaxis to Prevent Neonatal Morbidity/Mortality from PTB (Fetal Maturation)

Corticosteroids
Betamethasone, dexamethasone (only 2 corticosteroids that cross the placenta reliably).

Dose: One course: Betamethasone 12 mg SQ q24h × 2 doses or dexamethasone 6 mg SQ q12h × 4 doses (betamethasone, if available, should be preferred to dexamethasone—see below).

Mechanism of action: Enhanced maturational changes in lung architecture and induction of lung enzymes resulting in biochemical maturation.

Evidence for effectiveness: Corticosteroids given prior to PTB (either spontaneous or indicated) are effective in

Table 17.3 Estimated Incidences of Intramniotic Infection in Women in Different Clinical Scenarios

Condition	Percent
GA < 37 wk	
Asymptomatic 2nd trimester	0.5
PTL (intact membranes)	13
PPROM, no labor	25
PPROM, labor	39
Cervix $\geq$2 cm/80% in 2nd trimester	50
GA $\geq$37 weeks	
Labor	19
PROM	34

Abbreviations: GA, gestational age; PPROM, preterm premature rupture of membranes; PTL, preterm labor.

preventing RDS, IVH, and neonatal mortality (10). Antenatal administration of 24 mg of **betamethasone (12 mg intramuscularly q24h)**, or of 24 mg of **dexamethasone (6 mg intramuscularly q12h)**, to women expected to give birth preterm is associated with significant **41% reduction in neonatal mortality, 34% reduction in RDS and respiratory support, 46% reduction in IVH, 54% reduction in NEC, 20% reduction in intensive care admissions, and 44% reduction in systemic infections in the first 48 hours of life** in preterm infants. There are also decreased needs for surfactant, oxygen, and mechanical ventilation in the neonatal period. Treatment with antenatal corticosteroids does not increase risk to the mother of death, chorioamnionitis, or puerperal sepsis.

These benefits apply to **gestational ages of at least 24 to 33 6/7 weeks,** and are not limited by gender or race. There is insufficient data (no trial) to assess effect before or after these gestational ages. At 23 to 23 6/7 weeks, cohort studies have also shown benefit in decreasing neonatal death (11). The **effects are significant mostly at 48 hours to 7 days from first dose,** but treatment should not be withheld even if delivery appears imminent. Such steroids should therefore be administered to any woman at these gestational ages at significant PTB risk upon identification of the risk. Higher doses do not increase the benefits. Oral dexamethasone is less effective than intramuscular dexamethasone (12).

Type of steroid: There is **insufficient evidence to compare betamethasone and dexamethasone.** Dexamethasone may have some benefits compared with betamethasone, such as less IVH, although perhaps a higher rate of neonatal intensive care unit (NICU) admission (seen in only one RCT). Dexamethasone is associated with a decrease in the incidence of IVH compared with betamethasone (RR 0.44, 95% CI 0.21–0.92). No statistically significant differences are seen for RDS, bronchopulmonary dysplasia (BPD), severe IVH, periventricular leukomalacia, perinatal death, or mean birth weight. Results for biophysical parameters are inconsistent, but mostly no important differences were seen for these, or any other secondary outcome except for NICU admission. In one small RCT, significantly more infants in the dexamethasone group were admitted to NICU compared with the betamethasone group (RR 3.83, 95% CI 1.24–11.87) (13). Oral dexamethasone compared with intramuscular dexamethasone increased the incidence of neonatal sepsis (RR 8.48, 95% CI 1.11–64.93) in one trial of 183 infants. No statistically significant differences were seen for other outcomes reported. In one small trial of 69 infants comparing betamethasone acetate and phosphate with betamethasone phosphate, no differences were seen for any of the outcomes reported (13).

When RCTs that do not compare directly betamethasone to dexamethasone are evaluated, betamethasone treatment (RR 0.56, 95% CI 0.48–0.65) results in a greater reduction in RDS than dexamethasone treatment (RR 0.80, 95% CI 0.68–0.93). However, dexamethasone significantly increases the incidence of puerperal sepsis (RR 1.74, 95% CI 1.04–2.89, four studies, 536 women), while betamethasone does not (RR 1.00, 95% CI 0.58–1.72) (13). Betamethasone has been associated with less cystic periventricular leukomalacia, and possibly more substantial reduction in complications mentioned above, but this has not been confirmed by any trial. Hydrocortisone was not effective in a small trial (13). The results are in most part from singleton gestations, with insufficient data on multiple gestations.

Single "rescue" dose: As the effects of steroids for fetal maturation are best within 7 days before birth, timing the first single course of steroids is extremely important. **Rescue (one extra course) therapy should only be considered if multiple**

weeks have elapsed since the initial course of corticosteroids and a new episode of PTL or PPROM or impeding risk of PTB presents again at an early GA (14).

A single rescue course of betamethasone, two 12-mg dose 24 hours apart, received before 33 weeks at least 14 or more days after the first course, which was administered before 30 weeks, is associated with decreased RDS, ventilatory support, surfactant use, and composite neonatal morbidity (RR 0.65, 95% CI 0.44–0.97) (15,16). Instead, just one rescue "dose" is not associated with benefits in one RCT (17).

More than two courses of corticosteroids: More than two courses of corticosteroids for fetal maturity should probably be avoided until more long-term data are available on childhood outcomes. Treatment of women who remain at risk of PTB 7 or more days after an initial course of prenatal corticosteroids with repeat dose(s), compared with no repeat corticosteroid treatment, reduces the risk of their infants experiencing RDS (RR 0.83, CI 0.75–0.91) and serious infant outcome (RR 0.84, 95% CI 0.75–0.94). Treatment with repeat dose(s) of corticosteroid is associated with a reduction in mean birth weight (by about 76 g). However, outcomes that adjusted birth weight for GA do not differ between treatment groups (18). Some RCTs, including the largest one ever done, have also reported a smaller infant head size associated with repeated courses of steroids (19,20).

At early childhood follow-up, no statistically significant differences were seen for infants exposed to repeat prenatal corticosteroids compared with unexposed infants for the primary outcomes (total deaths; survival free of any disability or major disability; disability; or serious outcome) or in the secondary outcome growth assessments (18).

Contraindications: None.

Side effects: When used for only 1 course, no significant side effects are seen, except for transient maternal hyperglycemia from 12 hours to about 5 to 7 days after the dose. This effect results in false-positive glucose screening tests or difficulty in managing diabetes. There is no significant increase in maternal or fetal/neonatal infection. If ≥4 courses are used, there is an association with birth weight <10th percentile and probably with small (<10th percentile) neonatal head circumference, with evidence of some later "catch-up" (19,21). No adverse consequences of prophylactic corticosteroids for PTB in either the mothers or, most importantly, the infants, even at 10+ years follow-up, have been identified, but long-term follow-up is limited so far.

Thyrotropin-Releasing Hormone

Prenatal thyrotropin-releasing hormone (TRH), in addition to corticosteroids, given to women at risk of very PTB, does not improve infant outcomes and can cause maternal side effects (22). Overall, prenatal TRH, in addition to corticosteroids, does not reduce the risk of neonatal respiratory disease or chronic oxygen dependence, and does not improve any of the fetal, neonatal, or childhood outcomes. Indeed, prenatal TRH does have adverse effects for women and their infants. Side effects are more likely to occur in women receiving TRH. In the infants, prenatal TRH increases 16% the risk of needing ventilation, 48% having a low Apgar score at five minutes, and, for the two trials providing data, was associated with poorer outcomes at childhood follow-up (22).

Phenobarbital

The use of prophylactic maternal phenobarbital administration prior to preterm delivery does not prevent periventricular hemorrhage (PVH) or protect from neurological disability in preterm infants (23). Prenatal maternal phenobarbital is associated with a significant 35% reduction in the rates of all grades of PVH and 59% reduction in severe grades PVH (3 and 4) in the infants. These results are influenced by trials of poor quality that contribute excessive weight in the analysis due to their higher rates of severe PVH. When only the two higher quality trials were included (24,25), phenobarbital is not associated with any beneficial effects, including similar incidences of all grades of PVH and severe grades of PVH to placebo. No difference was found in the incidence of neurodevelopmental abnormalities at pediatric follow-up assessed between 18 to 36 months of age. Maternal sedation is more likely in women receiving phenobarbital (23).

Vitamin K

Vitamin K administered to women prior to very PTB has not been shown to significantly prevent PVHs or other neurodevelopmental abnormalities in preterm infants. Antenatal vitamin K is associated with a nonsignificant reduction in all grades of PVH (RR 0.76, 95% CI 0.54–1.06) and a significant reduction in severe PVH (grades 3 and 4) (RR 0.58, 95% CI 0.3–0.91) for babies receiving prenatal vitamin K compared with control babies. When the two quasi-randomized trials are excluded, antenatal vitamin K is associated with a nonsignificant reduction in all grades of PVH (RR 0.87, 95% CI 0.60–1.26) and a nonsignificant reduction in severe PVH (RR 0.82, 95% CI 0.49–1.36). Treatment with vitamin K results in a significant reduction in the Bayley Mental Development Index at 2 years of age; however, these results are derived from one trial with many participants lost to follow-up. No difference is found in the incidence of other neurodevelopmental abnormalities at pediatric follow-up at 18 to 24 months or 7 years of age between children born to mothers given vitamin K and children not so exposed (26).

Magnesium Sulfate for Neuroprotection

Antenatal magnesium sulfate therapy given to women at risk of PTB significantly reduces the risk of cerebral palsy in their child (RR 0.68, 95% CI 0.54–0.87). There was also a significant reduction in the rate of substantial gross motor dysfunction (RR 0.61, 95% CI 0.44–0.85). No statistically significant effect of antenatal magnesium sulfate therapy is detected on pediatric mortality (RR 1.04, 95% CI 0.92–1.17), or on other neurological impairments or disabilities in the first few years of life. There are higher rates of minor maternal side effects in the magnesium groups, but no significant effects on major maternal complications (27).

Magnesium sulfate should be therefore administered to singletons or twins at 24 0/7 through 31 6/7 weeks at high risk for spontaneous PTB because of PPROM or because of advanced PTL, with dilatation of 4 to 8 cm. Also eligible are women with an indicated PTB anticipated within 2 to 24 hours (e.g., for severe preeclampsia). Intravenous magnesium sulfate is administered with a loading dose of 6 g infused for 20 to 30 minutes, followed by a maintenance infusion of 2 g/hr (28). If delivery has not occurred after 12 hours and is no longer considered imminent (e.g., if the patient is not having regular uterine contractions), the infusion should be discontinued and resumed when delivery is deemed imminent again (e.g., when contractions develop). If at least 6 hours have passed since the discontinuation of the magnesium sulfate, another loading dose should be given. Administration of magnesium sulfate for prevention of cerebral palsy should not delay the delivery.

Nontocolytic Interventions in PTL

Bed Rest

Bed rest has never been tested in an RCT in singleton gestations complicated by PTL or PPROM. In twin pregnancies with cervical dilatation, bed rest in the hospital **did not decrease** PTB in one trial in Zimbabwe (29).

Hydration

There is **no advantage** of hydration compared with bed rest alone. Intravenous hydration does not seem to be beneficial, even during the period of evaluation soon after admission, in women with preterm labor. Women with evidence of dehydration may, however, benefit from the intervention. **Compared with bed rest alone, hydration is associated with similar incidences of PTB < 37 weeks, <34 weeks, or <32 weeks**, and **of admission to NICU** (30). Cost of treatment is slightly higher (US$39) in the hydration group for hospital costs during a visit of less than 24 hours. Women studied were at low risk, as about 30% of women required tocolysis, and <30% had PTB. No studies evaluated oral hydration (30).

Screen for Infections

Several infections are associated with a higher risk of PTL and PTB. These include chlamydia, gonorrhea, syphilis, trichomoniasis, and others, as well as bacterial vaginosis (see chap. 16) There is **insufficient evidence** to assess the effect of screening and treating for any of these infections in women with PTL, as no RCTs have been performed.

Antibiotics

There is **no clear overall benefit** or detriment from prophylactic antibiotic treatment for PTL with intact membranes on neonatal outcomes (31,32). PTB < 36 or 37 weeks is similar in antibiotics and placebo groups. There is **a trend for a 52% increase in neonatal mortality for those who received antibiotics** (RR 1.52, 95% CI 0.99–2.34), with similar overall perinatal mortality (RR 1.22, 95% CI 0.88–1.70) (31). The only benefit is a 26% reduction in maternal infection with the use of prophylactic antibiotics. Of the different antibiotics or combinations studied so far (macrolide antibiotics, beta-lactam antibiotics, a combination of beta-lactam and macrolide antibiotics, and antibiotics active against anaerobes), antibiotics active against anaerobes (clindamycin (33) and ampicillin-metronidazole) (34,35) show a 10-day increase in the interval from randomization to delivery, a 38% reduction in the number of women giving birth within 7 days of enrolment, and 37% fewer admissions to NICU in small trials. Follow-up at 7 years of the largest RCT showed **increased incidence of functional impairment associated with erythromycin,** and **increased incidence of cerebral palsy associated with either antibiotic studied (erythromycin or co-amoxiclav)** (36). Given these data, **antibiotics should not be used for prevention of PTB in women with PTL and intact membranes**.

Tocolysis

Principles

See Table 17.4.

Contraindications

See Table 17.5.

Primary Tocolysis—Single Agent
Betamimetics

Types: Ritodrine, terbutaline.

Dose: Ritodrine: 50 to 100 µg/min IV initial dose, increase 50 µg/min q10min (max 350 µg/min). [po: 1–20 mg po q2–4h] Terbutaline: 0.25 mg SQ q20min at first, then 2 to 3 hours; or 5 to 10 µg/min IV, max 80 µg/min; or 2.5 to 5 mg po q2–4h (hold for maternal HR > 120/min).

Mechanism of action: Stimulate B2 receptor through cyclic AMP, so no free calcium for myometrial contraction.

Evidence for effectiveness: (Table 17.6) **Compared with placebo, betamimetics are associated with a decrease in the number of women in PTL giving birth within 48 hours** (RR 0.63, 95% CI 0.53–0.75), but do not decrease the number of births within 7 days (37). No benefit is demonstrated for betamimetics on perinatal or neonatal death. No significant effect is demonstrated for RDS. A few trials reported the following outcomes, with no difference detected: cerebral palsy, infant death, and NEC. Betamimetics are significantly associated with the following side effects (see below): **withdrawal from treatment due to adverse effects, chest pain, dyspnea, tachycardia, palpitation, tremor, headaches, hypokalemia, hyperglycemia, nausea/vomiting, nasal stuffiness, and fetal tachycardia** (37). There is insufficient evidence to assess which of the studied betamimetics is most effective and/or associated with fewer

Table 17.4 Principles of Tocolytic Therapy

- **At 24–33 6/7 wk, steroids for fetal maturation should always be given if tocolysis is initiated.** Tocolytics should not be used without concomitant use of steroids for fetal maturation.
- Tocolysis is typically used for 48 hr to allow steroid effect. Given side effects, consider stopping tocolytic therapy at 48 hr after steroids given if PTL under control.
- **No tocolytic agent has been shown to improve perinatal mortality.**
- There is no tocolytic agent that is more safe and efficacious. **COX inhibitors** are the only class of primary tocolytics shown to decrease PTB < 37 wk compared with placebo. COX inhibitors and **ORA** have been shown to significantly prolong pregnancy at 48 hr and 7 days compared with placebo. COX inhibitors, **CCB**, and ORA, properly used, have significantly less side effects than betamimetics. Currently, **these three classes of tocolytics (CCB, COX, and ORA) are the ones best supported by evidence for safety and effectiveness.**
- There is no maintenance tocolytic that prevents PTB or perinatal morbidity/mortality, and therefore **maintenance tocolysis should not be used.** There is insufficient evidence to evaluate multiple tocolytic agents for primary tocolysis, refractory (primary agent is failing, so another is started) tocolysis, or repeated (after successful primary tocolysis) tocolysis.

Abbreviations: COX, cyclooxygenase; ORA, oxytocin receptor antagonists; CCB, calcium channel blockers; PTB preterm birth; PTL, preterm labor.

Table 17.5 Contraindications to Tocolytic Therapy

Maternal:
  Chorioamnionitis
  Severe vaginal bleeding/abruptio
  Preeclampsia
  Medical contraindications to specific tocolytic agent[a]
  Other maternal medical condition that makes continuing the pregnancy inadvisable

Fetal:
  Death
  Major (especially if lethal) fetal anomaly or chromosome abnormality
  Other fetal conditions in which prolongation of pregnancy is inadvisable
  Documented fetal maturity

[a]See text.

Table 17.6 Summary of the Evidence for Tocolytic Therapy

Tocolytics	48 hr	7 days	PTB < 32 wk	PTB < 37 wk	Perinatal mortality
PRIMARY—SINGLE AGENT VS. PLACEBO					
Betamimetics	**0.63 (0.53–0.75) [n = 1209]**	0.78 (0.68–1.10) [n = 911]	N/A	0.95 (0.88–1.03) [n = 1212]	0.84 (0.46–1.55) [n = 1174]
CCB	No RCT	No RCT	No RCT	No RCT	No RCT
COX	**0.19 (0.08–0.45) [n = 70][a]**	**0.43 (0.27–0.69) [n = 70][a]**	NC	**0.21 (0.07–0.62) [n = 36]**	0.80 (0.25–2.58) [n = 106]
Mg	0.57 (0.28–1.15) [n = 190]	NC	NC	0.92 (0.41–2.07) [n = 29]	1.74 (0.63–4.77) [n = 192]
ORA	**0.77 (0.61–0.97)** 86/302 vs. 115/311 [n = 613][a]	**0.74 (0.61–0.91)** 93/246 vs. 129/254 [n = 302][a]	1.33 (0.84–2.14) 35/153 vs. 23/134 [n = 287][a]	1.17 (0.99–1.37) [n = 501]	2.25 (0.79–6.40) [n = 583]
NOD	3.06 (0.74–12.63) [n = 33]	NC	NC	NC	0.94 (0.05–16.37) [n = 33] (neonatal)
Progesterone	N/A	N/A	N/A	N/A	N/A
COMPARISONS					
CCB vs. betamimetics	**0.72 (0.53–0.97) [n = 470]**	**0.76 (0.59–0.99) [n = 242]**	**0.79 (0.65–0.96) [n = 328] <34 wk**	0.89 (0.76–1.05) [n = 389]	1.20 (0.49–2.94) [n = 529] (excl. cong. anom.)
COX vs. betamimetics	**0.27 (0.08–0.96) [n = 100]**	0.88 (0.52–1.46) [n = 146]	NC	**0.53 (0.28–0.99) [n = 80]**	0.99 (0.27–3.57) [n = 237]
COX vs. CCB	No RCT	No RCT	No RCT	No RCT	No RCT
COX vs. Mg	0.75 (0.40–1.40) [n = 315]	NC	NC	0.55 (0.17–1.73) [n = 88]	2.31 (0.54–9.90) [n = 423]
Mg vs. betamimetics	1.08 (0.72–1.63) [n = 349]	NC	NC	0.85 (0.66–1.10) [n = 147]	1.19 (0.08–17.51) [n = 166]
Mg vs. CCB	1.20 (0.60–2.39) [n = 154]	NC	0.82 (0.45–1.50) [n = 80] <34 wk	1.04 (0.75–1.44) [n = 148]	0.19 (0.01–3.85) [n = 80]
Mg vs. COX	1.51 (0.53–4.30) [n = 101]	NC	NC	NC	0.98 (0.06–15.35) [n = 117]
ORA vs. betamimetics	0.98 (0.68–1.41) [n = 1033]	0.91 (0.69–1.20) [n = 731]	NC	0.90 (0.71–1.13) [n = 244]	0.66 (0.24–1.83) [n = 836]
ORA vs. CCB	No RCT	No RCT	No RCT	No RCT	No RCT
ORA vs. COX	No RCT	No RCT	No RCT	No RCT	No RCT
ORA vs. Mg	No RCT	No RCT	No RCT	No RCT	No RCT
NOD vs. betamimetics	1.43 (0.47–4.37) [n = 132]	1.10 (0.67–1.80) [n = 391]	1.00 (0.49–2.06) [n = 233]	**0.53 (0.35–0.81) [n = 391]**	1.03 (0.18–6.02) [n = 191]
NOD vs. Mg	N/A	N/A	N/A	N/A	N/A
PRIMARY—MULTIPLE AGENTS					
Indo and MgSO4 (vs. placebos)	N/A	N/A	N/A	1.35 (0.86–2.14) 23/43 vs. 17/43	∞ (0.51–∞) 2/47 vs. 0/45
Progesterone vs. placebo (all on ritodrine)	N/A	N/A	N/A	0.48 (0.14–1.44)	N/A
REFRACTORY					
Indo vs. sulindac	1.50 (0.32–7.17) [n = 36]	0.88 (0.40–1.88) [n = 36]	N/A	N/A	Not calculable 0/18 vs. 0/18
MAINTENANCE VS. PLACEBO					
Betamimetics (oral)	NC	NC	NC	NC	NC
Betamimetics (terb. pump) (vs. saline pump)	NC	NC	0.97 (0.51–1.84) [n = 52] <34 wk	1.17 (0.79–1.73) [n = 52]	NC
CCB (vs. no Rx)	NC	NC	NC	1.00 (0.73–1.37) [n = 74]	NC
COX	NC	NC	NC	NC	NC
Mg	NC	NC	NC	0.85 (0.47–1.51) [n = 50]	5.00 (0.25–99.17) [n = 50]
ORA	N/A	N/A	0.85 (0.47–1.54)[a] 19/158 vs. 18/127	0.89 (0.71–1.12)[a] 90/267 vs. 92/243	0.80 (0.23–2.72)[a] 4/252 vs. 5/251 (neonatal)
COMPARISONS					
Terb pump vs. po terb	NC	NC	NC	NC	NC

Data are shown as relative risk (95% confidence intervals). Significant results are shown in bold.

[a]Author's meta-analysis.

Abbreviations: PTB, preterm birth; N/A, not available in reports of studies; NC, not calculable from the available reports; no RCT, no randomized controlled trial reports on this comparison; CCB, calcium channel blocker; COX, cyclooxygenase; ORA, oxytocin receptor antagonists; NOD, nitric oxide donors; Terb, terbutaline; Mg, magnesium; Rx, therapy; excl. cong. anom, excluding congenital anomalies.

side effects, with most data reported for ritodrine. For comparison with other tocolytics, RCTS are too small and varied to make meaningful comparisons (37).

Specific contraindications: Cardiac arrhythmia or other significant cardiac disease, DM, poorly controlled thyroid disease (for ritodrine).

Side effects:

Maternal: Hyperglycemia (glucose 140–200 mg/dL in 20–50%; Mechanism: decreased peripheral insulin sensitivity and increased endogenous glucose production); hyperinsulinemia; hypokalemia ($K < 3$ mEq/L in 50%); tremors, nervousness, shortness of breath (10%), chest pain (5–10%), tachycardia/palpitations, arrhythmia (3%); EKG changes (2–3%); hypotension (2–3%); pulmonary edema (<1–5%; Mechanism: reduced sodium excretion—sodium and therefore fluid retention). Ritodrine: altered thyroid function, antidiuresis.

Fetal/Neonatal: Ritodrine: Neonatal tachycardia, hypoglycemia, hypocalcemia, hyperbilirubinemia, hypotension, IVH. Terbulatine: tachycardia, hyperinsulinemia, hyperglycemia, myocardial and septal hypertrophy, myocardial ischemia.

Calcium Channel Blockers (CCB)

Types: Nifedipine, nicardipine.

Dose: Nifedipine 20–30 mg × 1, then 10–20 mg q4–8h (max 90 mg/day) (nicardipine similar dosing).

Mechanism of action: Impair calcium channels, so inhibit influx of calcium into cell, and therefore myometrial contraction.

Evidence for effectiveness: (Table 17.6) **There are no studies of CCB compared with placebo for PTB prevention.**

When compared with any other tocolytic agent (mainly betamimetics, 9/12 trials), CCB reduce by 24% the number of women giving birth within 7 days of receiving treatment and by 17% PTB prior to 34 weeks' gestation (38). CCB show a trend to reduce PTB within 48 hours of initiation of treatment (RR 0.80, 95% CI 0.61–1.05), and PTB < 37 weeks' gestation (RR 0.95, 95% CI 0.83–1.09). **CCB also reduce by 37% the frequency of neonatal RDS, by 79% NEC, by 41% IVH, and by 27% neonatal jaundice. CCB also reduced the requirement for women to have treatment ceased for adverse drug reaction.** There are insufficient data regarding the effects of different dosage regimens and formulations of CCB on maternal and neonatal outcomes; the most studied is nifedipine, at dosage shown above. **CCB should be preferred to betamimetics for tocolysis.**

Specific contraindications: Cardiac disease; hypotension (<90/50); concominant use of magnesium; caution in renal disease.

Side effects:

Maternal: Flushing, headache, dizziness, nausea, transient hypotension. Caution in women with hypotension and renal disease, as well as women on magnesium (cardiovascular collapse).

Fetal/Neonatal: None.

Cyclooxygenase (COX) Inhibitors

Types: Nonselective COX inhibitors: indomethacin (indocin). Selective COX inhibitors (preferential COX-2 inhibitor): sulindac, rofecoxib (Vioxx), celecoxib, nimesulide.

Dose: Indomethacin: 50 to 100 mg loading dose (rectal or vaginal route preferred, oral otherwise), then 25–50 mg q6h **for 48 hours max,** and **always** <32 weeks. Sulindac 200 mg po q12h × 48 hours. Ketorolac: 60 mg IM, then 30 mg IM q6h × 48 hours.

Mechanism of action: COX inhibitors, so inhibit prostaglandin synthesis, therefore inhibit myometrial contraction.

Evidence for effectiveness: (Table 17.6) (The nonselective COX inhibitor, indomethacin, was used in most trials.)

When compared with placebo, COX inhibition (indomethacin only) results in a 79% reduction in PTB < 37 weeks' gestation in a small trial, an increase in GA of 3.5 weeks and a >700 g increase in birth weight (39). There is a trend toward a reduction in delivery within 48 hours of initiation of treatment (RR 0.20, 95% CI 0.03–1.28) and within 7 days (RR 0.41, 95% CI 0.10–1.66). No differences were detected in any other reported outcomes including perinatal mortality, RDS, etc.

Used for 48 hours only, the **intravaginal** route (100 mg q12h) decreases delivery at 48 hours and at <7 days compared to rectal/oral (100 mg rectally, followed by 25 mg po), with some improvement in neonatal morbidities in a small trial (40).

Compared with any other tocolytic, COX inhibition resulted in a 47% reduction in PTB < 37 weeks' gestation and a reduction in maternal drug reaction requiring cessation of treatment (39). No differences were detected in the fetal or neonatal outcomes such as perinatal mortality, RDS, intraventricular hemorrhage, NEC, premature closure of the ductus, persistent pulmonary hypertension of the newborn (PPHN).

Compared with **betamimetics**, COX inhibitors are associated with a **significant** 73% **reduction in the number of women delivering within 48 hours of initiation of treatment** (39).

Compared with **magnesium sulfate,** COX inhibitors are associated with trends for lower number of women delivering within 48 hours and lower PTB < 37 weeks (39).

A comparison of nonselective COX inhibitors versus selective COX-2 inhibitors does not demonstrate any differences in maternal or neonatal outcomes (41,42). Due to small numbers, all estimates of effect are imprecise and need to be interpreted with caution.

Specific contraindications: Renal or hepatic disease, active peptic ulcer disease, poorly controlled hypertension, nonsteroidal anti-inflammatory drug (NSAID)-sensitive asthma, coagulation disorders/thrombocytopenia.

Side effects: When used for only 48 hours, no serious maternal and fetal/neonatal side effects occur, and fetal surveillance is not indicated. Usually COX inhibitors are better tolerated by mother than other tocolytics such as magnesium and betamimetics.

Maternal: As with any NSAIDs, mild gastrointestinal (GI) upset—nausea, heartburn (take with some food/milk) (COX-1). GI bleeding (COX-1), coagulation, and platelet abnormalities (COX-1), asthma if ASA-sensitive. May obscure elevation in temperature. Long-term rofecoxib (Vioxx) use in adults has been associated with stroke, so this drug is now not available in many countries.

Fetal/neonatal: In trials, 403 women received short-term tocolysis (up to 48 hours) with COX inhibitors (mainly indomethacin) and there was only one case of antenatal **closure of the ductus arteriosus.** There was no increase in the incidence of patent ductus arteriosus (PDA) postnatally (eight treated with COX inhibitors versus eight treated with placebo or other tocolytics) (39). No difference in incidences of IVH, BPD, PDA, NEC, or perinatal mortality was noted in a review of trials aimed at evaluating safety (43). Use for **>48 hours,** especially ≥32 weeks, is associated with significant fetal effects such as constriction of the ductus arteriosus, which can lead to hydrops, pulmonary hypertension and death, and **renal insufficiency,** manifested in utero by oligohydramnios. Other effects with prolonged use such as hyperbilirubinemia, NEC, IVH have not been shown with <72 use. Selective COX-2 inhibitors have not been shown consistently to be any safer for the fetus/neonate than nonselective COX inhibitors such as indomethacin. Therefore, **continuous use of COX inhibitors for >48 hours and ≥32 weeks is contraindicated.**

Magnesium Sulfate (MgSO₄)

Dose: 40 g MgSO₄ in 1 L 1/2NS. Initial: 4 to 6 g/30 min, then 2 to 4 g/hr. A dose of 5 g/hr has not been shown beneficial in perinatal outcome compared with a dose of 2 g/hr, and is associated with significant side effects (44). Weaning MgSO₄ tocolysis has no benefits and a few harmful side effects compared with stopping MgSO₄ abruptly (45).

Mechanism of action: Intracellular calcium antagonist.

Evidence for effectiveness: (Table 17.6) Compared with placebo, there is **insufficient evidence** to show if MgSO₄ reduces the incidence of PTB or perinatal morbidity and mortality (46).

Compared with all controls (including other tocolytics), MgSO₄ did not prevent PTB at 48 hours, PTB < 37 weeks or < 32 weeks. Perinatal death was higher (only 2 perinatal deaths), while perinatal morbidities were similar. Dose of magnesium did not affect efficacy. Given these results, there is **no convincing evidence for recommending magnesium for tocolysis** (47).

Specific contraindications: Myasthenia gravis.

Management: Aim for 4 to 7 MgSO4 level. Monitor urinary output. Follow deep tendon reflexes: ↓ at level ≥8, absent ≥10. At ≥10, respiratory depression; at ≥ 15, risk of cardiac arrest.

Side effects:

Maternal: Flushing, lethargy, headache, muscle weakness, diplopia, dry mouth, pulmonary edema (1%; Mechanism: intravenous overhydration), cardiac arrest.

Fetal/Neonatal: Lethargy, hypotonia, hypocalcemia, respiratory depression. Prolonged use: demineralization.

Oxytocin Receptor Antagonists (ORA)

Types: Atosiban (Tractocile); barusiban.

Dose: Atosiban 6.75 mg bolus, then 300 µg/min IV × 3 hours, then 100 µg/min (max 45 hours).

Mechanism of action: Competitive inhibitor of oxytocin via blockade of oxytocin receptor.

Evidence for effectiveness: (Table 17.6) **Compared with placebo, atosiban does not reduce incidence of PTB or improve neonatal outcome** (48). In one trial, atosiban was associated with an increase in infant deaths at 12 months of age compared with placebo (49). However, this trial randomized significantly more women to atosiban before 26 weeks' gestation. Compared with placebo, use of atosiban results in about 140 g lower infant birth weight and more mild maternal adverse drug reactions (48). Compared with betamimetics, atosiban is associated with similar incidences of PTB and perinatal morbidity/mortality, and with fewer maternal drug reactions requiring treatment cessation (48). There is insufficient evidence to assess effectiveness of a different ORA, barusiban, as only one RCT has tested it against placebo at 34 to 35 weeks, with no changes in recorded outcomes (50). Therefore, **as per magnesium, the only evidence supporting use of oxytocin receptor agonists for primary tocolysis is that they have less side effects than the (effective) betamimetics.**

Side effects: Minimal to none.

Nitric Oxide Donors

Type: Nitroglycerine.

Dose: Nitroglycerine transdermal patch 0.4 mg/hr.

Mechanism of action: Direct relaxation of uterine muscle.

Evidence for effectiveness: (Table 17.6) There is currently **insufficient evidence** to support the routine administration of nitric oxide donors (NOD) for prevention of PTB in women with PTL (51). Compared with placebo, NOD do not prevent PTB or improve perinatal morbidity and mortality in a small trial (52). Compared with betamimetics, NOD are associated with a decreased PTB < 37 weeks. Incidences of PTB and perinatal mortality were not reported in the only trial comparing NOD to magnesium sulfate. While headaches are more common in women receiving NOD compared with controls, other side effects are less common compared with other tocolytics. Nitroglycerine has been the only NOD used in trials.

Progesterone

There is **insufficient data** to assess the efficacy for progesterone as primary tocolysis. The two RCTs to assess safety and efficacy of any type of progesterone as primary tocolysis (compared with no treatment or with other tocolytic) are small, in general of poor quality, over 20 years old, and at times did not report PTB outcomes (53). In one of these RCTs, in 57 women admitted between 13 and 36 weeks with contractions, progesterone 400 mg orally once was associated with a significant decrease in the frequency of contractions, but no PTB or neonatal outcomes were reported (54).

Primary Tocolysis—Multiple Agents Simultaneously

Indomethacin, ampicillin-sulbactam, and Magnesium Vs. Magnesium alone

Compared with placebos, indomethacin and ampicillin-sulbactam did not prevent PTB in women in PTL already receiving magnesium sulfate tocolysis (55).

Primary Tocolysis—Additional Agents Vs. One Agent Only

Progesterone Vs. Placebo, in Addition to Ritodrine

Compared with placebo, in women receiving ritodrine tocolysis, the addition of progesterone was not associated with a significant reduction in PTB < 37 weeks (16% vs. 33% in placebo) in a very small trial (53,56). In detail, in this RCT, in 44 women with mostly (>90%) singleton gestations and threatened PTL at less than 35 weeks treated with ritodrine, natural progesterone 400 mg orally q6h × 24 hours (then 400 mg q8h for next 24 hours, and then 300 mg q8h onward) was associated with similar incidence of PTB, with less quantity of ritodrine administered and shorter maternal hospital stay compared with placebo (56).

Refractory Tocolysis—Primary Agent Is Failing

Indomethacin is similar to sulindac in prevention of PTB in women failing primary magnesium sulfate tocolysis in a small trial (57).

Maintenance Tocolysis—After Successful Primary Tocolysis

Betamimetics (Oral)

Dose: Ritodrine: 1–20 mg po q2–4h. Terbutaline: 2.5–5 mg po q2–4h.

Evidence for effectiveness: Compared with **placebo**, oral betamimetic therapy for maintenance tocolysis **does not prevent PTB, recurrent PTL, recurrent hospitalizations, or perinatal morbidity and mortality** (58). Some adverse effects such as tachycardia are more frequent in the betamimetics group. Given this ample evidence from 13 trials, there is **absolutely no evidence** to support the use of oral betamimetics after PTL has resolved.

Terbutaline Pump
Dose: 0.05 mg/hr.
Evidence for effectiveness: Compared with **placebo,** terbutaline pump does not prevent PTB or improve perinatal morbidity and mortality. Side effects and costs associated with this therapy further **advice against its use** (59).

Calcium Channel Blockers
There is insufficient evidence to assess the efficacy of CCB maintenance therapy after successful tocolysis. In three small RCTs, the incidence of PTB < 37 weeks was similar to placebo (60), or no treatment (61,62).

COX Inhibitors
Compared with **placebo,** after successful tocolysis, oral sulindac either 200 mg q12h × 7 days or 100 mg q12h until 34 weeks does not reduce PTB compared with placebo (63,64). Given the association with fetal/neonatal complications with COX inhibitor use for >48 hours, COX inhibitors should not be used for maintenance tocolysis.

Compared with oral **terbutaline,** oral indomethacin is associated with a similar incidence of PTB when used for maintenance tocolysis after successful IV tocolysis, but indomethacin is associated with significant constriction of ductus arteriosus and oligohydramnios when used for >48 hours (65). Therefore, indomethacin should not be used for maintenance tocolysis, especially after 26 weeks.

Magnesium Sulfate
Compared with **placebo,** or **no treatment,** magnesium maintenance therapy **does not prevent PTB** (RR 1.05, 95% CI 0.80–1.40**) or affect perinatal morbidity and mortality** (mortality, RR 5.00, 95% CI 0.25–99.16) (66). It has also similar effect on PTB as alternative tocolytic drugs (RR 0.99, 95% CI 0.57–1.72) (i.e., it is equally ineffective). Therefore, magnesium sulfate should not be used as a maintenance tocolytic.

Oxytocin Receptor Antagonists
Compared with **placebo,** ORA (atosiban) maintenance therapy (30 μg/min) via pump up to 36 weeks does not prevent PTB or affect perinatal morbidity and mortality, with a 5 days (32.6 vs. 27.6, p = 0.02) longer interval to delivery in one trial (67). There are no side effects compared with placebo except for injection-site reactions. ORA are not available in oral form for maintenance.

Progesterone
Compared with identical placebo, progesterone IM injections did not prevent PTB in women discharged home after an episode of PTL in one old quasi-RCT (68). In a small RCT, compared with no 17P, 17P 341 mg IM twice a week at 25 to 33 weeks and then weekly until 36 weeks given after resolved PTL was associated with prevention of PTB (OR 0.15, 95% CI 0.04–0.58) and of cervical shortening (69). In another small RCT, compared with no vaginal progesterone, vaginal progesterone 400 mg daily until delivery was associated with longer latency to delivery and better neonatal outcomes (significantly less RDS) (70). In summary, **there is insufficient evidence to recommend progesterone for prevention of PTB in women who remain pregnant after an episode of PTL,** but recent evidence is encouraging.

PTL RESOLVED: HOME VS. IN-HOSPITAL CARE
After PTL has resolved (and cervical dilatation has not progressed ≥ 4 cm), **home management is associated with similar incidences of reaching ≥36 weeks compared with** hospital management (71,72). Hospitalization may increase maternal stress, vaginal examinations, time in recumbent position (and its consequences), and decreased plasma volume. **For the many women with arrested PTL, continued hospitalization after steroids administration seems unnecessary.**

PRECONCEPTION COUNSELING
Given its major impact of perinatal morbidity and mortality, it is important to **review risk factors for PTB in every pregnant woman.** In the woman with a risk factor (e.g., prior PTB), it is important to review prognosis, possible complications, and management of a future pregnancy (see above).

PRENATAL CARE
Preconception counseling as above, if not already done. Management should follow recommendations as above (Table 17.4). See also chapter 2.

ANTEPARTUM TESTING
No specific fetal testing is indicated. Home Uterine Activity Monitoring (HUAM), discussed in chapter 16, is not effective in preventing any complication.

DELIVERY
Mode
There is **insufficient evidence** to evaluate the use of a policy for uniform planned cesarean delivery (CD) compared with expectant management and selective CD for preterm (about 24–36 weeks) babies (73). Mothers in the planned CD group have more morbidity. Babies in the planned CD group show no statistical differences compared with expectant management, but trend to have less RDS, less neonatal seizures, and fewer deaths, although they were more likely to have a low cord pH immediately after delivery in the small trials that reported in these outcomes (73). Differentiation of data between breech and vertex presentations is difficult, with numbers too small for definite conclusions.

Delayed Cord Clamping
In preterm neonates, delayed cord clamping by about 30 to 60 seconds (120 maximum) is associated with fewer transfusions for anemia, less hypotension, and less intraventricular hemorrhage than early clamping at less than 30 seconds (74).

Milking of cord has been evaluated in two small RCTs in preterm neonates, so there is insufficient evidence for recommendation, even if it appears as beneficial as delayed cord clamping. Compared with no milking, milking of cord has been associated with less need for blood transfusions and less need for circulatory and respiratory support (75). Compared with 30-second delayed cord clamping, milking of cord four times achieved a similar amount of placento-fetal blood transfusion (76).

ANESTHESIA
No specific changes.

POSTPARTUM/BREASTFEEDING
As in other pregnancies, breastfeeding is encouraged as tolerated for the preterm infant. Extensive counseling should be provided regarding rate of recurrence of PTB, and future

management in pregnancy (see above). Treatment with antibiotics before pregnancy does not prevent recurrent PTB. **In women with a prior spontaneous PTB < 34 weeks, oral azythromycin and metronidazole every 4 months after the PTB and before the next conception does not significantly reduce subsequent PTB,** but is in fact associated with trends for earlier GA at delivery and lower birth weight (77) (see also chap. 16).

REFERENCES

1. Pereira L, Gould R, Pelham J, et al. Correlation between visual examination of the cervix and digital examination. J Matern Fetal Neonatal Med 2005; 17:223–227. [II-2]
2. Berghella V, Baxter JK, Hendrix NW. Cervical assessment by ultrasound for preventing preterm delivery. Cochrane Database of Syst Rev 2009; (3):CD007235. [Meta-analysis: 3 RCTs, n = 290]
3. Berghella V, Hayes E, Visintine J, et al. Fetal fibronectin testing for reducing the risk of preterm birth. Cochrane Database of Syst Rev 2008; (4):CD006843. [Meta-analysis: 5 RCTs, n = 474]
4. Ness A, Visintine J, Ricci E, et al. Does knowledge of cervical length and fetal fibronectin affect management of women with preterm labor? A randomized trial. Am J Obstet Gynecol 2007; 197(4):426.e1–426.e7. [RCT]
5. Horbar JD, Carpenter JH, Kenny M, eds. Vermont Oxford Network 2007 Very Low Birth Weight Summary. Burlington, VT: Vermont Oxford Network, 2008. [Epidemiologic data]
6. American College of Obstetricians and Gynecologists. ACOG Practice Bulletin, No. 38: Perinatal care at the threshold of viability. Washington, D.C.: ACOG, 2002. [Review]
7. Gomez R, Romero R, Medina L, et al. Cervicovaginal fibronectin improves the prediction of preterm delivery based on sonographic cervical length in patients with preterm uterine contractions and intact membranes. Am J Obstet Gynecol 2005; 192:350–359. [II-3]
8. American College of Obstetricians and Gynecologists. ACOG Practice Bulletin No. 43: Management of preterm labor. Washington, D.C.: ACOG, 2003. [Review]
9. Gomez R, Romero R, Nien JK, et al. A short cervix in women with preterm labor and intact membranes: a risk factor for microbial invasion of the amniotic cavity. Am J Obstet Gynecol 2005; 192:678–689. [II-3]
10. Roberts D, Dalziel SR. Antenatal corticosteroids for accelerating fetal lung maturation for women at risk of preterm birth. Cochrane Database Syst Rev 2006; (3):CD004454. [Meta-analysis: 18 RCTs, n >3700]
11. Hayes EJ, Paul DA, Stahl GE, et al. Effect of antenatal corticosteroids on survival of neonates born at 23 weeks of gestation. Obstet Gynecol 2008; 111:921–926. [II-1]
12. Egerman RS, Maercer BM, Doss JL, et al. A randomized controlled trial of oral and intramuscular dexamethasone in the prevention of neonatal respiratory distress syndrome. Am J Obstet Gynecol 1998; 179:1120–1126. [RCT, n = 170]
13. Brownfoot FC, Crowther CA, Middleton P. Different corticosteroids and regimens for accelerating fetal lung maturation for women at risk of preterm birth. Cochrane Database Syst Rev 2008; (4). [Meta-analysis: 10 RCTs, n = 1089]
14. Guinn DA, Atkinson MW, Sullivan L, et al. Single vs weekly courses of antenatal corticosteroids for women at risk of preterm delivery: a randomized trial. JAMA 2001; 286:1581. [RCT, n = 502]
15. Garite TJ, Kurtzman J, Maurel K, et al. Impact of a 'rescue course' of antenatal corticosteroids: a multicenter randomized placebo-controlled trial. Am J Obstet Gynecol 2009; 200:248. [RCT, n = 437].
16. McEvoy C, Schilling D, Peters D, et al. Respiratory compliance in preterm infants after a single rescue course of antenatal steroids: a randomized controlled trial. Am J Obstet Gynecol 2010; 202:544. [RCT, n = 44]
17. Peltoniemi OM, Kari MA, Tammela O, et al. Randomized trial of a single repeat dose of prenatal betamethasone treatment in imminent preterm birth. Pediatrics 2006; 119:290–298. [RCT, n = 249]
18. Crowther CA, McKinlay CJD, Middleton P, et al. Repeat doses of prenatal corticosteroids for women at risk of preterm birth for improving neonatal health outcomes. Cochrane Database Syst Rev 2011; (6). [Meta-analysis: 10 RCTs, n = 4730]
19. Wapner RJ for NICHD MFMU Network. A randomized trial of single versus weekly courses of corticosteroids. Am J Obstet Gynecol 2003; A2:S56. [RCT, n = 495]
20. Murphy KE, Hannah ME, Willan AR, et al. Multiple courses of antenatal corticosteroids for preterm birth (MACS): a randomized controlled trial. Lancet 2008; 372:2143–2151. [RCT, n = 1858]
21. Crowther CA, Harding J. Repeat doses of prenatal corticosteroids for women at risk of preterm birth for preventing neonatal respiratory disease. Cochrane Database Syst Rev 2005; (3). [Meta-analysis: 3 RCTs, n = 551]
22. Crowther CA, Alfirevic Z, Haslam RR. Thyrotropin-releasing hormone added to corticosteroids for women at risk of preterm birth for preventing neonatal respiratory disease. Cochrane Database Syst Rev 2005; (3). [Meta-analysis: 13 RCTs, n = >4600]
23. Crowther CA, Henderson-Smart DJ. Phenobarbital prior to preterm birth for preventing neonatal periventricular haemorrhage. Cochrane Database Syst Rev 2005; (3). [Meta-analysis: 9 RCTs, n = 1750]
24. Shankaran S, Papile L, Wright L, et al. The effects of antenatal phenobarbital therapy on neonatal intracranial haemorrhage in preterm infants. N Engl J Med 1997; 337:466–471. [RCT, n = 610]
25. Thorp JA, Ferrette-Smith D, Gaston L, et al. Antenatal vitamin K (VK) and phenobarbital (PH) for preventing intracranial hemorrhage (ICH) in the premature newborn: a randomized double blinded placebo controlled trial. Am J Obstet Gynecol 1995; 172:253. [RCT, n = 353]
26. Crowther CA, Crosby DD. Vitamin K prior to preterm birth for preventing neonatal periventricular haemorrhage. Cochrane Database Syst Rev 2010; (1):CD000229. [Meta-analysis: 8 RCTs, n = 843]
27. Doyle LW, Crowther CA, Middleton P, et al. Magnesium sulphate for women at risk of preterm birth for neuroprotection of the fetus. Cochrane Database Syst Rev 2009; (1):CD004661. [Meta-analysis: 5 RCTs, n = 6145]
28. Rouse D, Hirtz D, Thom E, et al. Magnesium sulfate for the prevention of cerebral palsy. N Engl J Med 2008; 359:895–905. [RCT, n = 2241]
29. Crowther CA, Neilson JP, Verkuyl DAA, et al. Preterm labour in twin pregnancies: can it be prevented by hospital admission? BJOG 1989; 96:850–853. [RCT, n = 139]
30. Stan C, Boulvain M, Hirsbrunner-Amagbaly P. et al. Hydration for treatment of preterm labour. Cochrane Database Syst Rev 2005; (3). [2 RCTs, n = 228]
31. King J, Flenady V. Prophylactic antibiotics for inhibiting preterm labour with intact membranes. Cochrane Database Syst Rev 2005; (3). [11 RCTs, n = 7428]
32. Kenyon SL, Taylor DJ, Tarnow-Mordi W. Broad-spectrum antibiotics for spontaneous preterm labour: the ORACLE II randomised trial. Lancet 2001; 357:991–996. [RCT, n = 6295. (i) 325 mg co-amoxiclav plus 250 mg erythromycin; (ii) 325 mg co-amoxiclav plus erythromycin placebo; (iii) 250 mg erythromycin plus co-amoxiclav placebo; (iv) co-amoxiclav placebo plus erythromycin placebo. All study medication was given orally every six hours for 10 days or until delivery.]
33. McGregor JA, French JI, Seo K. Adjunctive clindamycin therapy for preterm labor: results of a double-blind, placebo-controlled trial. Am J Obstet Gynecol 1991; 165(4):867–875. [RCT, n = 117. IV clindamycin 900 mg every 8 hours × 9 doses or identical placebo. IV therapy was followed by oral clindamycin 300 mg every 6 hours × 4 days VS identical placebo]
34. Norman K, Pattinson RC, de Souza J, et al. Ampicillin and metronidazole treatment in preterm labour: a multicentre, randomised controlled trial. BJOG 1994; 101:404–408. [RCT, n = 82. IV ampicillin 1 g every 6 hours × 4 doses followed by oral amoxicillin 500 mg every 8 hours × 5 days, plus metronidazole 1 g stat then 400 mg orally every 8 hours for 5 days, or corresponding placebos.]

35. Svare J, Langhoff-Roos J, Andersen LF, et al. Ampicillin-metronidazole treatment in idiopathic preterm labour: a randomised controlled multicentre trial. BJOG 1997; 104:892–897. [RCT, *n* = 112. IV ampicillin 2 g every 6 hours for 24 hours, followed by pivampicin 500 mg orally for 7 days, plus IV metronidazole 500 mg every 8 hours for 24 hours, followed by metronidazole 400 mg orally every 8 hours for 7 days, or identical placebo]

36. Childhood outcomes after prescription of antibiotics to pregnant women with spontaneous preterm labor: 7-year follow-up of the ORACLE II trial. Lancet 2008; 372:1319–1327. [RCT, *n* = 3196]

37. Anotayanonth S, Subhedar NV, Neilson JP, et al. Betamimetics for inhibiting preterm labour. Cochrane Database Syst Rev 2004; (4):CD004352. [Meta-analysis: 17 RCTs, *n* > 1332]

38. King JF, Flenady VJ, Papatsonis DNM, et al. Calcium channel blockers for inhibiting preterm labour. Cochrane Database Syst Rev 2005; (3). [Meta-analysis: 12 RCTs, *n* = 1029]

39. King J, Flenady V, Cole S, et al. Cyclo-oxygenase (COX) inhibitors for treating preterm labour. Cochrane Database Syst Rev 2005; (3): CD001992. [Meta-analysis: 13 RCTs, *n* = 713]

40. Abramov Y, Nadjari M, Weinstein D, et al. Indomethacin for preterm labor: a randomized comparison of vaginal and rectal routes. Obstet Gynecol 2000; 95:482–486. [RCT, *n* = 46].

41. Sawdy RJ, Lye S, Fisk NM, et al. A double-blind randomized study of fetal side effects during and after the short-term maternal administration of indomethacin, sulindac, and nimesulide for the treatment of preterm labor. Am J Obstet Gynecol 2003; 188:1046–1051. [RCT, *n* = 30. Sulindac 200 mg orally and a placebo suppository every 12 hours; vs. nimesulide 200 mg rectally and a placebo capsule orally every 12 hours; vs. indomethacin 100 mg rectally and a placebo capsule orally every 12 hours]

42. Stika CS, Gross GA, Leguizamon G, et al. A prospective randomized safety trial of celecoxib for treatment of preterm labor. Am J Obstet Gynecol 2002; 187(3):653–660. [RCT, *n* = 24. Indomethacin suppository 100 mg then 50 mg po q6h for 48 hours plus oral placebo vs. celecoxib po 100 mg initially then 100 mg q12h for 48 hours plus rectal and oral placebo]

43. Loe SM, Sanchez-Ramos L, Kaunitz A. Assessing the neonatal safety of indomethacon tocolysis: a systematic review with meta-analysis. Obstet Gynecol 2005; 106:173–179. [Meta-analysis of safety of indomethacin: *n* = 1621 fetuses exposed to indomethacin in RCTs and observational studies]

44. Terrone DA, Rinehart BK, Kimmel ES, et al. A prospective randomized controlled trial of high and low maintenance doses of magnesium sulfate for acute tocolysis. Am J Obstet Gynecol 2000; 182:1477–1482. [RCT, *n* = 160. All pts: MgSO₄ 4-g load, then RCT to 2 g vs. 5 g/hr]

45. Lewis DF, Bergstedt S, Edwards MS, et al. Successful magnesium sulfate tocolysis: is "weaning" the drug necessary? Am J Obstet Gynecol 1997; 177:742–745. [RCT, *n* = 140. Stop MgSO₄ abruptly vs. wean approx. 1 g q4h]

46. Crowther CA, Hiller JE, Doyle LW. Magnesium sulfate for preventing preterm birth in threatened preterm labour. Cochrane Database Syst Rev 2005; (3). [Meta-analysis: 23 RCTs, *n* = >2000]

47. Mercer BM, Merlino AA, for SMFM. Magnesium sulfate for preterm labor and preterm birth. Obstet Gynecol 2009; 114:650–668. [Meta-analysis: 19 RCTs]

48. Papatsonis D, Flenady V, Cole S, et al. Oxytocin receptor antagonists for inhibiting preterm labour. Cochrane Database Syst Rev 2005 (3):CD004452. [6 RCTs, *n* = 1695]

49. Romero R, Sibai BM, Sanchez-Ramos L, et al. An oxytocin receptor antagonist (atosiban) in the treatment of preterm labor: a randomized, double-blind, placebo-controlled trial with tocolytic rescue. Am J Obstet Gynecol 2000; 182(5):1173–1183. [RCT, *n* = 531. Atosiban group: initial bolus of 6.75 mg atosiban administered over 1 minute. Followed by an infusion of 300 µg/min for 3 hours followed by an infusion of 100 µg/min atosiban for 45 hours. When uterine quiescence was achieved maintenance therapy was continued subcutaneously with either atosiban or placebo until the end of the 36th week of gestation. Control: initial bolus or placebo administered over 1 minute. Followed by an

infusion of placebo for 48 hours. Maintenance therapy with subcutaneous placebo until 36 weeks]

50. Thornton S, Goodwin TM, Greisen G, et al. The effect of barusiban, a selective oxytocin antagonist, in threatened preterm labor at late gestational age: a randomized, double-blind, placebo-controlled trial. Am J Obstet Gynecol 2009; 200:627. [RCT, *n* = 163]

51. Durckitt K, Thornton S. Nitric oxide donors for the treatment of preterm labour. Cochrane Database Syst Rev 2005 (3). [Meta-analysis: 5 RCTs, *n* = 466]

52. Smith GN, Walker MC, McGrath MJ. Randomized double-blind, placebo controlled trial assessing nitroglycerin as a tocolytic. BJOG 1999; 106:736–739. [RCT, *n* = 33. GTN transdermal patch 9.6 mg/24 hour for 48 hours vs. placebo]

53. Su LL, Samuel M, Chong YS. Progestational agents for treating threatened or established preterm labour. Cochrane Database Syst Rev 2010; (1):CD006770. [2 RCTs on PTL; 1 RCT as adjuvant tocolysis; 1 RCT as maintenance tocolysis]

54. Erny R, Pigne A, Prouvost C, et al. The effects of oral administration of progesterone for premature labor. Am J Obstet Gynecol 1986; 154:525–529. [RCT, *n* = 57]

55. Newton ER, Shields L, Rigway LE, et al. Combination antibiotics and indomethacin in idiopathic preterm labor: a randomized double-blind study. Am J Obstet Gynecol 1991; 165:1753–1759. [RCT, *n* = 86]

56. Noblot G, Audra P, Dargent D, et al. The use of micronized progesterone in the treatment of menace of preterm delivery. Eur J Obstet Gynecol Reprod Biol 1991; 40:203–209. [RCT, *n* = 40 singletons]

57. Carlan S, O'Brien WF, O'Leary TD, et al. Randomized comparative trial of indomethacin and sulindac for the treatment of refractory preterm labor. Obstet Gynecol 1992; 79:223–228. [RCT, *n* = 36]

58. Dodd JM, Crowther CA, Dare MR, et al. Oral betamimetics for maintenance therapy after threatened preterm labour. Cochrane Database Syst Rev 2006; (1). [Meta-analysis: 13 RCTs, *n* = 1551]

59. Nanda K, Cook LA, Gallo MF, et al. Terbutaline pump maintenance therapy after threatened preterm labour for preventing preterm birth. Cochrane Database Syst Rev 2005; (3). [Meta-analysis: 2 RCTs, *n* = 94]

60. Carr DB, Clark AL, Kernek K, et al. Maintenance oral nifedipine for preterm labor: a randomized clinical trial. Am J Obstet Gynecol 1999; 181:822–827. [RCT, *n* = 74]

61. Lyell DJ, Pullen KM, Mannan J, et al. Maintenance nifedipine tocolysis compared with placebo—a randomized controlled trial. Obstet Gynecol 2008; 112:1221–1226. [RCT, *n* = 71]

62. Sayin NC, Varol FG, Balkanli-Kaplan P, et al. Oral nifedipine maintenance therapy after acute intravenous tocolysis in preterm labor. J Perinat Med 2004; 32:220–224. [RCT, *n* = 73]

63. Carlan SJ, O'Brien WF, Jones MH, et al. Outpatient oral sulindac to prevent recurrence of preterm labor. Obstet Gynecol 1995; 85:769–774. [RCT, *n* = 69; sulindac 200 mg × 7 day vs. placebo]

64. Humprey RG, Bartfield MC, Carlan SJ, et al. Sulindac to prevent recurrent preterm labor: a randomized controlled trial. Obstet Gynecol 2001; 98:555–562. [RCT, *n* = 95. Sulindac 100 mg until 34 w vs. placebo]

65. Bivins HA, Newman RB, Fyfe DA, et al. Randomized trial of oral indomethacin and terbutaline for the long-term suppression of preterm labor. Am J Obstet Gynecol 1993; 169:1065–1070. [RCT, *n* = 71]

66. Han S, Crowther CA, Moore V. Magnesium maintenance therapy for preventing preterm birth after threatened preterm labour. Cochrane Database Syst Rev 2010; (7):CD000940. [4 RCTs, *n* = 422]

67. Valenzuela GJ, Sanchez-Ramos L, Romero R, et al. Maintenance treatment of preterm labor with the oxytocin antagonist atosiban. Am J Obstet Gynecol 2000; 182:1184–1190. [RCT, *n* = 503]

68. Fuchs F, Stakeman G. Treatment of threatened premature labor with large doses of progesterone. Am J Obstet Gynecol 1960; 79:172–176. [RCT, *n* = 126]

69. Facchinetti F, Paganelli S, Comitini G, et al. Cervical length changes during preterm cervical ripening: effects of 17-alpha-

hydroxyprogesterone caproate. Am J Obstet Gynecol 2007; 196:453. [RCT, $n = 60$].

70. Borna S, Sahabi N. Progesterone for maintenance tocolytic therapy after threatened preterm labor: a randomized controlled trial. Austr NZ J Obstet Gynecol 2008; 48:58–63. [RCT, $n = 70$]

71. Yost NP, Bloom SL, McIntire DD, et al. Hospitalization for women with arrested preterm labor. Obstet Gynecol 2005; 106:14–18. [RCT, $n = 101$]

72. Goulet C, Gevry H, Lemay M, et al. A randomized clinical trial of care for women with preterm labour: home management versus hospital management. CMAJ 2001; 164:985–991. [RCT, $n = 250$]

73. Grant A, Glazener CMA. Elective caesarean section versus expectant management for delivery of the small baby. Cochrane Database Syst Rev 2005; (3). [Meta-analysis: 6 RCTs, $n = 122$]

74. Rabe H, Reynolds G, Diaz-Rossello J. Early versus delayed umbilical cord clamping in preterm infants. Cochrane Database Syst Rev 2010; (3). [7 RCTs, $n = 297$. All are small trials]

75. Hosono S, Mugishima H, Fijita H, etc. Umbilical cord milking reduces the need for red blood cell transfusions and improves neonatal adaptation in infants born at less than 29 weeks' gestation: a randomized controlled trial. Arch Dis Child Fetal Neonatal Ed 2008; 93:F14–F19. [RCT, $n = 40$].

76. Rabe H, Jewison A, Fernadez Alvarez R, et al. Milking compared to delayed cord clamping to increase placental transfusion in preterm neonates. Obstet Gynecol 2011; 117:205–211. [RCT, $n = 58$]

77. Andrews WW, Goldenberg RL, Hauth JC, et al. Interconceptional antibiotics to prevent spontaneous preterm birth: a randomized clinical trial. Am J Obstet Gynecol 2006; 194:617–623. [RCT, $n = 241$]

18

Preterm premature rupture of membranes

Anna Locatelli, Marianna Andreani, and Patrizia Vergani

KEY POINTS

- Definite diagnosis is by direct visualization of fluid ("**pooling**"), with **nitrazine** cervicovaginal swab and **ferning** as usual confirmatory tests.
- **Complications** of preterm premature rupture of membranes (PPROM) include **premature labor/delivery** with related complications of prematurity such as **respiratory distress syndrome (RDS), intraventricular hemorrhage (IVH) and periventricular leukomalacia (PVL), infection and necrotizing enterocolitis (NEC);** maternal or neonatal infections (**chorioamnionitis, endometritis, and sepsis); abruptio placentae, cord prolapse,** and, especially for PPROM <24 weeks, **perinatal death, pulmonary hypoplasia (PH), compression deformities, long-term infant morbidities, increased need for cesarean delivery (CD),** and **retained placenta**.
- If intrauterine infection, labor, or nonreassuring fetal heart rate tracing (NRFHT) is present, delivery is indicated.
- **Corticosteroids** should be administered in women with PPROM at 24 to 33 6/7 weeks, as this intervention is associated with **lower** incidences of **RDS, IVH, NEC,** and a trend for a lower **neonatal death rate.**
- **Antibiotics** (in particular **ampicillin and erythromycin** or **erythromycin alone)** are associated with less **chorioamnionitis, preterm birth (PTB) within 48 hours, PTB within 7 days, neonatal infection, surfactant use, oxygen therapy,** and **abnormal cerebral ultrasound scan** (including IVH). RDS and **NEC** are also decreased with ampicillin and erythromycin treatment.
- **Tocolytic therapy in women with PPROM is not associated with maternal or perinatal benefits** and should, in general, be avoided. Tocolysis may only be used in selected cases for ≤48 hours to allow administration of corticosteroids; such a regimen should always be accompanied by antibiotic prophylaxis.
- **Expectant management of PPROM in women with cerclage in place is associated with significantly increased maternal and fetal/neonatal infection risks. Therefore, the cerclage should, in general, be removed when the diagnosis of PPROM is made.** At maximum, cerclage might be left in place for <48 hours to allow steroid therapy.
- **See Figure 18.1 for management of PPROM. Before 34 weeks,** conservative management of PPROM is usually indicated, if possible. Delivery is indicated for NRFHT, preterm labor (PTL), chorioamnionitis, or ≥34 weeks.
- **The role of expectant management in women beyond 34 weeks or with proven fetal maturity is unproven.**
- There are no trials published to assess the benefit of interventions for PPROM <24 weeks.

DEFINITION

PPROM refers to chorioamniotic membrane rupture before the onset of labor in pregnancies at <37 weeks of gestation.

DIAGNOSIS

Definite diagnosis is by direct visualization of fluid (**pooling**) in the posterior vaginal fornix at sterile speculum examination. Confirmatory tests commonly done are **nitrazine** test on a cervicovaginal swab and the presence of arborization (**ferning**). History of persistent leakage of fluid and ultrasonographic diagnosis of oligohydramnios are two other confirmatory but not diagnostic findings. A negative fetal fibronectin assay after 21 weeks of gestation has a negative predictive value of only 81% to 99% and is not recommended. Although promising at preliminary studies, there is insufficient evidence to assess if the use of placental alpha-microglobulin-1 rapid immunoassay (AmniSure) and of an absorbent pad that changes color at pH > 5.2 (AmnioSense) significantly improve the accuracy provided by previous tests (1).

SYMPTOMS

Over 90% of women with PPROM report a history of "gush of fluid."

INCIDENCE

PPROM occurs in <1% at <24 weeks, and about 1% to 3% at 24 to 33 weeks, 3% to 5% at 34 to 36 weeks compared with about 8% to 10% for PROM at term. PPROM is responsible for 25% to 30% of all PTBs.

ETIOLOGY/BASIC PATHOPHYSIOLOGY

Etiology is complex and multifactorial (see chap. 16). Possible mechanisms leading to PPROM are choriodecidual infection, collagen degradation, decreased membrane collagen content, localized membrane defects, uterine overdistention, and programmed amniotic cell death (1). Evidence that supports a causal association between PPROM and infection is vast and includes the fact that microorganisms in the amniotic fluid are more frequently present and the rate of histological chorioamnionitis is higher in PPROM than in intact membranes preterm delivery and the frequency of PPROM is significantly higher in women with lower genital tract infections [e.g., group B streptococcus (GBS) and bacterial vaginosis]. Microorganisms that colonize the lower genital tract produce phospholipases, which can stimulate the production of prostaglandins and lead to uterine contractions; the immune response in endocervix and/or fetal membranes leads to the production of multiple inflammatory mediators (particularly matrix metalloproteinases) that can weaken membranes and result in PPROM (2).

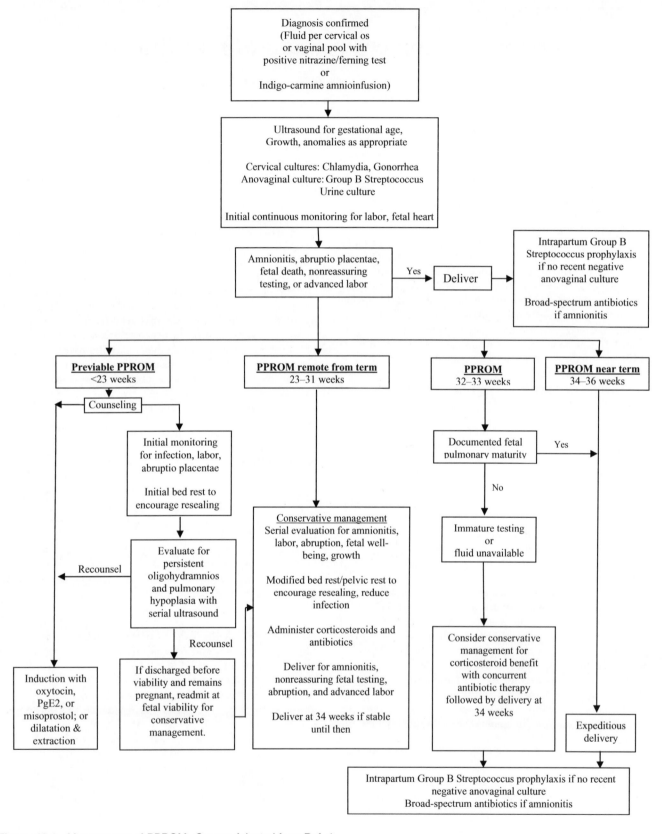

Figure 18.1 Management of PPROM. *Source*: Adapted from Ref. 4.

CLASSIFICATION

PPROM can be classified into **PPROM < 24 weeks** (usually 16–23 6/7 weeks, and called also previable or midtrimester or very early PPROM—see also end of this chapter) and PPROM at 24 0/7 to 36 6/7 weeks. PPROM at 24 to 36 weeks can be further subdivided into **PPROM at 24 to 33 6/7 weeks** (early PPROM) and **PPROM at 34 to 36 6/7** weeks (near-term PPROM—for management, see also chap. 19).

RISK FACTORS

See chapter 16. Transvaginal ultrasound **cervical length < 25 mm** is associated with a high rate of PPROM compared to PTL-related PTB.

COMPLICATIONS

Complications are inversely correlated with gestational age (GA) at PPROM and at delivery.

- **Premature labor/delivery**: In 50% of PPROM, labor occurs within 24 hours, and in 80% to 90% within 7 days. **Preterm delivery** and complications of prematurity are the most important causes of **perinatal mortality** and morbidity; complications decrease with advancing GA. Whether the PPROM has an independent effect on the neonatal prognosis in comparison with PTB deliveries with intact membranes is not clear (3,4).
- Most common neonatal morbidities are **RDS, IVH, PVL, and NEC.**
- **Infections: Mother** is at risk of **chorioamnionitis, endometritis, and sepsis.** Serious maternal consequences are uncommon. Mean incidence of chorioamnionitis is about 3% to 15%. Major **neonatal infections** occur in 5% of PPROM and 15% to 20% of cases developing chorioamnionitis. Fetal infection can precede clinically evident chorioamnionitis, resulting in neonatal pulmonary and cerebral morbidities.
- Other complications such as **abruptio placentae, cord prolapse, perinatal death, PH, compression syndrome, long-term infant morbidities, increased need for CD,** and **retained placenta** are most common at very early PPROM and are discussed more in detail for PPROM < 24 weeks.

MANAGEMENT (FIG. 18.1)
Prevention
See chapter 16.

Preconception Counseling
See chapters 1 and 16. Women with prior PPROM have a 20% to 30% chance of PTB, including a 15% to 20% chance of recurrent PPROM in the next pregnancy. Recurrence is higher in black race. These incidences are inversely related with GA at PPROM and interpregnancy interval. A double-blind, placebo-controlled trial involving pregnant women with a history of spontaneous PTB have demonstrated that weekly IM injections with 17α-hydroxyprogesterone caproate (250 mg) reduce by 34% the risk of recurrence (5).

Prenatal Counseling
Counseling regarding prognosis, possible complications, management, and expectations for neonatal outcome should be provided. Prognosis depends mostly on GA at PPROM and GA at delivery. Latency is inversely related with GA

Table 18.1 Latency Depending on Gestational Age at PPROM

GA at PPROM (wk)	Mean latency	Delivery		
		<48 hr	<7 days	<14 days
<24	7 days	20%	40–50%	70%
24–33 6/7	3–6 days	50%	70–80%	90%
34–36 6/7	24 hr	70–80%	90%	>95%

at PPROM (Table 18.1) and can be prolonged by some therapies (see below). No randomized study demonstrated that shortening or prolonging the latency period (interval between PPROM and delivery) before 34 weeks' gestation reduced neonatal mortality (6,7). Latency does not seem to differ for twin versus singleton gestations before 30 weeks but seems to be shorter for twins after 30 weeks. Fetal maturity depends on GA and is probably not enhanced or delayed by PPROM.

Workup
Speculum examination is necessary to confirm the diagnosis (see above), for direct visualization of leakage; for ferning; and for nitrazine tests. The nitrazine test can be falsely positive with blood or seminal fluid and has been associated with a 25% false-positive rate. Ferning can be falsely positive with highly estrogenized cervical mucus or extraneous saline and falsely negative at very early GA. Testing for gonorrhea and chlamydia is indicated, especially in high-risk groups. GBS culture should be sent from anorectal and vaginal areas. **Avoid** manual/digital examination of the cervix once PPROM is diagnosed by speculum examination. Digital examination is associated with shorter latency and higher incidences of infection.

Ultrasound should evaluate at least presentation, biometry for GA, anatomy, placenta and cord location, and amniotic fluid. The lower is the amniotic fluid volume [usually measured by amniotic fluid index (AFI) in most studies]; the higher is the incidence of perinatal infection and the shorter is the latency period.

Fifty to seventy percent of PPROM have low amniotic fluid volume on initial sonography. Low amniotic fluid volume is associated with an increased risk of umbilical cord compression and shorter latency but the predictive value is low (8). Patients with nonvertex presentations have in one study higher risk for prolapsed umbilical cord and of an unintended vaginal delivery when compared with vertex presentations (9).

See also chapter 16.

Infection Precautions
Women with active herpes simplex virus (HSV) infection or human immunodeficiency virus (HIV) with viral loads >1000 are **not,** in general, expectantly managed, especially if PPROM has occurred after 32 weeks (see chaps. 32 and 49 in *Maternal-Fetal Evidence Based Guidelines*). Management needs to be individualized with PPROM 24 to 30 weeks in the presence of these infections.

Amniocentesis
Amniocentesis can be of use for the evaluation of the following:

- The **diagnosis.** If diagnosis is in doubt, 1 mL of indigo carmine in 9 mL of normal saline can be injected into the amniotic cavity under continuous ultrasound guidance. Presence of blue on a pad worn on the perineum for 2 to 4 hours confirms the diagnosis.

- The **infectious** state of the amniotic cavity. Send amniotic fluid glucose (<15 mg/dL associated with positive culture), Gram stain, white blood cell count, and culture.
- The fetal **lung maturity.** Results of similar accuracy to amniocentesis can be obtained noninvasively by collecting vaginal fluid using a bedpan. Despite oligohydramnios, there is a 90% rate of success for transabdominal amniocentesis in PROM. There are insufficient data to assess the effect of amniocentesis on outcomes in PPROM. A small trial reported a **lower rate of NRFHT** in labor, **shorter neonatal stay,** and otherwise similar maternal and neonatal outcomes in a group randomized to amniocentesis compared with one expectantly managed (10).

Fetal Pulmonary Maturity Assessment

Assessment of fetal lung maturity can be obtained from amniotic fluid by amniocentesis or from the vaginal pool (see chap. 57 in *Maternal-Fetal Medicine Evidence Based Guidelines*). The predictive value of lung maturity tests is not modified by PPROM. Phosphatidylglycerol (PG), surfactant/albumin ratio (TDx/FLM), and lamellar body counts (LBC) are accurate when tested in the vaginal pool. PG is not accurate in the presence of meconium or blood, LBC is not accurate in the presence of meconium, while the **TDx/FLM is accurate with blood and/or meconium in the vaginal pool**, yielding results similar to those observed with samples obtained with amniocentesis.

Meconium

Meconium-stained amniotic fluid is associated with clinical chorioamnionitis and positive amniotic fluid cultures. In the absence of symptoms and signs of chorioamnionitis meconium alone is not an indication for intervention.

Hospitalization

There is **insufficient evidence** to compare hospital versus home management for PPROM. Home management can be offered only to consenting, reliable patients with the following: absence of infection, dependable transportation, living near hospital, evaluation in hospital before discharge, vertex presentation, vertical pocket of amniotic fluid >2 cm, home bed rest, recording of temperature and pulse every 6 hours, fetal movements count, twice-weekly nonstress tests (NST) and complete blood count, and weekly ultrasound. **Only 18% of patients with PPROM meet these criteria**, so that **most are managed in the hospital.** Eleven percent of women with PPROM managed at home **delivered unexpectedly at outside hospitals** (11). Women were **monitored for 48 to 72 hours** before randomization to hospitalization versus no hospitalization in the two RCTs on this subject (12).

Compared to hospitalization, no hospitalization was associated with similar incidences of perinatal mortality (RR 1.93, 95% CI 0.19–20.05), serious neonatal morbidity, chorioamnionitis, GA at delivery, birth weight and admission to neonatal intensive care unit, as well as CD (RR 0.28, 95% CI 0.07–1.15). There was no information on serious maternal morbidity or mortality. Mothers randomized to care at home spent approximately 10 fewer days as inpatients and were more satisfied with their care. Furthermore, home care was associated with reduced costs (12).

Maternal Surveillance

All women with PPROM should be monitored for signs of infection by assessment of clinical parameters (e.g., fever, maternal/fetal tachycardia, uterine tenderness, and purulent vaginal discharge). A diagnosis of chorioamnionitis is usually made by the presence of 2 or more of these criteria. The presence of a fever of unknown origin in the presence of PPROM is highly suspicious for chorioamnionitis, so that an amniocentesis should be considered if expectant management is still being considered.

There is no clear evidence to support the use of C-reactive protein (CRP) for the early diagnosis of chorioamnionitis. Maternal leukocytosis at admission is associated with higher adverse infant neurodevelopmental outcomes at 2 years of age in a study (13).

Fetal Surveillance (Antepartum Testing)

The two most common types of fetal surveillance are NST and biophysical profile (BPP) (14). Abnormalities of these tests can be somewhat predictive of fetal infection and umbilical cord compression related to oligohydramnios. There is insufficient evidence to assess the optimal type or frequency of testing. The NST or BPP performed daily have poor sensitivity (39% and 25%, respectively) and similar predictive values for predicting infection (6). No improvement in perinatal outcome has been reported in one trial (15). Given lower cost, the NST is usually suggested for daily to twice-a-week fetal surveillance. Monitoring may be more frequent with oligohydramnios, because it is associated with an increased risk of umbilical cord compression and shorter latency (8), with a preference for BPP as a backup if the NST is nonreassuring (5).

Amnioinfusion for Prolonging Latency

Compared with no amnioinfusion, **transabdominal** amnioinfusion with a 20-G needle for an average of 250 mL of isotonic sodium chloride solution enough to restore a normal AFI in women with PPROM at 24 to 32 6/7 weeks is associated with **increase in latency** from 9 to 21 days and a decrease in delivery within 7 days from 64% to 11% in a small trial. (16) This benefit is supported by case-control studies performed at lower GA (17). Transcervical amnioinfusion to prevent NRFHT is discussed below, under section "Delivery."

Corticosteroids for Fetal/Neonatal Maturation and Benefit

Antenatal steroid therapy should be administered in women with PPROM at 24 to 33 6/7 weeks, as this intervention is associated with **lower** neonatal complications: 44% less **RDS,** 53% less **IVH,** 79% less **NEC,** and a trend for a 32% lower incidence in **neonatal death,** without any increase in maternal or neonatal infection (8,18). Antenatal steroid therapy (24 mg of betamethasone—12 mg IM every 24 hours—or 24 mg of dexamethasone—6 mg IM every 12 hours) should not be repeated routinely in patients with PPROM, since weekly courses improve severe RDS, resulting in less composite neonatal morbidity among neonates delivered at 24 to 27 weeks but are associated with shorter latency, higher risks of chorioamnionitis and neonatal sepsis, and no improvement in overall composite neonatal morbidity (18,19). Rescue therapy can be considered if several weeks have elapsed since the initial course of antenatal corticosteroids (ACS) therapy and the delivery seems imminent with GA below 28 to 30 weeks. The National Institutes of Health consensus conference recommended steroid therapy for PPROM at <32 weeks of gestation without clinical chorioamnionitis (20). For patients admitted with PPROM at 32 to 34 weeks of gestation, if fetal lung maturity cannot be confirmed, a course of corticosteroids should be administered (14,18) (see also chap. 16).

Antibiotics for Prolongation of Latency and Fetal/Neonatal Benefit

Compared with placebo, antibiotics for women with PPROM are associated with short-term **benefits** for both women and neonates and should be routinely given (21–23). Benefits of maternal antibiotic therapy when there is PPROM are as follows:

- Maternal: 44% less **chorioamnionitis**
- Fetal/Neonatal:
  - Prolongation of pregnancy
  - 29% reduction in **PTB within 48 hours**
  - 21% reduction in **PTB within 7 days**
  - 33% reduction in **neonatal infection**
  - 17% reduction in use of **surfactant**
  - 12% reduction in **oxygen therapy**
  - 19% reduction in **abnormal cerebral ultrasound scan** (including IVH) prior to discharge from hospital
  - a 10% decreasing trend in perinatal mortality (RR 0.90, 95% CI 0.74–1.10)
  - **Decrease in RDS** and **NEC** with ampicillin and erythromycin treatment (see below) (21,22)

A meta-analysis limited to PPROM before 34 weeks shows similar results (24). ORACLE study evaluated the children's health at **7 years of age** and found no difference in any functional impairment after prescription of erythromycin, with or without co-amoxiclav, compared with those born to mothers who received no erythromycin; or after prescription of co-amoxiclav, with or without erythromycin, compared with those born to mothers who received no co-amoxiclav (25). **Long-term adverse effects** of antepartum prophylactic antibiotics for PPROM have not been observed in children followed to age 7 years (25). This finding is in contrast to the observation from the same authors that in patients with spontaneous PTL and intact membranes, the rate of cerebral palsy was increased in children exposed to antibiotics in utero (26). These results would suggest further caution should be used when considering the routine treatment of women with antibiotics if there is uncertainty about the diagnosis of PROM.

Benefits in short-term outcomes (prolongation of pregnancy, infection, need for respiratory therapy, less abnormal cerebral ultrasound before discharge from hospital, etc.) should be balanced against a lack of evidence of benefit for others, including perinatal mortality, and long-term outcomes.

Type

There is insufficient evidence on the optimal antibiotic type (and regimen) in women with PPROM. **Ampicillin and erythromycin** (22) or **erythromycin alone** (23) are associated with significant benefits in neonatal outcomes and should be used routinely in women with PPROM 24 to 34 weeks (24) (Table 18.2). A combination of ampicillin and erythromycin—for example, ampicillin 2 g and erythromycin 250 mg both IV every 6 hours for 48 hours, followed by amoxicillin 250 mg and erythromycin base 333 mg both orally (PO) every 8 hours for 5 days, for a total of 7 days—in women with PPROM with no concomitant steroids use showed an improvement in neonatal health by significantly reducing the rates of infants with one or more major infant morbidity (composite

Table 18.2 Possible Antibiotic Regimens

Antibiotic	Dose
Ampicillin	**2 g IV every 6 hr and**
Erythromycin	**250 mg IV every 6 hr for 48 hr followed by**
Amoxicillin	**250 mg PO every 8 hr and**
Erythromycin	**333 mg PO every 8 hr for 5 days.**
Ampicillin	1 or 2 g IV every 6 hr for 24 hr then 500 mg PO every 6 hr.
Erythromycin base	333 mg PO every 8 hr.
Piperacillin	3 g IV every 6 hr for 3 days.
Ampicillin-sulbactam	3 g every 6 hr for 7 days.
Ampicillin	2 g IV every 6 hr for 7 days.
Mezlocillin	3–4 g IV every 4–6 hr for 48 hr followed by
Ampicillin	2 g IV every 6 hr.
Gentamicin	90 mg IV initially, then 60 mg IV every 8 hr for 3 doses and 900 mg IV every 8 hr for 3 doses, followed by
Clindamycin	500 mg PO TID for 7 days.

In bold, suggested regimen.

morbidity: death, RDS, early sepsis, severe IVH, and severe NEC) from 53% to 44% (21). Compared with placebo, erythromycin 250 mg PO four times a day for 10 days is associated with decreases in neonatal death, chronic lung disease, major cerebral abnormalities, and prolongation of pregnancy in women with PPROM < 37 weeks who received steroids in >75% of cases (23). **Azythromycin** can be used instead of erythromycin, but there are less data on its efficacy in women with PPROM. In a large trial, amoxicillin/clavulanate was associated with an increased risk of neonatal NEC, although there is no consistent trend toward a positive or negative effect of broad-spectrum antibiotics for NEC in the literature (14,23). According to Cochrane review, co-amoxiclav should be avoided in women at risk of PTB due to increased risk of neonatal NEC (RR 4.72, 95% CI 1.57–14.23).

Possible antibiotic regimens are listed in Table 18.2.

Detection of specific cervicovaginal pathogens should be appropriately treated (see chaps. 32–37 of *Maternal-Fetal Evidence Based Guidelines*).

Clinical chorioamnionitis requires therapeutic antibiotics. For example, ampicillin (2 g IV every 6 hours) plus gentamicin (1.5 mg/kg IV every 8 hours or 5 mg/kg ideal body weight every 24 hours). If CD is performed, prophylactic antibiotics are indicated (see chap. 13). Intrapartum GBS prophylaxis should be given until culture results are available, and to carriers. There are insufficient data to assess the need for this intervention in women with PPROM in whom GBS is sensitive to antibiotics already given for PPROM, or if there has been no time for culture results. The suggested regimen is penicillin (5 million units IV, and then 2.5 million units every 4 hours), or (if unavailable) ampicillin (2 g IV, then 1 g every 4 hours).

Tocolysis for Prolongation of Latency and Fetal/Neonatal Benefit

Tocolytic therapy in women with PPROM is not associated with maternal or perinatal benefits and should, in general, be avoided. Most of the RCTs are small, did not use steroids for fetal maturation or antibiotics for increasing latency, and are in women without contractions (27–35).

Tocolysis may be considered for ≤48 hours with concurrent administration of antibiotic and corticosteroids for prolongation of pregnancy and achieving fetal maturity before 32 weeks in the presence of contractions and in the absence of contraindications to expectant management, but the **evidence for benefit of this management is insufficient to recommend it.**

Compared with short-term tocolysis to allow steroid effect, **long-term tocolysis >48 hours** is associated with a nonsignificant prolongation of pregnancy, no differences in neonatal complications, but increases in chorioamnionitis and postpartum endometritis. It **should** therefore **be avoided** (34).

Progesterone

Progesterone (17P) is not associated with increased latency versus placebo in women with PPROM (35). In women with singleton gestations and PPROM at 24 to 30 weeks, 17P 250 mg IM is associated with no effect on interval to delivery, GA at delivery, or neonatal mortality and morbidity in a small RCT (36). No RCT has evaluated the effect of vaginal progesterone in this population. In summary, there is **insufficient evidence** to assess effect of progesterone in women with PPROM. In a woman who has been receiving 17P for prior spontaneous PTB, in the absence of evidence to the contrary, it is reasonable to continue 17P once membranes have ruptured (37).

Vitamin C and E

There is **insufficient evidence** to assess the effect of vitamin supplementation in women with PPROM. In one small trial, compared with placebo, vitamin C 500 mg and vitamin E 400 IU daily in women with PPROM at 26 to 34 weeks were associated with 7-day prolongation in latency, but no other effects on maternal or neonatal morbidity and mortality (38).

Cerclage Removal

PPROM occurs in about 38% of women with cerclage in place (39). There is no trial to assess if cerclage should be removed or left in place in a woman with PPROM and cerclage in place. The prognosis of pregnancies with PPROM and immediate cerclage removal compared with those of PPROM without cerclage in place is similar (40,41). While leaving the cerclage in place >24 hours is associated with a longer latency >48 hours (94% vs. 51%; OR 16.1, 95% CI 3.7–71.3), **expectant management of PPROM, especially with cerclage in place, is associated with significantly increased maternal and fetal/ neonatal infection risks,** such as chorioamnionitis (43% vs. 20%; OR 2.9, 95% CI 1.7–5.0) and neonatal mortality from sepsis (12% vs. 1%; OR 13.2, 95% CI 1.6–108.3), and a trend for more neonatal sepsis (13% vs. 6%; OR 2.4, 95% CI 0.9–6.0) and neonatal mortality (17% vs. 10%; OR 2.0, 95% CI 0.9–4.3) (39,42–44). Therefore, **in most cases, cerclage should be removed in women with PPROM.**

If intrauterine infection, labor, or NRFHT is present, delivery is indicated in women with PPROM. At ≥30 weeks, cerclage should be immediately removed. At <28 to 30 weeks, it might be reasonable to administer steroids and antibiotics and remove the cerclage **at maximum after 48 hours** to allow the benefit of these interventions (Fig. 18.2).

Delivery

Timing
Once PPROM occurs, and steroids for fetal maturity have been administered, **the options for management include early delivery versus expectant management** until later in pregnancy. If expectant management is chosen, the issue is the

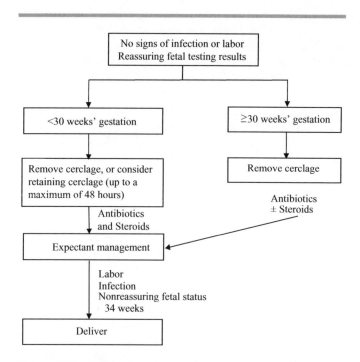

Figure 18.2 Timing of cerclage removal based on gestational age in women with PPROM.

following: until what GA? A longer latency is associated with higher rate of chorioamnionitis, a shorter latency with higher risk of severe prematurity.

Unfortunately, trials comparing immediate delivery to expectant management did not use steroids for fetal maturity, or tocolytics or antibiotics for pregnancy prolongation (45–48). As seen above, **steroids and antibiotics are associated with major perinatal benefits.** In these RCTs, which nowadays have therefore limited clinical validity, early delivery is associated with similar incidence of intrauterine deaths (RR 0.26, 95% CI 0.04–1.52), neonatal sepsis (RR 1.33, 95% CI 0.72–2.47), RDS (RR 0.98, 95% CI 0.74–1.29), cerebroventricular hemorrhage (RR 1.90 95% CI 0.52–6.92), NEC (RR 0.58, 95% CI 0.08–4.08), duration of neonatal hospitalization, neonatal deaths (RR 1.59, 95% CI 0.61–4.16), and perinatal mortality (RR 0.98, 95% CI 0.41–2.36), compared with expectant management. Regarding maternal outcomes, early delivery is associated with an increase in the incidence of CD (RR 1.51, 95% CI 1.08–2.10), endometritis (RR 2.32, 95% CI 1.33–4.07), and about 1 day less in duration of maternal hospital stay, but no effect on chorioamnionitis (RR 0.44, 95% CI 0.17–1.14) (49).

Delivery before 32 weeks is associated with risk of neonatal complications, including severe morbidity and death. Therefore, expectant management is indicated if possible before this GA, especially to allow steroid effect. The latency with PPROM >30 weeks is usually only 2 to 4 days.

There is no role of expectant management in any women beyond 34 weeks or with proven fetal maturity (45,47,48), since there are no fetal/neonatal benefits, whereas in all studies **maternal infection is increased with expectant management.** Two clinical trials, however, are under way on this topic. Between 32.0 and 33.6 weeks, delivery should be considered if a mature fetal lung test is available. If instead there is no amniotic fluid available for test or there is a negative test, expectant management with corticosteroids and antibiotic therapy are indicated. Antenatal magnesium sulfate therapy given to the mother before delivery of preterm babies improves chance of survival free of cerebral palsy (cumulative absolute risk reduction of 1.7%) in five studies (50). Results in PPROM cases were not reported separately in any study but constituted almost the 90% of the population in the largest study (51) (see Fig. 18.1).

Amnioinfusion for Preventing NRFHT
There is **insufficient evidence** to assess the effect of routine amnioinfusion in all women with PPROM, for prophylaxis either before labor or during labor. Prophylactic transabdominal amnioinfusion before labor to prolong pregnancy is discussed above.

Compared with no amnioinfusion, **transcervical amnioinfusion** (warmed saline at 10 mL/min for 1 hour, then 3 mL/min—total volume infused mean 1160 mL) at the time of labor for women with PPROM at 26 to 35 weeks is associated with statistically similar but more **favorable** incidences of CD, low Apgar scores, and neonatal death in one small trial (52). In the amnioinfusion group, the number of severe fetal heart rate decelerations per hour during the first stage of labor was reduced by just about one in this small trial. These outcomes are consistent with the benefits found for amnioinfusion for cord compression (see chap. 10).

Mode and Site of Delivery
Mode of delivery should not be altered solely for the presence of PPROM. Malpresentation is more common with PTB, with the incidence of malpresentation being indirectly related to weeks of GA (see chap. 22). Delivery should occur in a facility and by personnel capable of providing all the necessary support to the mother and fetus/neonate born preterm. **Transferring women** at risk of very PTB to perinatal centers for delivery **decreases the neonatal mortality rate considerably.** Predicting the time of delivery in PPROM is often impossible.

Anesthesia
No specific precautions.

Postpartum
See chapter 16. Women with PPROM are at high risk of recurrence in subsequent pregnancies, with an association between GA at the time of PPROM, latency period, interval between pregnancies, and PPROM recurrence. Patients with a history of cervical insufficiency and fetal loss/miscarriage should be considered at increased risk of midtrimester PPROM in the following pregnancy.

PPROM < 24 WEEKS
Definition
PROM <24 weeks or "previable PPROM" (arbitrary definition that varies among investigators and from year to year because of advances in neonatal intensive care) is a relevant and unique nosological entity because of its significant association with fetal and neonatal morbidity and mortality.

Incidence
The incidence is about 0.6% of pregnancies.

Etiology/Basic Pathophysiology
There are two different categories: spontaneous and iatrogenic. **Risk factors for spontaneous PPROM <24 weeks are similar to those for PTL and for PPROM later in pregnancy** (see

Table 16.1 in chap. 16). Fluid leakage or PPROM occurs in about 1% of genetic amniocenteses (53), 3% to 5% of diagnostic fetoscopies (40), and 10% of invasive fetoscopies (54).

Complications
Incidences of most complications are **inversely proportional to GA at PPROM, latency, residual amniotic fluid volume, and GA at delivery.**

Fetal/Neonatal
Neonatal death. Previable (<23 weeks) delivery in PPROM is usually lethal. Rates vary widely, depending on populations and range of GA studied, averaging for PROM <24 weeks approximately **60% to 70% or higher** (55–59). The mortality rate may be underestimated by including only patients continuing pregnancy or who have experienced initial latency. The most recent studies report 47% to 56% of perinatal survival in PROM <24 weeks routinely managed mostly with antibiotics, antenatal steroids, postnatal surfactant, and high-frequency ventilation (58,60).

Neonatal mortality is comparable to that in preterm deliveries matched for GA without PPROM.

Chorioamnionitis. Antenatal infection is the major complication limiting the latency interval. **If clinical infection occurs at any time during the latency period, delivery is indicated.** Chorioamnionitis complicates 24% to 77% of midtrimester PPROM, with an average of **40%** in most studies (38). Differences are mainly due to variability in criteria for infection diagnosis and antibiotic prophylaxis use. The occurrence of chorioamnionitis is higher early in the latency period; **more than 50% of cases occur within the first 7 days after rupture**, with the maximum clinical occurrence on 2 to 5 days (61,62). After the first week of latency, the incidence falls, suggesting that subclinical uterine or chorioamniotic infection that weakens membranes and causes rupture infection was probably present prior to membrane rupture, whereas bacteria migration is a less important component. The risk of chorioamnionitis is inversely proportional to residual amniotic fluid volume (63).

Placental abruption. Abruptio placentae is more frequent in pregnancies with midtrimester PPROM, occurring up to **44%** of cases compared with 0.8% of the general obstetric population (64). The risk is highest with lower GA at PPROM and with vaginal bleeding occurring prior to or after membrane rupture (64,65).

Cord prolapse. The incidence of cord prolapsed is about **2%** (51). The risk is higher (11% in one study) in the setting of nonvertex fetal presentations (9).

Fetal death. Fetal demise is primarily related to abruption, cord prolapse and compression, or infection. The average risk of fetal death after midtrimester PPROM is about **10%,** and is inversely related to GA at PPROM and residual amniotic fluid volume (65).

Pulmonary hypoplasia. PH is a decrease in the number of lung cells, airways, and alveoli, mainly due in PPROM to alterations of normal amniotic fluid pressure and egress of lung fluid during the canalicular stage of lung development (ending at nearly 24 weeks) (Fig. 18.3). The gold standard for the diagnosis of PH is lung weight by autopsy. The incidence of PH resulting from midtrimester PPROM varies from **13% to 28%** (55,57,65–67). The mortality rate in neonates with this condition is 70% to 95% (50,52–54). The main independent reported risk factors for development of PH are as follows: (*i*) early GA at membrane rupture (55,66–70); a risk of 50% to

Gestational age (weeks)	Stage of lung development	Description
4–6	EMBRIONIC	Lung bud arises
7–16	PSEUDOGLANDULAR	Nonrespiratory bronchi and bronchioles develop
17–24	CANALICULAR	First gas exchanging acini and pulmonary capillaries are forming
25–37	TERMINAL SAC	Subsaccules and alveoli develop with extensive capillary invasion and expansion of the alveolar blood barrier surface area
38 to age 3 years	ALVEOLAR	Subsaccules become alveoli

Figure 18.3 Phases of lung development.

60% was reported when PPROM occurs at 20 weeks or less; and (*ii*) low residual amniotic fluid volume (54,56,57,67). PH is more common among pregnancies with maximum pocket <2 cm or AFI <5, after controlling for GA at rupture (67,69). Incidences of PH with severe, moderate, and absent-to-mild oligohydramnios are 43%, 21%, and 7%, respectively (55).

Tests proposed to identify PH prenatally are ultrasound measurement of amniotic fluid, fetal breathing movements, fetal chest circumference, lung length, lung volume, Doppler studies of pulmonary vessels, and O_2 tests. In general, the predictive accuracy is poor and may be improved by combining tests (66,70).

Fetal compression syndrome. In early PPROM, asymmetric intrauterine pressure and restriction in fetal movement can lead to limb position deformities and craniofacial defects of variable severity, originally described in the context of renal agenesis. The mean frequency of skeletal deformities is **7%**. Duration of latency and severity of oligohydramnios independently increase the risk of skeletal abnormalities and act synergistically (68). The GA at PPROM is not a significant determinant due to the progressive and continuous development of the axial skeleton.

Increased likelihood of skeletal deformities observed among infants diagnosed with PH suggests that the two disorders share common risk factors. Surgical correction is not generally required as they resolve with postnatal growth and physiotherapy.

Other morbidities. Other neonatal morbidities are similar to that in PTB and are related to GA at PPROM. These include RDS, bronchopulmonary dysplasia (BPD), IVH, NEC, sepsis, and retinopathy of prematurity. The incidence of neonatal IVH and cystic PVL increases in cases complicated by clinical chorioamnionitis (71). Since midtrimester PPROM is associated with early delivery and infections, it constitutes a potential risk factor for long-term neurological morbidities. There may be a higher risk of PVL in infants born after prolonged PPROM compared with other types of prematurity (72). Prolonged latency in midtrimester PROM patients is not associated with an increasing frequency of abnormal neonatal cranial ultrasound examination (62).

Long-term morbidities. About 63% to 84% of survivors after midtrimester PPROM will be neurologically intact (57).

Maternal

Cesarean delivery. The CD rate increases secondary to more common fetal heart rate abnormalities (related to oligohydramnios and chorioamnionitis), malpresentation, and abruptio. A classical uterine incision may be required to reduce fetal trauma at early GA (oligohydramnios, fetal malpresentation, and lower uterine segment characteristics constitute risk factors).

Retained placenta. The risk of undergoing either uterine exploration or curettage is **9% to 18%,** and more likely if rupture occurs prior to 20 weeks of gestation.

Postpartum endometritis. This condition occurs in about **13%** of cases. Postpartum maternal **sepsis** (about 0.8%) and **death** (about 1/1000) are uncommon. The risk of maternal infection is inversely proportional to the latency period.

Management

Counseling

Parents should be counseled regarding the prognosis, complications, and management of PPROM <24 weeks. The **options** are **expectant management** or **delivery.** The impact of immediate delivery on neonatal outcome, and potential benefits and risks of conservative management, should be reviewed. PPROM related to genetic amniocentesis is associated with favorable outcomes even with expectant management (91–99% perinatal survival), which is very different than the prognosis with spontaneous PPROM <24 weeks.

Incidences of most complications are inversely proportional to **GA at PPROM, latency, residual amniotic fluid volume**, and **GA at delivery.**

The **latency** period between membrane rupture and delivery is critical in determining perinatal outcome.

Latency is indirectly correlated with GA at PPROM (Table 18.1) (73). While the mean latency is about 7 days, the median latency may be up to about 10 to 21 days because of the few pregnancies that gain a lot more than 14 days. **Up to 14%** of women with midtrimester PPROM **stop amniotic fluid loss,** presumably due to resealing of membranes (61,74). This subgroup of cases has outcomes similar to pregnancies uncomplicated by membrane rupture. In 10% to 20% of patients, amniotic fluid loss continues, but a partial reaccumulation during expectant management is observed (63,66).

Oligohydramnios (AFI <5 or deepest vertical pocket <2 cm) on admission, during latency period, or at the last ultra-sonographic examination is associated with shorter latency, and higher occurrences of PH, chorioamnionitis, and perinatal mortality (17,69,75). Conversely, adequate residual amniotic fluid volume identifies cases with elevated odds of perinatal survival (85–93%) and better long-term neurological outcomes (17,65).

Workup
See above.

Therapy
See Figure 18.1.
  Delivery in previable PPROM is **indicated in** the presence of

- **Intrauterine death**
- Spontaneous onset of **labor**
- Evidence of **maternal and/or or fetal infections**
- Any other obstetric **medical condition necessitating delivery** (e.g., abruptio placentae and preeclampsia)
- **Pregnancy termination request**

Delivery (termination) can be carried out usually by induction or by dilatation and extraction (D&X) by experienced operators, with no trials comparing these two modalities.

For management of women who elect **expectant management**, unfortunately there **are no trials on any interventions for PPROM <24 weeks**. There are therefore **insufficient data to assess the effect of any intervention studied for PPROM <24 weeks, such as hospitalization, steroids, antibiotics, tocolysis, or others**. Data for any benefit of these interventions are available only for PPROM diagnosed at ≥24 weeks, so these interventions should be used with caution before this GA, with the patients understanding these limitations in medical knowledge. If pregnancy continues, patients need to be counseled on clinical variables and complications that may affect outcome and treatment serially at diagnosis, during the latency period, and at delivery. Given the high incidence of infection, cerclage should be removed in women with cerclage in place at the time of PPROM <24 weeks. Use of intracervical tissue sealants with fibrin or a gelatin sponge (76,77), intra-amniotic injection of platelets and cryoprecipitate (i.e., amniopatch) (54), and serial amnioinfusions (17) has not been tested in any trials and should not be used in clinical practice outside of trials.

Proposed Management (see Fig. 18.1)
In women desiring expectant management, consider hospital bed rest during the first few days; administer an initial course of broad-spectrum antibiotic prophylaxis (7 days or until culture results). Take **urinary and anovaginal cultures on admission** and every 2 weeks (plus treatment of positive results for potentially pathogenic bacteria). **Avoid vaginal examination until labor or delivery.** During expectant management, monitor for the onset of infective complications, observing temperature, maternal or fetal tachycardia, uterine contractions or tenderness, purulent vaginal discharge, white blood cell counts, and CRP. As outpatient, instruct to maintain decreased activity, avoid intercourse, check temperature, and refer to hospital for vaginal bleeding and contractions. **At 24 weeks, suggest (re)admission to the hospital** and active expectant management, including administration of at least one course of steroids.

REFERENCES

1. Lee SE, Park JS, Norwitz ER, et al. Measurement of placental alpha-microglobulin-1 in cervicovaginal discharge to diagnose rupture of membranes. Obstet Gynecol 2007; 109:634–640. [II-3]
2. Canavan TP, Simhan HN, Caritis S. An evidence-based approach to the evaluation and treatment of premature rupture of membranes: part I. Obstet Gynecol Surv 2004; 59:669–677. [Review]
3. Melamed N, Ben-Haroush A, Pardo J, et al. Expectant management of preterm premature rupture of membranes: is it all about gestational age? Am J Obstet Gynecol 2011; 204:48.e1–48.e8. [Level III]
4. Blumenfeld YJ, Lee HC, Gould JB, et al. The effect of preterm premature rupture of membranes on neonatal mortality rates. Obstet Gynecol 2010; 116:1381–1386. [Level II-2]
5. Meis PJ, Klebanoff M, Thom E, et al.; National Institute of Child Health and Human Development Maternal. Fetal Medicine Units Network. Prevention of recurrent preterm delivery by 17 alpha-hydroxyprogesterone caproate. N Eng J Med 2003; 348:2379–2385. [RCT, *n* = 463] [Level I]
6. Pasquier JC, Bujold E, Rabilloud M, et al. Effect of latency period after premature rupture of membranes on 2 years infant mortality (DOMINOS study). Eur J Obstet Gynecol Reprod Biol 2007; 135:21–27. [Level II-2]
7. Manuck TA, Maclean CC, Silver RM, et al. Preterm premature rupture of membranes: does the duration of latency influence perinatal outcomes? Am J Obstet Gynecol 2009; 201:414.e1–414.e6. [Level II-2]
8. Mercer BM, Rabello YA, Thurnau GR, et al. The NICHD-MFMU antibiotic treatment of preterm PROM study: impact of initial amniotic fluid volume on pregnancy outcome. Am J Obstet Gynecol 2006; 194:438. [Level II-2]
9. Lewis DF, Robichaux AG, Jaekle RK, et al. Expectant management of preterm premature rupture of membranes and nonvertex presentation: what are the risks? Am J Obstet Gynecol 2007; 196:566. [Level III]
10. Cotton DB, Gonik B, Bottoms SF. Conservative versus aggressive management of preterm rupture of membranes: a randomized trial of amniocentesis. Am J Perinatol 1984; 1:322–324. [RCT, *n* = 47]
11. Carlan SJ, O'Brien WF, Parsons MT, et al. Preterm premature rupture of membranes: a randomized study of home versus hospital management. Obstet Gynecol 1993; 81:61–64. [RCT, *n* = 67]
12. Abou El, Senoun G, Dowswell T, et al. Planned home versus hospital care for preterm prelabour rupture of the membranes (PPROM) prior to 37 weeks' gestation. Cochrane Database Syst Rev 2010; (4):CD008053. [Meta-analysis: 2 RCTs, *n* = 116]
13. Pasquier JC, Picaud JC, Rabilloud M, et al. Maternal leukocytosis after preterm premature rupture of membranes and infant neuro-developmental outcome: a prospective, population-based study (DOMINOS Study). J Obstet Gynaecol Can 2007; 29:20–26. [Prospective cohort of 394 PPROM between 24 weeks and 33.6 weeks. Level II-2]
14. Mercer BM. Preterm premature rupture of membranes. Obstet Gynecol 2003; 101:178–193. [Review]
15. Lewis DF, Adair CD, Weeks JW, et al. A randomized clinical trial of daily nonstress testing versus biophysical profile in the management of preterm premature rupture of membranes. Am J Obstet Gynecol 1999; 181:1495–1499. [RCT, *n* = 135]
16. Tranquilli AL, Giannubilo SR, Bezzeccheri V, et al. Transabdominal amnioinfusion in preterm premature rupture of membranes: a randomized controlled trial. Br J Obstet Gynecol 2005; 112:759–763. [RCT, *n* = 34]
17. Locatelli A, Vergani P, Di Pirro G, et al. Role of amnioinfusion in the management of premature preterm rupture of membranes at <26 weeks gestation. Am J Obstet Gynecol 2000; 183:878–882. [Level II-2]
18. Harding JE, Pang JM, Knight DB, et al. Do antenatal corticosteroids help in the setting of preterm rupture of membranes? Am J Obstet Gynecol 2001; 184:131–139. [Meta-analysis: 15 RCTs, n = >1400]
19. Lee MJ, Davies J, Guinn D, et al. Single versus weekly courses of antenatal corticosteroids in preterm premature rupture of membranes. Obstet Gynecol 2004; 103:274–281. [RCT, *n* = 161 with PPROM]

20. Report on the Consensus Development Conference on the Effect of Corticosteroids for Fetal Maturation on Perinatal Outcomes. US Department of Health and Human Services, Public Health Service, NIH Pub No. 95–3784, November 1994. [Review]

21. Kenyon S, Boulvain M, Neilson JP. Antibiotics for preterm rupture of membranes. Cochrane Database Syst Rev 2010; (8): CD001058. [Metaanalysis: 22 RCTs, $n = 6800$]

22. Mercer BM, Miodovnik M, Thurnau GR, et al. Antibiotic therapy for reduction of infant morbidity after preterm premature rupture of the membranes: a randomized controlled trial. JAMA 1997; 278: 989–995. [RCT, $n = 614$]

23. Kenyon SL, Taylor DJ, Tarnow-Mordi W, ORACLE Collabrative Group. Broad-spectrum antibiotics for preterm, prelabour rupture of fetal membranes: the ORACLE I randomised trial. Lancet 2001; 357:979–988. [RCT, $n = 4826$]

24. Hutzal CE, Boyle EM, Kenyon SL, et al. Use of antibiotics for the treatment of preterm parturition and prevention of neonatal morbidity: a metaanalysis. Am J Obstet Gynecol 2008; 199:620. [Meta-analysis: 21 RCTs, $n = >4000$]

25. Kenyon S, Pike K, Jones DR, et al. Childhood outcomes after prescription of antibiotics to pregnant women with preterm rupture of the membranes: 7-year follow-up of the ORACLE I trial. Lancet 2008; 372:1310. [RCT, $n = 3298$]

26. Kenyon S, Pike K, Jones DR, et al. Childhood outcomes after prescription of antibiotics to pregnant women with spontaneous preterm labour: 7-year follow-up of the ORACLE II trial. Lancet 2008; 372:1319. [RCT, $n = 3196$]

27. Mackeen AD, Seibel-Seamon J, Grimes-Dennis J, et al. Tocolytics for preterm premature rupture of membranes. Cochrane Database Syst Rev 2011; (10):CD007062. [Metaanalysis: 8 RCTs, $n = 408$]

28. Christensen KK, Ingermarsson I, Leideman T, et al. Effect of ritodrine on labor after premature rupture of the membranes. Obstet Gynecol 1980; 55:187–190. [RCT, $n = 30$]

29. Levy DL, Warsof SL. Oral ritodrine and preterm premature rupture of membranes. Obstet Gynecol 1985; 66:621–623. [RCT, $n = 41$]

30. Garite TJ, Keegan KA, Freeman RK, et al. A randomized trial of ritodrine tocolysis in patients with preterm premature rupture of membranes. Am J Obstet Gynecol 1987; 157:388–393. [RCT, $n = 79$]

31. Dunlop P, Crowley PA, Lamont RF, et al. Preterm ruptured membranes, no contractions. J Obstet Gynecol 1988; 159:216. [RCT, $n = 48$]

32. Weiner CP, Renk K, Klugman M. The therapeutic efficacy and costeffectiveness of aggressive tocolysis for premature labor associated with premature rupture of the membranes. Am J Obstet Gynecol 1988; 159:216–222. [RCT, $n = 75$]

33. Matsuda Y, Ikenoue T, Hokanishi H. Premature rupture of membranes. Aggressive versus conservative approach: effect of tocolysis and antibiotic therapy. Gynecol Obstet Invest 1993; 36:102–107. [RCT, $n = 81$]

34. Decavalas G, Mastrogiannis D, Papadopoulos U, et al. Short term versus long-term prophylactic tocolysis in patient with preterm premature rupture of membranes. Eur J Obstet Gynecol Reprod Biol 1995; 59:143–147. [RCT, $n = 241$]

35. How HY, Cook CR, Cook VD, et al. Preterm premature rupture of membranes: aggressive tocolysis versus expectant management. J Matern Fetal Med 1998; 7:8–12. [RCT, $n = 145$]

36. Briery CM, Veillon EW, Klauser CK, et al. Women with preterm premature rupture of the membranes do not benefit from weekly progesterone. Am J Obstet Gynecol 2011; 204:54.e1–54.e5. [RCT, $n = 69$ (17P, $n = 33$; placebo, n = 36)]

37. Meis PJ; Society for Maternal-Fetal Medicine. 17 hydroxyprogesterone for theprevention of preterm delivery. Obstet Gynecol 2005; 105(5 pt 1):1128–1135. [Review]

38. Borna S, Borna H, Daneshbodie B. Vitamins C and E in the latency period in women with prterm premature rupture of membranes. Int J Gynaecol Obstet 2005; 90:16–20. [RCT, $n = 60$]

39. Giraldo-Isasa M, Berghella V. Cervical cerclage and preterm PPROM. Clin Obstet Gynecol 2011; 54:313–320. [Review]

40. Yeast JD, Garite TR. The role of cervical cerclage in the management of preterm premature rupture of membranes. Am J Obstet Gynecol 1988; 158:106–110. [II-2]

41. Blickstein I, Katz Z, Lancet M, et al. The outcome of pregnancies complicated by preterm rupture of the membranes with and without cerclage. Int J Gynaecol Obstet 1989; 28:237–242. [II-2]

42. Ludmir J, Bader T, Chen L, et al. Poor perinatal outcome associated with retained cerclage in patients with premature rupture of membranes. Obstet Gynecol 1994; 84:823–826. [II-2, $n = 30$]

43. Jenkins TM, Berghella V, Shlossman PA, et al. Timing of cerclage removal after preterm premature rupture of membranes: maternal and neonatal outcomes. Am J Obstet Gynecol 2000; 183:847–852. [II-2, $n = 62$]

44. McElrath TF, Norwitz ER, Lieberman ES, et al. Management of cervical cerclage and preterm premature rupture of the membranes: should the stitch be removed? Am J Obstet Gynecol 2000; 183:840–846. [II-2, $n = 81$]

45. Spinnato JA, Shaver DC, Bray EM, et al. Preterm premature rupture of the membranes with fetal pulmonary maturity present: a prospective study. Obstet Gynecol 1987; 69(2):196–201. [RCT, $n = 47$. PPROM at 25–36 weeks with L/S >2 or foam stability index >46. Tocolytics, steroids, or antibiotics were not used.]

46. Mercer BM, Crocker LG, Boe NM, et al. Induction versus expectant management in premature rupture of the membranes with mature amniotic fluid at 32 to 36 weeks: a randomized trial. Am J Obstet Gynecol 1993; 169: 775. [RCT, $n = 93$ women with PPROM at 32–36 6/7 weeks of gestation and a mature fetal lung profile. Tocolytics, steroids, or antibiotics were not used.]

47. Cox SM, Leveno KJ. Intentional delivery versus expectant management with preterm ruptured membranes at 30–34 weeks' gestation. Obstet Gynecol 1995; 86:875. [RCT, $n = 129$ women with PPROM at 30–34 weeks of gestation. Tocolytics, steroids, or antibiotics were not used. 3/62 (5%) neonatal death in intentional delivery, vs 1/69 (1.4%) fetal death in induction groups]

48. Naef RW III, Allbert JR, Ross EL, et al. Premature rupture of membranes at 34 to 37 weeks' gestation: aggressive versus conservative management. Am J Obstet Gynecol 1998; 178:126. [RCT, $n = 120$ women with PPROM at 34–36 weeks of gestation: chorioamnionitis 2% in induction vs. 16% in expectantly managed group. Tocolytics, steroids were not used; penicillin to all women for GBS prophylaxis]

49. Buchanan SL, Crowther CA, Levett KM, et al. Planned early birth versus expectant management for women with preterm prelabour rupture of membranes prior to 37 weeks' gestation for improving pregnancy outcome. Cochrane Database Syst Rev 2010; (3):CD004735. [Meta-analysis: 7 RCTs, $n = 690$]

50. Doyle LW, Crowther CA, Middleton P, et al. Magnesium sulphate for women at risk of preterm birth for neuroprotection of the fetus. Cochrane Database Syst Rev 2009; (1): CD004661. [Meta-analysis: 5 RCTs, $n = >6000$]

51. Rouse DJ, Hirtz DG, Thom E, et al. A randomized, controlled trial of magnesium sulfate for the prevention of cerebral palsy. N Engl J Med 2008; 359:895–905. [RCT, $n = 2241$]

52. Nageotte MP, Freeman RK, Garite TJ, et al. Prophylactic intrapartum amnioinfusion in patients with preterm premature rupture of membranes. Am J Obstet Gynecol 1985; 153:557–562. [RCT, $n = 61$]

53. Borgida AF, Mills AA, Feldman DM, et al. Outcome of pregnancies complicated by ruptured membranes after genetic amniocentesis. Am J Obstet Gynecol 2000; 183:937–939. [II-3]

54. Quintero RA, Morales WJ, Allen M, et al. Treatment of iatrogenic previable premature rupture of membranes with intra-amniotic injection of platelets and cryoprecipitate (amniopatch): preliminary experience. Am J Obstet Gynecol 1999; 181:744–749. [III]

55. Kilbride HW, Yeast J, Thibeault DW. Defining limits of survival: lethal pulmonary hypoplasia after midtrimester premature rupture of membranes. Am J Obstet Gynecol 1996; 175:675–681. [II-2]

56. Falk SJ, Campbell LJ, Lee-Parritz A, et al. Expectant management in spontaneous preterm premature rupture of membranes between 14 and 24 weeks' gestation. J Perinatol 2004; 24:611–616. [II-3]

57. Canavan TP, Simhan HN, Caritis S. An evidence based approach to the evaluation and treatment of premature rupture of membranes: Part II. Obstet Gynecol Surv 2004; 59:678–689. [Review]

58. Dinsmoor MJ, Bachman R, Haney EI, et al. Outcomes after expectant management of extremely preterm premature rupture of the membranes. Am J Obstet Gynecol 2004; 190:183–187. [II-3]

59. Carroll SG, Blott M, Nicolaides KH. Preterm prelabor amniorrhexis: outcome of live births. Obstet Gynecol 1995; 86:18–25. [II-3]

60. Manuck TA, Eller AG, Esplin MS, et al. Outcomes of expectantly managed preterm premature rupture of membranes occurring before 24 weeks of gestation. Obstet Gynecol 2009; 114:29–37. [II-2]

61. Beydoun SN, Yasin SY. Premature rupture of the membranes before 28 weeks: conservative management. Am J Obstet Gynecol 1986; 155:471–479. [II-3]

62. McElrath TF, Allred EN, Leviton A. Prolonged latency after preterm premature rupture of membranes: an evaluation of histologic condition and intracranial ultrasonic abnormality in the neonate born at <28 weeks of gestation. Am J Obstet Gynecol 2003; 189:794–798. [II-2]

63. Hadi HA, Hodson CA, Strickland D. Premature rupture of the membranes between 20 and 25 weeks' gestation: role of amniotic fluid volume in perinatal outcome. Am J Obstet Gynecol 1994; 170:1139–1144. [II-2]

64. Holmgren PA, Olofsson JI. Preterm premature rupture of membranes and the associated risk for placental abruption. Inverse correlation to gestational length. Acta Obstet Gynecol Scand 1997; 76:743–747. [II-2]

65. Farooqi A, Holmgren PA, Engberg S, et al. Survival and 2-year outcome with expectant management of second-trimester rupture of membranes. Obstet Gynecol 1998; 92:895–901. [II-3]

66. Winn HN, Chen M, Amon E, et al. Neonatal pulmonary hypoplasia and perinatal mortality in patients with midtrimester rupture of amniotic membranes—a critical analysis. Am J Obstet Gynecol 2000; 182:1638–1644. [II-3]

67. Vergani P, Ghidini A, Locatelli A, et al. Risk factors of pulmonary hypoplasia in second trimester premature rupture of membranes. Am J Obstet Gynecol 1994; 170:1359–1364. [II-2]

68. Rotschild A, Ling EW, Puterman ML, et al. Neonatal outcome after prolonged preterm rupture of the membranes. Am J Obstet Gynecol 1990; 162:46–52. [II-2]

69. Shumway JB, Al-Malt A, Amon E, et al. Impact of oligohydramnios on maternal and perinatal outcomes of spontaneous premature rupture of the membranes at 18–28 weeks. J Matern Fetal Med 1999; 8:20–23. [II-3]

70. Vergani P, Andreani M, Greco M, et al. Two- or three-dimensional ultrasonography: which is the best predictor of pulmonary hypoplasia? Prenat Diagn 2010; 30:834–838. [II-2]

71. Verma U, Tejani N, Klein S, et al. Obstetric antecedents of intraventricular hemorrhage and periventricular leukomalacia in the lowbirth—eight neonate. Am J Obstet Gynecol 1997; 176:275–281. [II-2]

72. Perlman JM, Risser R, Broyles S. Bilateral cystic periventricular leukomalacia in the premature infant: associated risk factors. Pediatrics 1996; 97:822–827. [II-2]

73. Schucker JL, Mercer BM. Midtrimester premature rupture of the membranes. Semin Perinatol 1996; 20:389–400. [Review]

74. Fortunato SJ, Welt SI, Eggleston MK Jr., et al. Active expectant management in very early gestations complicated by premature rupture of the fetal membranes. J Reprod Med 1994; 39:13–16. [II-3]

75. Vintzileos AM, Campbell WA, Nochimson DJ, et al. Degree of oligohydramnios and pregnancy outcome in patients with premature rupture of the membranes. Obstet Gynecol 1985; 66:162–167. [II-2]

76. O'Brien JM, Barton JR, Milligan DA. An aggressive interventional protocol for early midtrimester premature rupture of the membranes using gelatin sponge for cervical plugging. Am J Obstet Gynecol 2002; 187:1143–1146. [III]

77. Sciscione AC, Manley JS, Pollock M, et al. Intracervical fibrin sealants: a potential treatment for early preterm premature rupture of the membranes. Am J Obstet Gynecol 2001; 184:368–373. [III]

19

Premature rupture of membranes at or near term

Sally Segel

KEY POINTS

- **The diagnosis** of premature rupture of membranes (PROM) at term is based on **pooling, ferning**, and **nitrazine tests**. There is still insufficient information to assess if there are any effects of a rapid bedside immunoassay for placental alpha-microglobulin-1 for the diagnosis of PROM.
- The main **complication** is **intrauterine infection**; this incidence increases with duration of PROM, and, with longer latency, the risk of **neonatal infection** also increases.
- Women with PROM at term should be **hospitalized** and **induced** with **oxytocin** within 6 to 12 hours of PROM, as feasible. **Most women with PROM at term, if given a choice, prefer induction.** Oxytocin induction is safe, effective, and cost-effective. Misoprostol induction is an alternative that is just as effective when 25 µg every 4 hour dosing is used, but there is limited data regarding its safety. Foley catheter ripening is another safe and efficacious alternative, especially in cases of unfavorable cervical exam.
- Antibiotics are recommended only if the patient is group B streptococcus (GBS) positive, or complications (chorioamnionitis, PROM >18 hours) develop during labor.

DEFINITION

Premature rupture of membranes is rupture of fetal membranes prior to the onset of labor (1). Preterm premature rupture of membranes (PPROM) is premature rupture of fetal membranes ≤37 weeks (1). This chapter includes guidance for near-term (34–36 6/7 weeks) as well as term (≥37 weeks) PROM. For PPROM < 34 weeks, see chapter 18.

DIAGNOSIS

The diagnosis of PROM and PPROM is based on history and physical examination findings (see also chap. 18). A maternal history suggestive of PROM includes a gush of fluid soaking clothes or a constant trickle of fluid that does not stop. Physical exam for PROM starts with a **sterile speculum** examination (1–3). **Visualization of amniotic fluid passing from the cervical canal is diagnostic** of this condition (1–3).

Another helpful test is the **nitrazine test**. The pH of the vagina is usually 4.5 to 6.0, whereas amniotic fluid has a pH 7.0 to 7.7; nitrazine paper turns blue with pH > 6.5 (1,2). A false positive nitrazine test can be caused from blood, semen, alkaline antiseptic, or bacterial vaginosis. A false-negative nitrazine test can be caused by prolonged leaking of amniotic fluid or minimal residual fluid. The sensitivity of nitrazine is 90.2% (81.3–100%) and the specificity is 79.3% (16–100%) (2).

A third helpful test is called "**ferning**." A swab of vaginal fluid from the posterior fornix is placed on a slide and allowed to air dry. Arborization (ferning) under microscopic visualization suggests rupture of membranes. Ferning has a sensitivity of 90.8% (62.0–98.5%) and a specificity of 95.3% (88.2–100%) (2).

The combination of vaginal pool of fluid, nitrazine, and ferning has a sensitivity of 90.8% and a specificity of 95.6% (2). These tests are more accurate when patients present in labor and less accurate when nonlaboring (3). If these tests are equivocal, an ultrasound can be performed to evaluate for amniotic fluid, but oligohydramnios is not diagnostic of PROM, since it can be associated with other etiologies, such as placental insufficiency.

Placental alpha-microglobulin-1 is a 34-kDa glycoprotein abundant in amniotic fluid (2000–25,000 ng/mL) and there is a negligible amount in vaginal fluid with intact fetal membranes (0.05–2.0 ng/mL) (2,4,5). AmniSure is a bedside immunoassay that uses the delta in concentration of placental alpha-microglobulin-1 for diagnostic accuracy. AmniSure has a sensitivity of 98.7% to 98.9% and a specificity of 87.5% to 100% (4,5). Further studies are needed to assess reliability with special attention paid to time of presumed membrane rupture (2,3).

INCIDENCE

PROM complicates approximately 8% of all term deliveries (1).

ETIOLOGY

The etiology of PROM without signs of infection or bleeding is often unknown, and this should be considered a physiologic, not pathologic, event.

RISK FACTORS

The risk factors associated with rupture of fetal membranes include low socioeconomic status, low BMI < 19.8 kg/m^2, nutritional deficiencies of ascorbic acid and cooper, connective tissue disorders, smoking, cold knife cone biopsy, cervical cerclage, pulmonary disease, uterine overdistension, and amniocentesis (1). In addition, pregnant women with a previous preterm birth, midtrimester short cervix, and preterm labor are at increased risk for PROM; however, the majority of cases have no identifiable cause (1).

COMPLICATIONS

The most common complications of PROM are **chorioamnionitis, endomyometritis, and postpartum hemorrhage**. With increasing time interval from rupture of membranes, there is a significant increase in these complications: about 12 hours for chorioamnionitis, 16 hours for endometritis, and 8 hours for postpartum hemorrhage (6). As the latency from ROM to delivery increases, so does the risk for neonatal infection. Maternal GBS colonization also increases the risk for neonatal infection. Incidence of cesarean delivery is not affected by management with either induction or expectant management, but depends on other risk factors (e.g., nulliparity) (7).

MANAGEMENT
Initial Evaluation
Initial evaluation of PROM involves confirmation of the diagnosis. **Digital examination** can increase the risk of infection and as a result **should be avoided** (7). The cervix can be visually assessed for dilation and effacement (8). Fetal presentation should be confirmed by ultrasound. Fetal well being and the presence of uterine contractions should be assessed by external monitoring.

Counseling
Risk factors, complications, and management of PROM should be reviewed with the patient. About 50% of women with PROM at term deliver within 6 to 12 hours and 95% of women will deliver within 28 hours of membrane rupture (1,7). Principles of management can be reviewed (Table 19.1).

Hospitalization
Compared with management in the hospital, management of PPROM at term at **home** is associated with a 52% increase in **need for maternal antibiotics** for nulliparas and 97% more **neonatal infections** (9). **PROM at term should be managed in hospital**.

Delivery Vs. Expectant Management
Women with PROM ≥ 34 weeks should be delivered (see also chap. 18). Induction of labor with oxytocin has been shown to **decrease the rate of maternal chorioamnionitis and postpartum fevers** without significantly affecting the rate of cesarean delivery, compared with expectant management (7). In most RCTs, induction was with oxytocin or prostaglandin, with one trial using homeopathic caulophyllum. Overall, no differences are detected for mode of birth between induced and expectant groups: cesarean (RR 0.94, 95% CI 0.82–1.08); operative vaginal birth (RR 0.98, 95% 0.84–1.16). Significantly fewer women in the induced compared with expectant management groups have chorioamnionitis (RR 0.74, 95% CI 0.56–0.97) or endometritis (RR 0.30, 95% CI 0.12–0.74). No difference is seen for neonatal infection (RR 0.83, 95% CI 0.61–1.12). However, fewer infants under induced management went to neonatal intensive or special care compared with expectant management (RR 0.72, 95% CI 0.57–0.92, number needed to treat 20) (10).

Table 19.1   Management of PPROM at ≥34 Weeks

- Deliver
- Manage in hospital
- There is insufficient evidence to recommend one induction agent over another, but oxytocin has been the best studied for safety and effectiveness
- Antibiotics are recommended only if the patient is GBS positive, or complications (chorioamnionitis, PROM > 18 hours) develop during labor

Abbreviations: PPROM, preterm premature rupture of membranes; GBS, group B streptococcus.

Compared with expectant management, induction of labor by **oxytocin** is associated with a 37% **decrease** in risk of **maternal infection**, 28% in **endometritis**, and 36% in **neonatal infection** (10). Based on one trial, women were more likely to view their care positively if labor was induced with oxytocin (7). Cesarean delivery rates are similar between groups. Oxytocin is associated with more frequent use of pain relief and internal fetal heart rate monitoring. Perinatal mortality rates are low and not significantly different between groups, although the **trend** is toward **fewer perinatal deaths** with induction of labor by oxytocin (10).

Compared with placebo or no treatment, both **vaginal prostaglandin E2 (PGE2) and F2a (PGF2a)** reduce the likelihood of vaginal delivery not being achieved within 24 hours, with no evidence of a difference in cesarean delivery (10). Induction of labor by prostaglandins is associated with a decrease by 23% in risk of chorioamnionitis and by 21% in admission to neonatal intensive care. Induction by prostaglandins is associated with a more frequent maternal diarrhea and use of anesthesia and/or analgesia (10). There is insufficient data to make meaningful conclusions for the comparison of vaginal PGE2 and PGF2a. PGE2 tablet, gel, and pessary appear to be as efficacious as each other. Lower-dose regimens appear as efficacious as higher dose regimens (10).

Medications for Induction
Immediate induction of labor with intravenous **oxytocin** has been shown to decrease the rate of maternal infection without increasing the rate of cesarean section (7). Please see above data on individual agents for induction compared with placebo or no treatment.

Currently, there have been no studies that demonstrate misoprostol or PGE2 are superior to intravenous oxytocin even in women with an unfavorable cervix (11). However, when misoprostol is compared with PGE2, length of labor is shorter but there is increased uterine tachysystole (11).

Compared with **prostaglandins**, induction with **oxytocin** is associated with **decrease** in maternal nausea and/or vomiting, numerous vaginal examinations, **chorioamnionitis** and **neonatal infections**, neonatal antibiotic therapy, and **admission to neonatal intensive care unit (NICU)**, but increase in epidural analgesia and internal fetal heart rate monitoring. Cesarean delivery, endometritis, and perinatal mortality are not significantly different between the groups (10). Cost is less with oxytocin induction.

Vaginal **misoprostol** in doses above 25 μg every 4 hours is more effective than PGE2, intracervical PGE2, and oxytocin (or obviously expectant management) in achieving vaginal delivery (10,12). **Compared with oxytocin, misoprostol** was associated with a decrease in CD from 51% to 20% in a small trial in women with an unfavorable cervix and from 14% to 11% in other women (10,12). If a dose of 50 μg of vaginal misoprostol is used, in 85% of cases only one dose is needed for induction with term PROM, but this is associated with a higher rate of uterine tachysystole compared with oxytocin, with similar maternal and neonatal outcomes (13). However, the studies reviewed were not large enough to exclude the possibility of serious adverse events with misoprostol including neonatal complications from uterine hyperstimulation. Lower doses of vaginal misoprostol were similar to other methods in effectiveness and risk. Oral misoprostol appears to be an effective means of labor induction comparable to oxytocin, but again the studies reviewed were not large enough to exclude the possibility of serious adverse events with misoprostol (14–16).

There is insufficient evidence to assess if the combination of dinoprostone (PGE2) together with oxytocin is superior to oxytocin alone (17).

The safety and efficacy of **Foley bulb** or other mechanical means of induction in women with PROM has been evaluated, and Foley appears to be both safe and efficacious for cervical ripening of women with PPROM $\geq$ 34 weeks and unfavorable cervical exam (see also chap. 20).

In summary, in patients with PROM at term, once the diagnosis has been confirmed, **induction of labor is recommended.** Induction should probably occur at least within 6 to 12 hours of PPROM, or earlier if feasible. **Currently, oxytocin is the recommended induction medication, as it is safe, effective, and cost-effective**. Vaginal and oral misoprostol are also safe and effective but have not been proven to be superior to oxytocin when appropriate doses (e.g., 25 µg for vaginal misoprostol) are used (11). With increasing latency from PROM to delivery, there is an increased risk for chorioamnionitis, endomyometritis, and postpartum hemorrhage (6). Women should be counseled to initiate induction of labor in order to decrease the risk of these complications.

Antibiotics

GBS positive: In women with a positive GBS culture, antibiotics should be administered according to the new CDC guideline (18) (see chap. 37 in *Maternal-Fetal Evidence Based Guidelines*). **Women who are GBS positive with PROM at ≥34 weeks are treated with penicillin in labor**. Ampicillin is a reasonable alternative. If the patient is penicillin-allergic but not at high risk for anaphylaxis, cefazolin is the agent of choice. For women at high risk for anaphylaxis, GBS isolate should be tested for susceptibility to clindamycin and erythromycin. Vancomycin is recommended if isolate is resistant to either clindamycin or erythromycin. Intrapartum treatment for chorioamnionitis is recommended regardless of GBS maternal status.

In these revised recommendations, 4 hours of intravenous antibiotics are considered adequate treatment for a neonate; however, no medically necessary obstetric procedure should be delayed to achieve 4 hours of intravenous antibiotic therapy (18). If a patient presents with PROM at term, antibiotics can be administered and induction of labor can begin concurrently. In addition, if a woman is scheduled for a repeat cesarean section and presents with PROM, GBS antibiotic prophylaxis should be administered while arranging for the repeat cesarean section (18).

GBS negative: There is **insufficient evidence** to recommend for or against antibiotics in GBS-negative women with PROM at ≥34 weeks. Routine antibiotics for women with PROM are associated with a **significant decrease in maternal infectious morbidity (chorioamnionitis or endometritis**: RR 0.43, 95% CI 0.23–0.82), but there is insufficient evidence to evaluate the fetal and neonatal effects. As a result, the final conclusions recommend that further randomized controlled trials need to be performed to adequately evaluate the effects of antibiotics in PPROM (19).

GBS status unknown: If the patient has no risk factors (previous infant with GBS sepsis, <37 weeks, rupture of membranes >18 hours, chorioamnionitis), there is usually no need for GBS prophylaxis and/or antibiotics. In PROM 34 to 36 6/7 weeks, if the patient has no GBS culture from the previous 5 weeks, antibiotics can be administered per protocol or a rapid GBS test can be performed. If the rapid GBS result is negative, antibiotics can be withheld unless other risk factors develop (chorioamnionitis or rupture of fetal membranes greater than 18 hours) (18).

In summary, for PROM at ≥34 weeks, antibiotics should be withheld unless the patient is GBS+ or infectious complications develop during labor (19). Given the low rate of maternal infection in the control population (~7%), it is not justifiable to expose all women with term PROM to antibiotics when treatment can be restricted to those who develop clinical indications for antibiotic treatment.

Special Considerations for PPROM at 34 to 36 Weeks' Gestation

Management of PPROM from 34 0/7 to 36 6/7 weeks is based on extrapolation from a few small studies (20–23), and therefore the scientific evidence is limited. These studies were performed before a standardized therapy for PPROM was developed, and corticosteroids and antibiotics were not routinely used. The current American College of Obstetrics and Gynecology Practice Bulletin states that **"delivery is recommended when PROM occurs at or beyond 34 weeks of gestation"** (1).

Since 1990, the rate of **late PTB** (34–36 6/7 weeks) has increased 25%, to 9.15% in 2007 (24). This increase in late PTB represents approximately 75% of the increase in PTB rate in the United States. Recent studies have called attention to the neonatal complications of late PTB, which include respiratory complications, sepsis evaluations, hyperbilirubinemia requiring phototherapy, and death. This combination of potential complications has lead to an increase in NICU admissions, increasing length of stay, urgent hospital visits, and hospital readmissions (25–32).

The original research determining the best antenatal approach to PPROM including the late preterm period studied patients with documented fetal lung maturity (20,23). Spinnato et al. randomized 47 nonlaboring PPROM patient to either delivery or expectant management with hospitalization and intensive antenatal surveillance. There was a statistically significant increase in chorioamnionitis or postpartum endometritis in expectant management group; however, neonatal morbidity and mortality were similar between groups (23). Mercer et al. also randomized 93 PPROM patients from 32 to 36 weeks' gestation with fetal lung maturity to immediate induction of labor or expectant management. Women randomized to expectant management had a significant increase in chorioamnionitis and fetal heart rate abnormalities in labor (20). In addition, neonates from the expectant management group had a significant increase in the initiation and length of antibiotic treatment for presumed neonatal infection (20). These two trials had significant similarities in that the expectant management group was hospitalized with intensive surveillance and antibiotics were only administered for chorioamnionitis. Overall their results demonstrated that expectant management in PPROM patients, including the late preterm period and with fetal lung maturity, had longer latencies and increased maternal infection without significant neonatal benefit. Naef et al. also performed a randomized trial of 120 PPROM patients in the late preterm period. Women in the expectant management group received GBS prophylaxis during their hospitalization (21). Even with the addition of GBS prophylaxis, women randomized to the expectant management group had a significant increase in chorioamnionitis and their neonates had a significant increase in NICU admission with a trend toward an increase in culture-proven sepsis (21). Overall, these studies found that **expectant management produced longer latencies; however, there was a significant increase in maternal infection without demonstration of neonatal benefit** (20,21,23).

Currently there are two international RCTs examining the best management strategy for PPROM in the late preterm period (33,34). These international RCTs will examine the rate of neonatal sepsis, neonatal morbidity and mortality, and maternal complications when immediate delivery is compared with expectant management in PPROM patients from 34 0/7 to 36 6/7 weeks' gestation. In both of these RCTs, latency antibiotics will be administered in the expectant management group in accordance with the policy of the local participating center. See chapter 18 for other details on management for women with PPROM < 37 weeks (35).

REFERENCES

1. American College of Obstetricians and Gynecologists. ACOG Practice Bulletin No. 80: Premature rupture of membranes. Washington, D.C.: ACOG, 2007. [Review]
2. El-Messidi A, Cameron A. Diagnosis of premature rupture of membranes: inspiration from the past and insights for the future. J Obstet Gynaecol Can 2010; 32(6):561–569. [Review]
3. Strevens H, Allen K, Thornton JG. Management of premature prelabor rupture of the membranes. Ann N Y Acad Sci 2010; 1205:123–129. [Review; 44 refs]
4. Lee SE, Park JS, Norwitz ER, et al. Measurement of placental alpha-microglobulin-1 in cervicovaginal discharge to diagnose rupture of membranes. Obstet Gynecol 2007; 109(3):634–640. [II-2]
5. Cousins LM, Smok DP, Lovett SM, et al. AmniSure placental alpha microglobulin-1 rapid immunoassay versus standard diagnostic methods for detection of rupture of membranes. Am J Perinatol 2005; 22(6):317–320. [II-3]
6. Tran SH, Cheng YW, Kaimal AJ, et al. Length of rupture of membranes in the setting of premature rupture of membranes at term and infectious maternal morbidity. Am J Obstet Gynecol 2008; 198(6):700.e1–700.e5. [II-2]
7. Hannah ME, Ohlsson A, Farine D, et al. Induction of labor compared with expectant management for prelabor rupture of the membranes at term. N Engl J Med 1996; 334:1005–1010. [RCT, n = 5041]
8. Pereira L, Gould R, Pelham J, et al. Correlation between visual examination of the cervix and digital examination. J Matern Fetal Neonatal Med 2005; 17(3):223–227. [II-2]
9. Hannah ME, Hodnett ED, Willan A, et al. Prelabor rupture of the membranes at term: expectant management at home or in the hospital? Obstet Gynecol 2000; 96:533–538. [RCT secondary analysis, n = 1670]. .
10. Dare MR, Middleton P, Crowther CA, et al. Planned early birth versus expectant management (waiting) for prelabour rupture of membranes at term (37 weeks or more). Cochrane Database Syst Rev 2006; (1):CD005302. [Meta-analysis: 12 RCTs, n = 6814]
11. Mozurkewich E. Prelabor rupture of membranes at term: induction techniques. Clin Obstet Gynecol 2006; 49(3):672–683. [Review]
12. Hofmeyr GJ, Gülmezoglu AM, Pileggi C. Vaginal misoprostol for cervical ripening and induction of labour. Cochrane Database Syst Rev 2010; (10):CD000941. [Meta-analysis]
13. Sanchez-Ramos L, Chen AH, Kaunitz AM, et al. Labor induction with intravaginal misoprostol in term premature rupture of membranes: a randomized study. Obstet Gynecol 1997; 89:909–912. [RCT, n = 141]
14. Butt KD, Bennett KA, Crane JMG, et al. Randomized comparison of oral misoprostol and oxytocin for labor induction in term prelabor membranes rupture. Obstet Gynecol 1999; 94:994–999. [RCT, n = 108]
15. Ngai SW, Chan YM, Lam SW, et al. Labour characteristics and uterine activity: misoprostol compared to oxytocin in women at term with prelabour rupture of membranes. Br J Obstet Gynecol 2000; 107:222–227. [RCT, n = 80]
16. Mozurkewich E, Horrocks J, Daley S, et al.; MisoPROM study. The MisoPROM study: a multicenter randomized comparison of oral misoprostol and oxytocin for premature rupture of membranes at term. Am J Obstet Gynecol 2003; 189:1026–1030. [RCT, n = 305]
17. Tan PC, Daoud SA, Omar SZ. Concurrent dinoprostone and oxytocin for labor induction in term premature rupture of membranes. Obstet Gynecol 2009; 113:1059–1065. [RCT, n = 114]
18. Revised Guidelines from CDC. Prevention of perinatal group B streptococcal disease. MMWR Morb Mortal Wkly Rep 2010; 59 (RR10):1–32. [Epidemiologic data]
19. Flenady V, King J. Antibiotics for prelabour rupture of membranes at or near term. Cochrane Database Syst Rev 2009; (2). [Meta-analysis: 2 RCTs, n = 838]
20. Mercer BM, Crocker LG, Boe NM, et al. Induction versus expectant management in premature rupture of the membranes with mature amniotic fluid at 32 to 36 weeks: a randomized trial. Am J Obstet Gynecol 1993; 169(4):775–782. [RCT]
21. Naef RW III, Allbert JR, Ross EL, et al. Premature rupture of membranes at 34 to 37 weeks' gestation: aggressive versus conservative management. Am J Obstet Gynecol 1998; 178(1 pt 1):126–130. [RCT]
22. Neerhof MG, Cravello C, Haney EI, et al. Timing of labor induction after premature rupture of membranes between 32 and 36 weeks' gestation. Am J Obstet Gynecol 1999; 180(2 pt 1):349–352. [RCT]
23. Spinnato JA, Shaver DC, Bray EM, et al. Preterm premature rupture of the membranes with fetal pulmonary maturity present: a prospective study. Obstet Gynecol 1987; 69(2):196–201. [RCT]
24. Martin JA, Hamilton BE, Sutton PD, et al. Centers for Disease Control and Prevention National Center for Health Statistics National Vital Statistics System. Natl Vital Stat Rep 2009; 57 (7):1–102. [Epidemiologic data]
25. Bhutani VK, Johnson L. Kernicterus in late preterm infants cared for as term healthy infants. Semin Perinatol 2006; 30(2):89–97. [II-3]
26. Clark RH. The epidemiology of respiratory failure in neonates born at an estimated gestational age of 34 weeks or more. J Perinatol 2005; 25(4):251–257. [II-3]
27. Jain L, Eaton DC. Physiology of fetal lung fluid clearance and the effect of labor. Semin Perinatol 2006; 30(1):34–43. [II-3]
28. Laptook A, Jackson GL. Cold stress and hypoglycemia in the late preterm ("near-term") infant: impact on nursery of admission. Semin Perinatol 2006; 30(1):24–27. [II-3]
29. McIntire DD, Leveno KJ. Neonatal mortality and morbidity rates in late preterm births compared with births at term. Obstet Gynecol 2008; 111(1):35–41. [II-2]
30. Shapiro-Mendoza CK, Tomashek KM, Kotelchuck M, et al. Risk factors for neonatal morbidity and mortality among "healthy," late preterm newborns. Semin Perinatol 2006; 30(2):54–60. [II-3]
31. Tomashek KM, Shapiro-Mendoza CK, Weiss J, et al. Early discharge among late preterm and term newborns and risk of neonatal morbidity. Semin Perinatol 2006; 30(2):61–68. [II-3]
32. Wang ML, Dorer DJ, Fleming MP, et al. Clinical outcomes of near-term infants. Pediatrics 2004; 114(2):372–376. [II-3]
33. Morris JM, Roberts CL, Crowther CA, et al. Protocol for the immediate delivery versus expectant care of women with preterm prelabour rupture of membranes close to term (PPROMT). BMC Pregnancy Childbirth 2006; 6:9. [Review]
34. van der Ham DP, Nijhuis JG, Mol BWJ, et al. Induction of labour versus expectant management in women with preterm prelabour rupture of membranes between 34 and 37 weeks (the PPROMEXIL-trial). BMC Pregnancy Childbirth 2007; 7:11. [Planned RCT]
35. Buchanan SL, Crowther, CA, Levett KM, et al. Planned early birth versus expectant management for women with preterm prelabour rupture of membranes prior to 37 weeks' gestation for improving pregnancy outcome. Cochrane Pregnancy Childbirth Group Cochrane Database Syst Rev 2010; (6). [Meta-analysis]

20

Induction of labor

Kelly E. Ruhstaller and Anthony C. Sciscione

KEY POINTS

- **Complications** of induction of labor at term include **prolonged first stage of labor, operative vaginal and cesarean delivery (CD),** and their risks.
- **An ultrasound examination** (usually <20 weeks) determining accurate gestational age is associated with a **reduction in the rates of induction of labor for postterm pregnancy**.
- **Gestational age** should be **documented accurately** before considering induction.
- **Possible indications** for induction of labor, and suggested best gestational age for induction, are listed in Table 20.1.
- **Without indications, induction before 39 weeks should be avoided.** An induction based solely on maternal request should be designated as such (induction for maternal request), with counseling regarding the possible maternal and perinatal consequences of induction.
- **Contraindications** to induction of labor include transverse or oblique fetal lie, umbilical cord prolapse, previous classical uterine incision or transfundal uterine surgery (e.g., from myomectomy), placenta or vasa previa, active genital herpes infection, and any contraindications to vaginal delivery, or indication for CD (Table 20.2).
- **Misoprostol should not be used for cervical ripening or labor induction in women with prior uterine incisions, given the >5% risk of uterine rupture.** In women with prior uterine incisions, **prostaglandin E2 (PGE2)** for cervical ripening is associated with approximately **1.4% to 2.5% risk of rupture;** oxytocin has a **1.1% risk.** Cervical ripening with the Foley catheter is not associated with any additional risk of uterine rupture in patients undergoing a trial of labor after cesarean section.
- A Bishop score of ≥9 is usually associated with the **probability of vaginal delivery** after labor induction **similar to that after spontaneous labor.**
- In women with **an unfavorable** (Bishop score <5, or even <9) cervical exam:
  - **Sweeping of membranes** at term doubles the rate of onset of labor (to approximately **36%) in the next 48 hours,** without major complications.
  - **The Foley balloon** is associated with **less hyperstimulation accompanied by fetal heart rate (FHR) changes, and increased use of oxytocin,** but results in the same number of vaginal deliveries and the same number of women delivered within 24 hours as all of the locally applied prostaglandins [prostaglandin E1 and E2 (PGE1 and PGE2)]. It is therefore **one of the preferred methods for labor induction** when the cervix is <3 cm dilated.

- **Vaginal misoprostol 25 μg every 3 to 6 hours** is the preferred safe dosage, as effective as PGE2 or any other method; this is also a preferred method of labor induction.
- PGE2 tablet, gel, and insert appear to be as safe and efficacious as each other in terms of tachysystole, CD rates, and neonatal outcomes.
- Other cervical ripening or induction agents are either not sufficiently studied, unsafe, or not as effective as the agents already mentioned.
- In women with **favorable** cervical exam:
  - Oxytocin is safe and effective for induction of labor in these women.
- There are insufficient safety data for **outpatient use** of pharmacologic cervical ripening or induction agents. However, there is emerging evidence that the Foley catheter may be an effective and safe method for outpatient cervical ripening.
- Contraction pressures of ≥**200 Montevideo units** should be targeted in induction or augmentation of laboring patients to achieve **adequate labor.** While the definition of a failed induction of labor is elusive, a **failed induction** should not be diagnosed until after **12 hours of oxytocin after membrane rupture in the active phase (usually ≥6 cm in nulliparous women),** assuming reassuring fetal heart pattern.
- **Induced labor should be managed, in general, as for spontaneous labor.**

DEFINITIONS

Induction of labor is the stimulation of uterine contractions prior to spontaneous labor in order to achieve childbirth. **Cervical ripening** is a process that occurs prior to labor in which the cervix is softened, thinned, and dilated.

INCIDENCE/EPIDEMIOLOGY

Of the 4,265,555 U.S. births reported in 2006, 22.5% were the result of induced labor; this represents an induction rate more than double that of the 9.0% reported in 1989. From 1990 to 2006, induction rates increased for all gestational ages. Since 2003, the rate of reported preterm inductions has increased, while inductions after 37 weeks also continue to increase; the rate is much slower than in the 1990s (1). One explanation for increasing induction rates is that inductions without medical or obstetric indication are on the rise, representing 25% of all inductions in a report (2). However, it has been shown that using birth certificate data overestimates the number of nonmedically indicated inductions by 11-fold (3).

Table 20.1 Common Indications for Possible Induction of Labor (Suggested Timing of Delivery for Selected Conditions)

Placental and uterine issues	Gestational age[a] for delivery
• Placenta previa[b]	36–37 wk
• Placenta accreta/increta/percreta with placenta previa	34–35 wk
• Prior classical cesarean (upper segment uterine incision)	36–37 wk
• Prior myomectomy requiring cesarean delivery	37–38 wk (Situations with more extensive or complicated procedures may require earlier delivery, similar to prior classical cesarean)
• Prior uterine rupture	36–37 wk
• Abruptio placentae	At detection (see chap. 26)
• Intrauterine infection (e.g., chorioamnionitis)	At detection
Fetal issues	
• Fetal growth restriction—singleton	38–39 wk: • Otherwise uncomplicated, no concurrent findings 34–37 wk: • Concurrent conditions (e.g., abnormal umbilical artery Dopplers) Expeditious delivery regardless of gestational age • Persistent abnormal fetal surveillance suggesting imminent fetal jeopardy
• Fetal growth restriction—twin gestation	36–37 wk: • Dichorionic-diamniotic twins with isolated fetal growth restriction 32–34 wk: • Monochorionic-diamniotic twins with isolated fetal growth restriction • Concurrent conditions (e.g. abnormal umbilical artery Dopplers) Expeditious delivery regardless of gestational age • Persistent abnormal fetal surveillance suggesting imminent fetal jeopardy
• Fetal congenital malformations	• 34–39 wk: • Suspected worsening of fetal organ damage • Potential for fetal intracranial hemorrhage (e.g., Vein of Galen aneurysm and NAIT) • When delivery prior to labor is preferred (e.g., EXIT procedure) • Previous fetal intervention • Concurrent maternal disease (e.g., preeclampsia and chronic hypertension) • Potential for adverse maternal effect from fetal condition Expeditious delivery regardless of gestational age • When intervention is expected to be beneficial • Fetal complications develop (abnormal fetal surveillance, new onset hydrops fetalis, and progressive/new-onset organ injury) • Maternal complications develop (mirror syndrome)
• Multiple gestations: dichorionic/diamniotic[b]	38 wk
• Multiple gestations: monochorionic/diamniotic[b]	34–37 wk
• Multiple gestations: di/di or mono/di with single fetal death[b]	If occurs at or after 34 wk, consider delivery. If occurs before 34 wk, individualize based on concurrent maternal/fetal conditions.
• Multiple gestations: monochorionic/monoamnioticb	32–34 wk
• Multiple gestations: monochorionic/monoamniotic with single fetal death[b]	Consider delivery; individualized according to gestational age and concurrent complications.
• Oligohydramnios (MVP <2 cm)—isolated but persistent[b]	37 wk
• Nonreassuring fetal heart testing (e.g., category III FHR tracing)	At detection (see chap. 10)
• Fetal death	At detection (see chap. 10)
Maternal and obstetrical issues **Maternal issues**	
• Chronic hypertension—no medications[b]	38–39 wk
• Chronic hypertension—controlled on medications[b]	37–39 wk
• Chronic hypertension—difficult to control (requiring frequent medication adjustments)[b]	36–37 wk
• Gestational hypertension[c]	38 wk
• Preeclampsia—severe	At diagnosis (recommendations limited to pregnancies at or after 34 wk)
• Preeclampsia—mild	**37 weeks**
• Eclampsia	At detection
• Diabetes—pregestational well-controlled[b]	39–40 wk
• Diabetes—pregestational with vascular disease	37–39 wk
• Diabetes—pregestational, poorly controlled	34–39 wk (individualized to situation)
• Diabetes—gestational well-controlled on diet[b]	Induction before 40 wk not recommended
• Diabetes—gestational well-controlled on medication[b]	39–40 wk

Table 20.1   Common Indications for Possible Induction of Labor (Suggested Timing of Delivery for Selected Conditions) (*Continued*)

• Diabetes—gestational poorly controlled on medication[b]	34–39 wk individualized to situation
• Cardiac disease	39 wk (individualize depending on type and severity)
Obstetrical issues	
• Prior stillbirth—unexplained	39 wk Consider amniocentesis for fetal pulmonary maturity if delivery planned before 38 wk
• Spontaneous PPROM	**34 wk**
• Spontaneous preterm labor	Delivery at 34–36 wk if progressive labor or additional maternal/fetal indication
• Prolonged pregnancy	**≥41 wk**

Bold: level 1 evidence for delivery.
[a]Gestational age is in completed weeks, thus "34 weeks" includes 34 weeks and 0 days through 34 weeks and 6 days.
[b]Uncomplicated, thus no FGR, superimposed preeclampsia, etc. If these are present, then the complicating conditions take precedence and earlier delivery may be indicated.
[c]Maintenance antihypertensive therapy should in general not be used to treat gestational hypertension.
Abbreviations: PPROM, preterm premature rupture of membranes; NAIT, neonatal alloimmune thrombocytopenia; MVP, maximum vertical pocket; FHR, fetal heart rate; FGR, fetal growth restriction.
Source: Modified from Ref. 10.

Table 20.2   Contraindications to Induction of Labor

- Transverse or oblique fetal lie
- Umbilical cord prolapse
- Previous classical uterine incision or transfundal uterine surgery (e.g., from myomectomy)
- Placenta or vasa previa
- Active genital herpes infection
- Any contraindications to vaginal delivery, or indication for cesarean delivery

BASIC PATHOPHYSIOLOGY

The cervix functions as the gatekeeper to parturition maintaining a fine balance between the integrity of the pregnancy and delivery. Histologically, the cervix is composed of mostly collagen, with some smooth muscle; the stability of these components and the ability to become dynamic when stressed on a physical and molecular level are what changes the cervical status. This cervical status prior to induction is predictive of induction success, as described below (4).

RISK FACTORS/ASSOCIATIONS

Factors that may increase the risk for complications associated with induction are nulliparity, no prior vaginal delivery, unfavorable cervical exam, postterm, and a large fetus.

COMPLICATIONS

Complications of inductions include **prolonged first stage of labor** (especially latent phase); **operative vaginal and CD** (5). Preterm (<37 weeks) induction is associated with prematurity risks.

PREGNANCY CONSIDERATIONS

The risks and complications of induction of labor should be weighed against the possible benefits. A **successful induction** has been defined in many different ways but usually is one that achieves an uncomplicated vaginal delivery within 24 hours. If active phase is not achieved within 24 hours, this is not a reason per se for CD. Compared with a shorter induction-to-delivery interval, an induction lasting greater than 24 hours is associated with a higher risk for adverse outcomes, with a higher (e.g., 50%) risk of CD (6). A **failed induction** should not be diagnosed until after 12 hours of oxytocin after membrane rupture in the active phase (usually >6 cm in nulliparous women), assuming reassuring fetal heart pattern (7).

PREVENTION

A routine (i.e., performed on every pregnant woman) ultrasound examination is associated with a 39% **reduction in the incidence of postterm pregnancies and rates of induction of labor for postterm pregnancy,** by allowing a more precise estimation of exact gestational age. An ultrasound performed in the first trimester (6–14 weeks) provides the best estimate of gestational age and the most benefit in terms of avoiding induction for postterm pregnancy (8) (see also chap. 4).

CRITERIA FOR INDUCTION
Workup/Counseling

Gestational age should be **documented accurately** before considering induction, to avoid inadvertent postterm and preterm deliveries. Indications and contraindications need to be carefully reviewed. Women requesting an induction based only on their request should be particularly aware of the risks of the induction of labor. Counseling with the patient should include discussion of specific indications, risks (possible complications), and benefits of induction.

Indications

Once a term gestation has been confirmed, possible **indications for induction and suggested best timing** are shown in Table 20.1 (9,10).

For more details on the indications, see each specific guideline [e.g., chap. 24 "Postterm Pregnancy," chap. 18 "Preterm Premature Rupture of Membranes," chap. 14 "Trial of Labor After Cesarean" in this volume; and chap. 4 "Pregestational Diabetes," chap. 5 "Gestational Diabetes," chap. 45 "Fetal

Macrosomia," chap. 43 "Multiple Gestations," and chap. 10 "Intrahepatic Cholestasis of Pregnancy" in *Maternal-Fetal Evidence Based Guidelines*]. The term *elective* induction should be avoided, as an induction should be performed upon a precise and accepted indication (11). An induction based solely on maternal request should be designated as such.

Gestational Age of Induction

The gestational age at which the induction is being considered is very important. There are some indications for induction before 39 weeks (Table 20.1), but **without indications induction before 39 weeks should be avoided** (12). In this chapter, induction and ripening in the third trimester, and usually at or near term, is reviewed. For second-trimester induction and ripening, see chapter 29. For induction for gestational age ≥41 weeks, see chapter 24.

Some have advocated induction at about 39 0/7 to 40 6/7 weeks, even without medical indications. In a meta-analysis including 11 randomized control trials (RCTs) and 25 observational studies evaluating pregnancies at **37 0/7 to 41 6/7 weeks**, **compared with "elective" induction, expectant management was associated with higher incidence of CD** (OR 1.22, 95% CI 1.07–1.39), and **higher incidence of meconium** (OR 2.04, 95% CI 1.34–3.09), but otherwise similar maternal and perinatal outcomes (13). These results are driven mostly by data at 41 weeks or more, when induction is indicated (see chap. 24). An RCT on induction based on risk-based induction of labor at 38 to 40 6/7 weeks was associated with similar incidence of CD and less neonatal intensive care unit (NICU) admission compared with expectant management (14). **There are insufficient data to evaluate the safety and effectiveness of induction without a medical indication at 39 to 40 6/7 weeks.**

Contraindications

Induction of labor is **contraindicated** in the situations shown in Table 20.2 (12). The attending physician should use his or her own discretion in the event of multifetal pregnancy, polyhydramnios, maternal heart disease, prior low-transverse CD, severe hypertension, abnormal FHR patterns not necessitating emergent delivery, or when the presenting part is above the pelvic inlet.

Induction of Labor after Cesarean

The **risk of uterine rupture** after induction in **women with a prior CD** deserves special attention (see chap. 14). Misoprostol induction in women with a prior CD was associated with a 5.6% risk of uterine rupture in one of the largest series (15). **Therefore misoprostol should not be used for cervical ripening or labor induction in women with prior uterine incisions except under very unusual circumstances.** According to retrospective studies, using PGE2 for cervical ripening in women who have a history of previous cesarean also increases the risk of uterine rupture (16–19). Risk of uterine rupture is approx-

imately **1.4 to 2.5 with PGE2** use (with or without oxytocin) (18,19), and about **1.1 with oxytocin alone** (19). Alternatively, **cervical ripening with the Foley catheter is not associated with any additional risk of uterine rupture in patients undergoing a trial of labor after cesarean section** (20). A patient who has a prior CD, no previous vaginal delivery, and an unfavorable Bishop score up to 39 to 40 weeks has more risks (e.g., septicemia, uterine rupture, and hysterectomy) from induction of labor; these women may elect for repeat CD after counseling (16–19) (see chap. 14).

Time of Day for Induction

Spontaneous labor has been shown to have a circadian rhythm with a higher occurrence at night due to a higher concentration of myometrial oxytocin receptors and maternal oxytocin concentrations. One RCT showed no difference in outcomes for women induced in the morning versus the evening (21). Another RCT showed no differences in outcomes in women induced in the morning versus the evening, except for less oxytocin required in the morning group and less operative vaginal delivery in the morning nulliparas group (22).

PREDICTION OF SUCCESSFUL INDUCTION
Maternal Characteristics

There are certain maternal characteristics that have been shown to favorably predict successful induction of labor. A secondary analysis of a study investigating vaginal misoprostol versus vaginal dinoprostone showed that prior vaginal delivery, lower maternal BMI, tall maternal stature, and neonatal birth weight <4000 g were associated with a higher likelihood of a vaginal delivery, independent of method. Race was also predictive, with Hispanic race being a positive predictor of successful induction and African-American race being associated with a lower likelihood of successful induction of labor (23).

Bishop Score

In 1964, Bishop reported that his pelvic score (Table 20.3) is inversely proportional to the time from examination to time at which spontaneous labor begins (4). **Unfavorable (<5) Bishop scores at admission for induction of labor are associated with two- to threefold increased risk of CD** when compared to spontaneous onset of labor (4,5,24). Data show a score of ≥9 to predict a short time until onset of spontaneous labor and, therefore, indicate favorability for induction (23). A simplified Bishop score might also be considered (25). A Bishop score of ≥9 is usually associated with a **probability of vaginal delivery** after labor induction **similar to that after spontaneous labor** (12).

Transvaginal Cervical Length

Compared with using a Bishop score <5 for defining an unfavorable cervix, using a transvaginal ultrasound (TVU) cervical length (CL) >27 mm is associated with a reduced

Table 20.3 Bishop Score for Cervical Favorability

Score	Dilation (cm)	Effacement (%)	Station	Cervical consistency	Position of cervix
0	Closed	0–30	−3	Firm	Posterior
1	1–2	40–50	−2	Medium	Midposition
2	3–4	60–70	−1,0	Soft	Anterior
3	5–6	80	+1,+2	–	–

Source: Modified from Ref. 4.

need for prostaglandins without affecting the outcome of the induction in one RCT (26). In a systematic review of mostly observational studies, a CL of <30 mm did not predict vaginal delivery; a CL >30 mm did not predict cesarean section (27). When compared with Bishop score, there was no significant difference in prediction of successful labor induction, mode of delivery, vaginal delivery within 24 hours of starting induction, or achievement of the active stage of labor. Cervical wedging/funneling has been investigated in several studies and associated with prediction of labor induction success, but there is need of further investigation. Additionally, 3D cervical imaging has shown promise for prediction of successful labor (27).

Fetal Fibronectin

Testing for the presence of fetal fibronectin has become an important tool in our ability to anticipate the likelihood of preterm labor. However, two studies that examined the utility of fetal fibronectin for predicting successful induction of labor have had conflicting results (28,29). As such, there are **insufficient data to recommend routine use of fetal fibronectin in order to predict which patient's labor induction will result in a successful vaginal delivery**.

INDUCTION/RIPENING METHODS

Induction of labor is one of the most-studied interventions in obstetrics, with hundreds of trials reported. Cervical ripening/ induction agents can be functionally divided into two methods: **mechanical** and **pharmacologic**. Mechanical methods have been utilized since the days of Hippocrates, 460 to 360 B.C. Many methods have been compared not only to placebo or no treatment but also among themselves, in different populations and clinical settings, making for an extensive experience.

Mechanical Methods

Mechanical methods include the following: hygroscopic dilators (laminaria, lamicel, or dilapan); balloon (e.g., Foley catheter); and balloon with extra-amniotic infusion. Other methods reviewed under this category are membrane stripping and amniotomy.

Hygroscopic (Osmotic) Dilators (Laminaria, Lamicel, or Dilapan)
Hygroscopic devices are made either from synthetic or from organic material. The **laminaria** are the organic hygroscopic devices, which are made from cold water seaweed. Under direct visualization facilitated by a vaginal speculum, laminaria are placed in the cervical canal. Once in the cervix, the device absorbs water from surrounding tissues causing it to slowly swell, dilating the cervix. Generally the laminaria are left in place for 6 to 12 hours.

Currently, **no evidence exists to support using laminaria to decrease either the interval from induction to delivery or the rate of CD**. However, their use may cause an increase in maternal endometritis and neonatal sepsis likely due to the inability to reliably ensure sterility in this organic product (30). In attempt to avoid problems associated with lack of sterility, polyvinyl alcohol polymer–magnesium sulfate (**lamicel**) and polyacrylonitrile (**dilapan**) were developed as synthetic hygroscopic devices. Like the laminaria, they are inserted in the same manner and function by attracting water from the surrounding tissue to achieve cervical softening, effacement, and dilation. However, lamicel and dilapan may be delivered sterilely.

Compared with placebo/no treatment, laminaria are associated with similar incidence of CD (30). Similarly, no differences were noted between lack of treatment and dilapan in one trial (31).

Compared with any prostaglandins (vaginal PGE2, intracervical PGE2, or misoprostol), laminaria are also associated with similar incidence of CD, but less tachysystole with FHR changes. Serious maternal or perinatal morbidity is infrequent (30).

Compared with oxytocin, laminaria are associated with similar incidence of CD (30).

Compared with **extra-amniotic induction**, laminaria are associated with similar outcomes (30).

Compared with prostaglandin alone, the addition of laminaria is not associated with significant benefit (30).

Compared with **oxytocin alone**, there is insufficient evidence (1 trial only) but no evidence of benefit from the addition of laminaria (30).

Foley Catheter
In 1853, Kraus first described a balloon device for preinduction cervical ripening. Much like the placement of laminaria, a vaginal speculum is often utilized to insert the Foley catheter in the cervical os; however, placement via a digital examination is becoming more common. Optimally, the catheter is placed at a level above the internal cervical os sometimes with the assistance of forceps or a clamp to guide the catheter. The Foley catheter affects cervical ripening in two ways: (*i*) gradual mechanical dilation and (*ii*) separation of the decidua from the amnion, stimulating prostaglandin release. Many studies have demonstrated the Foley catheter to be an effective tool for achieving a favorable cervix (30,32–37).

There is some evidence to assess the type of Foley catheter to use. Various sizes and balloon capacities have been investigated and used; these include a range from 25- to 80-mL balloons with 14- to 18-F catheters. **Filling the balloon to 80 mL versus 30 mL resulted in an increased rate of delivery within 24 hours, increase in vaginal delivery rate, decreased need for oxytocin, and higher rate of postripening dilation of 3 cm or more** (38–40). Also, a double balloon has been used, but there is insufficient evidence on its safety and efficacy (41).

Once placed above the internal os, the operator uses sterile saline or water to inflate the catheter's balloon. Correct placement is verified by gentle traction on the catheter until the inflated balloon meets the resistance of the internal os. Once the location is verified, gentle traction is applied by taping the distal end of the catheter to the patient's inner thigh. The cervix dilates as the balloon is expelled. After expulsion, a favorable Bishop score is most often achieved and induction may begin. If the Foley is not expulsed within 12 hours, consideration should be given to removing it, as leaving it in 24 hours is associated with longer inductions (42).

Compared with no treatment, one trial reported Foley catheters to have no effect in the risk of CD (30).

Compared with all locally applied prostaglandins (LAPG), including PGE2 and misoprostol, the rate of CDs is the same. LAPG were associated with a higher rate of excessive uterine activity and Foley catheter was associated with an increased need for oxytocin augmentation in labor, according to a meta-analysis of 27 trials (34). Obviously this analysis is not very clinically helpful, as comparison group should not mix PGE1 and PGE2.

Compared with vaginal misoprostol, transcervical Foley catheter has been demonstrated to be **equivalent** for cervical ripening, with **no significant difference in time to delivery** (1 hour less for misoprostol, but not statistically significant), **similar rates of chorioamnionitis and other maternal and perinatal outcomes, except a higher incidence of tachysystole associated with misoprostol** (RR 2.9, 95% CI 1.39–5.81) (37,43).

Compared with use with oxytocin for cervical ripening, Foley use without oxytocin was associated with a similar rate of vaginal delivery in 24 hours and CD rate. Patients treated with oxytocin required increased use of pain control (44).

Compared with use with extra-amniotic saline infusion (EASI) and oxytocin, Foley use with only oxytocin had a similar rate of delivery within 24 hours and the safety profiles between the two regimens were similar. Overall, there were no significant differences between the treatment groups (45).

Compared with prostaglandin alone, the **addition of a Foley** catheter to prostaglandin increases the likelihood of vaginal delivery within 24 hours, in one trial, with a lower likelihood of observing no cervical change when a balloon catheter is used (30).

Foley bulbs were equally effective ripening agents in both **outpatient** and inpatient settings per the results of one trial (46).

In women with a singleton gestation who undergo term induction with the intracervical Foley catheter, **early amniotomy after expulsion of catheter** is associated with similar labor length but **higher incidence of CD and CD for dystocia** compared with oxytocin and late amniotomy (47).

Foley catheter has been associated with certain complications: bleeding, fever, displacement of the presenting part, and premature rupture of membranes (PROM). Foley should not be used in women with low-lying placentas. However, no randomized trial has shown an increase in these complications in comparison to other methods, as they are infrequent occurrences. Overall, **the Foley catheter is an inexpensive, safe, well-tolerated, and easy tool for cervical dilation** (32–36). In a recent review of over 1200 low-risk women who received the intracervical Foley catheter for cervical ripening in our institution, there were no adverse events necessitating delivery in the preinduction ripening period (48). **Foley is as effective as other methods, including misoprostol, and possibly safer than pharmaceutical methods, and should be considered as first line in all inductions, including those with PROM** (see chap. 19).

Extra-Amniotic Saline Infusion
EASI involves, as the term states, infusing usually saline through the cervix by a Foley balloon. For infusion of PGE2, see subsection "Extra-Amniotic Prostaglandins."

Compared with PGE2, EASI with an intracervical Foley balloon is associated with **shorter time intervals to yield a favorable Bishop score**, and similar incidence of CD (49–51).

Compared with vaginal misoprostol, EASI with an intracervical Foley balloon and oxytocin is associated with shorter induction-to-delivery interval, and less nonreassuring fetal heart testing (NRFHT), but similar incidence of CD in one trial (52).

Compared with laminaria, EASI with an intracervical Foley balloon is associated with **shorter induction-to-delivery interval** and less **CD for failed induction** in one trial (52).

Compared with Foley only, EASI with Foley catheters has been associated with shorter induction-to-delivery interval in one RCT (53) but not in another larger RCT (54).

In summary, **there is insufficient evidence to use EASI instead of Foley balloon for cervical ripening**.

Membrane Stripping (or Sweeping)
Membrane stripping is the practice of inserting a finger through the internal os and sweeping to separate the membranes from the lower uterine segment. This technique stimulates prostaglandin release as plasma prostaglandin levels have been observed to increase poststripping. Sweeping the membranes promotes the onset of labor.

Compared with no sweeping, **sweeping of the membranes**, performed as a general policy in women at term (e.g., weekly starting at 38 weeks), **is associated with reduced duration of pregnancy** and **reduced frequency of pregnancy continuing beyond 41 weeks** (RR 0.59, 95% CI 0.46–0.74) **and 42 weeks** (RR 0.28, 95% CI 0.15–0.50) (55–57). To avoid one formal induction of labor, sweeping of membranes must be performed in eight women. **Rate of CD and maternal or neonatal infection are similar**. Discomfort during vaginal examination and other adverse effects (bleeding and irregular contractions) are more frequently reported by women allocated to sweeping, but not associated with complications. Studies comparing sweeping with prostaglandin administration are of limited sample size and do not provide evidence of benefit.

When used as a means for induction of labor, the woman should be counseled that her chance of going to spontaneous labor after one sweeping at term is about **36% in the next 48 hours**, versus 17% without sweeping (so doubling the rate of onset of labor) (55,56). Possible complications such as bleeding, infection, and ruptured membranes are not found to be increased with stripping (55,56).

In nulliparas being induced with PGE2 and oxytocin, the **addition of membrane sweeping** is associated with **shorter induction-to-delivery interval and increased vaginal delivery rates** in one trial (57). There were no differences noted in nulliparas with favorable cervices or in multiparas.

Amniotomy
Amniotomy—artificial rupture of the membranes—is another technique used in labor induction. There is **insufficient evidence** to assess the effectiveness of amniotomy alone (58). No trials compared amniotomy alone with intracervical prostaglandins. If performed without cervical ripening or achieving a favorable cervix, amniotomy may be followed by long intervals before onset of labor. Although early amniotomy may be associated with **shorter labor**, it is also associated with an **increase in nonreassuring fetal heart rate (NRFHR) patterns consistent with cord compression and chorioamnionitis** (59).

Compared with **placebo**, amniotomy and intravenous (IV) oxytocin are associated with significantly fewer instrumental vaginal deliveries than placebo. Compared with **vaginal prostaglandins**, amniotomy and IV oxytocin result in **more postpartum hemorrhage** and **more dissatisfaction in women** (58,60).

Pharmacologic Methods
Pharmacologic methods include the prostaglandins—E1: misoprostol; E2: dinoprostone; and F2α—as well as mifepristone, estrogen, relaxin, oxytocin, etc.

Misoprostol
Misoprostol (Cytotec™) is PGE1, which is an endogenously produced hormone that acts locally on surrounding tissues. Through complex molecular actions, PGE1 stimulates uterine contractions and cervical dilation in a manner akin to the onset of spontaneous labor. More specifically, PGE1 potentiates

calcium ion transport across the cellular membrane and regulates cyclic adenosine monophosphate (AMP) within the uterine smooth muscle cells to trigger contractions. Additionally PGE1 facilitates cervical ripening by stimulating the pathway leading to the activation of collagenases. Collagenases, in turn, break down the structural collagen network of the cervix yielding a softer, thinner cervix.

Although it is currently on the market as a 100-μg tablet to prevent peptic ulcers, misoprostol is available and widely used in an "off label" form for preinduction cervical ripening and induction. **Misoprostol should not be used for cervical ripening or labor induction in women with prior uterine incisions** (e.g., prior CD) **after 28 weeks** (12,15). For use of misoprostol for induction in the second trimester, see chapter 29 and chapter 54 in *Maternal-Fetal Evidence Based Guidelines*. Misoprostol can be administered vaginally, orally (buccal), or sublingually.

Vaginal misoprostol suppository. Vaginal misoprostol is most commonly administered by placing a tablet in the **posterior fornix of the vagina**. Several studies have focused on the dose administered. **Vaginal misoprostol in doses above 25 μg every 4 hour is more effective** (higher success rate for vaginal delivery within 24 hours of induction, decrease need for oxytocin, and decrease induction-to-delivery intervals) **than conventional methods of labor induction, but with more uterine hyperstimulation. Lower doses (25 μg) are similar to conventional methods in effectiveness and risks**. Lower doses of misoprostol compared with higher doses were associated with more need for oxytocin augmentation and less uterine tachysystole, with and without FHR changes, and less meconium aspiration (52). Therefore, **25 μg of misoprostol** (one-quarter of a 100-μg tablet) **given not more frequently than every 3 to 6 hours has been recommended** by the American College of Obstetricians and Gynecologists (12).

Compared with placebo, misoprostol is associated with reduced failure to achieve vaginal delivery within 24 hours (RR 0.51, 95% CI 0.37–0.71), and with increased uterine tachysystole without FHR changes (RR 3.52, 95% CI 1.78–6.99) (52).

Compared with vaginal PGE2, intracervical PGE2, and oxytocin, vaginal misoprostol is associated with less epidural analgesia use, **fewer failures to achieve vaginal delivery within 24 hours**, and **more uterine tachysystole** (52).

Compared with vaginal or intracervical PGE2, oxytocin augmentation was less common with misoprostol, and meconium-stained liquor more common (52,61).

Compared with vaginal PGE2 only, a meta-analysis of 11 RCTs showed that vaginal misoprostol was associated with a higher likelihood of vaginal delivery within 12 and 24 hours and lower use of oxytocin augmentation. There was no difference between the groups in relation to rate of CD, or incidence of tachysystole. Additionally, the cost of a 25-μg pill of misoprostol is approximately $2 compared to the dinoprostone vaginal insert at approximately $168 (62).

In summary, **vaginal misoprostol 25 μg every 4 to 6 hours is a safe, effective means for cervical ripening, more effective than PGE2.**

Vaginal misoprostol insert. A phase III clinical trial of a 50- and 100-μg vaginal insert (which is equivalent to a 25-μg tablet fragment being inserted every 6 hours) showed that the 100-μg vaginal insert had equal median times to vaginal delivery as the 10-mg dinoprostone vaginal insert. The 50-μg and 100-μg misoprostol inserts and the 10-mg dinoprostone insert all had comparable rates of CD and safety profile (63). In women with a modified Bishop score <5, doses of misoprostol vaginal insert of 50 μg, 100 μg, and 200 μg were associated with similar

proportion of delivery within 24 hours, but less induction time was associated with the 100- and 200-μg doses, and more tachysystole and CD for NRFHT associated with the 200-μg dose, making the 50- or 100-μg doses the most applicable to future use (64). In summary, **there is still insufficient evidence for clinical use of misoprostol vaginal insert, but the data so far are promising.**

Oral misoprostol. Studies that examine patient satisfaction have shown a definite preference toward oral administration (65,66).

Compared with placebo in women with PROM, women who received oral misoprostol had a higher likelihood to deliver vaginally within 24 hours (RR 0.16, 95% CI 0.05–0.49), needed less oxytocin (RR 0.35, 95% CI 0.28–0.44), and had a lower cesarean section rate (RR 0.61, 95% CI 0.41–0.93) (66).

Compared with vaginal PGE2 prostaglandins, low-dose oral misoprostol (e.g., 20 μg) administered every 2 hours had the same rate of vaginal delivery in 24 hours and a significantly lower rate of CD (65). Women given oral misoprostol were also less likely to need a cesarean section (RR 0.87, 95% CI 0.77–0.98). There was some evidence that they had slower inductions, but there were no other significant differences (66).

Compared with oxytocin, the only difference associated with oral misoprostol was an increase in meconium-stained liquor in women with ruptured membranes (RR 1.72, 95% CI 1.08–2.74) (66).

Compared with vaginal misoprostol, oral misoprostol appeared to be less effective in seven trials. More women in the oral misoprostol group did not achieve vaginal delivery within 24 hours of randomization (50%) compared with 40% in the vaginal misoprostol group (55). The **cesarean section rate is lower in the oral misoprostol** group (16.7%) compared with 21.7% in the vaginal misoprostol group. There was **no difference in uterine tachysystole with FHR changes** (8.5% vs. 7.4%). There were no reported cases of severe neonatal and maternal morbidity, except there were fewer babies born with a low Apgar score in the oral misoprostol group (RR 0.65, 95% CI 0.44–0.97). The data on optimal regimens and safety are lacking. It is possible that effective oral regimens may have an unacceptably high incidence of complications such as uterine tachysystole and possibly uterine rupture (66).

Compared with vaginal misoprostol, low-dose oral misoprostol (20–25 μg) given every 2 hours was shown in a review of two trials to cause fewer incidences of uterine tachysystole with FHR changes. There were no other differences between the groups. When examining frequently titrated doses of oral misoprostol to vaginal misoprostol, the oral misoprostol group had a higher rate of vaginal delivery in 24 hours (65).

Sublingual misoprostol. Based on only three small trials, **sublingual** misoprostol appears to be at least as effective as when the same dose is administered orally, but there are **inadequate data** to assess safety, optimal dose, and side effects (67). When the same dosage (50 μg) is used sublingually versus orally, the sublingual route is associated with less failure to achieve vaginal delivery within 24 hours, reduced oxytocin augmentation, and reduced cesarean section in a small trial, but the differences are not statistically significant. When a smaller dose was used sublingually than orally, there were no differences in any of the outcomes.

Prostaglandin E2 (Dinoprostone)
PGE2 is an endogenously produced hormone that acts locally on surrounding tissues. Such effect is manifested in the smooth muscle of the uterus and gastrointestinal tract.

PGE2 can be used for induction of labor via different routes of administration, such as vaginal, extra-amniotic, oral, and intravenous. The vaginal route is the most common route of administration of PGE2 for labor induction. It can be given in different forms, such as tablet, gel, and insert.

All PGE2 vaginal forms. **Compared with placebo or no treatment**, **vaginal PGE2 (all forms)** is associated with a **higher likelihood of vaginal delivery within 24 hours** (18% vs. 99%), no difference in CD rates, and an increase in the risk of uterine tachysystole with FHR changes (4.4% vs. 0.5%) (60). PGE2 tablet, gel, and pessary appear to be as efficacious as each other (60).

PGE2 vaginal gel. Dinoprostone gel (Prepidil) is packaged as a 0.5-mg dose in a 2.5-mL syringe. A shielded catheter is added to the syringe end to facilitate safe injection, usually intracervical. Under direct visualization using a speculum, the syringe contents should be injected into the endocervical canal using sterile technique. The patient should remain supine for 30 minutes to minimize leakage from the canal. An alternative method for administering the gel is to inject into the posterior fornix or intravaginal administration. Until achieving a favorable cervix, dinoprostone 0.5 mg may be repeated every 6 hours up to a maximum dose of 1.5 mg in a 24-hour period. Once the cervix is favorable, oxytocin may be initiated for induction 6 hours after the last dose.

Compared with PGE2 tablets, PGE2 gel is associated with a **lower need for oxytocin** (60). Cervical ripening with dinoprostone gel has been shown to be an effective method for preinduction cervical ripening in randomized trials (60).

Compared with placebo, intracervical PGE2 is associated with decreased risk of not achieving vaginal delivery within 24 hours (RR 0.61, 95% CI 0.47–0.79). There was a small, and statistically nonsignificant, reduction of the risk of cesarean section when PGE2 was used (RR 0.88, 95% CI 0.77–1.00). The finding was statistically significant in a subgroup of women with intact membranes and unfavorable cervix only (RR 0.82, 95% CI 0.68–0.98). The risk of tachysystole with FHR changes was not significantly increased (RR 1.21, 95% CI 0.72–2.05). However, the risk of tachysystole without FHR changes was significantly increased (RR 1.59, 95% CI 1.09–2.33) (68,69).

PGE2 vaginal insert. PGE2 vaginal insert (Cervidil) (also called slow-release pessary) is a thin, vaginal insert containing 10 mg of dinoprostone and delivers roughly 0.3 mg of dinoprostone each hour over a 24-hour period. The insert is placed in the posterior fornix of the vagina and left in place until the desired ripening has occurred when the insert is removed. Removal should occur at least 30 minutes prior to starting oxytocin. Cervidil use is indicated for cervical ripening and induction of labor in patients who have a medical indication for induction at or near term. However, it should be used with caution in the following situations: fetal malpresentation, previous uterine or cervical surgery, cephalopelvic disproportion, nonreassuring fetal heart tones, current pelvic inflammatory disease, multiple gestation, when labor has begun, patients with more than three term deliveries, or any other contraindication to vaginal delivery (68).

Compared with PGE2 gel, PGE2 insert is associated with an increased risk of not achieving a vaginal delivery within 24 hours (RR 1.26, 95% CI 1.12–1.41). There was no change in the risk of cesarean section (RR 1.07, 95% CI 0.93–1.22). The risks of tachysystole with FHR changes (RR 0.76, 95% CI 0.39–1.49) and without FHR changes (RR 0.80, 95% CI 0.56–1.15) were nonsignificantly different with the two methods of PGE2 administration. Only one trial with a small sample size reported on women's views, with no difference between

groups (68–72). The use of sustained-release PGE2 inserts is associated with a reduction in instrumental vaginal delivery rates (9.9% vs. 19.5%; RR 0.51, 95% CI 0.35–0.76, NNT 10) when compared to vaginal PGE2 gel or tablet (60). Therefore, the common use of PGE2 insert can be also associated with its ease of use by the practitioner.

Compared with intracervical PGE2 low dose, intracervical PGE2 high dose has been insufficiently studied to provide any useful information (68).

Compared with Cervidil followed by oxytocin, Cervidil started concurrently with oxytocin is associated with a shorter induction-to-delivery interval and higher incidence of vaginal deliveries within 24 hours in one small trial (73).

Extra-amniotic prostaglandins. There is **insufficient evidence** to fully assess the effectiveness of extra-amniotic prostaglandins for induction of labor, with enough evidence to discourage its use compared with other methods (see also subsection "Extra-Amniotic Saline Infusion"). Extra-amniotic placement of prostaglandins was first undertaken in the early 1970s and has been largely replaced with cervical or vaginal placement. Most of the studies used PGE2 [the minority prostaglandin F2α (PGF2α)] and gel preparations. Of the primary outcomes, there were significantly fewer women delivered vaginally within 24 hours among those induced with extra-amniotic PGF2α compared with vaginal misoprostol (RR 2.43, 95% CI 1.42–4.15). No other differences between groups for primary outcomes were found to be statistically significant. Oxytocin was used to initiate or augment labor significantly less frequently with extra-amniotic prostaglandins when compared with placebo (RR 0.51, 95% CI 0.39–0.67) but significantly more frequently when compared with vaginal misoprostol (RR 1.73, 95% CI 1.20–2.49). When extra-amniotic PGE2 was compared with Foley catheter only, the only difference between groups was that there were fewer cases of unfavorable cervix at 12 to 24 hours following treatment (RR 0.59, 95% CI 0.41–0.86). Women receiving extra-amniotic prostaglandin were more likely to be satisfied and less likely to be embarrassed by the treatment compared with vaginal PGE2. There were no other significant differences when extra-amniotic prostaglandins were compared with other methods of cervical ripening or induction of labor. Although this could suggest that extra-amniotic prostaglandins are as effective as other agents, the findings are difficult to interpret because they are based on very small numbers and may lack the power to show a real difference (74).

Oral prostaglandins. Compared with placebo or no treatment, PGE2 is associated with a 54% decrease in CD. Otherwise, there were no significant differences between PGE2 and other interventions for this outcome (75).

Compared to vaginal prostaglandins, there is insufficient evidence, but no gross differences in three small trials (75).

Compared with all oxytocin treatments, oral PGE2 is associated with a trend for a lower incidence of vaginal delivery not achieved within 24 hours (RR 1.97, 95% CI 0.86–4.48).

Oral prostaglandin was associated with **vomiting** across all comparison groups. There are **no clear advantages** to oral prostaglandin over other methods of induction of labor.

Intravenous prostaglandins. IV prostaglandins **should not be used** for induction or cervical ripening, as they are no more efficient than IV oxytocin for the induction of labor, but their use is associated with higher rates of maternal side effects and uterine tachysystole. Compared with oxytocin, IV prostaglandins are associated with **higher rates of uterine tachysystole** both with and without changes in the FHR, and similar incidence of vaginal delivery (76). Use of IV prostaglandins is also

Table 20.4   Labor Stimulation with Oxytocin: Examples of Low- and High-Dose Oxytocin Protocols

Regimen	Starting dose	Incremental increase (mU/min)	Dosage interval (min)
Low dose	0.5–1	1	30–40
	1–2	2	15
High dose	~6	~6	15
	6	6[a],3,1	20–40

[a]The incremental increase is reduced to 3 mU/min in presence of tachysystole and reduced to 1 mU/min with recurrent tachysystole.

associated with significantly **more maternal side effects** (gastrointestinal, thrombophlebitis, and pyrexia). No significant differences emerged from subgroup analysis or from the trials comparing combination oxytocin/PGF2α and oxytocin or extra-amniotic versus IV PGE2 (76). There is insufficient information to assess a combination of PGF2α and oxytocin compared with oxytocin alone or extra-amniotic and IV PGE2.

Oxytocin
In 1948, the posterior pituitary extract, oxytocin, was first used for labor induction via IV drip. Oxytocin was then synthesized by du Vigneaud and associates in 1953; this accomplishment won the Nobel Prize in chemistry in 1955. Oxytocin is now widely utilized worldwide. Oxytocin is routinely utilized as it is the drug of choice also for augmentation of labor. While induction of labor is the stimulation of contractions before the spontaneous onset of labor, augmentation is the stimulation of contractions in the face of inadequate contractions following the spontaneous onset of labor.

By increasing intracellular calcium concentration, oxytocin stimulates the smooth muscle cells of breast, vessels, and, moreover, the uterus. Receptors for oxytocin are expressed in cells of the endometrium, liver, pancreas, and breast tissue. After the 13th week of gestation, myometrial cells express oxytocin receptors as well. Peak expression by the myometrium and endometrium occurs at term. Oxytocin increases both the amplitude and frequency of contractions, making labor effective. When continuously administered IV, oxytocin affects uterine response within 1 minute. Steady-state plasma concentrations are obtained within 40 minutes.

Overall, comparison of oxytocin with either intravaginal or intracervical PGE2 reveals that the **prostaglandin agents probably increase the chances of achieving vaginal birth within 24 hours**. Oxytocin induction may increase the rate of interventions in labor. In women with ruptured membranes induction can be recommended by either method, and in women with intact membranes there is insufficient information to make firm recommendations (77).

Compared with expectant management, oxytocin alone inductions are associated with fewer women failing to deliver vaginally within 24 hours (8% vs. 54%; RR 0.16, 95% CI 0.10–0.25), with the cesarean section rate slightly increased (10.4% vs. 8.9%). There is a significant increase in the number of women requiring epidural analgesia (RR 1.10, 95% CI 1.04–1.17). Fewer women are dissatisfied with oxytocin induction in one trial reporting this outcome (5.9% vs. 13.7%; RR 0.43, 95% CI 0.33–0.56) (77).

Compared with vaginal prostaglandins, oxytocin alone is associated with an **increase in unsuccessful vaginal delivery within 24 hours** (70% vs. 21%; RR 3.33, 95% CI 1.61–6.89), irrespective of membrane status, but there was no difference in cesarean section rates.

There was a small increase in epidurals when oxytocin alone was used (RR 1.09, 95% CI 1.01–1.17). Most of the studies included women with ruptured membranes, and there was some evidence that oxytocin decreased infection in mothers (chorioamnionitis; RR 0.66, 95% CI 0.47–0.92) and babies (use of antibiotics; RR 0.68, 95% CI 0.53–0.87). These data should be interpreted cautiously as infection was not prespecified in the original review protocol (77).

Compared with intracervical PGE2 prostaglandins, oxytocin alone is associated with an **increase in unsuccessful vaginal delivery within 24 hours** (50% vs. 35%; RR 1.47, 95% CI 1.10–1.96). For all women with an unfavorable cervix regardless of membrane status, the cesarean section rate is increased (19% vs. 13%; RR 1.37, 95% CI 1.08–1.74) (77,78).

Oxytocin seems to be as effective as prostaglandins in women with PROM (78) (see chap. 19).

Either low- or high-dose oxytocin regimens are reasonable (12,78–83). Table 20.4 shows examples of each regimen (see also chap. 7). Compared with low-dose oxytocin, **high-dose oxytocin** has been associated in some studies with **shorter average time from admission to delivery, higher incidence of uterine tachysystole**, but with similar incidences of cesarean section (lower incidence of CD for failed induction) and **similar neonatal outcomes** (78–83).

Prostaglandin F2α
Compared with placebo, vaginal PGF2α is associated with improved cervical score (60% vs. 15%), reduced need for oxytocin augmentation (54% vs. 89%), and similar cesarean section rates (69). There were insufficient data to make meaningful conclusions for the comparison of vaginal PGE2 and PGF2-α (69). There is therefore **insufficient data** to assess the safety and efficacy of PGF2-α for induction.

Mifepristone
There is **insufficient information** available from clinical trials to support the use of mifepristone to induce labor. **Compared with placebo**, mifepristone-treated women were more likely to be in labor or to have a favorable cervix at 48 hours (RR 2.41, 95% CI 1.70–3.42) and this effect persisted at 96 hours (RR 3.40, 95% CI 1.96–5.92). They were less likely to need augmentation with oxytocin (RR 0.80, 95% CI 0.66–0.97). Mifepristone-treated women were less likely to undergo cesarean section (RR 0.74, 95% CI 0.60–0.92) but more likely to have an instrumental delivery (RR 1.43, 95% CI 1.04–1.96). Women receiving mifepristone were less likely to undergo a cesarean section as a result of failure to induce labor (RR 0.40, 95% CI 0.20–0.80) (84).

There is insufficient evidence to support a particular dose but a single dose of 200-mg mifepristone appears to be the lowest effective dose for cervical ripening: increased likelihood of cervical ripening at 72 hours (RR 2.13, 95% CI 1.15–3.97). Abnormal FHR patterns were more common after mifepristone treatment (RR 1.85, 95% CI 1.17–2.93), but there was no evidence of differences in other neonatal outcomes (84). However there is some concern about changes in fetal aldosterone levels (85). There is insufficient information on the occurrence of uterine rupture/dehiscence in the reviewed studies. Similarly, there is little information about maternal side effects although some nausea and vomiting were reported in one trial. There is very limited information comparing mifepristone with alternative methods of inducing labor, for example, prostaglandins (84).

Estrogen

Several studies have shown that estradiol given via a variety of routes has the ability to achieve some degree of improved cervical ripening with minimal myometrial stimulation (85). However, on a whole there were **insufficient data** to draw any conclusions regarding the efficacy of estrogen as an induction agent, given small, differing trials with different controls and different outcomes reported (86).

Relaxin

There is **insufficient evidence** to assess the safety and efficacy of relaxin as an intervention for induction of labor. There are no reported cases of uterine tachysystole with NRFHT in any of the four small trials (87). Compared with placebo, relaxin is not associated with differences in CD, but there is a reduction in the risk of the cervix remaining unfavorable or unchanged with induction with relaxin (22% vs. 49%) (87).

Dehydroepiandrosterone Sulfate

Dehydroepiandrosterone sulfate (DHEAS) is converted to estrogen by the fetoplacental unit, and it was investigated as a possible mechanism for cervical ripening without myometrial contractions. There is **insufficient evidence** on its efficacy as one trial that investigated its use showed poor results when compared with placebo (85).

Dexamethasone Sulfate

There is **insufficient evidence** to assess the safety and efficacy of steroids as inductions agents. Compared with oxytocin alone, dexamethasone IM and oxytocin are not associated with significant effects in maternal and perinatal outcomes in one small RCT (88).

Hyaluronidase

There is **insufficient evidence** to assess the safety and efficacy of intracervical injections of hyaluronidase for cervical ripening. It is not common practice, and it is an invasive procedure that women may find unacceptable in the presence of less invasive methods. In one RCT, when compared with placebo for cervical ripening, intracervical injections of hyaluronidase resulted in women receiving significantly fewer cesarean sections (18% vs. 49%; RR 0.37, 95% CI 0.22–0.61), less need for oxytocin augmentation (10% vs. 47%; RR 0.20, 95% CI 0.10–0.41), and increased cervical favorability after 24 hours (60% vs. 98%; RR 0.62, 95% CI 0.52–0.74). No side effects for mother or baby were reported in this trial (89).

Nitric Oxide Donors

Nitric oxide (NO) donors **do not appear currently to be a useful tool** in the process of induction of labor. Included studies compared NO donors with placebo, vaginal PGE2, intracervical PGE2, and vaginal misoprostol. There are very limited data available to compare NO donors to any other induction agent. There is no evidence of any difference between any of the prespecified outcomes when comparing NO donors with other induction agents, with the exception of an increase in maternal side effects. More studies are required to examine how NO donors may work alongside established induction of labor protocols, especially those based in outpatient settings (90).

Other Methods

Acupuncture

There is insufficient and conflicting evidence to assess the efficacy of acupuncture for induction of labor. Compared with a sham procedure, **the use of acupuncture prior to a scheduled induction is not associated with any difference in the need for induction agents or duration of labor in women with a postterm pregnancy** (83,91,92). A Cochrane review showed a decreased need for induction methods in women receiving acupuncture; however, the two largest latest studies were not yet included, and the studies involved had a small sample size and patients were not blinded to their treatment (83).

Breast Stimulation

Compared with no intervention, breast stimulation is associated with a significant **reduction in the number of women not in labor at 72 hours** (63% vs. 94%). This result is not significant in women with an unfavorable cervix. The rate of postpartum hemorrhage is reduced (0.7% vs. 6%). There is no significant difference in the cesarean section rate, in the rate of meconium staining or uterine tachysystole. The three perinatal deaths were associated just with breast stimulation (1.8% vs. 0%) (93).

Compared with oxytocin alone, breast stimulation is associated with a higher number of women not in labor after 72 hours (59% vs. 25%), and similar cesarean section rates, and meconium staining. Three of the four perinatal deaths were in high-risk women in the breast stimulation group (17.6% vs. 5%) (93). Until **safety issues** have been fully evaluated, breast stimulation should not be used in high-risk women (93).

Castor Oil

Castor oil **should not be used for induction of labor** (94). Compared with no treatment, a single dose of castor oil is associated with similar cesarean section rates, meconium-stained liquor or Apgar score <7 at 5 minutes (85). There is insufficient evidence on neonatal or maternal mortality or morbidity. The number of participants was small; hence only large differences in outcomes could have been detected. All women who ingested castor oil felt nauseous (94).

Homeopathy

There is insufficient evidence to recommend the use of homeopathy (e.g., with caulophyllum) as a method of induction. **No benefits** were seen in the two small, poor-quality trials (95).

Sexual Intercourse

There is **insufficient evidence** to assess the efficacy of sexual intercourse for induction of labor. A "coital diary" prospective study showed no difference in the incidence of spontaneous labor in the "advised-coitus" group despite 1.5 times as many participants in that group reporting intercourse. There was also no difference in the rate of cesarean section or adverse outcomes (96). One RCT is too small for meaningful guidance (97). In another RCT, compared with no such advice, advice for coitus was associated with more coital activity (60% vs. 40%), but similar rates of spontaneous labor (56% vs. 52%) (98).

There are no trials on enemas, baths, or other methods for induction of labor.

ANTEPARTUM TESTING DURING CERVICAL RIPENING

Fetal heart monitoring during cervical ripening depends on the agent used. There are no trials to assess the effectiveness and best modality for monitoring. In general, a nonstress test (NST) should be obtained before any induction or cervical ripening agent is used to assure fetal well-being. After administration of **PGE2 gel or tablet**, the fetal heart can be monitored continuously for about 0.5 to 2 hours, although the proper amount of time for monitoring is unclear. After administration of **PGE2 insert**, the fetal heart can be monitored continuously for the duration of the insertion (99). After administration of **misoprostol**, the fetal heart should be monitored continuously, given the higher chance of contractions, and uterine tachysystole with related NRFHT.

OUTPATIENT VS. INPATIENT

Induction of labor in outpatient settings appears **feasible, but the evidence is still insufficient for routine use.** Important **adverse events are rare** (100). There is **insufficient evidence to know which induction agents are most effective and safe to use in outpatient setting.** Studies examined **vaginal and intracervical PGE2, isosorbide mononitrate** (for these three agents there is most evidence of safety, $n \geq 500$ each), Foley (47), vaginal and oral misoprostol, mifepristone, estrogens, and acupuncture (very limited evidence for these other agents) (101). There **is insufficient evidence to assess the safety of outpatient misoprostol** for induction of labor. While effective in decreasing the length of gestation and induction-to-delivery interval, the safety of this approach, even at low (25 µg) doses, is still unproven in the three small trials (101–103).

There was no strong evidence that agents used to induce labor in outpatient settings had an impact (positive or negative) on maternal or neonatal health. There was some evidence that, compared with placebo or no treatment, **induction agents reduced the need for further interventions to induce labor and shortened the interval from intervention to birth.** There was no evidence that induction agents increased interventions in labor such as operative deliveries. Only two studies provided information on women's views about the induction process, and overall there was very little information on the costs to health service providers of different methods of labor induction in outpatient settings (100,104).

Labor Management with Induction
The patterns by which labor progresses in spontaneous labor and electively induced labor are significantly different (24). Latent and early active phases proceed **slower** than a spontaneous labor in induced labor in which cervical ripening was necessary. Induction nonnecessitating cervical ripening may be associated with a quicker labor course from 4 to 10 cm (24). The risk of **CD** is increased during the first stage of labor of an induction needing cervical ripening, mainly because of dystocia. Induction without need for cervical ripening may have no or only a minor effect on the risk of cesarean (24). Applying the same standards of spontaneous labor curves (e.g., Friedman's curve) to induced patients may lead to an increase cesarean section rate in induction (78) (see also chaps. 7 and 8).

When administering oxytocin, the target is to stimulate uterine activity that is sufficient to effect cervical change as well as fetal descent without compromising the fetus. Minimal criteria for effective uterine activity are 3 contractions per 10 minutes averaging greater than 25 mmHg above baseline, with 5 contractions in 10 minutes. The Montevideo unit was created in 1957 to describe the summation of the amplitudes of all contractions in a 10-minute window. Uterine tachysystole is defined as >5 contractions in 10 minutes. During induction with oxytocin, 91% of patients delivered vaginally achieved 200 Montevideo units without neonatal morbidity in one retrospective study (105). Contraction pressures of ≥ 200 Montevideo units should be targeted in induction or augmentation of laboring patients to achieve adequate labor (105,106). **Induced labor should be managed, in general, as for spontaneous labor** (see chaps. 7 and 8). If active phase is not achieved within 24 hours, this is not a reason per se for CD. A **failed induction** should not be diagnosed until after **12 hours of oxytocin after membrane rupture in the active phase** (usually 6 cm in a nulliparous patient), assuming reassuring fetal heart pattern (7,24).

REFERENCES

1. Martin JA, Hamilton BE, Sutton PD, et al. National Vital Statistics Reports. Vol. 57, No. 7. Hyattsville, MD: National Center for Health Statistics, 2009. [Epidemiologic data report]
2. Glantz JC. Labor induction rate variation in upstate New York: what is the difference? Birth 2003; 30(3):168–174. [II-2]
3. Bailit JL, Gregory KD, Reddy UM, et al. Maternal and neonatal outcomes by labor onset type and gestational age. Am J Obstet Gynecol 2010; 202(3):245.e1–245.e12.
4. Bishop EH. Pelvic scoring for elective induction. Obstet Gynecol 1964; 24:266–268. [II-3]
5. Vrouenraets FP, Roumen FJ, Dehing CJ, et al. Bishop score and risk of cesarean delivery after induction of labor in nulliparous women. Obstet Gynecol 2005; 105:690–697. [II-2, n = 765]
6. Sciscione AC, Zhang J, Laughon K, et al. The duration of labor induction and maternal and neonatal outcomes. Poster Presentation. SMFM Annual Meeting, San Francisco, CA, February 2011. [II-2]
7. Rouse DJ, Owen J, Hauth JC. Criteria for failed labor induction: prospective evaluation of a standardized protocol. Obstet Gynecol 2000; 96:671–677. [II-3, n = 509]
8. Neilson JP. Ultrasound for fetal assessment in early pregnancy. Cochrane Database Syst Rev 2005;(3). [Meta-analysis: 9 RCTs, n = >24,000]
9. Mozurkewich E, Chilimigras J, Koepke E, et al. Indications for induction of labour: a best evidence review. BJOG 2009; 116:626–636. [Review]
10. Spong CY, Mercer BM, D'alton M, et al. Timing of indicated late-preterm and early-term birth. Obstet Gynecol 2011; 118(2 pt 1): 323–333. [Review]
11. Berghella V, Blackwell SC, Ramin SM, et al. Use and misuse of the term "elective" in obstetrics. Obstet Gynecol 2011; 117(2 pt 1): 372–376. [Review]
12. American College of Obstetricians and Gynecologists. ACOG Practice Bulletin No. 107: Induction of labor. Obstet Gynecol 2009; 114:386–397. [Review]
13. Caughey AB, Sundaram V, Kaimal AJ, et al. Systematic review elective induction of labor versus expectant management of pregnancy. Ann Int Med 2009; 151:252–263. [Systematic review]
14. Nicholson JM, Parry S, Caughey AB, et al. The impact of the active management of risk in pregnancy at term on birth outcomes a randomized clinical trial. Am J Obstet Gynecol 2008; 198:e511–e515. [RCT, n = 270]
15. Plaut MM, Schwartz ML, Lubarsky SL. Uterine rupture associated with the use of misoprostol in the gravid patient with a previous cesarean section. Am J Obstet Gynecol 1999; 180:1535–1542. [II-2, n = 512]
16. Hoffman MK, Sciscione AC, Srinivasana M, et al. Uterine rupture in patients with a prior cesarean delivery: the impact of cervical ripening. Am J Perinatol 2004; 21:217–222. [II-2, n = 972]
17. Bujold E, Blackwell SC, Hendler I, et al. Modified Bishop's score and induction of labor with patients with previous cesarean delivery. Am J Obstet Gynecol 2004; 191:1644–1648. [II-2, n = 685]

18. Landon MB, Hauth JC, Leveno KJ, et al. Maternal and perinatal outcomes associated with a trial of labor after prior cesarean delivery. N Engl J Med 2004; 351(25):2581–2589. [II-2; prospective; *n* = 33,699]

19. Lyndon-Rochelle M, Holt VL, Easterling TR, et al. Risk of uterine rupture during labor among women with a prior cesarean delivery. N Engl J Med 2001; 345(1):3–8. [II-2, *n* = 20,095]

20. Bujold E, Blackwell SC, Gauthier RJ. Cervical ripening with transcervical Foley catheter and the risk of uterine rupture. Obstet Gynecol 2004; 103:18–23. [II-2, *n* = 2479]

21. Bakker JJ, De Vos R, Pel M, et al. Start of Induction of labour with oxytocin in the morning or in the evening. A randomized controlled trial. BJOG 2009; 116:562–568. [RCT, *n* = 371]

22. Dodd JM, Crowther CA, Robinson JS. Morning compared with evening induction of labor—a nested randomized controlled trial. Obstet Gynecol 2006; 108:350–360. [RCT, *n* = 620]

23. Pevzner L, Rayburn WF, Rumney P, et al. Factors predicting successful labor and induction with dinoprostone and misoprostol vaginal inserts. Obstet Gynecol 2009; 114:261–267. [II-2, *n* = 1274]

24. Vahration A, Zhang J, Troendle JF, et al. Labor progression and risk of cesarean delivery in electively induced nulliparas. Obstet Gynecol 2005; 105:698–704. [II-2, *n* = 429]

25. Laughton SK, Zhang J, Troendle J, et al. Using a simplified Bishop score to predict vaginal delivery. Obstet Gynecol 2011; 117(4):805–811. [II-2]

26. Park KH, Kim SN, Lee SY, et al. Comparison between sonographic cervical length and Bishop score in preinduction cervical assessment: a randomized trial. Ultrasound Obstet Gynecol 2011; 38:198–204. [RCT, *n* = 154]

27. Hatfield AS, Sanchez-Ramos L, Kaunitz AM. Sonographic cervical assessment to predict the success of labor induction: a systematic review with metaanalysis. Am J Obstet Gynecol 2007; 197:186–192. [Review]

28. Garite TJ, Carcia-Alonso A, Kreaden U, et al. Fetal fibronectin: a new tool for the prediction of successful induction of labor. Am J Obstet Gynecol 1996; 175:1516–1521. [II-2]

29. Sciscione AC, Hoffman MK, DeLuca S, et al. Fetal fibronectin as a predictor of vaginal birth in nulliparas undergoing preinduction cervical ripening. Obstet Gynecol 2005; 106:980–985. [II-2, *n* = 241]

30. Boulvain M, Kelly AJ, Lohse C, et al. Mechanical methods for induction of labour. Cochrane Database Syst Rev 2001; (4): CD001233. [Meta-analysis: 45 RCTs, *n* = >5000]

31. Gilson GJ, Russell DJ, Izquierdo LA, et al. A prospective, randomized evaluation of a hygroscopic cervical dilator, Dilapan, in the preinduction ripening of patients undergoing induction of labor. Am J Obstet Gynecol 1996; 175:145–149. [RCT, *n* = 240]

32. Sciscione AC, McCullough H, Manley JS, et al. A prospective, randomized comparison of Foley catheter insertion versus intracervical prostaglandin E2 gel for preinduction cervical ripening. Am J Obstet Gynecol 1999; 180:55–59. [RCT, *n* = 149]

33. Thomas IL, Chenowith JN, Tronc GN, et al. Preparation for induction of labour of the unfavourable cervix with Foley catheter compared with vaginal prostaglandin. Aust NZ J Obstet Gynaecol 1986; 26:30–35. [RCT, *n* = 57]

34. Orhue A. Induction of labour at term in primigravidae with low Bishop's score: a comparison of three methods. Eur J Obstet Gynecol Reprod Biol 1995; 58:119–125. [RCT, *n* = 90]

35. St. Onge RD, Conners GT. Preinduction cervical ripening: a comparison of intracervical prostaglandin E2 gel versus the Foley catheter. Am J Obstet Gynecol 1995; 172:687–690. [RCT, *n* = 66]

36. Lieberman JR, Piura B, Choim W, et al. The cervical balloon method for induction of labor. Acta Obstet Gynecol Scand 1977; 56:499–503. [RCT, *n* = 194]

37. Sciscione AC, Ngyuen L, Manley J, et al. A randomized comparison of transcervical Foley catheter to intravaginal misoprostol for preinduction cervical ripening. Obstet Gynecol 2001; 97:603–607. [RCT, *n* = 111]

38. Delaney S, Shaffer BL, Yvonne CW, et al. Labor induction with a Foley balloon inflated to 30 mL compared with 60 mL. Obstet Gynecol 2010; 115:1239–1245. [I, *n* = 192]

39. Levy R, Kanengiser B, Furman B, et al. A randomized trial comparing a 30-mL and an 80-mL Foley catheter balloon for preinduction cervical ripening. Am J Obstet Gynecol 2004; 191:1632–1636. [RCT]

40. Kashanian M, Nazemi M, Malakzadegan A. Comparison of 30-mL and 80-mL Foley catheter balloons and oxytocin for preinduction cervical ripening. Int J Gynaecol Obstet 2009; 105:174–175. [RCT]

41. Yuen PM, Pang HYY, Chung T, et al. Cervical ripening before induction of labour in patients with an unfavourable cervix: a comparative randomized study of the Atad Ripener Device, prostaglandin E2 vaginal pessary, and prostaglandin E2 intracervical gel. Aust NZ J Obstet Gynaecol 1996; 36(3):291–295. [RCT, *n* = 114]

42. Cromi A, Ghezzi F, Agosti M, et al. Is transcervical Foley catheter actually slower than prostaglandins in ripening the cervix? A randomized study. Am J Obstet Gynecol 2011; 204:338.e1–338.e7. [RCT, *n* = 397]

43. Fox NS, Saltzman DH, Roman AS, et al. Intravaginal misoprostol versus Foley catheter for labour induction: a meta-analysis. BJOG 2011; 118(6):647–654. [Meta-analysis: 9 RCTs, *n* = 1603]

44. Vaknin Z, Kurzweil Y, Sherman D. Foley catheter balloon vs locally applied prostaglandins for cervical ripening and labor induction: a systematic review and metaanalysis. Am J Obstet Gynecol 2010; 204:418–429. [Meta-analysis]

45. Pettker C, Pocock SB, Smok DB, et al. Transcervical Foley catheter with and without oxytocin for cervical ripening: a randomized controlled trial. Obstet Gynecol 2008; 111:1320–1326. [I, *n* = 183]

46. Lin MG, Reid KJ, Treaster MR, et al. Transcervical Foley catheter with and without extraamniotic saline infusion for labor induction: a randomized controlled trial. Obstet Gynecol, 2007; 110:558–565. [I, *n* = 181]

47. Sciscione AC, Muench M, Pollock M, et al. Transcervical Foley catheter for preinduction cervical ripening in an outpatient versus inpatient setting. Obstet Gynecol 2001; 98:5(1):751–756. [RCT, *n* = 111]

48. Sciscione AC, Hoffman MK, Bedder CL, et al. The safety of the Foley catheter for preinduction cervical ripening in a low risk population. Poster Presentation. SMFM Annual Meeting, San Francisco, CA, February 2011. [II-1]

49. Schreyer P, Sherman DJ, Ariely S, et al. Ripening the highly unfavorable cervix with extra-amniotic saline instillation or vaginal prostaglandin E2 application. Obstet Gynecol 1898; 73:938–941. [RCT, *n* = 106]

50. Rouben D, Arias F. A randomized trial of extra-amniotic saline infusion plus intracervical Foley catheter balloon versus prostaglandin E2 vaginal gel for ripening the cervix and inducing labor in patients with unfavorable cervices. Obstet Gynecol 1993; 82:290–294. [RCT, *n* = 112]

51. Goldman JB, Wigton TR. A randomized comparison of extra-amniotic saline infusion and intracervical dinoprostone gel for cervical ripening. Obstet Gynecol 1999; 93:271–274. [RCT, *n* = 52]

52. Mullin PM, House M, Paul RH, et al. A comparison of vaginally administered misoprostol with extra-amniotic saline infusion for cervical ripening and labor induction. Am J Obstet Gynecol 2002; 187:847–852. [RCT, *n* = 200]

53. Karyane NW, Brock EL, Walsh SW. Induction of labor using a Foley balloon, with and without extra-amniotic saline infusion. Obstet Gynecol 2006; 107:234–239. [RCT, *n* = 120]

54. Lin MG, Reid KJ, Treaster MR, et al. Transcervical Foley catheter with and without extraamniotic saline infusion for labor induction. Obstet Gynecol 2007; 110:558–565. [RCT, *n* = 188]

55. Boulvain M, Stan CM, Irion O. Membrane sweeping for induction of labour. Cochrane Database Syst Rev 2005; (1):CD000451. [Meta-analysis: 22 RCTs, *n* = 2797]

56. Berghella V, Rogers RA, Lescale K. Stripping of membranes as a safe method to reduce prolonged pregnancies. Obstet Gynecol 1996; 87(6):927–929. [RCT, *n* = 142]

57. Foong LC, Vanaja K, Tan G, et al. Membranes sweeping in conjunction with labor induction. Obstet Gynecol 2000; 96:539–542. [RCT, *n* = 248 (*n* = 130 nulliparas)]

58. Bricker L, Luckas M. Amniotomy alone for induction of labour. Cochrane Database Syst Rev 2000; (4):CD002862. [Meta-analysis: 2 RCTs, *n* = 310]

59. Mercer BM, McNanley T, O'Brien JM, et al. Early versus late amniotomy for labor induction: a randomized trial. Am J Obstet Gynecol 1995; 173:1371. [RCT, *n* = 209]

60. Howarth G, Botha DJ. Amniotomy plus intravenous oxytocin for induction of labour. Cochrane Database Syst Rev 2001; (3): CD003250. [Meta-analysis: 17 RCTs, *n* = 2566]

61. Hofmeyr GJ, Gülmezoglu AM, Pileggi C. Vaginal misoprostol for cervical ripening and induction of labour. Cochrane Database Syst Rev 2010; (10):CD000941. [Meta-analysis: 121 RCTs, *n* = >10,000]

62. Austin SC, Sanchez-Ramos L, Adair CD. Labor Induction with intravaginal misoprostol compared with dinoprostone vaginal insert: a systematic review and meta-analysis. Am J Obstet Gynecol 2010; 202:624.e1–624.e9. [Meta-analysis: 11 RCTs, *n* = 1572]

63. Wing DA; Misoprostol Vaginal Insert Consortium. Misoprostol vaginal insert compared with dinoprostone vaginal insert: a randomized controlled trial. Obstet Gynecol 2008; 112:801–812. [RCT, *n* = 1308]

64. Wing DA, Miller H, Parker L, et al. Misoprostol vaginal insert for successful labor induction—a randomized controlled trial. Obstet Gynecol 2011; 117:533–541. [RCT, *n* = 374]

65. Kundodyiwa TW, Alfirevic Z, Weeks AD. Low-dose oral misoprostol for induction of labor: a systematic review. Obstet Gynecol 2009; 113:374–383. [Meta-analysis, *n* = 2937]

66. Alfirevic Z, Weeks A. Oral misoprostol for induction of labour. Cochrane Database Syst Rev 2006; (2):CD001338. [Meta-analysis: vs. placebo: 7 RCTs, *n* = 669; vs. vaginal PGE2: 10 RCTs, *n* = 3368; IV oxytocin: 8 RCTs, *n* = 1026; vaginal misoprostol: 26 RCTs, *n* = 5096]

67. Muzonzini G, Hofmeyr GJ. Buccal or sublingual misoprostol for cervical ripening and induction of labour. Cochrane Database Syst Rev 2004; (4):CD004221. [Meta-analysis: 3 RCTs, *n* = 502]

68. Boulvain M, Kelly AJ, Irion O. Intracervical prostaglandins for induction of labour. Cochrane Database Syst Rev 2008; (1): CD006971. [Meta-analysis: 56 RCTs, *n* = 7738; intracervical PGE2 with placebo/no treatment: 28 trials, 3764 women; intra-cervical PGE2 with intravaginal PGE2: 29 trials, 3881 women]

69. Kelly AJ, Malik S, Smith L, et al. Vaginal prostaglandin (PGE2 and PGF2a) for induction of labour at term. Cochrane Database Syst Rev 2009; (4):CD003101. [Meta-analysis: 63 RCTs, *n* = 10,441]

70. Chyu J, Strassner HT. Prostaglandin E2 for cervical ripening: a randomized comparison of Cervidil versus Prepidil. Am J Obstet Gynecol 1997; 177:606–611. [RCT, *n* = 73]

71. Smith CV, Rayburn WF, Miller AM. Intravaginal prostaglandin E2 for cervical ripening and initiation of labor. Comparison of a multidose gel and single, controlled-release pessary. J Reprod Med 1994; 39(5):381–384. [RCT, *n* = 121]

72. Perryman D, Yeast J, Holst V. Cervical ripening: a randomized study comparing prostaglandin E2 gel to prostaglandin E2 suppositories. Obstet Gynecol 1992; 79:670–672. [RCT, *n* = 90]

73. Christensen FC, Tehranifar M, Gonzalez JL, et al. Randomized trial of concurrent oxytocin with a sustained-release dinoprostone vaginal insert for labor induction at term. Am J Obstet Gynecol 2002; 186:61–65. [RCT, *n* = 71]

74. Hutton EK, Mozurkewich EL. Extra-amniotic prostaglandin for induction of labour. Cochrane Database Syst Rev 2001; (2): CD003092. [Meta-analysis: 12 RCTs]

75. French L. Oral prostaglandin E2 for induction of labour. Cochrane Database Syst Rev 2001; (2):CD003098. [Meta-analysis: 15 RCTs, *n* = >500]

76. Luckas M, Bricker L. Intravenous prostaglandin for induction of labour. Cochrane Database Syst Rev 2000; (4):CD002864. [Meta-analysis: 13 RCTs, *n* = 1165]

77. Alfirevic Z, Kelly AJ, Dowswell T. Intravenous oxytocin alone for cervical ripening and induction of labour. Cochrane Database Syst Rev 2009; (4):CD003246. [Meta-analysis: 61 RCTs, *n* = 12,819]

78. Satin AJ, Leveno KJ, Sherman ML, et al. High- versus low-dose oxytocin for labour stimulation. Obstet Gynecol 1992, 80:111–116. [II-1, *n* = 1112]

79. Cummiskey KC, Dawood MY. Induction of labor with pulsatile oxytocin. Am J Obstet Gynecol 1990; 163:1868–1874. [RCT, *n* = 106]

80. Blakemore KJ, Qin NG, Petrie RH, et al. A prospective comparison of hourly and quarter-hourly oxytocin dose increase intervals for the induction of labor at term. Obstet Gynecol 1990; 75:757–761. [RCT, *n* = 52]

81. Mercer B, Pilgrim P, Sibai B. Labor induction with continuous low-dose oxytocin infusion: a randomized trial. Obstet Gynecol 1991; 77:659–663. [RCT, *n* = 123]

82. Muller PR, Stubbs TM, Laurent SL. A prospective randomized clinical trial comparing two oxytocin induction protocols. Am J Obstet Gynecol 1992; 167:373–381. [RCT, *n* = 151]

83. Smith CA, Crowther CA. Acupuncture for induction of labour. Cochrane Database Syst Rev 2004; (1):CD002962. [Meta-analysis: 3 RCTs, *n* = 212]

84. Hapangama D, Neilson JP. Mifepristone for induction of labour. Cochrane Database Syst Rev 2009; (3):CD002865. [Meta-analysis: 10 RCTs, *n* = 1108]

85. MacKenzie IZ. Induction of labour at the start of the new millennium. Reproduction 2006; 131:989–998. [Review]

86. Thomas J, Kelly AJ, Kavanagh J. Oestrogens alone or with amniotomy for cervical ripening or induction of labour. Cochrane Database Syst Rev 2001; (4):CD003393. [Meta-analysis: 8 RCTs, *n* = 421]

87. Kelly AJ, Kavanagh J, Thomas J. Relaxin for cervical ripening and induction of labour. Cochrane Database Syst Rev 2001; (2): CD003103. [Meta-analysis: 4 RCTs, *n* = 267]

88. Ziaei S, Rosebehani N, Kazeminejad A, et al. The effects of intramuscular administration of corticosteroids on the induction of parturition. J Perinat Med 2003; 31:134–139. [RCT, *n* = 66]

89. Spallicci MDB, Bittar RE. Randomized double blind study of ripening the cervix with hyaluronidase in term gestations [Estudo clinico aleatorizado com grupo controle e mascaramento duplo da maturacao do colo uterino pela hialuronidase em gestacoes a termo]. Rev Bras Ginecol Obstet 2003; 25:67. [RCT, *n* = 168]

90. Kelly AJ, Munson C, Minden L. Nitric oxide donors for cervical ripening and induction of labour. Cochrane Database Syst Rev 2011; (6):CD006901. [Meta-analysis: 10 RCTs, *n* = 1889]

91. Modlock J, Nielsen BB, Uldbjerg N. Acupuncture for the induction of labor: a double-blind randomized controlled study. BJOG 2010; 117:1255–1261. [RCT, *n* = 125]

92. Smith CA, Crowther CA, Collins CT, et al. Acupuncture to induce labor – a randomized controlled trial. Obstet Gynecol 2008; 112:1067–1074. [RCT, *n* = 364]

93. Kavanagh J, Kelly AJ, Thomas J. Breast stimulation for cervical ripening and induction of labour. Cochrane Database Syst Rev 2005; (3):CD003392. [Meta-analysis: 6 RCTs, *n* = 719]

94. Garry D, Figueroa R, Guillaume J, Cucco V. Use of castor oil in pregnancies at term. Altern Ther Health Med 2000; 6:77–79. [RCT, *n* = 100]

95. Smith CA. Homoeopathy for induction of labour. Cochrane Database Syst Rev 2003; (4):CD003399. [Meta-analysis: 2 RCTs, *n* = 133]

96. Tan PC, Anggeriana M, Azmi N, et al. Effect of coitus at term on length of gestation, induction of labor and mode of delivery. Obstet Gynecol 2006; 134–140. [II-2]

97. Bendvold E. Coitus and induction of labour [Samleie og induksjon av fodsel]. Tidsskrift for Jordmodre 1990; 96:6–8. [RCT, *n* = 28]

98. Tan PC, Yow CM, Omar SZ. Effect of coital activity on onset of labor in women scheduled for labor induction. Obstet Gynecol 2007; 110:820–826. [RCT, *n* = 210]

99. American College of Obstetricians and Gynecologists. ACOG Committee Opinion No. 209: Monitoring during induction of labor with dinoprostone. Washington, D.C.: ACOG, 1998. [Review]

100. Dowswell T, Kelly AJ, Livio S, et al. Different methods for the induction of labour in outpatient settings. Cochrane Database Syst Rev 2010; (8):CD007701. [Meta-analysis: 28 RCTs, $n = 2616$]

101. McKenna DS, Ester JB, Proffitt M, et al. Misoprostol outpatient cervical ripening without subsequent induction of labor: a randomized trial. Obstet Gynecol 2004; 104:579–584. [RCT, $n = 33$]

102. Stitely ML, Browning J, Fowler M, et al. Outpatient cervical ripening with intravaginal misoprostol. Obstet Gynecol 2000; 96:684–688. [RCT, $n = 60$]

103. Incerpi MH, Fassett MJ, Kjos SL, et al. Vaginally administered misoprostol for outpatient cervical ripening in pregnancies complicated by diabetes mellitus. Am J Obstet Gynecol 2001; 185:916–919. [RCT, $n = 120$]

104. Kelly AJ, Alfirevic Z, Dowswell T. Outpatient versus inpatient induction of labour for improving birth outcomes. Cochrane Database Syst Rev 2009; (2):CD007372. [Meta-analysis: 3 RCTs, $n = 612$]

105. Hauth JC, Hankins GD, Gilstrap LC III, Strickland DM. Uterine contraction pressures with oxytocin induction/augmentation. Obstet Gynecol 1986; 68:305–309. [II-2, $n = 109$]

106. American College of Obstetricians and Gynecologists. ACOG Practice Bulletin No. 49: Dystocia and augmentation of labor. Washington, D.C.: ACOG, 2003. [Review]

21

Meconium

Sarah Poggi and Alessandro Ghidini

KEY POINTS

- **Fetal passage of meconium is common (12%),** usually after 34 weeks and especially postterm. In a minority of cases, the association of meconium with fetal hypoxia may be secondary to the fact that **fetal hypoxic stress may stimulate colonic activity, and may also stimulate fetal gasping leading to meconium aspiration. Therefore, meconium may not be causative, but just associated with fetal hypoxia and its complications.**

- Prevention of meconium passage and of meconium aspiration syndrome (MAS) may be accomplished by reducing the rate of postterm deliveries.

- **Amnioinfusion for meconium-stained amniotic fluid (MSAF) is associated with improvements in perinatal outcome, particularly in settings where facilities for perinatal surveillance are limited.** Under **standard perinatal surveillance,** compared with no amnioinfusion, **amnioinfusion** for MSAF (usually thick) is associated with significant **reductions in MAS; heavy meconium staining of the liquor; variable fetal heart rate deceleration;** and cesarean delivery **(CD) for nonreassuring fetal heart tracing (NRFHT).** Under **limited perinatal surveillance,** compared with no amnioinfusion, **amnioinfusion** for MSAF (usually thick) is associated with significant **reductions in MAS; 5-minute Apgar <7; neonatal hypoxic-ischemic encephalopathy; neonatal ventilation or intensive care unit admission; overall CD rate, and CD for NRFHT. No increased maternal risk** has been consistently demonstrated.

- **Oro- and nasopharyngeal suctioning** before delivery of the shoulder **does not decrease the incidence of MAS, need for mechanical ventilation for MAS, any other associated morbidities, or neonatal mortality.**

- **Routine endotracheal intubation** at birth in meconium-stained neonates who are otherwise vigorous **does not improve neonatal outcomes over routine resuscitation.**

HISTORIC NOTES

Meconium is a term derived from the Greek "mekoni," which means poppy juice or opium. Confirming previous clinical impressions, meconium passage was formally recognized to be associated with increased perinatal morbidity and mortality in the 1975 Collaborative Study of Cerebral Palsy.

DIAGNOSES/DEFINITIONS

Meconium is the intestinal content of the fetus and is variably composed of mucopolysaccharides, blood byproducts, hair, and squamous cells. Diagnosis of MSAF is made clinically on the basis of appearance (greenish or brownish staining) or by histopathologic examination of the placenta. Particularly in the preterm (<33 week) gestation, a clinical impression of MSAF may be false and instead reflect staining by another mechanism (i.e., hemosiderin). The diagnosis of MAS is respiratory distress requiring supplemental oxygen usually in the first 4 hours of life in the presence of meconium in a neonate without other causes of respiratory distress, and classified as shown below.

EPIDEMIOLOGY/INCIDENCE

MSAF occurs in about 17% to 19% of term placentas, and about **12%** (7–22%) of term pregnancies. **MAS** happens in about **5% of these cases,** and, **of these, approximately 4% die.** The incidence of MSAF increases with term/postdates pregnancies: about 10% of 39- to 41-week gestations, 18% of >41-week gestations.

ETIOLOGY/BASIC PATHOPHYSIOLOGY

The fetal hormone motilin promotes peristalsis. Motilin is not present in significant quantity in the extremely preterm (i.e., mid-trimester) fetus to cause in utero defecation. In later preterm, term, and postdates fetuses, increased motilin levels leading to meconium passage may be mediated by fetal stress from hypoxia, infection, or cord compression. However, particularly in the postterm fetus, passage may simply indicate gastrointestinal maturation (1–5). Chronic or acute asphyxia and intrauterine infection are more likely sources of respiratory compromise in the presence of meconium than meconium aspiration itself (1). **Fetal hypoxic stress may stimulate colonic activity, and may also stimulate fetal gasping leading to meconium aspiration. Therefore, meconium may not be causative, but just associated with fetal hypoxia and its complications.** Meconium is associated with a chemical pneumonitis in neonatal lungs, which is associated then with inhibition of surfactant function, inflammation, and obstruction, leading to MAS.

SYMPTOMS

Symptoms of neonatal **MAS** include respiratory compromise, with tachypnea, cyanosis, and reduced pulmonary compliance. In some cases, pulmonary hypertension develops.

CLASSIFICATION (OF MECONIUM ASPIRATION SYNDROME)

- Mild: supplemental oxygen <40% for <48 hours
- Moderate: supplemental oxygen ≥40% or for ≥48 hours
- Severe: need for intubation (or primary pulmonary hypertension)

RISK FACTORS

Postterm pregnancy and **fetal acidemia** (association, not necessarily causative).

COMPLICATIONS

MSAF is associated with **fetal acidemia, neonatal seizures, neonatal intensive care unit (NICU) admission, respiratory distress, long-term sequela of cerebral palsy (but not necessarily causative)** (1–5).

PREGNANCY MANAGEMENT
Meconium at Genetic Amniocentesis

Suspicion of MSAF in the extremely preterm fetus (i.e., at genetic amniocentesis) should prompt **evaluation for other causes of discolored amniotic fluid** (e.g., infection and/or abruption workup).

Meconium in Later Preterm and Term Fetus <39 Weeks

MSAF in the later preterm and term fetus <39 weeks should prompt evaluation for **infection and fetal hypoxia** as the finding may not be attributable to normal physiology alone at this gestation.

Meconium at ≥39 Weeks

MSAF in the full term or postdates fetus ≥39 weeks may reflect normal physiology and maturation of the gastrointestinal tract only, but cannot exclude the possibilities of infection or hypoxia as etiologies. Progression in meconium consistency in labor from no/little meconium to presence of thicker meconium should elicit particular concern as this may be associated with higher rates of fetal acidemia.

PREVENTION

Prevention of meconium passage and of MAS may be accomplished by reducing the rate of postterm deliveries. Early ultrasound dating and stripping of membranes at ≥38 weeks both decrease the incidence of postterm pregnancies (see chap. 24).

MANAGEMENT TECHNIQUES USED IN THE SETTING OF MECONIUM-STAINED AMNIOTIC FLUID
Fetal

Amnioinfusion

The efficacy of amnioinfusion to "dilute" meconium and reduce associated neonatal morbidity has historically been controversial (6). Smaller randomized trials in some settings have shown benefit in terms of MAS, NICU admission, and neonatal hypoxic-ischemic encephalopathy (7–18), though a landmark, well-powered study failed to demonstrate a benefit (19). The most recent meta-analysis includes 15 total RCTs (7–23). Results are reported separately for sites with standard versus those with limited perinatal surveillance. The main outcome in the RCTs was usually MAS.

Under **standard perinatal surveillance**, compared with no amnioinfusion, **amnioinfusion** for MSAF (usually thick) is associated with significant **reductions in MAS** (47% reduction: RR 0.53, 95% CI 0.29–0.98) (23,24); **heavy meconium staining of the liquor** (97% reduction); **variable fetal heart rate deceleration** (33%); and **CD for fetal distress** (18%), as well as trends to reduction in overall CD rate (RR 0.78, 95% CI 0.60–1.02), NICU admission (55%), and **pH < 7.20** (38%) (6–24). There were no statistically significant differences in the rates of 5-minute Apgar <7 and perinatal death.

Under **limited perinatal surveillance**, compared with no amnioinfusion, **amnioinfusion** for MSAF (usually thick) is associated with significant **reductions in MAS** (75% reduction; RR 0.25, 95% CI 0.13–0.47); 5-minute Apgar <7 (64%); **neonatal hypoxic ischemic encephalopathy** (93%) and **neonatal ventilation or NICU admission** (48%); **overall CD rate** (30%), and **CD for NRFHT** (50%). Furthermore, there is a trend toward reduced **perinatal mortality** (RR 0.37, 95% CI 0.13–1.01) (6–22).

No increased maternal risk has been consistently demonstrated. There is no difference seen in the rates of maternal endometritis, and the trials reviewed are too small to address the possibility of rare but serious maternal adverse effects of amnioinfusion. (6–22).

In summary, **amnioinfusion for MSAF is associated with improvements in perinatal outcome, particularly in settings where facilities for perinatal surveillance are limited**. In general, amnioinfusion is offered at ≥34 weeks. There are many variations of the amnioinfusion technique, but a "typical" protocol calls for infusion via an intrauterine pressure catheter (obviously in a woman with dilated cervix and ruptured membranes) of **500 mL of normal saline over a period of 30 minutes**. See also chapter 10.

For amnioinfusion in presence of variable decelerations, see chapter 10; for amnioinfusion for oligohydramnios without PPROM, see chapter 56 in *Maternal-Fetal Evidence Based Guidelines*; for amnioinfusion for PPROM, see chapter 18.

Antibiotics

There is **insufficient evidence** to assess the effectiveness of antibiotics for women with meconium in labor, as there is only one small RCT on this topic. Compared with normal saline, ampicillin-salbactam are associated with no statistically significant reduction in the incidence of neonatal sepsis (RR 1.00, 95% CI 0.21–4.76), NICU admission (RR 0.83, 95% CI 0.39–1.78), and postpartum endometritis (RR 0.50, 95% CI 0.18–1.38), but a significant decrease in the risk of chorioamnionitis (RR 0.29, 95% CI 0.10–0.82) in women with MSAF. No serious adverse effects were reported (25).

Oro- and Nasopharyngeal Suctioning

Suctioning of the oro- and nasopharynx before delivery of the shoulder or the "first cry" **does not decrease the incidence of MAS, need for mechanical ventilation for MAS, any other associated morbidities, or neonatal mortality** (26,27).

Neonatal

Endotracheal Intubation

A policy of routine endotracheal intubation at birth in meconium-stained babies who are otherwise vigorous **does not improve neonatal outcomes over routine resuscitation** (28). For depressed or nonvigorous newborns, endotracheal intubation and suctioning may still be performed in infants born through MSAF (28).

REFERENCES

1. Ghidini A, Spong C. Severe meconium aspiration is not caused by aspiration of meconium. Obstet Gynecol 2001; 185:931–938. [Review]
2. Locatelli A, Regalia AL, Patregnani C, et al. Prognostic value of change in amniotic fluid color during labor. Fetal Diagn Ther 2005; 20(1):5–9. [II-2]
3. Nathan L, Leveno KJ, Carmody TJ III, et al. Meconium: a 1990s perspective on an old obstetric hazard. Obstet Gynecol 1994; 83(3):329–332. [review]

4. Rossi EM, Philipson EH, Williams TG, et al. Meconium aspiration syndrome: intrapartum and neonatal attributes. Am J Obstet Gynecol 1989; 161:1106–1110. [II-3]

5. Usher RH, Boyd ME, McLean FH, et al. Assessment of fetal risk in postdate pregnancies. Am J Obstet Gynecol 158:259:1988. [II-2]

6. Hofmeyr GJ, Xu H. Amnioinfusion for meconium-stained liquor in labor (review). Cochrane Database Syst Rev 2010; CD000014. [Meta-analysis: 15 RCT, n = 4998, ref. 7–22]

7. Adam K, Cano L, Moise KJ. The effect of intrapartum amnioinfusion on the outcome of the fetus with heavy meconium stained amniotic fluid. Proceedings of 9th Annual Meeting of the Society of Perinatal Obstetricians, New Orleans, Louisiana, U.S.A. 1989; 438. [RCT]

8. Alvarez M, Puertas A, Suarez AM, et al. Transcervical amnioinfusion in deliveries with meconium-stained amniotic fluid. Amnioinfusion transcervical en partos con liquido amniotico tenido de meconio. Prog Obstet Ginecol 1999; 42:365–372. [RCT]

9. Cialone PR, Sherer DM, Ryan RM, et al. Amnioinfusion during labor complicated by particulate meconium-stained amniotic fluid decreases neonatal morbidity. Am J Obstet Gynecol 1994; 170:842–849. [RCT]

10. Eriksen N, Hostetter M, Parisi V. Prophylactic amnioinfusion in pregnancies complicated by thick meconium. Am J Obstet Gynecol. 1994; 170:344. [RCT]

11. Hofmeyr GJ, Gulmezoglu AM, Buchmann E, et al. The Collaborative Randomised Amnioinfusion for Meconium Project (CRAMP): 1. South Africa. Br J Obstet Gynaecol 1998; 105:304–308. [RCT]

12. Ilagan NB, Kazzi GM, Shankaran S, et al. Transcervical amnioinfusion for the prevention of neonatal meconium aspiration. Pediatr Res 1992; 31(4):205A. [RCT]

13. Macri CJ, Schrimmer DB, Leung A, et al. Prophylactic amnioinfusion improves outcome of pregnancy complicated by thick meconium and oligohydramnios. Am J Obstet Gynecol 1992; 67:117–1121. [RCT]

14. Mahomed K, Mulambo T, Woelk G, et al. The Collaborative Randomised Amnioinfusion for Meconium Project (CRAMP): 2. Zimbabwe. Br J Obstet Gynaecol 1998; 105:309–313. [RCT]

15. Moodley J, Matchaba P, Payne AJ. Intrapartum amnioinfusion for meconium-stained liquor in developing countries. Trop Doct 1998; 28:31–34. [RCT]

16. Sadovsky Y, Amon E, Bade ME, et al. Prophylactic amnioinfusion during labor complicated by meconium: a preliminary report. Am J Obstet Gynecol 1989; 61:613–617. [RCT]

17. Spong CY, Ogunipe OA, Ross MG. Prophylactic amnioinfusion for meconium-stained amniotic fluid. Am J Obstet Gynecol 1994; 171:931–935. [RCT]

18. Wenstrom KD, Parsons MT. The prevention of meconium aspiration in labor using amnioinfusion. Obstet Gynecol 1989; 73:647–651. [RCT]

19. Fraser WD, Hofmeyr J, Lede R, et al. for the amnioinfusion trial group. Amnioinfusion for the prevention of the meconium aspiration syndrome. N Engl J Med 2005; 353:909–917. [RCT, n = 1998]

20. Puertas A, Paz Carrillo M, Molto L, et al. Meconium-stained amniotic fluid in labor: a randomized trial of prophylactic amnioinfusion. Eur J Obstet Gynecol Reprod Biol 2001; 99:33–37. [RCT]

21. Rathor AM, Singh R, Ramji S, et al. Randomised trial of amnioinfusion during labour with meconium stained amniotic fluid. Br J Obstet Gynecol 2002; 109(1):17–20. [RCT]

22. Sood M, Charulata, Dimple D, et al. Amnioinfusion in thick meconium. Indian J Pediatr 2004; 71:677–681. [RCT, n = 196]

23. Sanchez-Ramos L. Intrapartum Amnioinfusion for meconium-stained amniotic fluid: a systematic review of randomized controlled trials. Br J Obstet Gynecol 2010; 115:409–410. [Letter to editor]

24. Steer PJ. How much weight should we put on the conclusions of meta-analyses? Br J Obstet Gynecol 2008; 115(3):299–300. [Editorial]

25. Adair CD, Ernest JM, Sanchez-Ramos L, et al. Meconium-stained amniotic fluid-associated infectious morbidity: a randomized, double-blind trial of ampicillin-sulbactam prophylaxis. Obstet Gynecol 1996; 88(2):216–220. [RCT, n = 120]

26. Falciglia HS, Henderschott C, Potter P, et al. Does DeLee suction at the perineum prevent meconium aspiration syndrome? Am J Obstet Gynecol 1992; 167(5):1243–1249. [II-2]

27. Vain NE, Szyld EG, Prudent LM, et al. Oropharyngeal and nasopharyngeal suctioning of meconium-stained neonates before delivery of their shoulders: multicentre, randomized controlled trial. Lancet 2004; 364:597–602. [RCT, n = 2514]

28. Halliday HL, Sweet D. Endotracheal intubation at birth for preventing morbidity and mortality in vigorous, meconium stained infants born at term. Cochrane Database Syst Rev 2001; (1):CD000500. [Meta-analysis: 4 RCTs, n = 2884]

22

Malpresentation and malposition

Candice T. Tong

KEY POINTS

- **Malpresentation** is **associated** with **uterine anomalies, fibroids, placenta previa, grand multiparity, contracted maternal pelvis, pelvic tumors, prematurity** (the earlier the gestational age, the higher the incidence of malpresentation), **multiple gestation, polyhydramnios, short umbilical cord, fetal anomalies** (e.g., anencephaly, hydrocephalus), **abnormal fetal motor ability, and prior breech delivery.**
- **Complications** of breech presentation are **congenital anomalies, preterm birth (PTB), birth trauma, low Apgar scores, and lower pH**, mostly regardless of mode of delivery. **Cord prolapse, head hyperextension,** and **head or arm entrapment** are more common with vaginal breech delivery.
- **External cephalic version** (ECV) is a safe and effective intervention. **Urgent cesarean delivery (CD)** for nonreassuring fetal heart rate tracing (NRFHT) and placental **abruption** occur in <0.5% of ECV.
- **ECV** is avoided with **any contraindications to vaginal delivery** such as placenta **previa**, or **prior classical uterine incision**, and, relatively, with rupture of membranes, oligohydramnios, known uterine or fetal anomaly, unexplained uterine bleeding, or active phase of labor.
- **ECV reduces the incidences of noncephalic birth by 54%** and **CD by 37%.** Because ECV is associated with a very low incidence of adverse events and with a significant decrease in CD, **all women at or near term with nonvertex presentations should be offered an ECV attempt. Success rates** range roughly average **50% to 70%.** Success is increased with **higher parity, transverse or oblique lie, nonengagement of the breech, a relaxed uterus, a palpable fetal head, and maternal weight less than 65 kg.**
- There is **insufficient evidence to assess the best gestational age** at which to perform ECV. **Compared with ECV at term, ECV before term (e.g., 34–35 weeks) reduces noncephalic presentation at birth but does not reduce the rate of CD, and may be associated with an increase in the incidence of PTB.** About **36 weeks is generally considered to be the optimal time for attempted version.**
- Tocolysis with **betamimetics** prior to attempt at ECV is associated with **fewer failures of ECV**, and **less CDs.**
- **Anesthetic dose neuraxial blockade (usually with spinal) is associated with a 44% increase in the success rate of external fetal version.**
- ECV should be performed in a facility with ready availability for emergency CD, after appropriate counseling and consent, with ultrasound availability.
- **There is inconsistent evidence that moxibustion** at point BL67, alone or in combination with acupuncture, **is associated with higher rates of cephalic version**, especially when performed in China.

- Compared with planned vaginal delivery, **planned CD** for the **term breech** fetus is associated with **decrease in perinatal or neonatal death or serious neonatal morbidity, but no difference in death or neurodevelopmental delay at 2 years after delivery.**
- There is **insufficient evidence** to assess if outcomes of the **preterm** fetus presenting breech are affected by mode of delivery.
- There is **insufficient evidence** to assess the best mode of delivery for the **nonvertex second twin**. Vaginal delivery of the second nonvertex twin may be a reasonable management option by expert operator, possibly by breech extraction.
- There is insufficient evidence to assess any intervention for malposition.

DEFINITIONS

Presentation: Fetal body part that is in the lower uterine segment (lowest in the uterus and closest to the cervix).

Malpresentation: Fetus presenting with the fetal head not in the lower uterine segment.

Position: Relationship of presenting part (usually occiput for head) to pelvic outlet.

Malposition: Fetal position that is not occiput-anterior.

MALPRESENTATION
Symptoms

Maternal impression of fetal presentation based on fetal movement is suggestive but overall unreliable for predicting fetal presentation.

Epidemiology/Incidence

Breech presentation complicates **3% to 4%** of all pregnancies at term ($\geq$37 weeks) (1). Its incidence is inversely proportional to gestational age, with an incidence of about 25% at 28 weeks, of 11% at 32 weeks, and of 5% at 34 weeks (2). In 1990, 90% of these presentations resulted in CD (compared with 11.6% in 1970), accounting for 15% of all cesarean sections, and adding 1.4 billion dollars to U.S. obstetrical costs (3).

Classifications

Breech

Fetus presents in longitudinal lie with head not in the lower uterine segment.

Fetal breech presentation is further classified as follows:

- *Complete*—Flexion of the fetal hips and knees
- *Incomplete*—Extension of one or both hips (includes footling)
- *Frank*—Flexion at the hips and extension at the knees

Transverse

The fetal longitudinal axis is perpendicular to the long axis of the uterus. The fetus can either present "back up" (fetal small parts present to the cervix), or "back down" (fetal spine or shoulder present to the cervix).

Oblique

The fetal longitudinal axis is diagonal to the long axis of the uterus.

Face

The fetal head is hyperextended so that the fetal occiput is in contact with the fetal back and the mentum (chin) is presenting. The fetal chin may be anterior or posterior relative to the maternal pubic symphysis.

Brow

The presenting part is the portion of the fetal head between the orbital ridge and the anterior fontanel. The fetal head is in position midway between full flexion and extension.

Compound

Simultaneous presentation of a prolapsing fetal extremity and the presenting part.

Risk Factors/Associations

Both maternal and fetal factors can lead to this presentation, including **uterine anomalies, fibroids, placenta previa, grand multiparity, contracted maternal pelvis, pelvic tumors, prematurity** (the earlier the gestational age, the higher the incidence of malpresentation), **multiple gestation, polyhydramnios, short umbilical cord, fetal anomalies** (e.g., anencephaly, hydrocephalus), **abnormal fetal motor ability, and prior breech delivery**. Prior breech delivery gives a 9% risk of recurrence in subsequent pregnancies.

Complications

Incidence of **congenital anomalies** (up to 6%), **PTB, birth trauma, low Apgar scores, and lower pH** are higher with a breech presentation compared with a vertex presentation, **mostly regardless of mode of delivery**. Breech presentation may be a sign and a consequence of fetal compromise, again regardless of delivery mode. Incidence of **cord prolapse** is about the same with frank breech as with vertex presentations (<1%), 5% with complete breech, up to 15% with footling, and is inversely proportional to gestational age (GA). **Head hyperextension** (associated with spinal cord injury) and **head or arm entrapment** are all associated with breech presentation, and especially with vaginal delivery. Presentation at birth does not seem to affect adult intellectual performance. Cesarean or vaginal delivery for breech presentation does not seem to differ in terms of long-term adult intellectual performance (4).

Workup

Fetal presentation should be assessed by Leopold's maneuvers at each visit starting at ≥34 weeks of gestation. If the clinician is unsure, a vaginal examination, or even better, if still unclear, an ultrasound is indicated to assess fetal presentation.

External cephalic version (Fig 22.1)

Definition. Procedure performed by application of pressure and maneuvers to the maternal abdomen with the goal to turn the fetus to a cephalic presentation, thus increasing the likelihood of vaginal delivery (1).

Complications. While the rate of short-term fetal bradycardia is as high as 20% or more, the rate of need for **urgent CD** for NRFHT after an ECV is about 1/600 (5). Placental **abruption** (<1%) and **onset of labor** are uncommon complications. Rare fetal deaths following attempts at version have not been felt to be a result of the procedure (1). Femur fracture has been reported. In a meta-analysis, there was a **risk of 4.7% for transient abnormal cardiotocography, 0.21% risk of abnormal cardiotocography leading to emergency CD** but with good neonatal outcomes, and **0.35% risk of emergency CD**. Other risks included 0.24% risk of stillbirth, 0.18% risk of placental abruption, 0.18% risk of cord prolapse, and 0.19% risk of fetal death. These complications were not found to be directly related to the ECV procedure. Vaginal bleeding related to ECV occurred in 0.34% of patients and rupture of membranes related to ECV occurred in 0.22% of patients (6).

Contraindications. Any **contraindications to vaginal delivery** such as placenta **previa** or **prior classical uterine incision** are also generally considered contraindications to ECV. There are no trials on ECV in **multiple gestations**, so the safety and efficacy of this procedure cannot be assessed. Relative contraindications are **rupture of membranes, oligohydramnios, known uterine or fetal anomaly, unexplained uterine bleeding, or active phase of labor** (1,7). ECV in women with prior cesarean deliveries are associated with comparable success rates to those of women without prior cesarean deliveries, but there is insufficient data to assess the safety of this management (8).

Efficacy. Compared with no ECV, **ECV at term** is associated with a statistically significant and clinically meaningful 54% (RR 0.46, 95% CI 0.31–0.66) **reduction in noncephalic birth** and a 37% (RR 0.63, 95% CI 0.44–0.90) **decrease in CD** (9). There are no significant differences in the incidence of Apgar score ratings <7 at 5 minutes (RR 0.76, 95% CI 0.32–1.77), low umbilical artery pH levels (RR 0.65, 95% CI 0.17–2.44), neonatal admission (RR 0.36, 95% CI 0.04–3.24), perinatal death (RR 0.34, 95% CI 0.05–2.12), nor time from enrollment to delivery (9). Because ECV is associated with a very low incidence of adverse events and with a significant decrease in CD, **all women at or near term with nonvertex presentations should be offered an ECV attempt**.

Success rates are about **58%**, with a range of 25% to 80% (1). Success is increased with **higher parity**, and **transverse or oblique lie** (vs. breech). Lower amniotic fluid volume, anterior placenta, and high maternal BMI might decrease the success rate (1). Also a meta-analysis showed that **multiparity, nonengagement of the breech, a relaxed uterus, a palpable fetal head, and maternal weight less than 65 kg** were predictors of successful ECV (10). There is no scoring system to accurately predict the probability of success of ECV. After successful ECV, the chance of spontaneous version to breech is low but understudied. The chance of spontaneous version after failed ECV is about 6.6% in one study (11).

Timing of version. Compared with no ECV attempt, **ECV before term reduces noncephalic births** (12–15). A more important comparison, though, is between term (≥37 weeks) and preterm (<37 weeks) timing for ECV.

Compared with ECV at term, **ECV before term reduces noncephalic presentation at birth, but does not reduce the rate of CD, and may be associated with an increase in the incidence of PTB.** There is **insufficient evidence to assess the best gestational age** at which to perform ECV. In general, the later the gestational age, the lower the success rate, but

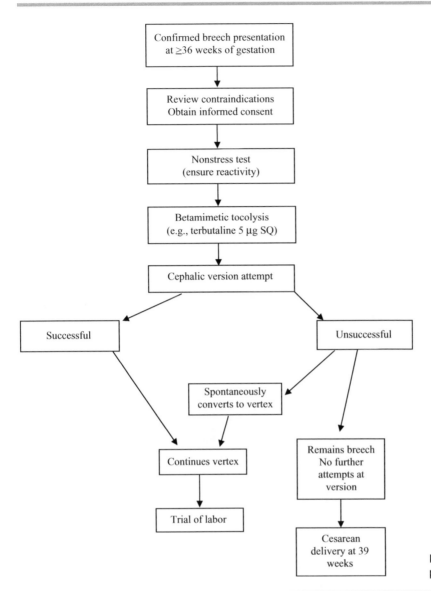

Figure 22.1 Suggested management of breech presentation. *Source*: Adapted from Ref. 1.

there are reports of successful ECV in women in term labor. About **36 weeks is generally considered to be the optimal time for attempted version**. At this gestational age there is felt to be adequate room to turn the fetus while minimizing the risk of reversion to breech after a successful version. At the same time, if delivery becomes necessary, a 36-week infant has a low rate of respiratory distress syndrome or other complications of prematurity. Compared with ECV at 37 0/7 to 38 0/7 weeks, ECV at 34 0/7 to 36 0/7 weeks is associated with nonsignificant trends for slightly lower (57% vs. 66%) noncephalic presentation at birth and slightly lower (65% vs. 72%) CD (12–15). In the largest RCT so far, compared with ECV at ≥37 weeks, ECV at 34 0/7 to 35 6/7 weeks was associated with a decrease in the incidence of noncephalic presentation at birth (41% vs. 49%; RR 0.84, 95% CI 0.75–0.94), but no difference in rates of CD (52% vs. 56%; RR 0.93, 95% CI 0.85–1.02) and in risk of PTB (6.5% vs. 4.4%; RR 1.48, 95% CI 0.97–2.26) (16).

Tocolysis. Tocolysis with **betamimetics** prior to attempt at ECV is associated with 26% **fewer failures of ECV**, a nonsignificant reduction in noncephalic presentations at birth, and 15% **less cesarean deliveries** (17). A common type and dose is terbutaline 5 mg subcutaneously once, 10 to

15 minutes before ECV, but different betamimetics have been used, with no evidence as to the best one or its dosage/timing (17). One recent RCT of adjusted doses of intravenous salbutamol tocolysis prior to ECV increased success rates, decreased CD rate, and was well tolerated (18). Tocolysis can be used with success also in a second ECV attempt after a first ECV attempt has failed (19).

Nitroglycerin has been studied as an agent to improve version success rates. In four small trials, sublingual nitroglycerin was associated with significant side effects and was **not** found to be **effective** (17). One randomized control trial demonstrated that treatment with intravenous nitroglycerin increased the rate of successful ECV in nulliparous women (24% compared to 8%, p = 0.04) but not in multiparous women (20). The terbutaline 25 μg subcutaneous 5 minutes prior group was found to have a significantly higher ECV success rate than the nitroglycerin group in one trial (21).

Nifedipine as a uterine relaxant for ECV has also been evaluated in RCTs. In a randomized, double-blind, placebo-controlled trial of 320 participants, nifedipine **did not significantly improve the success of ECV** (22). In two RCTs evaluating oral nifedipine versus subcutaneous terbutaline tocolysis for

ECV, there was a higher ECV rate with terbutaline (52.2–58.1% for terbutaline vs. 34.1–39.5% for nifedipine), less cesarean sections, no difference in neonatal outcomes, although more side effects (maternal palpitations and tachycardia) (23–25).

Fetal acoustic stimulation. Fetal acoustic stimulation to the fetal head for 1 to 3 seconds in midline fetal spine positions is associated with fewer failures of ECV at term in a very small study (17,26). Eleven of 12 versions were successful following stimulation (26). The crossover arm (patients who failed version without stimulation) were then stimulated, and 8 of 10 patients were successfully verted, for a total of 19 of 22 successful versions (86%) (26). The success rate in the control group of this study was much lower than expected (8%) (26). The **evidence is insufficient** to make a recommendation.

Anesthesia. There is **limited convincing evidence** that regional anesthesia affects ECV success. ECV failure, noncephalic births, and cesarean sections were reduced in two trials with epidural but not in three with spinal analgesia (17). ECV success rates increased from 33% to 59% with epidural in one study and from 32% to 69% in another (3,27). Potential bias in both studies lies in that the care provider was not blinded to placement of epidural (3,27). It is important to note that **the control groups had lower success rates than expected**, as the average success rate in the literature, which is mostly without anesthesia, is about 58%, as shown above. All patients in both studies received terbutaline prior to attempt at version. Some have postulated that large volume preloading with epidural may have increased the amniotic fluid volume (17). The use of spinal anesthesia has not been associated with any benefit in the success of ECV in some individual RCTs (7,17). However, a meta-analysis including seven RCTs, of which five used spinal and two used epidural anesthesia for ECV versus controls, demonstrated **anesthetic dose neuraxial blockade (usually spinal) is associated with a 44% increase in the success rate of external fetal version** (28). There are no trials to evaluate the potential effects of hydration or transabdominal amnioinfusion on the success rate of spontaneous version or ECV.

ECV procedure. Given the possible complications, it is prudent to perform ECV in a **facility** with ready availability for emergency CD. **Consent** should be obtained after **counseling** regarding possible complications, other options (CD), prognosis, and some explanation of the actual procedure. A **nonstress test** should be performed before and after the procedure. Anesthesia is usually not necessary, and has not been absolutely proven to benefit outcomes. **Betamimetic** prophylactic tocolysis should be given (e.g., terbutaline 5 μg subcutaneously 5 to 10 minutes prior to procedure). There is no trial to compare other technical aspects of ECV. The technique using one or two operators can be used. Frequent if not continuous **ultrasound** guidance to assess for fetal well-being and presentation is suggested. Rh-negative women can receive anti-D immunoglobulin. There is no evidence to support immediate induction after successful ECV.

Moxibustion and/or acupuncture

Moxibustion is a form of traditional Chinese medicine that uses heat generated by burning herbs, most often *Artemisia vulgaris*, to stimulate the acupuncture point BL67 (Zhiyin in Chinese) (29–33). There is **inconsistent evidence** to assess if the use of moxibustion significantly converts a breech to a cephalic presentation. There have been differences in interventions (e.g., moxibustion alone or with acupuncture) making it not appropriate to perform a satisfactory meta-analysis. Moxibustion may reduce the need for ECV by 53%, the incidence of nonvertex presentation at term by 35% to 70%, but

mainly in the Chinese trials (30,31). In the two trials performed in Italy, moxibustion was either not well tolerated by 22% of women and therefore not effective (32), or effective when used with acupuncture (33). Moxibustion may decrease the use of oxytocin before or during labor for women who had vaginal deliveries (29). It might be that acupuncture and not moxibustion (especially not at home) is beneficial (33). A meta-analysis performed compiling data from six studies of both Western and Chinese databases shows that **moxibustion at point BL67, alone or in combination with acupuncture, is associated with higher rates of cephalic version** of 72.5%, compared with 53.2% in the control group (RR 1.36, 95% CI 1.17–1.58). This data should be viewed with caution given the high degree of heterogeneity of the studies (34). Also, there were no significant differences found in safety of moxibustion compared with other techniques. A more recent small RCT, not yet included in any meta-analysis, reported **no beneficial effect of moxibustion to facilitate ECV** with the percentage of versions similar between moxibustion (18%) and controls (16%). Women did have a positive opinion of the intervention (35).

Maternal change in posture

Maternal change in position such as knee-chest and others has been suggested as a means to correct breech presentation in pregnancy. There is **insufficient evidence** from the small trials reported so far to support the use of postural management for breech presentation (36). Meta-analysis of these data could not be done as study designs and outcomes measured were different (37). Postural management is not associated with a significant effect on the rate of noncephalic births, either for the subgroup in which no ECV was attempted, or for the group overall (RR 0.98, 95% CI 0.84–1.15). No differences were detected for cesarean sections (RR 1.10, 95% CI 0.89–1.37). As such **there is no solid evidence for this practice** (36,37).

Delivery outcomes

It is important to note that the rate of CD after ECV is still about double that of pregnancies presenting with spontaneous cephalic presentation because of higher incidences of dystocia and NRFHT after successful ECV (38).

MODE OF DELIVERY
Singleton
Term

Term breech. Three RCTs (39), including one large study (40), have compared a policy of planned CD to a policy of planned trial of labor to attempt a vaginal delivery. CD occurs in about 45% of those women allocated to a vaginal delivery protocol and >90% in those allocated to a CD protocol.

At 4 to 6 weeks after delivery, compared with planned vaginal delivery, **planned CD** is associated with a 67% (RR 0.33, 95% CI 0.19–0.56) **decrease in perinatal or neonatal death** (excluding fetal anomalies) **or serious neonatal morbidity** (39). This reduction is (surprisingly) less for countries with high national perinatal mortality rates (40). Planned CD is associated with a 71% reduction (from 1.15% to 0.26%) in perinatal or neonatal death (excluding fetal anomalies) (39). This reduction was similar for countries with low and high national perinatal mortality rates. One death would be prevented for every 112 cesarean sections planned (39). A secondary analysis (41) of the short-term outcomes of the Term Breech Trial (40) looked at factors associated with adverse outcomes. The lowest morbidity was found in patients with planned section prior to the onset of labor. If vaginal birth is the desired route, labor augmentation and a second stage greater than 60 minutes are associated with poorer outcomes (41). Factors not shown to affect outcome included induction, parity, use of continuous electronic fetal monitoring, or epidural (41). A skilled clinician at the delivery was associated with lower adverse outcomes. "Skilled clinician" was best described by the clinician themselves rather than by years of experience or being a licensed obstetrician (41).

At three months after delivery, women allocated to the planned cesarean section group reported 38% **less urinary incontinence**; 89% **more abdominal pain**; and 68% **less perineal pain** (42).

At 2 years after delivery, there was **no difference in the combined outcome "death or neurodevelopmental delay."** Of 463 vaginal delivery patients followed at 2 years, there were only 6 deaths and 7 neurodevelopmental delays (2.8%), compared with 2 and 12 of 457 patients (3.1%) in the cesarean section group (43). The disappearance at 2 years of age of the difference seen at neonatal follow-up is because most children with serious neonatal morbidity survive and develop normally. Moreover, there might still not be a sample size big enough to detect small differences for the 2 years of data (43). **Maternal outcomes at 2 years** were also very **similar,** with **constipation** significantly more **common** in the **CD** group (27% vs. 20%), while self-reported incontinence was nonsignificantly different (18% vs. 22%) (44). Incontinence was different (16% vs. 25%) if comparing women who actually planned and had a cesarean versus those who planned and had a vaginal delivery (44).

All these results are mostly from the Term Breech Trial (40) and its secondary analyses and follow-up (41–44). Also important to note is that these outcomes are based on deliveries done by "clinicians who were regarded as experienced at vaginal breech delivery" (40–44). As the number of breech vaginal deliveries decreases, physician skill to do this will continue to diminish, with the potential to make vaginal delivery less safe. While it is estimated that >90% of babies presenting nonvertex are currently delivered by cesarean, there might still be a small role for vaginal delivery for the woman who declines scheduled cesarean or presents in advanced labor. Still, **all women with breech presentation with a large fetus (>3500 g estimation), unfavorable pelvis, hyperextended head, incomplete or footling breech presentation, NRFHT, severe fetal growth restriction, or lack of experienced obstetrical and anesthesiological operators should absolutely have a CD.**

Technical aspects.

Cesarean breech delivery: There are no trials to assess technical aspects of breech (or other malpresentation) CD. There is insufficient evidence to assess if intra-abdominal version during CD before uterine incision affects outcomes.

Vaginal breech delivery: There are several technical suggestions for assisting a vaginal breech delivery. None are based on trials. There is insufficient evidence to assess if clinical/radiologic pelvimetry affects outcomes in the management of breech presentation. Usually a double setup is suggested, so that an attempt at vaginal delivery should be organized in the operating room and ready for possible CD.

Some other suggestions are as follows: minimal intervention at least until the abdomen, up to the umbilical cord, is delivered; prevention of head extension, with prophylactic Mauriceau maneuver; and proper use of Pipers forceps, if necessary. There is not enough evidence to evaluate the effects of expedited vaginal breech delivery (breech delivery from

umbilicus to delivery of the head within one contraction) on perinatal outcomes (45).

Term transverse or oblique
The same management options exist for transverse/oblique lie as for breech. Fetal version and CD are the standards of care, with lack of trial evidence.

Preterm
The premature breech
There is **insufficient evidence** to assess if outcomes of the preterm fetus presenting breech are affected by mode of delivery. Very little prospective data, mostly nonrandomized, exists regarding vaginal versus CD of the premature breech infant (1). Two trials aimed to assess this question failed to randomize the planned sample sizes. After 17 months of patient recruiting at 26 different hospitals, only 13 women had been randomized making it impossible to confer any conclusions in one study (46). The Iowa premature breech trial was somewhat more successful, recruiting 38 patients over 5 years, but had insufficient data for meaningful conclusions (47). Outcomes in premature breech infants are mainly related to prematurity and/or fetal anomaly, with unclear effect of mode of delivery (48).

Twins
Breech Second Twin (See Also Chapter 43 in Maternal-Fetal Evidence Based Guidelines)
Pregnancies at 35 to 43 weeks with vertex/breech presentation in twin gestations <7 cm dilated have similar Apgar scores or incidence of neonatal morbidity in the second twin if delivered by vaginal or cesarean birth in a very small trial (49). There was no incidence of birth trauma or IVH in any of the 27 breech deliveries (49). Maternal febrile morbidity and length of stay was increased in the cesarean group (49). As such, **vaginal delivery of the second nonvertex twin is a reasonable management option.** Attempt at vaginal twin delivery has been supported, especially for twins with an estimated fetal weight (EFW) of >1500 g, and can only be performed with adequate experience of the obstetrician, as well as continuous availability of expert anesthesia, usually in or very close to an operating room. **Total breech extraction** is associated with shorter maternal stay and lower neonatal pulmonary disease, infection, and ICN stay compared with cephalic version in retrospective studies (49,50). There are no trials for twins presenting with **first twin nonvertex** (about 26%), with recommendation for CD based mostly on data from singleton gestations. Because vaginal delivery of **triplets** is usually associated with an increased risk for stillbirth or neonatal and infant deaths as compared with CD, **cesarean section is the route of choice**, even if some small series have recently reported similar outcomes for trial of labor or CD for triplets.

MALPOSITION
Diagnosis
Fetal malposition can be detected by provider digital exam as well as by ultrasound. There is insufficient evidence on the topic but one prospective RCT found a difference in digital vaginal examination and transabdominal ultrasonographic examination of fetal head position during the second stage of labor in 20% of the cases evaluated, promoting the use of abdominal ultrasound to locate the fetal head (51).

Management

Hands and Knees Posture

There is **insufficient evidence** for assessing the effect of **hands and knees posture** to correct malposition. This has been evaluated **both before (for prevention) and during labor.**

There are two trials on the effect of hands and knees posture **before labor** (52). Compared to a sitting position, 10 minutes in the hands and knees position is associated with a lower likelihood of malposition of the presenting part of the fetus in a small trial, but advice to assume the hands and knees posture for 10 minutes twice daily in the last weeks of pregnancy had **no effect on the baby's position at delivery** or any of the other pregnancy outcomes measured in a larger trial (52).

One study evaluated the use of hands and knees position **in labor** involving 147 women in labor at term who assumed the position for a period of at least 30 minutes. There was **no significant reduction** in occiput-posterior or occiput-transverse positions at delivery or reduction of operative deliveries. However, there was a significant reduction in back pain (53).

Manual Rotation

Persistent fetal occiput-posterior position is a risk factor for prolonged labor and higher rate of CD. There is **insufficient evidence** evaluating the use of manual (also called digital) rotation in reducing the prevalence of persistent occiput-posterior position and its consequences. In a retrospective cohort study, in women with a fetus in persistent occiput-posterior or transverse position in the second stage of labor, manual rotation was associated with lower rates of CD, perineal lacerations, postpartum hemorrhage, and chorioamnionitis, but a higher rate of cervical lacerations (54). A prospective (but not randomized) study of singletons with occiput-posterior position reported an increase in fetuses delivered in occiput-anterior position (93% vs. 15%) and in spontaneous vaginal delivery (77% vs. 27%) compared with no manual rotation, using historic controls (55) (see chap. 8).

ANESTHESIA

For vaginal breech delivery, an anesthesiologist skilled at the pharmacology of uterine relaxation (e.g., nitric oxide) should be present.

POSTPARTUM/BREASTFEEDING

No specific recommendations.

REFERENCES

1. American College of Obstetricians and Gynecologists. ACOG Clinical Management Guidelines for Obstetrician-Gynecologists Number 13: External cephalic version. Washington, D.C.: ACOG, 2000. [Review]
2. Hill LM. Prevalence of breech presentation by gestational age. Am J Perinatol 1990; 7(1):92–93. [II-3]
3. Mancuso KM, Yancey MK, et al. Epidural analgesia for cephalic version: a randomized trial. Obstet Gynecol 2000; 95(5):648–651. [RCT, *n* = 108]
4. Eide MG, Oyen N, Skjaerven R, et al. Breech delivery and intelligence: a population-based study of 8,738 breech infants. Obstet Gynecol 2005; 105(1):4–11. [II-2]
5. Dyson DC, Ferguson JE, Hensleigh P. Antepartum external cephalic version under tocolysis. Obstet Gynecol 1986; 67(1):63–68. [II-2]
6. Grootscholten K, Kok M, Oei SG, et al. External cephalic version-related risks: a meta-analysis. Obstet Gynecol 2008; 112(5):1143–1151. [Meta-analysis, 84 studies, *n* = 12,955]
7. Dugoff L, Stamm CA, Jones OW, et al. The effect of spinal anesthesia on the success rate of external cephalic version: a randomized trial. Obstet Gynecol 1999; 93(3):345–349. [RCT, *n* = 102]
8. Flamm BL, Fried MW, Lonky NM, et al. External cephalic version after previous cesarean section. Am J Obstet Gynecol 1991; 165 (2):370–372. [II-2]
9. Hofmeyr GJ, Kulier R. External cephalic version for breech presentation at term. Cochrane Database Syst Rev 2000; (2): CD000083. [5 RCTs, *n* = 533]
10. Kok M, Cnossen J, Gravendeel L, et al. Clinical factors to predict the outcome of external cephalic version: a metaanalysis. Am J Obstet Gynecol 2008; 199(6):630.e1–630.e7. [Meta-analysis, 53 studies, *n* = 10,149]
11. Ben-Meir A, Elram T, Tsafrir A, et al. The incidence of spontaneous version after failed external cephalic version. Am J Obstet Gynecol 2007; 196(2):157.e1–157.e3. [II-2]
12. Hutton EK, Hofmeyr GJ. External cephalic version for breech presentation before term. Cochrane Database Syst Rev 2006; (1): CD000084. [Meta-analysis: 7 RCTs, *n* = 1235]
13. Hutton EK, Kaufman K, Hodnett E, et al. External cephalic version beginning at 34 weeks' gestation versus 37 weeks' gestation: a randomized multicenter trial. Am J Obstet Gynecol 2003; 189(1):245–254. [RCT, *n* = 233]
14. Mensink WF, Huisjes HJ. Is external version useful in breech presentation? Ned Tijdschr Geneeskd 1980; 124(43):1828–1831. [RCT, *n* = 102]
15. Van Veelen AJ, Van Cappellen AW, Flu PK, et al. Effect of external cephalic version in late pregnancy on presentation at delivery: a randomized controlled trial. Br J Obst Gynaecol 1989; 96(8):916–921. [RCT, *n* = 180]
16. Hutton EK, Hannah ME, Ross SJ, et al. Early ECV2 Trial Collaborative Group. The Early External Cephalic Version (ECV) 2 Trial: an international multicentre randomised controlled trial of timing of ECV for breech pregnancies. Br J Obstet Gynecol 2011; 118 (5):564–577. [RCT, *n* = 1543]
17. Hofmeyr GJ. Interventions to help external cephalic version for breech presentation at term. Cochrane Database Syst Rev 2004; (1):CD000184. [6 RCTs betamimetic tocolysis, *n* = 617; 4 RCTs nitric oxide donors, *n* = >100; 1 acoustic stimulation, *n* = 26]
18. Vani S, Lau SY, Lim BK, et al. Intravenous salbutamol for external cephalic version. Int J Gynaecol Obstet 2009; 104(1):28–31. [RCT, *n* = 114]
19. Impey L, Pandit M. Tocolysis for repeat external cephalic version in breech presentation at term: a randomised, double-blinded, placebo-controlled trial. Br J Obstet Gynecol 2005; 112(5):627–631. [RCT, *n* = 124]
20. Hilton J, Allan B, Swaby C, et al. Intravenous nitroglycerin for external cephalic version: a randomized controlled trial. Obstet Gynecol 2009; 114(3):560–567. [RCT, *n* = 82]
21. El-Sayed YY, Pullen K, Riley ET, et al. Randomized comparison of intravenous nitroglycerin and subcutaneous terbutaline for external cephalic version under tocolysis. Am J Obstet Gynecol 2004; 191(6):2051–2055. [RCT, *n* = 59]
22. Kok M, Bais JM, van Lith JM, et al. Nifedipine as a uterine relaxant for external cephalic version: a randomized controlled trial. Obstet Gynecol 2008; 112(2 pt 1):271–276. [RCT, *n* = 32]
23. Mohamed Ismail NA, Ibrahim M, Mohd Naim N, et al. Nifedipine versus terbutaline for tocolysis in external cephalic version. Int J Gynaecol Obstet 2008; 102(3):263–266. [RCT, *n* = 86]
24. Collaris R, Tan PC. Oral nifedipine versus subcutaneous terbutaline tocolysis for external cephalic version: a double-blind randomised trial. Br J Obstet Gynecol 2009; 116(1):74–80. [RCT, *n* = 90]
25. Wilcox CB, Nassar N, Roberts CL. Effectiveness of nifedipine tocolysis to facilitate external cephalic version: a systematic review. Br J Obstet Gynecol 2011; 118(4):423–428. [3 RCTs, *n* = 496]
26. Johnson RL, Strong TH, Radin TG, et al. Fetal acoustic stimulation as an adjunct to external cephalic version. J Reprod Med 1995; 40 (10):696–698. [II-3]
27. Schorr SJ, Speights SE, Ross EL, et al. A randomized trial of epidural anesthesia to improve external cephalic version success. Am J Obstet Gynecol 1997; 177(5):1133–1137. [RCT, *n* = 69]
28. Lavoie A, Guay J. Anesthetic dose neuraxial blockade increases the success rate of external fetal version: a meta-analysis. Can J Anesth 2010; 57(5):408–414. [Meta-analysis, 7 RCT, *n* = 681]

29. Coyle ME, Smith CA, Peat B. Cephalic version by moxibustion for breech presentation. Cochrane Database Syst Rev 2005; (2): CD003928. [Meta-analysis: 3 RCTs, *n* = 597]

30. Cardini F, Weixin H. Moxibustion for correction of breech presentation: a randomized controlled trial. JAMA 1998; 280 (18):1580–1584. [RCT, *n* = 260, in China]

31. Li Q, Wang L. Clinical observation on correcting malposition of fetus by electro-acupuncture. J Tradit Chin Med 1996; 16 (4):260–262. [RCT, *n* = 111]

32. Cardini F, Lombardo P, Regalia AL, et al. A randomised controlled trial of moxibustion for breech presentation. Br J Obstet Gynecol 2005; 112(6):743–747. [RCT, *n* = 123, in Italy]

33. Neri I, Airola G, Contu G, et al. Acupuncture plus moxibustion to resolve breech presentation: a randomized controlled study. J Matern Fetal Neonatal Med 2004; 15(4):247–252. [RCT, *n* = 240, in Italy]

34. Vas J, Aranda JM, Nishishinya B, et al. Correction of nonvertex presentation with moxibustion: a systematic review and metaanalysis. Am J Obstet Gynecol 2009; 201(3):241–259. [Meta-analysis: 6 RCTs, *n* = 1087]

35. Guittier MJ, Pichon M, Dong H, et al. Moxibustion for breech version: a randomized controlled trial. Obstet Gynecol 2009; 114 (5):1034–1040. [RCT, *n* = 106]

36. Hofmeyr GJ, Kulier R. Cephalic version by postural management for breech presentation. Cochrane Database Syst Rev 2000; (3): CD000051. [Meta-analysis: 6 RCTs, *n* = 417]

37. Founds SA. Maternal posture for cephalic version of breech presentation: a review of the evidence. Birth 2005; 32(2):137–144. [Meta-analysis: 4 RCTs, *n* = 346, but could not be performed because of flaws in RCTs]

38. Vezina Y, Bujold E, Varin J, et al. Cesarean delivery after successful external cephalic version of breech presentation at term: a comparative study. Am J Obstet Gynecol 2004; 190(3):763–768. [II-2, *n* = 602]

39. Hofmeyr GJ, Hannah ME. Planned caesarean section for term breech delivery. Cochrane Database Syst Rev 2003; (3):CD000166. [Meta-analysis: 3 RCTs, *n* = 2396]

40. Hannah ME, Hannah WJ, Hewson SA, et al. Term Breech Trial Collaborative Group. Planned caesarean section versus planned vaginal birth for the breech presentation at term: a randomised multicentre trial. Lancet 2000; 356(9239):1375–1383. [RCT, *n* = 2088]

41. Su M, McCleod L, Ross S, et al. Term Breech Trial Collaborative Group. Factors associated with adverse perinatal outcome in the Term Breech Trial. Am J Obstet Gynecol 2003; 189(3):740–745. [Secondary analysis of RCT, *n* = 2083]

42. Hannah ME, Hannah WJ, Hodnett ED, et al. Term Breech Trial 3-Month Follow-up Collaborative Group. Outcomes at 3 months after planned cesarean vs planned vaginal delivery for breech presentation at term: the international randomized Term Breech Trial. JAMA 2002; 287(14):1822–1831. [RCT analysis of 3-months questionnaire follow-up, *n* = 1596]

43. Whyte H, Hannah ME, Saigal S, et al. Term Breech Trial Collaborative Group. Outcomes of children at 2 years after planned cesarean birth versus planned vaginal birth for breech presentation at term: the international Randomized Term Breech Trial. Am J Obstet Gynecol 2004; 191(3):864–871. [2-year follow-up of children of RCT, *n* = 923]

44. Hannah ME, Whyte H, Hannah WJ, et al. Term Breech Trial Collaborative Group. Maternal outcomes at 2 years after planned cesarean section versus planned vaginal birth for breech presentation at term: the international Term Breech Trial. Am J Obstet Gynecol 2004; 191(3):917–927. [2-year maternal follow-up of RCT, *n* = 917]

45. Hofmeyr GJ, Kulier R. Expedited versus conservative approaches for vaginal delivery in breech presentation. Cochrane Database Syst Rev 2000; (2):CD000082. [Meta-analysis: no RCTs]

46. Penn ZJ, Steer PJ, Grant A. A multicentre randomised controlled trial comparing elective and selective caesarean section for the delivery of the preterm breech infant. Br J Obstet Gynecol 1996; 103(7):684–689. [RCT, *n* = 13; stopped recruitment]

47. Zlatnik FJ. The Iowa premature breech trial. Am J Perinatol 1993; 10(1):60–63. [RCT, *n* = 38]

48. Cibils LA, Karrison T, Brown L. Factors influencing neonatal outcomes in the very-low-birth-weight fetus (<1500 grams) with a breech presentation. Am J Obstet Gynecol 1994; 171(1):35–42. [II-2]

49. Rabinovici J, Barkai G, Reichman B, et al. Randomized management of the second nonvertex twin: vaginal delivery or cesarean section. Am J Obstet Gynecol 1987; 156(1):52–56. [RCT, *n* = 60]

50. Mauldin JG, Newman RB, Mauldin PD. Cost-effective delivery management of the vertex and nonvertex twin gestation. Am J Obstet Gynecol 1998; 179(4):864–869. [II-2]

51. Dupuis O, Ruimark S, Corinne D, et al. Fetal head position during the second stage of labor: comparison of digital vaginal examination and transabdominal ultrasonographic examination. Eur J Obstet Gynecol Reprod Biol 2005; 123(2):193–197. [II-2]

52. Hofmeyr GJ, Kulier R. Hands and knees posture in late pregnancy or labour for fetal malposition (lateral or posterior). Cochrane Database Syst Rev 2005; (2):CD001063. [Meta-analysis: 2 RCTs, *n* = 2647]

53. Hunter S, Hofmeyr GJ, Kulier R. Hands and knees posture in late pregnancy or labour for fetal malposition (lateral or posterior). Cochrane Database Syst Rev 2007; (4):CD001063. [Meta-analysis: 3 RCT, *n* = 2794]

54. Shaffer BL, Cheng YW, Vargas JE, et al. Manual rotation to reduce caesarean delivery in persistent occiput posterior or transverse position. J Matern Fetal Neonatal Med 2011; 24(1):65–72. [II-2]

55. Reichman O, Gdansky E, Latinsky B, et al. Digital rotation from occipito-posterior to occipito-anterior decreases the need for cesarean section. Eur J Obstet Gynecol Reprod Biol 2008; 136 (1):25–28. [RCT, *n* = 61]

23

Shoulder dystocia

Sean C. Blackwell

KEY POINTS

- Risk factors for shoulder dystocia include prior shoulder dystocia (recurrence risk ∼1–15%); fetal macrosomia, diabetes mellitus, obesity, postterm, labor induction, epidural anesthesia, labor abnormalities (e.g., prolonged second stage), and operative vaginal delivery (Table 23.1).
- In 50% of shoulder dystocia cases, no risk factors are identified. Therefore clinicians should be ready for possible shoulder dystocia at every delivery.
- In 40% to 60% of shoulder dystocia cases, birth weight is <4000 g.
- Maternal complications of shoulder dystocia include serious vaginal laceration (third or fourth degree) and postpartum hemorrhage.
- A perinatal complication of shoulder dystocia is brachial plexus impairment (BPI), which occurs in 4% to 40% of shoulder dystocia cases; over 90% are transient. Approximately one-half of cases of BPI occur without documented shoulder dystocia.
- Other perinatal complications of shoulder dystocia include fractures, hypoxic-ischemic encephalopathy, long-term neurologic disability, and even death.
- Preconception prevention of maternal obesity and diabetes, as well as prenatal prevention of excessive weight gain, decrease the incidence of shoulder dystocia, mainly by prevention of fetal macrosomia.
- In women with **prior shoulder dystocia**, clinicians should review recurrence risk (7–15%), which risk factors (Table 23.1) are present in the current pregnancy, and also possible complications. If several significant risk factors are still present, the woman may opt for cesarean delivery. If risk factors are not present (except for prior shoulder dystocia), the woman may decide after counseling for either trial of labor or cesarean delivery.
- In pregnancies with estimated fetal weights (EFW) **>5000 g in nondiabetic and >4500 g in diabetic women**, American College of Obstetrician and Gynecologists (ACOG) **suggests planned cesarean delivery (without labor attempt) may be considered to avoid shoulder dystocia.**
- In women with EFW > 3800 g, prophylactic McRobert's maneuver and suprapubic pressure are associated in one randomized controlled trial (RCT) with **significantly fewer instances of shoulder dystocia.**
- Initial responses to shoulder dystocia involve asking for help, and, as first maneuvers, use of McRobert's maneuver and suprapubic pressure (Fig. 23.1).
- Second-line maneuvers include direct fetal manipulation such as delivery of the posterior arm, or then rotation of fetal shoulders. One-third of shoulder dystocia cases require use of more than two maneuvers. See Figure 23.1 for suggested management of shoulder dystocia.

DIAGNOSIS/DEFINITION

Shoulder dystocia is diagnosed when additional obstetrical maneuvers are required following failure of gentle downward traction on the fetal head to effect delivery of the shoulders (1). Shoulder dystocia pertains only to vertex presentation.

A quantitative definition of shoulder dystocia has been proposed as a prolonged head-to-body delivery time >60 seconds (2). This definition categorized 10% of vaginal deliveries as having shoulder dystocia, while only 25% to 45% of these cases were diagnosed as such by the delivery provider (3). However, these diagnostic criteria have not been adopted, and shoulder dystocia remains a subjective clinical diagnosis by the delivery provider. This may account for some of the variability in the frequency of reported shoulder dystocia across various populations and different studies.

SIGNS

- Retraction of the delivered fetal head against the maternal perineum ("turtle sign")
- Inability to deliver the fetal shoulders with routine traction in the "axial" direction

EPIDEMIOLOGY/INCIDENCE

The incidence of shoulder dystocia is about 1% (range 0.6–1.4%, depending on definition used).

ETIOLOGY/BASIC PATHOPHYSIOLOGY

Shoulder dystocia results from size discrepancy between the fetal shoulders and the pelvic inlet that results in impaction of the anterior shoulders behind the maternal pubis symphysis or the posterior shoulder on the sacral promontory (uncommon), or both (rare) (4). Persistent anterior-posterior location of the fetal shoulders at the pelvic brim occurs most often due to the following: increased resistance between the fetal skin and vaginal walls (e.g., fetal macrosomia), a large fetal chest relative to the biparietal diameter (e.g., infants of diabetic mothers), and when truncal rotation does not occur (e.g., precipitous labor).

RISK FACTORS/ASSOCIATIONS

Table 23.1 lists antepartum and intrapartum risk factors associated with shoulder dystocia. These risk factors have poor predictive value (whether in isolation or in combination with other factors), making them not very useful for clinical decision-making. In 50% of cases of shoulder dystocia, no risk factors are identified.

The two risks factors for shoulder dystocia most studied are **maternal diabetes and fetal macrosomia**. The frequency

Table 23.1 Factors Associated with Shoulder Dystocia

Antepartum	Intrapartum
Multiparity	Labor induction and/or augmentation
Postterm gestation	
Maternal obesity	Labor abnormalities
Maternal diabetes	Prolonged first stage
Prior shoulder dystocia	Prolonged second stage
Prior macrosomic child	Epidural
Excessive gestational weight gain	Operative vaginal delivery (forceps or vacuum)
Fetal macrosomia	

Source: From Ref. 1.

Table 23.2 Relationship Between Increasing Birth Weight and Maternal Diabetes and the Development of Shoulder Dystocia

Birth weight (g)	No diabetes (%)	Maternal diabetes (%)
4000–4250	5.25	12.2
4250–4500	9.1	16.7
4500–4750	14.3	27.3
4750–5000	21.1	34.8

Source: From Ref. 5.

of shoulder dystocia increases with higher birth weight (5) (Table 23.2).

Although there is a consistent relationship regarding birth weight and the risk for shoulder dystocia, it should also be remembered that 40% to 60% of cases occur with birth weight <4000 g, and of deliveries with birth weight >4000 g only 3.3% develop shoulder dystocia (4,6,7).

Although recognized as a risk factor associated with shoulder dystocia, multiple studies including those using advanced statistical models and techniques have been unable to discriminate labor patterns (e.g., prolonged first and/or second stage) in a manner that improves intrapartum management to predict and avoid shoulder dystocia (8–12).

COMPLICATIONS
Maternal

Although maternal complications can occur, these are most often mild and not associated with long-term morbidities. The most common complications involve postpartum blood loss and vaginal laceration (Table 23.3).

Perinatal

The most common major complication of shoulder dystocia is **neonatal BPI**, which occurs in 4% to 40% of cases of shoulder dystocia. In one of the largest series, the rate was 16.8% (see Table 23.3) (13). Most cases of BPI are unilateral (right > left) and involve the C5-C6 roots (Erb–Duchenne's palsy) (Table 23.4). Most bony injuries (clavicle or humerus), although always concerning, are not serious and heal promptly without long-term sequelae. Approximately one-third of BPIs have a concomitant bony fracture. Fortunately <10% of BPIs are permanent. Most fully recover with physical therapy and, in some situations, respond to neurosurgical treatment. **Permanent BPI is very rare and occurs in 1 to 2 out of every 10,000 births.** Signs and symptoms are a limp or unmoving paralyzed arm; lack of muscle control in the arm, hand, or wrist; and lack of feeling or sensation in the arm or hand. Neonatal BPIs can occur without shoulder dystocia. In fact, it is estimated that one-half of all BPIs occur in the absence of shoulder dystocia and up to 4% of BPIs are associated with cesarean delivery (14,15). **These BPIs are most likely due to mechanisms unrelated to clinician-applied traction and**

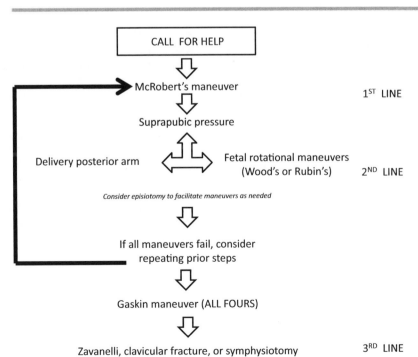

Figure 23.1 Management algorithm for shoulder dystocia.

Table 23.3 Maternal and Newborn Complications of Shoulder Dystocia Reported at Single Large Tertiary Care Center

Complication	Frequency (%)
Maternal	
Postpartum hemorrhage	11
Fourth-degree laceration (either extension of episiotomy or extension of laceration)	3.8
Vaginal lacerations	19.3
Cervical tear	2
Perinatal	
Any fetal injury	24.9
Brachial plexus injury	16.8
Clavicular fracture	9.5
Humeral fracture	4.2

Source: From Refs. 7,13.

Table 23.4 Types of Brachial Plexus Impairments

Palsy	Description	Level	Frequency (%)
Erb's palsy (also known as Erb–Duchenne's palsy)	Paralysis of flexion, abduction, and internal and external rotation of the forearm	C5, C6	>98
Klumpke's palsy	Paralysis of the thumb, fingers, and pronation of the forearm	C8, T1	<1
Complete brachial plexus palsy	Both Erb's and Klumpke's	C5, T1	<1

rather due to endogenous labor forces and/or in utero compression or maladaptation (16,17). External maneuvers and forces at vaginal delivery may not be responsible for injury from shoulder dystocia (6). In fact, the estimated pressures from endogenous forces are four to nine times greater than those calculated for clinician-applied forces (18).

Fractures of the clavicle and humerus have also been associated with shoulder dystocia, and the maneuvers to resolve it. Hypoxic-ischemic encephalopathy (HIE) and neurologic disability related to shoulder dystocia are very rare (<5%). The approximate incidence of fatal shoulder dystocia is 0.025 per 1000 deliveries.

MANAGEMENT
Principles
Shoulder dystocia is an obstetrical emergency and cannot be predicted. Thus, prompt recognition and response are essential for optimizing outcomes once it develops. Obstetricians should be trained and ready to manage this complication at every delivery. Therefore, it is imperative that shoulder dystocia training occurs early, and that at least one clinician experienced in the management of shoulder dystocia is present at every delivery.

Prevention
Preconception
Preconception prevention of maternal obesity and diabetes, as well as prenatal prevention of excessive weight gain, decreases

the incidence of shoulder dystocia, mainly by prevention of fetal macrosomia.

Antepartum
Since clinical risk factors (Table 23.1) do not accurately predict who will develop shoulder dystocia, few preventive strategies have been proven effective. Women with **prior shoulder dystocia** have about a 1% to 15% (19,20) risk of recurrence. In women with a prior shoulder dystocia, counseling should include review of prior delivery events including severity of injury of prior child, which risk factors (Table 23.1) are present in the current pregnancy, and also possible short-term and long-term complications of cesarean delivery. If several significant risk factors are still present, the woman may opt for cesarean delivery. However, given at least 85% of women will not have a recurrent shoulder dystocia and cesarean delivery does have certain surgical risks (especially in setting of maternal comorbidities), a woman with a prior shoulder dystocia after counseling may choose to pursue vaginal delivery (1).

Strategies to perform **cesarean delivery** without a labor attempt, due solely to suspected fetal macrosomia, are neither cost-effective nor practical due to poor prediction abilities (21,22). This is complicated by the known limitations of prenatal ultrasound to accurately estimate fetal weight, especially with increased fetal size (23,24). Only at very high EFW (>5000 g in nondiabetic and >4500 g in diabetic women), ACOG does suggest planned cesarean delivery (without labor attempt) may be considered to avoid shoulder dystocia (23).

Labor induction for women with suspected macrosomia does not decrease the rate of shoulder dystocia (25–27). However, labor induction in women with insulin-requiring diabetes did decrease the rate of shoulder dystocia but did not reduce neonatal morbidities (28) (see chaps. 4 and 5 in *Maternal-Fetal Evidence Based Guidelines*).

Intrapartum
Prophylactic McRobert's maneuver, prior to the development of shoulder dystocia, has not been shown to decrease subsequent shoulder dystocia in women at low risk for this complication (29). In a small RCT, in 40 women, compared with lithotomy position, the use of the McRobert's maneuver was associated with the same incidence (7.1% vs. 7.7%) of shoulder dystocia in both prophylactic and lithotomy groups. The force used in traction of the fetal head during vaginal delivery was the same in each group (29).

In another RCT, in 185 women likely to give birth to a large baby (EFW > 3800 g), compared with no prophylactic maneuvers, the McRobert's maneuver and suprapubic pressure were associated with a **trend for a lower rate of shoulder dystocia** compared with controls (9% vs. 21%; RR 0.44, 95% CI 0.17–1.14). There were significantly more cesarean sections in the prophylactic group, and when these were included in the results, **significantly fewer instances of shoulder dystocia were seen in the prophylactic group** (RR 0.33, 95% CI 0.12–0.86). In this study, 13 (18%) women in the control group required therapeutic maneuvers after delivery of the fetal head compared with 3 (5%) in the treatment group (RR 0.31, 95% CI 0.09–1.02). One infant in the control group had a brachial plexus injury (RR 0.44, 95% CI 0.02–10.61), and one infant had a 5-minute Apgar score <7 (RR 0.44, 95% CI 0.02–10.61) (30,31).

Training
Two nonrandomized studies that used historic controls have shown benefits of shoulder dystocia training. A "before and

Table 23.5 Description of Various Obstetrical Maneuvers to Resolve Shoulder Dystocia

Maneuver	Maternal or fetal manipulation	Type	Description
	Characteristics		
McRobert's	Maternal	First line	Hyperflexion and abduction of the maternal hips (knee-to-abdomen position). This causes cephalad rotation of the symphysis pubis, and flattening of the lumbar lordosis, freeing the impacted shoulder.
Suprapubic pressure	Maternal	First line	Pressure directed posteriorly in an attempt to force the anterior shoulder under the symphysis pubis. It also may include lateral pressure from either side of the maternal abdomen or alternating between sides using a rocking pressure. It works by reducing the fetal bisacromial diameter and rotating the anterior shoulder into oblique pelvic diameter.
Rubin's	Fetal	Second line	Pressure is applied to the posterior surface of the most accessible part of the fetal shoulder to effect shoulder adduction. It works by rotating the fetal shoulder into the oblique pelvic diameter.
Wood's	Fetal	Second line	Pressure is applied onto the anterior surface of the posterior shoulder in order to abduct the posterior shoulder. It works by rotating the fetal shoulder into the oblique pelvic diameter.
Delivery of posterior arm	Fetal	Second line	The delivery attendant places his/her hands in the vagina and applies pressure at the antecubital fossa in order to flex the fetal forearm. The arm is subsequently swept out over the infant's chest and delivered over the perineum. Rotation of the fetal trunk to bring the posterior arm anteriorly is sometimes required. Fracture of the humerus can occur with grasping and pulling directly on the fetal arm, as well as application of pressure onto the midhumeral shaft.
Gaskin (knee-chest or all fours)	Maternal	Second line	Patient is rolled from her existing position onto her hands and knees. It works through the downward force of gravity and/or a favorable change in pelvic diameters that causes disimpaction of the fetal shoulder.
Intentional fracture of clavicle	Fetal	Third line	This works by decreasing the fetal bisacromial diameter.
Zavanelli (cephalad replacement)		Third line	Cephalic replacement of the fetal head from the vagina back into the uterus and then delivery by cesarean section.
Symphysiotomy	Maternal	Third line	Surgical or traumatic separation of the pubis symphysis to facilitate disimpaction of the fetal shoulders.

after" study showed that training decreased the rate of BPI (0.4% vs. 0.15%; $p < 0.01$) even after adjusting for confounding factors (32). Another before and after study in the United Kingdom showed a reduction in neonatal injury at birth after shoulder dystocia: (9.3% vs. 2.3%; RR 0.25, 95% CI 0.11–0.57) (33). Both the Joint Commission in the United States and the Royal College recommend such training.

Recognition
After diagnosis of shoulder dystocia, whether done via recognition of the turtle sign or lack of fetal progression with gentle traction, the delivery provider should "**call for help**." This includes utilizing the assistance of other caregivers present in the delivery room as well as alerting other obstetrical, pediatric, and/or anesthesia providers on the labor and delivery unit.

Therapy
There are no interventional trials in human subjects that compare the safety or effectiveness of various shoulder dystocia therapeutic maneuvers (31). Thus, guidelines are based on observational data and/or expert opinion. The most important feature of the response to shoulder dystocia is that it should be a coordinated and orderly application and progression of obstetrical maneuvers (Fig. 23.1) (1,34). Table 23.5 describes maneuvers employed to relieve shoulder dystocia (4,35).

Most authorities recommend **McRobert's as the initial maneuver** since it is easy to perform, is effective, and has a low complication rate. McRobert's alone is effective in 40% to 90% of cases. Suprapubic pressure is often done in direct conjunction by nursing personnel.

If McRobert's combined with suprapubic pressure is not successful, direct fetal manipulation is attempted next. In a very large series, delivery of the posterior shoulder was associated with the highest rate of delivery (84%) compared with all other maneuvers (24–72%) (36). These authors have suggested considering using delivery of the posterior arm if delivery is not achieved with McRobert's maneuver and suprapubic pressure. Since shoulder dystocia is a bony dystocia, routine episiotomy is not advised. In situations where delivery of the posterior arm is being tried, episiotomy or proctoepisiotomy may give the delivery attendant additional room to grab the posterior fetal arm. Other helpful fetal manipulation interventions are either the Wood's corkscrew (Fig. 23.2) or Rubin's maneuver (Fig. 23.3).

In a series, more than one-third of patients required more than two maneuvers to relieve the shoulder dystocia (37). The need of additional maneuvers is associated with higher rates of neonatal injury (36).

If these steps all fail, one can repeat the sequence of initial maneuvers and/or attempt placement of the patient in the "ALL FOURS" position (Gaskin maneuver) (Fig. 23.1). More aggressive maneuvers, "heroic" maneuvers that have very high frequency of maternal and fetal complications, may be considered after repeat failure of these first- and second-line interventions. Third-line maneuvers include intentional fracture of the fetal clavicle, Zavanelli (cephalic replacement), and symphysiotomy. Fundal pressure should always be avoided

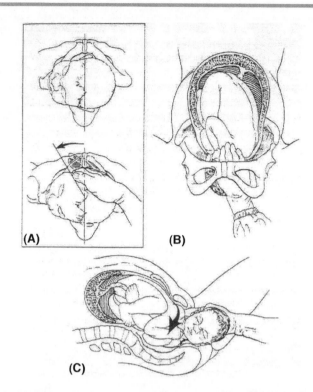

Figure 23.3 Rubin's maneuver: **(A)** and **(B)** Pressure is exerted on the posterior surface of the most accessible part of the shoulder to facilitate abduction and disimpaction of the anterior shoulder. **(C)** Further rotation and adduction toward the fetal chest reduce the bisacromial diameter and result in the movement of the shoulders in a transverse position, facilitating passage of the anterior side of the shoulder beneath the pubic arch. *Source*: From Ref. 5.

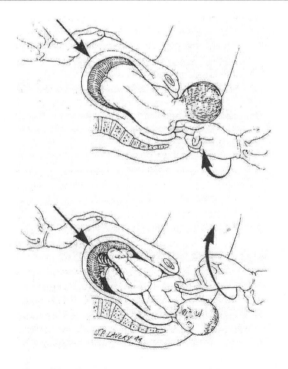

Figure 23.2 Wood's corkscrew maneuver. Initial pressure exerted on the anterior surface of the posterior shoulder facilitates rotation of the posterior shoulder anteriorly (*upper*). With concurrent synchronized downward pressure, the shoulder "screws" through the maternal pelvis, disimpacting the previously impacted shoulder (*lower*). *Source*: From Ref. 5.

in shoulder dystocia, as it may worsen impaction of fetal shoulder(s).

COUNSELING AND DOCUMENTATION

After completion of all necessary medical interventions (e.g., repair of maternal lacerations or treatment of hemorrhage), the delivery provider should sit down with patient and her family to review the delivery events, the management steps performed, and need for close newborn follow-up to evaluate for any neonatal injuries, especially bony fracture and symptoms of BPI. Open and honest communication with the mother and family after delivery is recommended.

It is important to document in the medical record all maneuvers used in detail, including which shoulder was anterior, and the time from delivery of head to complete delivery of the body (Fig. 23.4) (38,39).

ANESTHESIA

An anesthesiologist should be present during cases of shoulder dystocia to ensure adequate analgesia and prompt preparation for cesarean delivery if needed.

NEONATAL/INFANT FOLLOW-UP

It is important for the obstetrician, midwife, and delivery staff to follow up with the family regarding the outcome of the

Shoulder Dystocia Delivery Note Addendum

1. Antepartum documentation:
   a. Prior shoulder dystocia? Yes   no
   b. Estimated fetal weight _____
2. Mode of vaginal delivery
   a. Spontaneous
   b. Vacuum
   c. Forceps
3. How was the shoulder dystocia diagnosed? Turtle sign
   Failure to deliver shoulders with gentle downward pressure
   Other _____

4. Time fetal head delivered? _____

5. Time body delivered? _____

6. Total duration of shoulder dystocia (in minutes and seconds): _____

7. What shoulder was under the pubis symphysis (anterior) at delivery: Left   Right   Unknown

8. Please describe the obstetrical maneuvers were attempted, their order, and who performed:

Maneuver	Order	By whom
McRobert's (Hip flection)	1 2 3 4 5 6 7 8	_____
Suprapubic	1 2 3 4 5 6 7 8	_____
Delivery of posterior arm	1 2 3 4 5 6 7 8	_____
Rubin's (Anterior scapula)	1 2 3 4 5 6 7 8	_____
Wood's (Posterior scapula)	1 2 3 4 5 6 7 8	_____
Episiotomy	1 2 3 4 5 6 7 8	_____
Extension of Episiotomy	1 2 3 4 5 6 7 8	_____
Gaskin's (Knee-chest, all fours)	1 2 3 4 5 6 7 8	_____
Other _____	1 2 3 4 5 6 7 8	_____
Other _____	1 2 3 4 5 6 7 8	_____
Other _____	1 2 3 4 5 6 7 8	_____

Additional delivery comments: _____
_____

9. Was fundal pressure performed: Yes   NO

If yes, by whom and what was reason: _____

10. Who were the health care providers present at delivery?

Primary delivery attendant: _____
CNM: _____
Resident (s) [include PGY year]: _____
Nurse 1: _____
Nurse 2: _____
Nurse 3: _____
Pediatrician: _____
Anesthesiology: _____
Other providers (please add name and role): _____

11. Birth weight (grams)_____
12. Was baby moving his/her extremities: Left   right   Comment: _____
13. Was XRAY ordered for evaluation any bony fractures?   YES   NO
14. Were umbilical cord gases ordered?   YES   NO
15. Confirm that notes (e.g. medical, nursing, anesthesia, etc) are consistent   YES   NO
16. Has delivery note been dictated?   YES   NO
17. Family counseled   YES   NO
18. Debriefing with appropriate personnel involved   YES   NO
19. Follow-up about condition of neonate in nursery   YES   NO

Signatures:

_____   _____   _____
Primary Delivery Provider   Primary delivery nurse   Other care providers in attendance

Figure 23.4 Checklist for documentation of delivery complicated by shoulder dystocia.

infant born after shoulder dystocia. Table 23.4 describes most common palsies associated with shoulder dystocia. Erb's palsy is by far the most common and the one with the best prognosis. Occasionally BPI occurs on the posterior shoulder. Over 90% of neonates with Erb's palsy with shoulder dystocia recover within 1 year, with most recovery already evident at 3 to 6 months. Erb's palsy without shoulder dystocia has only a 60% recovery rate, and in about 68% of cases involves the posterior shoulder. Only about 40% of babies with Klumpke's palsy recover by 1 year. If permanent injury (5–8%) occurs, there is insufficient evidence to assess if surgery is effective.

REFERENCES

1. ACOG Committee on Practice Bulletins–Gynecology, the American College of Obstetrician and Gynecologists. ACOG practice bulletin clinical management guidelines for obstetrician-gynecologists. Obstet Gynecol 2002; 100(5 pt 1):1045–1050. [Practice guideline; Latest practice guideline for United States.]
2. Spong CY, Beall M, Rodrigues D, et al. An objective definition of shoulder dystocia: prolonged head-to-body delivery intervals and/or the use of ancillary obstetric maneuvers. Obstet Gynecol 1995; 86(3):433–436. [II-2]
3. Beall MH, Spong C, McKay J, et al. Objective definition of shoulder dystocia: a prospective evaluation. Am J Obstet Gynecol 1998; 179(4):934–937. [II-2]
4. Gherman RB, Chauhan S, Ouzounian JG, et al. Shoulder dystocia: the unpreventable obstetric emergency with empiric management guidelines. Am J Obstet Gynecol 2006; 195(3):657–672. [III; An excellent review article from experts in the field.]
5. Nesbitt TS, Gilbert WM, Herrchen B. Shoulder dystocia and associated risk factors with macrosomic infants born in California. Am J Obstet Gynecol 1998; 179(2):476–480. [II-2]
6. Gherman RB, Ouzounian JG, Goodwin TM. Brachial plexus palsy: an in utero injury? Am J Obstet Gynecol 1999; 180 (5):1303–1307. [II-2]
7. Gherman RB, Goodwin TM, Souter I, et al. The McRoberts' maneuver for the alleviation of shoulder dystocia: how successful is it? Am J Obstet Gynecol 1997; 176(3):656–661. [II-2]
8. McFarland M, Hod M, Piper JM, et al. Are labor abnormalities more common in shoulder dystocia? Am J Obstet Gynecol 1995; 173(4):1211–1214. [II-2]
9. Gemer O, Bergman M, Segal S. Labor abnormalities as a risk factor for shoulder dystocia. Acta Obstet Gynecol Scand 1999; 78 (8):735–736. [II-2]
10. Lurie S, Levy R, Ben-Arie A, et al. Shoulder dystocia: could it be deduced from the labor partogram? Am J Perinatol 1995; 12 (1):61–62. [II-2]
11. Mehta SH, Bujold E, Blackwell SC, et al. Is abnormal labor associated with shoulder dystocia in nulliparous women? Am J Obstet Gynecol 2004; 190(6):1604–1607; discussion 1607–1609. [II-2]
12. Dyachenko A, Ciampi A, Fahey J, et al. Prediction of risk for shoulder dystocia with neonatal injury. Am J Obstet Gynecol 2006; 195(6):1544–1549. [II-2]
13. Gherman RB, Ouzounian JG, Goodwin TM. Obstetric maneuvers for shoulder dystocia and associated fetal morbidity. Am J Obstet Gynecol 1998; 178(6):1126–1130. [II-2]
14. Gherman RB, Ouzounian JG, Miller DA, et al. Spontaneous vaginal delivery: a risk factor for Erb's palsy? Am J Obstet Gynecol 1998; 178(3):423–427. [II-2]
15. Sandmire HF, DeMott RK. Erb's palsy without shoulder dystocia. Int J Gynaecol Obstet 2002; 78(3):253–256. [Review; Along with references #16 and #17, a fascinating and compelling review regarding causation of brachial plexus impairment including non-traction-associated injuries.]
16. Sandmire HF, Demott RK. Controversies surrounding the causes of brachial plexus injury. Int J Gynaecol Obstet 2009; 104(1):9–13. [Review]
17. Sandmire HF, DeMott RK. Erb's palsy causation: iatrogenic or resulting from labor forces? J Reprod Med 2005; 50(8):563–566. [Review]
18. Gonik B, Walker A, Grimm M. Mathematic modeling of forces associated with shoulder dystocia: a comparison of endogenous and exogenous sources. Am J Obstet Gynecol 2000; 182(3):689–691. [Computer modeling experiment]
19. Bingham J, Chauhan SP, Hayes E, et al. Recurrent shoulder dystocia: a review. Obstet Gynecol Surv 2010; 65(3):183–188. [Review; Recent review that summarizes the literature of the reoccurrence rate of shoulder dystocia.]
20. Mehta SH, Sokol RJ. Risk of shoulder dystocia in second delivery: does a history of shoulder dystocia matter? Am J Obstet Gynecol 2010; 202(3):e11–e12; author reply e12. [II-2]
21. Rouse DJ, Owen J, Goldenberg RL, et al. The effectiveness and costs of elective cesarean delivery for fetal macrosomia diagnosed by ultrasound. JAMA 1996; 276(18):1480–1486. [Cost-effectiveness analysis; Classic study that defined the utility and costs of planned cesarean delivery to prevent shoulder dystocia.]
22. Rouse DJ, Owen J. Prophylactic cesarean delivery for fetal macrosomia diagnosed by means of ultrasonography—A Faustian bargain? Am J Obstet Gynecol 1999; 181(2):332–338. [Review]
23. American College of Obstetrician and Gynecologists. ACOG Technical Bulletin No. 159—September 1991: Fetal macrosomia. Int J Gynaecol Obstet 1992; 39(4):341–345. [Practice guideline; Practice bulletin that defines the EFW thresholds for consideration of offering cesarean delivery without labor attempt to avoid shoulder dystocia.]
24. Mehta SH, Blackwell SC, Hendler I, et al. Accuracy of estimated fetal weight in shoulder dystocia and neonatal birth injury. Am J Obstet Gynecol 2005; 192(6):1877–1880; discussion 1880–1881. [II-2]
25. Irion O, Boulvain M. Induction of labour for suspected fetal macrosomia. Cochrane Database Syst Rev 2000; (2):CD000938. [Meta-analysis]
26. Gonen O, Rosen DJ, Dolfin Z, et al. Induction of labor versus expectant management in macrosomia: a randomized study. Obstet Gynecol 1997; 89(6):913–917. [I]
27. Leaphart WL, Meyer MC, Capeless EL. Labor induction with a prenatal diagnosis of fetal macrosomia. J Matern Fetal Med 1997; 6(2):99–102. [II-2]
28. Boulvain M, Stan C, Irion O. Elective delivery in diabetic pregnant women. Cochrane Database Syst Rev 2001; (2):CD001997. [Meta-analysis]
29. Poggi SH, Allen RH, Patel CR, et al. Randomized trial of McRoberts versus lithotomy positioning to decrease the force that is applied to the fetus during delivery. Am J Obstet Gynecol 2004; 191(3):874–878. [I]
30. Beall MH, Spong CY, Ross MG. A randomized controlled trial of prophylactic maneuvers to reduce head-to-body delivery time in patients at risk for shoulder dystocia. Obstet Gynecol 2003; 102 (1):31–35. [RCT, *n* = 185]
31. Athukorala C, Middleton P, Crowther CA. Intrapartum interventions for preventing shoulder dystocia. Cochrane Database Syst Rev 2006; (4):CD005543. [Meta-analysis: 2 RCTs, *n* = 225; Systematic review shows the paucity of interventional trial to treat shoulder dystocia and the lack of high-quality data.]
32. Inglis SR, Feier N, Chetiyaar JB, et al. Effects of shoulder dystocia training on the incidence of brachial plexus injury. Am J Obstet Gynecol 2011; 204(4): 322.e1–322.e6. [II-3]
33. Draycott TJ, Crofts JF, Ash JP, et al. Improving neonatal outcome through practical shoulder dystocia training. Obstet Gynecol 2008; 112(1):14–20. [II-3]
34. Royal College of Obstetrians and Gynecologists. RCOG Guideline No. 42: Shoulder dystocia. London: RCOG Press, 2005:1–13. [Practice guideline; Practice guideline from RCOG. Provides evidence-based algorithm for management of shoulder dystocia].
35. Gherman RB. Shoulder dystocia: prevention and management. Obstet Gynecol Clin North Am 2005; 32(2):297–305. [Review]

36. Hoffman MK, Bailit JL, Branch DW, et al. A comparison of obstetric maneuvers for the acute management of shoulder dystocia. Obstet Gynecol 2011; 117(6):1272–1278. [II-2]

37. Stallings SP, Edwards RK, Johnson JW. Correlation of head-to-body delivery intervals in shoulder dystocia and umbilical artery acidosis. Am J Obstet Gynecol 2001; 185(2):268–274. [II-2]

38. Grobman WA, Hornbogen A, Burke C, et al. Development and implementation of a team-centered shoulder dystocia protocol. Simul Healthc 2010; 5(4):199–203. [II-2]

39. Deering SH, Tobler K, Cypher R. Improvement in documentation using an electronic checklist for shoulder dystocia deliveries. Obstet Gynecol 2010; 116(1):63–66. [II-2]

24

Postterm pregnancy

Sandra D. Dayaratna

KEY POINTS

- **Postterm pregnancy** is defined as a **singleton** pregnancy that has lasted until **≥42 weeks, or ≥294 days.**
- **Complications** for the baby include increased incidence of **meconium aspiration, intrauterine infection, oligohydramnios, macrosomia, nonreassuring fetal heart testing (NRFHT), low umbilical artery pH, low 5-minute Apgar score, dysmaturity syndrome**, and **perinatal mortality. Complications** for the mother include increased risk of **labor dystocia, perineal injury**, and **cesarean delivery.**
- **Pregnancies with risk factors** such as maternal (e.g., hypertension and diabetes) and fetal (growth restriction, etc.) diseases should be delivered at term or as described in the **pertinent guidelines.**
- **Prevention** of postterm pregnancy can be achieved with accurate dating by **routine first-trimester ultrasound** and with serial membrane stripping starting at term (e.g., 38 weeks).
- There is insufficient evidence to assess the efficacy of antepartum testing for pregnancies after their due date. Twice-weekly fetal testing with nonstress test (NST), or NST and amniotic fluid volume (AFV), or biophysical profile (BPP), has been proposed, starting at 41 weeks.
- Routine **induction of labor at ≥41 weeks reduces perinatal mortality**, due to a **decrease in fetal and neonatal deaths**. Routine induction of labor in this setting is associated with no change **in the incidence of cesarean delivery**.
- In women with a prior cesarean delivery, induction of labor is associated with an increase in uterine rupture in comparison to an unscarred uterus and in comparison to spontaneous labor.

DIAGNOSIS/DEFINITION

Postterm pregnancy is defined as pregnancy that has lasted until ≥42 weeks, or ≥294 days, or ≥14 days after the due date [estimated date of confinement (EDC)] (1). Prolonged pregnancy can be defined as a pregnancy that has lasted until ≥41 weeks, or ≥287 days, or ≥7 days after the due date (EDC) (2). The term "postdates" can signify a pregnancy that lasted until ≥40 weeks, or ≥280 days, but is often defined differently in the literature and should be avoided (1). All these definitions may have slightly different meanings in the literature, so it is important to be clear when using these terms. These definitions and this guideline pertain to **singleton gestations**. For multiple gestations, please refer to chapter 43 in *Maternal-Fetal Evidence Based Guidelines*.

EPIDEMIOLOGY/INCIDENCE

The **incidence** of postterm pregnancy is about 7% (1).

ETIOLOGY/BASIC PATHOPHYSIOLOGY

The most frequent cause of postterm pregnancy is an **error in dating** (1,3). See chapter 4 for accurate dating criteria and their benefits, as well as the following sections.

RISK FACTORS/ASSOCIATIONS

Poor (wrong) dating; prior postterm pregnancy; obesity; nulliparity; long (>28 days) cycles without early ultrasound; placental sulfatase deficiency; anencephaly; and male fetus. Obesity appears to be one modifiable risk factor for postterm pregnancy (2).

COMPLICATIONS
Perinatal

Many epidemiological studies have shown that fetal and neonatal complications increase with gestational age after 41 weeks. **Meconium aspiration, intrauterine infection, oligohydramnios, macrosomia, NRFHT, low umbilical artery pH**, and **low 5-minute Apgar score** have all been associated with postterm pregnancy. **Perinatal mortality** (fetal and neonatal deaths) is twice as high at ≥42 weeks and 6 times as high at ≥43 weeks compared with the rate for pregnancies delivered between 39 and 40 weeks (1,4).

Two markers of **immediate neonatal morbidity**, umbilical artery pH <7 and base excess <−12, have been shown to increase in a continuous manner in pregnancies beyond 40 weeks, and increase by odds ratio (OR) 1.65 for pH <7 for pregnancies between 41 and 42 weeks (5).

Neonatal mortality of normal-weight infants appears to be higher for infants born between 41 and 0 days and 41 weeks and 6 days compared with infants born between 38 weeks and 40 weeks and 6 days (OR 1.37, 95% CI 1.08–1.73) (6).

These data are, however, mixed and may vary based on whether risk factors such as intrauterine growth restriction (IUGR) are included in the analysis. In a review of all epidemiological studies published after 1990, 7 out of 11 studies demonstrated an increased stillbirth risk with postterm pregnancies and 4 suggested that other issues such as IUGR or fetal anomalies had a greater contribution to the stillbirth rate than did prolonged pregnancy (7).

Dysmaturity syndrome is present in about 20% of neonates born postterm and has some of the characteristics mentioned above, as well as possibly hypoglycemia, seizures, from uteroplacental insufficiency, and unclear long-term outcomes with an increased risk of infant death (1).

Maternal

Women giving birth postterm are at increased risk of **labor dystocia, perineal injury**, and **cesarean delivery**, with their complications (1).

PREGNANCY CONSIDERATIONS

Every woman should be counseled early in pregnancy that up to 50% of gestations, especially in nulliparous women, last until past the due date. This is physiologic and natural for humans. The incidence of fetal death is significantly higher than that of neonatal death at $\geq$283 days ($\geq$40 weeks and 3 days) (8). In large series, delivery at 38 weeks is associated with the lowest risk of perinatal death, but this risk is low at <1 to 2/1000 up to 41 weeks and 6 days (9). **It is important to identify maternal (e.g., hypertension and diabetes) and fetal (e.g. growth restriction) risk factors that would necessitate special management**, as described in the specific chapters in *Maternal-Fetal Evidence Based Guidelines*. The OR for stillbirths and neonatal mortality increases in gestations from 40 weeks onward, and this increase is compounded 7- to 10-fold when the fetus is growth restricted (10).

MANAGEMENT (FIG. 24.1)
Preconception Counseling

Women with prior posterm pregnancy are at increased risk for recurrent postterm pregnancy. Prevention strategies including weight loss for obese women, appropriate weight gain during the pregnancy, early initiation of prenatal care, and early ultrasound screening should be discussed (2).

Prevention

Routine Early Ultrasound to Reduce Postterm Pregnancies
Accurate assessment of gestational age is extremely important in improving perinatal morbidity and mortality. **First-trimester ultrasound** is the most accurate for pregnancy dating. Early ultrasound also reduces the number of postterm inductions.

Over 40% of women randomized to undergo first-trimester screening had their gestational age adjusted based on the ultrasound measurement of crown-rump length, whereas the corresponding number was only 10.9% for women assigned to second-trimester ultrasound. Furthermore, 4.8% in the first-trimester screening group compared with 13% in the second-trimester ultrasound group had labor induced for a postterm pregnancy (RR 0.37, 95% CI 0.14–0.96), which is a **63% reduction in the induction rate for postterm pregnancy** (11,12). Compared with no routine early ultrasound, **routine early pregnancy (<20 weeks) ultrasound reduces by 32% to 39% the incidence of postterm pregnancy and of induction for postterm pregnancy** (3,11,12) (see also chap. 4).

Stripping/Sweeping of Membranes
Compared with no sweeping, **sweeping of the membranes**, performed weekly as a general policy in women at term (e.g., weekly starting at 38 weeks), **is associated with reduced duration of pregnancy** and **reduced frequency of pregnancy continuing beyond 41 and 42 weeks** (13,14). To avoid one formal induction of labor, sweeping of membranes must be performed in eight women. **Risk of cesarean section, maternal, or neonatal infection is similar. Serial sweeping of membranes starting at 41 weeks every 48 hours** also **decreases the risk of postterm pregnancy** from 41% to 23%, with efficacy both in nulliparous and multiparous women (15). Discomfort during vaginal examination and other adverse effects (bleeding and irregular contractions) are more frequently reported by women allocated to sweeping, but its safety has been confirmed in multiple studies (13–16) (see also chap. 20).

Breast and Nipple Stimulation to Reduce Postterm Pregnancies
Breast and nipple stimulation daily starting at 39 weeks has not been sufficiently studied to ascertain safety, but it does

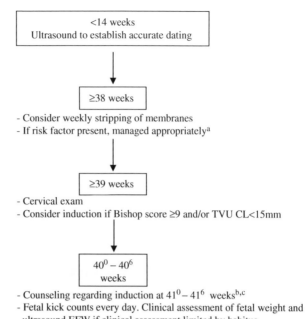

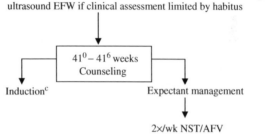

^aRisk factor examples include hypertension, diabetes mellitus, FGR, multiple gestation, etc. Please see chapter in *Maternal-Fetal Evidence Based Guidelines* pertinent to specific risk factor for management.
^bSuggest induction for all women between 41^0 and 41^6 weeks.
^cSee chapter 20 for effective induction management.

Figure 24.1 Management of postterm pregnancy. *Abbreviations*: TVU, transvaginal ultrasound; CL, cervical length; 2×/wk; twice per week; NST, nonstress test; AFV, amniotic fluid volume assessment; FGR, fetal growth restriction.

appear to reduce the incidence of postterm pregnancy by 48% (17,18).

Antepartum Testing

There are insufficient data to assess the best mode of fetal monitoring after the due date, as there are **no trials** to assess the effect of antepartum testing on these pregnancies compared with no testing. Since fetal death rates incrementally increase after the due date, it seems reasonable to test fetuses to assure well-being, especially at $\geq$41 weeks (1,3,8). The most used options include NST (also called cardiography), BPP, and modified BPP. Modified BPP includes NST and ultrasound measurement of maximum vertical depth (MVP) of AFV. Others have been described, with even less evidence for efficacy. Doppler of any vessel, including the umbilical artery, is not effective in the management of postterm pregnancy.

Compared with fetal monitoring using NST and AFV, BPP (computerized cardiotocography, amniotic fluid index, fetal breathing, fetal tone, and fetal body movements) is associated with increased incidence of inductions and similar outcomes in a small trial in women ≥42 weeks (19). At ≥41 weeks, **twice-weekly testing** (e.g., with NST and MVP) is recommended (1), but not based on trials (see also chap. 55 in *Maternal-Fetal Evidence Based Guidelines*). In addition, an effort should be made to **assess fetal weight**, either clinically or, if this assessment is limited, by ultrasound, as the known increase in fetal and neonatal mortality in pregnancies beyond their due date is even higher in IUGR fetuses (10,20).

Interventions

Routine Induction of Labor at ≥41 Weeks

A policy of **labor induction at 41 completed weeks (41–41 6/7) or beyond is associated with significantly less perinatal deaths** (1/2986 vs. 9/2953; RR 0.30, 95% CI 0.09–0.99) compared with expectant management, with induction not before 42 weeks (20,21). If deaths due to congenital abnormality are excluded, no deaths remain in the labor induction group and seven deaths remain in the no induction group. There is **no significant difference in the risk of cesarean section** (RR 0.92, 95% CI 0.76–1.12; RR 0.97, 95% CI 0.72–1.31) for women induced at 41 and 42 completed weeks, respectively (20–22). **Labor induction at 41 weeks also significantly reduces the risk of perinatal meconium aspiration syndrome** compared with expectant management (RR 0.29, 95% CI 0.12–0.68). It is important to recognize, however, that in general the outcomes are very good with both expectant management and induction, with the absolute perinatal death rate/1000 ongoing pregnancies no higher than 1.2/1000 at 42 weeks, increasing up to 6/1000 ongoing pregnancies at 43 weeks (23). About 527 inductions (95% CI 4.57–6.12) would need to be done at 41 weeks in order to prevent one perinatal death (23). In order to prevent one stillbirth at 41 weeks, 671 inductions (95% CI 5.71–7.94) would need to be done (23,24).

The use of analgesia, NRFHT, operative vaginal delivery rates, and other neonatal outcome measures are similar with induction or expectant management. **Routine induction is more cost-effective than expectant management** (21). Several studies have shown that **patient satisfaction is higher with induction of labor** and cesarean rates are either lower or the same as the expectant management group (20,21). Iatrogenic prematurity should be avoided by careful assessment of gestational age. This risk should be minimal with the advent of widespread early ultrasound use to confirm pregnancy dating. See also chapter 20 for other induction risks and benefits, as well as management of induction.

Women with a favorable cervix. No trials have focused on or included in sufficient numbers pregnancies ≥41 weeks with a favorable cervix (i.e., Bishop score ≥9 or TVU CL <15 mm). As the complications of induction, particularly a failed induction and unnecessary subsequent cesarean section, are low in women with a favorable cervix, and there appears to be a trend toward decreased perinatal deaths and a statistically significant reduction in meconium aspiration, it seems reasonable to at least **offer, if not recommend, induction by 41 weeks** (41 and 0/7 days) for these women (20,21).

Women with an unfavorable cervix. Cervical ripening is recommended for women with unfavorable cervix prior to labor induction. **If cervical ripening is used, there is no difference in the incidence of cesarean** section in women who were induced or expectantly managed (1,21,24). A discussion about induction of labor after 41 weeks versus expectant management should occur with the patient, and management should include consideration for patient preference and access to antenatal testing (see also chap. 20).

Induction should absolutely be recommended for all patients by 42 0/7 weeks. One hundred and ninety-five inductions would prevent one perinatal death in this group (23).

Women with a prior cesarean delivery. In women with a prior cesarean delivery, induction is associated with a higher incidence of uterine rupture, especially in the nulliparous woman with an unfavorable cervix. The rate of uterine rupture is about 0.4% to 0.5% for spontaneous labor, 0.8% for labor induced without prostaglandins, and 2.2% for prostaglandin-induced labor (25). Prostaglandins should, in general, not be used for cervical ripening in a woman with a prior cesarean section. If the woman desires vaginal birth after cesarean (VBAC), it seems reasonable to wait until 40 to 41 weeks for spontaneous labor. There are insufficient data to assess the risks of trial of labor after cesarean section in a postterm gestation, but if the cervix is favorable, induction can be performed after through discussion of the risks and benefits. If the cervix is unfavorable, the patient should be apprised of the higher risks of uterine rupture, as well as the risks of a failed induction with an unfavorable cervix. A repeat cesarean section can be offered to decrease these risks (1,26) (see also chap. 14).

REFERENCES

1. American College of Obstetricians and Gynecologists. ACOG Practice Bulletin No. 55: Management of postterm pregnancy. Obstet Gynecol 2004; 104:639–646. [Review]
2. Caughey AB, Stotland NE, Washington AE, et al. Who is at risk for prolonged and postterm pregnancy? Am J Obstet Gynecol 2009; 200:683.e1–683.e5. [II-3, $n = 119,162$]
3. Neilson JP. Ultrasound for fetal assessment in early pregnancy. Cochrane Database Syst Rev 2005;; (3). [Meta-analysis: 9 RCTs, $n = >24,000$]
4. Myers ER, Blumrick R, Christian Al, Management of Prolonged Pregnancy. Rockville, MD: Agency for Healthcare Research and Quality (US), 2002. [Review]
5. Caughey AB, Washington AE, Laros RK. Neonatal complications of term pregnancy: rates by gestational age increase in a continuous, not threshold, fashion. Am J Obstet Gynecol 2005; 192:185–190. [II-3, $n = 32,679$]
6. Bruckner TA, Cheng YW, Caughey AB. Increased neonatal mortality among normal-weight births beyond 41 weeks of gestation in California. Am J Obstet Gynecol 2008; 199:421.e1–421.e7. [II-3, $n = 1,815,811$]
7. Mandruzzato G, Alfirevic Z, Chervenak F, et al. World Association of Perinatal Medicine. Guidelines for the management of postterm pregnancy. J Perinatal Med 2010; 38:111–119. [Meta-analysis]
8. Divon MY, Ferber A, Sanderson M, et al. A functional definition of prolonged pregnancy based on daily fetal and neonatal mortality rates. Ultrasound Obstet Gynecol 2004; 23:423–426. [II-2, $n = 656,134$]
9. Smith GCS. Life-table analysis of the risk of perinatal death at term and post term in singleton pregnancies. Am J Obstet Gynecol 2001; 184:489–496. [II-2, $n = 700,878$]
10. Divon M, Haglund B, Nisell H. Fetal and neonatal mortality in the postterm pregnancy: the impact of gestational age and fetal growth restriction. Am J Obstet Gynecol 1998; 178:726–731. [II-2, $n = 181,524$]
11. Crowley, P. Interventions for preventing or improving the outcome of delivery at or beyond term. Cochrane Database Syst Rev 2005; (4):CD000331. [Meta-analysis: 26 RCTs (variable quality), $n = >25,000$; early ultrasound: 4 RCTs, $n = 21,776$; induction at ≥41 weeks: 19 RCTs, $n = 7925$]

12. Bennett K, Crane J, O'Shea P, et al. First trimester ultrasound screening is effective in reducing postterm labor induction rates: a randomized controlled trial. Am J Obstet Gynecol 2003; 190:1077–1081. [RCT, $n = 218$]

13. Berghella V, Rogers RA, Lescale K. Stripping of membranes as a safe method to reduce prolonged pregnancies. Obstet Gynecol 1996; 87(6):927–929. [RCT, $n = 142$]

14. Boulvain M, Stan C, Irion O. Membrane sweeping for induction of labour. Cochrane Database Syst Rev 2005; (4):CD000451. [Meta-analysis: 22 RCTs, $n = 2797$]

15. de Miranda E, van der Bom JG, Bonsel GJ, et al. Membrane sweeping and prevention of post-term pregnancy in low-risk pregnancies: a randomized controlled trial. Br J Obstet Gynecol 2006; 113:402–408. [RCT, $n= 742$]

16. Kashanian M, Akbarian A, Baradaran H, et al. Effect of membrane sweeping at term pregnancy on duration of pregnancy and labor induction: a randomized trial. Gynecol Obstet Invest 2006; 62:41–44. [RCT, $n = 122$]

17. Elliott JP, Flaherty JF. The use of breast stimulation to prevent postdate pregnancy. Am J Obstet Gynecol 1984; 149:628–632. [RCT]

18. Kadar N, Tapp A, Wong A. The influence of nipple stimulation at term on the duration of pregnancy. J Perinatol 1990; 10:164–166. [RCT]

19. Alfirevic Z, Walkinshaw SA. A randomized controlled trial of simple compared with complex antenatal fetal monitoring after 42 weeks of gestation. Br J Obstet Gynaecol 1995; 102:638–643. [RCT]

20. Gulmezoglu AM, Crowther CA, Middleton P. Induction of labour for improving birth outcomes for women at or beyond term. Cochrane Database Syst Rev 2009; (4). [Meta-analysis: 19 RCTs, $n = 7984$]

21. Hannah ME, Hannah WJ, Hellman J, et al. Canadian Multicenter Post-Term Pregnancy Trial Group. Induction of labour as compared with serial antenatal monitoring in post-term pregnancy. A randomized controlled trial. N Engl J Med 1992; 326:1587–1592. [RCT, $n = 3407$]

22. Wennerholm U, Hagberg H, Brorsson B, et al. Induction of labor versus expectant management for post-date pregnancy: is there sufficient evidence for a change in clinical practice? Acta Obstet Gynecol 2009; 88:6–17. [Meta-analysis: 14 RCTs, 3 systematic reviews, $n = 6617$]

23. Heimstad R, Romundstad P, Salvesen K. Induction of labour for post-term pregnancy and risk estimates for intrauterine and perinatal death. Acta Obstet Gynecol 2008; 87:247–249. [II-3, $n = 408,631$]

24. Heimstad R, Skogvall E, Mattsson L, et al. Induction of labor and serial antenatal fetal monitoring in postterm pregnancy. A randomized controlled trial. Obstet Gynecol 2007; 109:609–617. [RCT, $n = 508$]

25. Lydon-Rochelle M, Holt VL, Easterling TR, et al. Risk of uterine rupture during labor among women with a prior cesarean delivery. N Engl J Med 2001; 345:3–8. [II-2]

26. American College of Obstetricians and Gynecologists. ACOG Practice Bulletin No. 115: Vaginal birth after previous cesarean delivery. Obstet Gynecol 2010; 116:450–463. [Review]

25

Placental disorders[a]

William Grobman

KEY POINTS
Placenta Previa

- **Placenta previa** is defined as a placenta that covers the internal os.
- **Low-lying placenta** is defined as a placenta that comes within 0.1 to 2.0 cm of the internal os but does not cover it.
- **Placental location should be assessed when the fetal anatomic survey ultrasound (usually 18–24 weeks) is performed.** If a placenta previa is suspected on transabdominal ultrasound, a **transvaginal ultrasound (TVU) should be performed** to confirm the diagnosis.
- The risk that a placenta previa diagnosed in the antepartum period remains a placenta previa at the time of delivery depends on several factors, especially gestational age (GA) at detection, the placental distance from or extent of overlap of the internal os, and the a priori risk of placenta previa related to other risk factors (e.g., prior cesarean delivery). **Most placenta previas diagnosed before the third trimester do not remain placenta previas at the time of delivery.**
- Women who have the inferior edge of the placenta ≥ 1 cm **from the internal os at around 20 weeks usually do not require further ultrasounds for placental location.**
- **All patients with the inferior placenta edge <1 cm from the internal os or overlying the os at around 20 weeks should be rescanned at least once at approximately 32 to 35 weeks' gestation** to reassess for placental location.
- All patients with **prior cesarean delivery and placenta previa** that extends anteriorly should have evidence of **placenta accreta** assessed ultrasonographically.
- Women with a **placenta previa** should be delivered by **cesarean**. If the placental lower edge is **within 1 to 20 mm of the internal os**, a **trial of labor** can be attempted, but the risk of significant bleeding during labor may be higher, especially in those with a distance of only 1 to 10 mm.
- The optimal GA for delivery of an asymptomatic woman (i.e., a woman without acute bleeding) with placenta previa is unknown, but **many experts recommend delivery at approximately 37 weeks.**

Placenta Accreta

- **Risk factors for placenta accreta** include **prior cesarean delivery; placenta previa; prior uterine surgery (e.g., prior myomectomy or prior multiple D&Es); Asherman's syndrome; submucous leiomyomata; maternal age ≥ 35 years; multiparity; and smoking.**

- **Maternal complications** of placenta accreta include **hysterectomy, injury to other organs, blood transfusion, disseminated intravascular coagulation (DIC), infection,** and **death.** Fetal complications include **preterm birth (PTB) and small for gestational age (SGA).**
- There are **no randomized trials** to assess efficacy of different surgical interventions in or the approaches to the management of placenta accreta. Planned hysterectomy may be beneficial in cases in which the diagnosis is highly suspected, especially for the woman who does not desire further fertility.

Vasa Previa

- **Vasa previa** exists when umbilical vessels, unprotected by the umbilical cord, run through the membranes and over the internal os. In this circumstance, rupture of the membranes can lead to rupture of these fetal vessels, with a significant possibility of fetal death. Women with risk factors, such as a velamentous cord insertion or a succenturiate or bilobed placenta in which intervening vessels may cross the cervix, should have a TVU to detect vasa previa.

PLACENTA PREVIA
Diagnoses/Definitions

Placenta previa is defined as **a placenta that covers the internal os**. The diagnosis of placenta previa is established by TVU. The terms partial, marginal, complete, or incomplete placenta previa are rooted in preultrasound physical examinations, have been used to signify different conditions, and therefore should be avoided. Moreover, many studies have used these terms to signify different conditions. When the placenta does not cover the internal os, rather than use ambiguous language, it is best to describe the distance of the tip of the placenta from the internal os. **Low-lying placenta** is defined as a placenta that comes within 0.1 to 2.0 cm of the internal os but does not cover it.

Symptoms

Approximately two-thirds of women with placenta previas have antepartum vaginal bleeding. Therefore, about 33% do not have any symptoms before delivery.

Epidemiology/Incidence

The incidence of placenta previa at term is approximately **0.5%** (1). The frequency of placenta previa is higher earlier in gestation, but many of these cases will resolve. The likelihood of resolution is inversely proportional to GA at the time of examination (Table 25.1) (2).

---

[a]Includes placenta previa, placenta accreta, and vasa previa. For normal or abnormal third stage, including postpartum hemorrhage, retained placenta, and uterine inversion, see chapter 9.

Table 25.1   Persistence of Placenta Previa until Delivery Stratified by Gestational Age at Ultrasound Detection, Type of Previa, and Prior Cesarean Delivery

GA at detection (wk)	15–19	20–23	24–27	28–31	32–35
Incomplete previa,[a] no prior cesarean	6	11	12	35	39
Incomplete previa,[a] prior cesarean	7	50	40	38	63
Complete previa, no prior cesarean	20	45	56	89	90
Complete previa, prior cesarean	41	73	84	88	89

All data presented as %.
[a]Incomplete previa defined as inferior edge of the placenta partially covering or reaching the margin of the internal os.
Abbreviation: GA, gestational age.
Source: From Refs. 2,7,10.

Table 25.2   Risk of Placenta Previa and/or Accreta Stratified by Number of Prior Cesarean Deliveries

	1st CD	2nd CD	3rd CD	4th CD	5th CD	≥6th CD
Previa	6.4	1.3	1.1	2.3	2.3	3.4
Accreta (*no previa*)	0.03	0.2	0.1	0.8	0.8	4.7
Accreta (*previa*)	3.3	11	40	61	67	67

All data presented as %.
Abbreviation: CD, cesarean delivery.
Source: From Ref. 5.

Risk Factors/Associations

Prior cesarean delivery (Table 25.2), any other uterine surgery (e.g., myomectomy, D&E, D&C, and hysteroscopy) involving the uterine cavity, prior placenta previa, and multiparity (3–5).

Complications

Placenta accreta, antepartum and/or postpartum hemorrhage, PTB, and perinatal death (6).

Management

Principles

Placenta location should be assessed at the time of the fetal anatomic survey (usually 18–24 weeks). If placenta previa is suspected by transabdominal examination, a **TVU should be performed for confirmation of the diagnosis** (Fig. 25.1). A single antenatal ultrasound that detects a placenta previa, however, may not indicate that a placenta previa will be

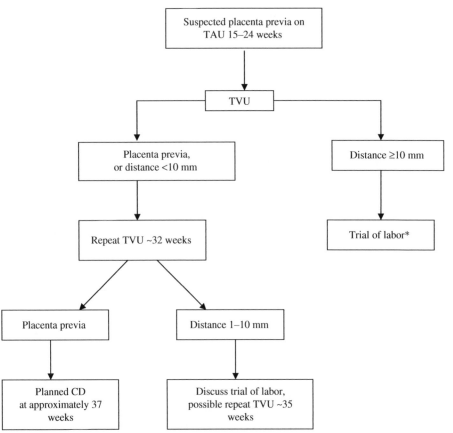

*After discussion with the couple and if no contraindication.

Figure 25.1 Management of suspected placenta previa. *Abbreviations*: Distance: distance between placental edge to internal cervical os; TAU, transabdominal ultrasound; TVU, transvaginal ultrasound; CD, cesarean delivery.

present at delivery, as the relative position of the placenta with respect to the internal os will change as gestation progresses (2). The reason for this change in relative position is not placental migration but likely due to the growth and development of the lower uterine segment. Atrophy of placental cells overlying the os also has been postulated as a contributing factor to this apparent positional change. This phenomenon has been cited as the reason that **vasa previa** can be seen in this setting (i.e., when an initially diagnosed placenta previa resolves).

Workup

Examination. Because of the reliability of ultrasound for diagnosis of previa, the technique of double setup examination is unnecessary. If employed, double setup examination should be performed in a setting with the ability to proceed in a prompt fashion with cesarean delivery if indicated.

Ultrasound. TVU is the **gold standard for the diagnosis of placenta previa**. It is very safe in these women (3). The risk that a placenta previa that is diagnosed with ultrasound is present at delivery depends on several factors, including GA at detection, the placental distance from or extent of overlap of the internal os, as well as a woman's a priori risk of placenta previa (e.g., related to a prior cesarean delivery). **Most previas diagnosed before the third trimester resolve** (Table 25.1) (2,7). If a placenta previa "resolves" but remains proximate to the internal cervical os, a woman still may have an increased risk of third-trimester bleeding, intrapartum hemorrhage, and cesarean delivery (8,9).

Women who have the inferior edge of the placenta $\geq$**1 cm from the internal os at around 20 weeks usually do not require further ultrasounds for placental location** as they are exceedingly unlikely to have a placenta that is low-lying or a previa at delivery. Women who have the inferior placental edge **overlapping the internal os by** $\geq$**25 mm at around 20 weeks** have been reported to **usually have persistence of previa even by term** (10,11) (Table 25.1).

All patients with suspected placenta previa in the second trimester should be **rescanned at** approximately **32 to 35 weeks'** gestation to assess for persistence of placenta previa (Fig. 25.1). Additionally, even if a placenta previa is no longer present, **measuring the distance from the placental edge to the internal os in the third trimester can help estimate the risk of bleeding with a trial of labor** (8,9).

All patients with **prior cesarean delivery and placenta previa** that extends anteriorly should have evidence of **placenta accreta assessed ultrasonographically** (5,6) (see section "Placenta Accreta").

Prenatal Care

All patients with **placenta previa** and **antenatal bleeding** in the third trimester should be advised about **pelvic rest (no vaginal penetration)**. Pelvic rest recommendations in women with previa placenta that is near but not overlapping the internal os should be individualized and based on bleeding during the pregnancy as well as the distance between the placenta and the internal os. There is insufficient evidence to support the use of routine bed rest in women with placenta previa or to be certain who are optimal candidates, when asymptomatic, for hospitalization (12). There is no evidence to support the use of autologous blood donation/transfusion for placenta previa (13).

Therapy/Interventions

Management at home vs. hospitalization. There has been no evidence of any clear advantage to a policy of home versus routine hospital care, with **similar maternal and fetal outcomes** demonstrated in the trials that do exist. The only difference is that, compared to hospitalization, management at home, not surprisingly, has been associated with a reduced length of stay in the hospital (12). There are no data to allow certainty as to who are the optimal candidates for inpatient management. Women who, traditionally, have been **more likely to be managed in the hospital** even though they are not acutely symptomatic are those who **have had recurrent episodes of antepartum hemorrhage (e.g., three or more episodes of bleeding); have other medical complications that increase their risks (e.g., congenital cardiac disease); or are unable to easily access the hospital in an emergency (e.g., lack of telephone at home and far distance from an adequate care facility)**.

Often, after an initial antenatal bleeding episode related to placenta previa, if several days of no further bleeding have occurred and there is no other indication for hospitalization, women may be managed as outpatients.

Cervical cerclage. Cervical cerclage has not been proven to be an effective intervention for women with placenta previa (12). Although the meta-analysis in the Cochrane review that evaluated cervical cerclage in the setting of placenta previa revealed that women randomized to cerclage had a reduced length of inpatient hospitalization, as well as reduced risks of an SGA birth or delivery <34 weeks, the benefits were evident in studies with lower methodological quality, and thus there is not yet sufficient evidence to justify this intervention.

Tocolysis. There is insufficient evidence to assess the benefits of tocolysis for treatment of preterm labor (PTL) specifically in women with a placenta previa. It is reasonable to consider tocolysis, as for women without a placenta previa, if PTL is diagnosed and a course of steroids has not yet been administered (14). Acute bleeding with instability of the mother or fetus is considered a contraindication to tocolysis.

Antepartum testing. There are insufficient data to assess the usefulness of routine antenatal testing in improving outcomes, and this strategy is presently not indicated.

Delivery.

Timing. There is insufficient evidence to be certain of the optimal GA of delivery for women with placenta previa who are not acutely bleeding, although experts have recommended approximately **37 weeks** (15,16) (Fig. 25.1). In the setting of acute bleeding, the timing of delivery depends upon individualization of patient circumstances, taking into account GA, amount of bleeding, and other comorbidities.

Mode. Delivery of women with a placenta previa should be by **cesarean**. Those with a placenta not covering the internal os but in the lower segment may have a trial if labor offered, with individual circumstances (e.g., the presence of antepartum bleeding) and the risk of bleeding at delivery taken into consideration. In a recent series, 26/28 (93%) women who had a placental edge to cervical os distance of 1 to 20 mm and who underwent a trial of labor delivered vaginally (8,17). Women with a placental edge that is within 1 cm of the internal os can have uncomplicated vaginal deliveries, although their risk of bleeding and requiring a cesarean is higher than in those women whose placenta is 10 to 20 mm distant from the os (risks of cesarean 75% and 31%, respectively) (8) (Table 25.3). As such, depending upon the distance of the placental edge from the internal os as well as other factors, these patients (i.e., those with a placenta not covering the internal os but that is 2 cm or less from the internal os prior to delivery) should have

Table 25.3 Selected Outcomes with Low-Lying Placenta According to Placental Edge to Internal Os Distance

	Distance between placental edge and internal cervical os	
	1–10 mm	11–20 mm
Cesarean delivery	75%	31%
Antepartum hemorrhage	29%	3%
Postpartum hemorrhage	21%	10%
Postpartum hemorrhage >1000 mL	8%	10%

Source: From Ref. 17.

their circumstances discussed and be delivered in facilities with the capacity to perform emergent operative delivery if necessary (18). In women with the placenta 2 cm from the internal os, a trial of labor should be encouraged.

PLACENTA ACCRETA
Diagnosis/Definition

Placenta accreta is defined as a placenta that is abnormally adherent to the uterus. The diagnosis of this condition can be quite difficult, as full ascertainment would require postpartum histologic examination of the entire uteroplacental interface with both placenta and uterus available. Since this is not typically possible, in cases of clinically suspected placenta accreta, failure to demonstrate abnormal villous invasion by pathologic examination cannot always be used to exclude this diagnosis (19). Therefore, **the diagnosis is often made clinically at delivery**. The antenatal suspicion of placenta accreta can be based on history (e.g., prior cesarean delivery and an anterior placenta previa) or imaging findings (e.g., by ultrasound or MRI), but no method can provide 100% accuracy in antenatal diagnosis.

Epidemiology/Incidence

Traditionally 1/2500 deliveries, although evidence of increasing frequency (3/1000 or more), thought to be related to the increased rate of cesarean delivery, has been reported (20,21).

Etiology/Pathophysiology

Abnormal adherence of chorionic villi to myometrium, associated with total or partial lack of the decidua basalis layer.

Classification

Abnormally invasive placentas may be categorized according to the depth of their invasion (22).

- **Placenta accreta:** Chorionic villi are attached directly to, but do not invade, the myometrium.
- **Placenta increta:** Placental villi invade into the myometrium.
- **Placenta percreta:** Placental villi invade through the myometrium into the uterine serosa; adjacent organs (e.g., the bladder) may be involved, but this extension is not necessary for the diagnosis.

Risk Factors/Associations

Prior cesarean delivery; placenta **previa** (Table 25.2); **prior uterine surgery involving the cavity** (e.g., prior myomectomy; D&Es); **Asherman's syndrome; and submucous leiomyomata** (5,6,22).

Table 25.4 Ultrasonographic Signs Associated with Placenta Accreta

Loss of retroplacental hypoechoic zone
Retroplacental myometrial thickness <1 mm
Multiple placental lakes
Blood vessels or placental tissue bridging uterine-placental margin, myometrial-bladder interface, or crossing uterine serosa

Source: From Refs. 22,26–28.

Complications

Maternal: blood transfusion, infection, DIC, **injury to other organs, hysterectomy, venous thromboembolism, and death** (5,6)

  Perinatal: **PTB and SGA** (23)

Management

There are **no trials** to assess the comparative effectiveness of different interventions (e.g., planned hysterectomy vs. attempted placental extraction for suspected placenta accreta; and preoperative placement vs. no preoperative placement of catheters to allow the inflation for internal iliac balloons) in the management of placenta accreta.

Workup

No one imaging modality has been shown to be able to accurately diagnose placenta accreta with 100% sensitivity or specificity. Given the frequency of ultrasonographic imaging during pregnancy, this modality has been most frequently assessed with regard to attempting an antepartum diagnosis. Ultrasonographic findings that have been reported in association with placenta accreta are shown in Table 25.4 (22,24–28). However, even the combination of all these signs is not 100% sensitive for the diagnosis of accreta, and the sensitivity, specificity, positive and negative predictive values for individual signs and combinations of signs have varied substantially in published studies, but have been commonly reported to be about >80% (22). Further imaging modalities to evaluate the possibility of placenta accreta include **MRI** (especially T-2 images), which may be informative but also is not considered to be completely diagnostic (27,28). Cystoscopy can be considered as an adjunctive tool to assess for the possibility of placenta percreta in cases where bladder invasion is highly suspected due to radiologic studies or to signs such as frank blood in the urine.

Preparations and Plans for Delivery

If placenta accreta is suspected, appropriate counseling and preparations should be made (Table 25.5) (22). Labor and delivery staff (nursing and anesthesia) as well as blood bank should be notified regarding delivery plans, and the delivery should occur in a location that has the capacity to provide large volumes of blood transfusion and emergent surgery (including hysterectomy). It should be considered whether the particular circumstances would suggest the need for additional surgical services (e.g., gynecologic oncology, urology, general surgery, and vascular surgery). Another potential adjunctive strategy that may be considered is the cell saver. Although multiple other strategies (e.g., ureteral stents, preoperative placement of pelvic artery catheters for potential postpartum embolization and/or balloon inflation) have been utilized, these strategies have not been shown in either prospective trials or

Table 25.5   Sample of Possible Medical Record List Including Considerations for Preparations in Cases of Suspected Placenta Accreta

Patient name

....

Medical record number

....

Estimated due date

....

Preoperative diagnosis of accreta; specify: accreta/increta/percreta

....

Placenta location

....

Relevant ultrasound findings

....

Relevant MRI findings

....

Obstetric history

....

No. of prior cesarean deliveries

....

Other prior uterine surgery

....

Blood type

....

Antibody screen

....

Date and value of most recent hematocrit/hemoglobin

....

Date and value of most recent creatinine

....

Iron supplementation; if yes, specify type, dose yes/no

....

Epogen in this pregnancy; if yes, give dates yes/no

....

Transfusion in this pregnancy; if yes, give dates yes/no

....

Date of planned surgery

....

(Continued)

Table 25.5 Sample of Possible Medical Record List Including Considerations for Preparations in Cases of Suspected Placenta Accreta (*Continued*)

Planned surgery location and contact number

....

Gestational age at planned delivery

....

Antenatal glucocorticoids; if yes, give dates yes/no

....

Primary obstetrician; list name and contact number

....

Preoperative consultations and notifications; if yes, list name and contact number

....

Obstetric anesthesiologist/Anesthesiologist no/yes _____

....

Maternal-fetal medicine specialist no/yes _____

....

Neonatologist/Pediatrician no/yes _____

....

Gynecologic oncologist/Pelvic surgeon no/yes _____

....

Urologist no/yes _____

....

General surgeon no/yes _____

....

Vascular surgeon no/yes _____

....

Interventional radiologist no/yes _____

....

Blood bank specialist/Hematologist no/yes _____

....

Cell saver specialist no/yes _____

....

Intensive care specialist no/yes _____

....

Individual practices and circumstances will vary. This example does not indicate that certain evaluations or consultations are anticipated or expected in all cases.
Abbreviation: MRI, magnetic resonance imaging.
Source: From Ref. 22.

retrospective studies to have clear benefits that outweigh risks (22,29–31).

The patient (and family members if available) should be counseled regarding risks, complications, and management. The possible need for **hysterectomy** as a life-saving procedure should be **discussed** with the patient. Plans for future reproduction should be discussed and weighted against the risk of retaining the uterus. Other preventive or therapeutic interventions as described above and below should be discussed.

Delivery

Timing. The **optimal GA** for delivery of a woman with placenta accreta is **uncertain**. Many authors recommend a delivery prior to 39 weeks (e.g., 36–37 weeks) in order to avoid an unscheduled delivery and to optimize the capacity for preparation. Fetal maturity testing has been advocated by some and not by others, and one recent decision analysis suggests that it does not help to improve overall health outcomes. This analysis also suggests that in certain high-risk cases (e.g., intermittently bleeding placenta previa with suspected placenta percreta) even earlier delivery (e.g., **34–35 weeks**) may be acceptable (1,16,22,32). The final timing for delivery will need to be individualized, and take into account the risks of prematurity to the infant and the risks of major morbidity to the mother.

Technique. General intraoperative considerations include the possibility of a planned vertical skin incision. The uterine incision should be made, if possible, away from the placenta, the position of which can be determined by ultrasound beforehand. **Intraoperative ultrasound** with a sterile cover over the probe placed on the exposed uterus may be helpful if preoperative ultrasound is not informative.

The two most common approaches to management of suspected placenta accreta are hysterectomy without attempt at placental removal versus attempt at placental removal. While there are different potential approaches for managing placenta accreta after delivery of the baby by cesarean, many experts would recommend that **if there is proven placenta accreta** (e.g., placenta directly visualized in the serosa), **highly suspected** accreta by history and radiologic studies (e.g., multiple prior cesarean deliveries, placenta previa, and several ultrasonographic findings of placenta accreta), **or if the mother plans no more childbearing** (e.g., has requested tubal ligation), a reasonable course of action is to **avoid disturbing the implantation of the placenta and proceed with a hysterectomy** while the placenta remains attached (33). In these controlled situations, maternal morbidity of gravid hysterectomy may be decreased, but fertility is lost.

During hysterectomy, **the uterine serosa overlying the placenta should not be dissected**, including trying to avoid bladder dissection. The blood supply to the placenta is not just from the uterine arteries but also from many collateral vessels. Care should be given to dissection of this extensive blood supply by attempting uterine artery dissection laterally, and then continuing down without incising the placenta. **Total hysterectomy is generally necessary**, as subtotal hysterectomy may leave in part of the lower segment, where the placenta is abnormally attached and causing bleeding if a previa is present.

If the diagnosis is possible but not certain, and the patient desires to make attempts at avoiding hysterectomy despite having been counseled regarding risks, it is not unreasonable to wait for signs of placental separation, although abnormal adherence or significant hemorrhage should be ascertained and acted upon promptly. If spontaneous placental delivery fails, the operator must decide if either manual placental removal in pieces or hysterectomy is the next intervention, based on several factors, including the degree of invasiveness and amount of bleeding.

If only a small area of the placenta is adherent and a focal area of the placental bed is bleeding, sewing over this area with **sutures can be considered**, but usually these are in the very low uterine segment and cervix and often continue to bleed despite suturing or **uterotonics**. Some have suggested **ligation** of pelvic vessels (such as the internal iliac artery) in the setting of significant hemorrhage, although this may not be beneficial, given the many collateral vessels, and may incur risks as well. Pelvic **packing** has been used in some cases as a measure to temporarily lessen bleeding and allow attainment of hemodynamic stability. Hysterectomy may be necessary if uterine bleeding cannot be controlled, hopefully before massive blood loss and cardiovascular instability. When bleeding is from the lower part of the uterus in the setting of an accreta and placenta implanted low in the uterus (e.g., a previa), total hysterectomy is desirable as subtotal hysterectomy may not control bleeding. Gravid hysterectomy has been associated with an incidence of maternal mortality of up to 7%, with a 90% incidence of transfusion, 28% incidence of postoperative transfusion, and a 5% incidence of ureteral injuries or fistula formation (19,34).

In some cases, a woman who has not completed childbearing may strongly want to avoid hysterectomy. There are several case reports of expectant or medical management in the setting of placenta accreta. In these circumstances, the placenta is left in situ and the cord ligated close to its origin, either with no therapy or with an adjunctive therapy such as **methotrexate and/or arterial embolization**. Antibiotic prophylaxis has been suggested given the risk of infection, as have short-term uterotonics for postpartum hemorrhage prevention, but there are no trials of these interventions. Follow-up is also not based on good evidence, but serial ultrasounds (to monitor involution and decrease in placental vascularity) and quantitative human chorionic gonadotrophin (HCG) levels have been proposed. If HCG levels plateau, or uterine size or placental vascularity does not decrease by 72 hours, methotrexate has been given as 1 mg/kg on alternate days for a total of 4 to 6 doses, or according to HCG levels and ultrasonographic findings (35). Women on methotrexate should be monitored with liver function tests (LFTs), platelet counts, and creatinine levels. However, **this type of management has been associated with significant morbidity, including infection and delayed hemorrhage** (36–38), and should be considered only when the woman has been fully apprised of the risks and when no active uterine bleeding is present.

Postpartum
Consider reservation of intensive care unit bed for postpartum care.

VASA PREVIA
Diagnosis/Definition
Umbilical vessels, unprotected by the umbilical cord, that run through the membranes and over the internal os.

Symptoms
Asymptomatic unless membranes rupture, at which time vaginal bleeding may be noted.

Epidemiology/Incidence

Approximately 1/2500 deliveries (1).

Risk Factors/Associations

Placenta in the lower uterine segment, velamentous cord insertion, and succenturiate or bilobed placenta.

Complications

Perinatal morbidity (e.g., neonatal anemia) and mortality (up to 56%) due to acute hemorrhage (39).

Management

Principles

Timing of bleeding with antenatally diagnosed vasa previa is variable and impossible to predict. Rupture of membranes may result in rapid fetal exsanguination.

Workup

TVU with color Doppler is the standard for diagnosis of vasa previa. Women with risk factors that are judged to increase their risk of vasa previa (see above) should be screened with TVU for this condition. Not all vasa previa can be detected, even by adequate examinations and experienced operators using color Doppler. Women whose vasa previa has been diagnosed prenatally have been reported to have lower perinatal mortality than those with vasa previas that are undiagnosed (3% vs. 56%) (39).

The Apt test may be used to distinguish between fetal and maternal sources of vaginal bleeding, although this test may be of little use in many clinical situations with bleeding from a vasa previa, as bleeding can lead to rapid deterioration of the fetal status and require urgent delivery before an Apt test can be completed.

Therapy

Level 1 data to guide the management of antenatally diagnosed vasa previa are currently lacking. While some experts suggest that hospitalization at some time after viability may be reasonable, this strategy is unsupported by any adequately powered trials. **Women with vasa previa should be delivered by cesarean.** Timing of delivery is controversial, with suggestions for cesarean delivery anywhere between 34 and 37 weeks, although earlier when preterm premature rupture of membranes (PPROM), PTL, or significant bleeding occurs (1).

REFERENCES

1. Oyelese Y, Smulian JC. Placenta previa, placenta accreta, and vasa previa. Obstet Gynecol 2006; 107:927–941. [Review]
2. Dashe JS, McIntire DD, Ramus RM, et al. Persistence of placenta previa according to gestational age at ultrasound detection. Obstet Gynecol 2002; 99:692–697. [II-2]
3. Ananth CV, Smulian JC, Vintzileos AM. The association of placenta previa with history of cesarean delivery and abortion: a metaanalysis. Am J Obstet Gynecol 1997; 177:1071–1078. [Meta-analysis]
4. Gilliam M, Rosenberg D, Davis F. The likelihood of placenta previa with greater number of cesarean deliveries and higher parity. Obstet Gynecol 2002; 99:976–980. [II-2]
5. Silver RM, Landon MB, Rouse DJ, et al. Maternal morbidity associated with multiple repeat cesarean deliveries. Obstet Gynecol 2006; 107:1226–1232. [II-2]
6. Grobman WA, Lai Y, Landon MB, et al. Pregnancy outcomes for women with placenta previa in relation to the number of prior cesareans. Obstet Gynecol 2007; 110:1249–1255. [II-2]
7. Becker RH, Vonk R, Mende BC, et al. The relevance of placental location at 20-23 weeks gestational weeks for prediction of placenta previa at delivery: evaluation of 8650 cases. Ultrasound Obstet Gynecol 2001; 17:496–501. [II-2]
8. Vergani P, Ornaghi S, Pozzi I, et al. Placenta previa: distance to internal os and mode of delivery. Am J Obstet Gynecol 2009; 201:266.e1–266.e5. [II-2]
9. Bronsteen R, Valice R, Lee W, et al. Effect of a low-lying placenta on delivery outcome. Ultrasound Obstet Gynecol 2009; 33:204–208. [II-2]
10. Oppenheimer L, Simpson P, Holmes N, et al. Diagnosis of low-lying placenta: can migration in the third trimester predict outcome? Ultrasound Obstet Gynecol 2001; 18:100–102. [II-2]
11. Oyalese Y. Placenta previa and vasa previa: time to leave the Dark Ages. Ultrasound Obstet Gynecol 2001; 18:96–99. [Review]
12. Neilson JP. Interventions for suspected placenta praevia. Cochrane Database Syst Rev 2010. [Meta-analysis]
13. Dinsmoor MJ, Hogg BB. Autologous blood donation with placenta previa: is it feasible? Am J Perinatol 1995; 12:382–384. [II-2]
14. Sharma A, Suri V, Gupta I. Tocolytic therapy in conservative management of symptomatic placenta previa. Int J Gynaecol Obstet 2004; 84:109–113. [II-2]
15. Zlatnick MG, Little SE, Kohli P, et al. When should women with placenta previa be delivered? J Reprod Med 2010; 55:373–381. [Decision analysis]
16. Spong CY, Mercer BM, D'alton M, et al. Timing of indicated late-preterm and early-term birth. Obstet Gynecol 2011; 118(2pt 1):323–333. [Review]
17. Vergani P, Ornaghi S, Ghidini A. Placenta previa (reply). Am J Obstet Gynecol 2010; 202(6):e10; author reply e10. [Letter to the Editor]
18. Royal College of Obstetricians and Gynaecologists. Clinical Green-Top Guideline No. 27. Placenta praevia: diagnosis and management. London: RCOG Press, 2001. [Guideline]
19. Jacques SM, Qureshi F, Trent VS et al. Placenta accreta: mild cases diagnosed by placental examinationy. Int J Gynecol Pathol 1996; 15:28–33. [II-2]
20. Miller DA, Chollet JA, Goodwin TM. Clinical risk factors for placenta previa-placenta accreta. Am J Obstet Gynecol 1997; 177:210–214. [II-2]
21. Wu S, Kocherginsky M, Hibbard JU,. Abnormal placentation: twenty-year analysis. Am J Obstet Gynecol 2005; 192:1458–1461. [II-2]
22. Publications Committee, Society for Maternal-Fetal Medicine, Belford MA. Placenta accreta. Am J Obstet Gynecol 2010; 203:430–439. [Review]
23. Gielchinsky Y, Mankuta D, Rojansky N, et al. Perinatal outcome of pregnancies complicated by placenta accreta. Obstet Gynecol 2004; 104:527–530. [II-2]
24. Chou MM, Ho ES, Lee YH. Prenatal diagnosis of placenta previa accreta by transabdominal color Doppler ultrasound. Ultrasound Obstet Gynecol 2000; 15:28–35. [II-2]
25. Comstock CH, Love JJ Jr., Bronsteen RA, et al. Sonographic detection of placenta accreta in the second and third trimesters of pregnancy. Am J Obstet Gynecol 2004; 190:1135–1140. [II-2]
26. Twickler DM, Lucas MJ, Balis AB, et al. Color flow mapping for myometrial invasion in women with a prior cesarean delivery. J Matern Fetal Med 2000; 9:330–335. [II-2].
27. Palacios Jaraquemada JM, Bruno CH. Magnetic resonance imaging in 300 cases of placenta accreta: surgical correlation of new findings. Acta Obstet Gynecol Scand 2005; 84:716–724. [II-2]
28. Warshak CR, Eskander R, Hull AD, et al. Accuracy of ultrasonography and magnetic resonance imaging in the diagnosis of placenta accreta. Obstet Gynecol 2006; 108:573–581. [II-2]
29. Levine AB, Kuhlman K, Bonn J. Placenta accreta: comparison of cases managed with and without pelvic artery balloon catheters. J Mat Fetal Med 1999; 8:173–176. [II-2]
30. Greenberg JI, Suliman A, Iranpour P, et al. Prophylactic balloon occlusion of the internal iliac arteries to treat abnormal placentation a cautionary case. Am J Obstet Gynecol 2007; 197:470.e1–470.e4. [III]

31. Sewell MF, Rosenblum D, Ehrenberg H. Arterial embolus during common iliac balloon catheterization at cesarean hysterectomy. Obstet Gynecol 2006; 108:746–748. [III]

32. Robinson BK, Grobman WA. Effectiveness of timing strategies for delivery of patients with placenta previa and accreta. Obstet Gynecol 2010; 116(4):835–842. [Decision analysis]

33. American College of Obstetricians and Gynecologists. ACOG Committee Opinion No. 266: Placenta accreta. Int J Gynaecol Obstet 2002; 77(1):77–78. [Review]

34. O'Brien JM, et al. The management of placenta percreta: conservative and operative strategies. Am J Obstet Gynecol 1996; 175:1632–1638. [II-2]

35. Hundley AF, Lee-Parrotz A. Managing placenta accreta. OBG Management 2002; 14(8):18–33. [Review]

36. Alkazaleh F, Geary M, Kingdom J, et al. Elective non-removal of the placenta and prophylactic uterine artery embolization postpartum as a diagnostic imaging approach for the management of placenta percreta: a case report. J Obstet Gynaecol Can 2004; 26:743–746. [III]

37. Butt K, Gagnon A, Delisle MF. Failure of methotrexate and internal iliac balloon catheterization to manage placenta percreta. Obstet Gynecol 2002; 99:981–982. [III]

38. Teo SB, Kanagalingam D, Tan HK, et al. Massive postpartum hemorrhage after uterus-conserving surgery in placenta percreta: the danger of the partial placenta percreta. Br J Obstet Gynecol 2008; 115:789–792. [III]

39. Oyelese Y, Catanzarite V, Prefumo F, et al. Vasa previa: the impact of prenatal diagnosis on outcomes. Obstet Gynecol 2004; 103:937–942. [II-2]

26

Abruptio placentae

John F. Visintine

KEY POINTS
- Approximately 1% of all pregnancies are complicated by placental abruption.
- Nearly 50% of women with placental abruption have no identifiable risk factors. Risk factors include **abruption in a prior pregnancy**, maternal **hypertensive disorders, smoking, cocaine, polyhydramnios, multiple gestation, preterm and term premature rupture of membrane, chorioamnionitis, elevated maternal serum alpha-fetoprotein (MS-AFP), leiomyoma, subchorionic hematoma, vaginal bleeding <20 weeks, previous cesarean delivery**, and **abdominal trauma**. Association with thrombophilias has for the most part not been confirmed by prospective studies.
- **Complications** include **antepartum and postpartum hemorrhage, disseminated intravascular coagulopathy (DIC)**, and **acute renal failure**, as well as **perinatal mortality, preterm delivery, fetal hypoxia** and/or **exsanguination**, and **growth restriction**.
- The diagnosis of placental abruption is primarily a clinical one. **History, physical exam**, and **laboratory** and **ultrasonographic studies** guide management. Ultrasound is primarily useful in ruling out other causes of third-trimester bleeding.
- There are no trials to assess any intervention for prevention of abruption or its complications.
- Prompt **delivery** is indicated **if the pregnancy is near term**. However, if less than 34 weeks, expectant management for mild (grade 1) abruptions may allow time for glucocorticoid administration. Maternal or fetal compromise may necessitate delivery. A decision-to-delivery interval of 20 minutes or less is associated with a substantial reduction of neonatal morbidity and mortality in placental abruption with nonreassuring fetal heart testing.
- Mode of delivery is dependent primarily on the condition of the mother and fetus.
  - In most cases, for mild abruption (grade 1, no evidence of maternal or fetal compromise), **vaginal delivery** is indicated.
  - For moderate abruption (grade 2, evidence of fetal nonreassuring testing), rapid delivery typically by **cesarean** is indicated.
  - For severe abruption (grade 3, fetal demise, often with DIC), **vaginal delivery** is indicated.

DEFINITION
Placental abruption (also known as abruptio placentae) is defined as a premature separation of a normally implanted placenta.

SIGNS AND SYMPTOMS
Signs and symptoms are shown in Table 26.1 (1). About 10% of abruption present with only concealed (occult) bleeding. Occasionally the presenting sign is fetal death.

EPIDEMIOLOGY/INCIDENCE
- Approximately **0.5% to 1%** of all pregnancies are complicated by placental abruption (2). The incidence in the United States has recently increased, especially in the African-American population, the ethnic group at highest risk, in particular for severe (or grade 3) abruption (2).
- About 60% of abruptions occur preterm, and 50% occur prior to labor.
- The incidence of abruption is possibly highest at 24 to 26 weeks (up to 9 per 100 births) (3).

GENETICS
The association with thrombophilias has not been confirmed in prospective studies. See subsection "Risk Factors/Associations" and chapter 27 in *Maternal-Fetal Evidence Based Guidelines*.

ETIOLOGY/BASIC PATHOPHYSIOLOGY
The etiology is not completely understood but appears to occur as the result of two mechanisms: mechanical separation or as the end result of **defective deep placentation** (4). Placental separation occurring in association with **mechanical trauma or rapid decompression of a distended uterus** is believed to occur due to shearing forces resulting from a change in surface area of a relatively elastic uterine wall in relation to an inelastic placenta. Blunt trauma to the uterus resulting in abruption or rupture of membranes with rapid decompression of an over distended uterus resulting in abruption are examples of this mechanism.

Evidence in support of a defective deep placentation mechanism comes from placental bed biopsies from cases of placental abruption, which show an **absence of physiologic trophoblastic invasion, dilated vessels, and recent thrombosis of spiral arteries** (5). These changes are seen not only in abruption but also in preeclampsia, intrauterine growth restriction (IUGR), and preterm premature rupture of membranes (PPROM), suggesting that placental abruption represents one manifestation of a long-standing pregnancy disorder (4). Moreover, abnormalities in circulating angiogenic factors have been observed in women who subsequently developed placental abruption. In a nested case-control study, serum levels of the proangiogenic factor placental growth factor (PlGF) were lower, and levels of the potent inhibitor of PlGF, soluble fms-like tyrosine kinase 1 (sFlt-1), were increased (6).

Gross pathology findings associated with placental abruption include **adherent retroplacental clot with depression or disruption of the underlying placental tissue**. Microscopic changes associated with abruption resulting in perinatal mortality include **thrombosed arteries and necrosis of the deciduas basalis, and large recent infarcts and stromal fibrosis** in the terminal villi of the placental parenchyma (7).

Table 26.1 Clinical Findings in Women with Placental Abruption

Clinical findings	%
Vaginal bleeding	78
Fetal nonreassuring testing	60
Uterine-abdominal tenderness/Back pain	66
Uterine contractions (>5/10 min)	17
Uterine hypertonus	17

Source: From Ref. 1.

Severe cases of abruption can result in hemorrhagic infiltration between myometrial fibers that extends to the serosal surface giving the uterus a **dark purple discoloration, also known as Couvelaire uterus** in honor of the French obstetrician who first described this pathologic finding in the early 20th century (8).

CLASSIFICATION (TABLE 26.2)

A uniformly accepted classification system for placental abruption does not exist. The clinical classification system originally published by Page in 1954 has been used by subsequent authors as a means of grouping placental abruptions in those that can be potentially managed conservatively (grade 1) and those that require more aggressive management (grades 2 and 3) (9).

RISK FACTORS/ASSOCIATIONS (TABLE 26.3)

Nearly 50% of women with placental abruption have no identifiable risk factors (10).

- History of an **abruption in a prior pregnancy**: The risk of recurrence is about 5% to 17% (11). After two abruptions, the risk of recurrence is about 25%.
- Maternal **hypertensive disorders**: associated with up to almost 50% of grade 3 abruption cases. In particular, chronic hypertension (incidence 1.5–2.5%, OR 2.8), superimposed preeclampsia (about 3%), and severe preeclampsia (OR 4.1) are associated with placental abruption (12,13).
- **Abdominal trauma** is a recognized cause of placental abruption but is responsible for only 1% of cases (14). See also chapter 29 in *Maternal-Fetal Evidence Based Guidelines*.
- **Smoking:** 90% increase in abruption in women who smoke compared with controls. Smoking is responsible for 15% to 25% of episodes of abruption (12).
- **Cocaine:** 1.9% rate of abruption (15).
- **Previous cesarean** delivery is associated with an increased risk of abruption in subsequent pregnancies (OR 1.3) (16).
- **Polyhydramnios** has been associated with placental abruptions in patients >37 weeks' gestation (17).
- **Multiple gestation:** 1.2% risk of abruption in twins, 1.5% in triplets (18).
- **PPROM**: OR 3.5 (19). Evidence of old decidual hemorrhage can be found in nearly 40% of placentas from patients with PPROM (20).

Table 26.3 Risk Factors for Placental Abruption

Prior abruption
Chronic hypertension
Severe preeclampsia
Smoking
Cocaine
Chorioamnionitis
Unexplained elevated MS-AFP
(P)PROM
Subchorionic hemorrhage
Leiomyoma
Vaginal bleeding <20 wk
Polyhydramnios
Multiple gestation
Trauma
Prior cesarean delivery

- **Chorioamnionitis:** OR 9 (19). Neutrophil infiltration of the fetal membranes and cervix is seen in premature rupture of membranes (PROM), and chorioamnionitis is associated with placental abruption (21).
- **Leiomyomas** detected at second-trimester ultrasound are associated with a small increase in the risk of abruption (OR 2.1) (22).
- **Ultrasound-detected subchorionic hemorrhage** before 22 weeks of gestation results in an increased risk of placental abruption (OR 2.6) (23).
- **Vaginal bleeding <20 weeks** is associated with an increased risk of abruption (RR 1.6) (24).
- Unexplained **elevated MS-AFP** in the second trimester: OR 6 to 10 for placental abruption (25,26).
- **Inherited thrombophilias** have been associated with abruption in case-control studies (27,28). However **most prospective studies have shown no increased risk of abruption** (29–31). A retrospective cohort study comparing thromboprophylaxis with heparin for women with an inherited thrombophilia demonstrated no difference in rates of abruption or other adverse outcomes regardless of treatment (32). But **one large prospective cohort study did demonstrate an increased risk of abruption for women with the prothrombin gene mutation 20210A** (OR 12), but not for factor V Leiden mutation, MTHFR C677T or A1298C mutations, or the thrombomodulin gene mutation (33).
- **Advanced maternal age:** It is unclear if there is an association with abruption, as the data are conflicting (34,35).

COMPLICATIONS

- **Maternal**
  - **Antepartum hemorrhage** remains a leading cause of maternal mortality. For pregnancies ending in stillbirth, hemorrhage related to abruptio placenta is the leading cause of maternal mortality (36).
  - DIC was first reported to occur in association with placental abruption by De Lee in 1901 (37). The

Table 26.2 Classification of Placental Abruption

Grade[a]	Clinically evident bleeding	Uterine tenderness/Tetany	Maternal hypotension	Maternal coagulopathy	Fetal distress
0	No	No	No	No	No
1	Yes	Yes or No	No	No	No
2	Yes or No	Yes	No	Rare	Yes
3	Yes or No	Yes	Yes	Often	Death

[a]Grade 0: Diagnosis based on examination of the placenta.
Source: Adapted from Ref. 6.

development of DIC is thought to be due to a release of thromboplastins, as well as consumption of coagulation factors secondary to an enlarging hematoma. Nearly 30% of patients who present with a severe (grade 3) abruption develop DIC.

- **Acute renal failure** is a potential maternal complication associated with abruption. Fortunately the incidence of acute renal failure appears to be decreasing, possibly due to improved medical management.
- **Postpartum hemorrhage secondary to uterine atony** is associated with abruption, as is postpartum **anemia** and **infection**.

- Perinatal
  - **Perinatal mortality** (both fetal and neonatal deaths) varies from 4 to 12/1000 (38). This high perinatal mortality with abruption is attributable, in part, to its association with **preterm delivery**.
  - Of the excess perinatal deaths, about 55% can be attributed to prematurity. The other is associated with **fetal hypoxia** and/or **exsanguination**, or **growth restriction**.
  - Among abruption cases from a large multicenter case-control study, 60% were found to be small for gestational age; the authors concluded that this association was primarily due to preterm birth (39).
  - Of children with spastic quadriplegic or dyskinetic cerebral palsy, 5.7% are associated with placental abruption (40).

MANAGEMENT (FIG. 26.1)

Unfortunately there are **no trials to assess any intervention for management of abruption or its complications**. Recommendations for management are primarily based on expert opinion or at best retrospective case-control studies.

Prevention

Smoking cessation counseling, avoidance of cocaine, and, if possible, avoidance of other risk factors may prevent abruptio placentae.

Preconception Counseling

Women with risk factors should be counseled regarding the risk and complications of placental abruption, as well as interventions for its prevention.

Workup

- The **diagnosis** of abruption is usually made **clinically** and confirmed by gross or histologic examination of the placenta. However, placental abruptions may be occult. At times presenting as preterm labor, they may go undiagnosed until after delivery. Using the clinical criteria listed in Table 26.1, as well as ultrasound evaluation, the diagnosis of placental abruption is made prior to delivery in only 62% of cases (1), so that >30% of cases of abruption may go undiagnosed until examination of the placenta after delivery.
- **History and physical exam**, as well as appropriate **laboratory and ultrasonographic studies,** guide management. Routine assessment should be conducted including **vital signs, oxygenation status, and urine output. Laboratory** assessment may include a **hematocrit, platelet count, coagulation studies** [prothrombin time **(PT)**, partial

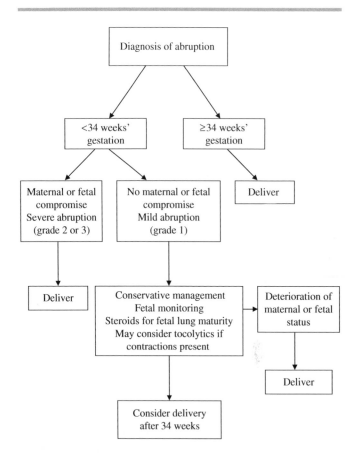

Figure 26.1 Management of abruption placentae.

thromboplastin time **(PTT), and fibrinogen], blood type and screen, or cross-match, serum creatinine, and a drug screen**. Other causes of third-trimester bleeding must be excluded. The **differential diagnosis** includes placenta previa, vasa previa, cervical lesions (for example, malignancy) and vaginal lesions.

- An **ultrasound examination** is useful primarily in the exclusion of placenta previa or vasa previa. The sensitivity and specificity of ultrasound in the diagnosis of placental abruption were 24% and 96%, respectively, in one study (41). So while ultrasound is very helpful in ruling out other causes of third-trimester bleeding, it lacks the sensitivity needed to reliably detect placental abruption (41). The echogenicity of the collection of blood of an abruption depends on the time the ultrasound was performed relative to the onset of symptoms (42). Acute hemorrhage is hyperechoic to isoechoic compared with the placenta. Resolving hematomas become hypoechoic within 1 week and sonolucent within 2 weeks.
- Computed tomography (CT) has been found to be a reliable method of detecting abruption in pregnant trauma patients. A retrospective study of pregnant trauma patients who were evaluated with CT found a high sensitivity (86%) and specificity (98%) in the detection of placental abruption (43).
- A **vaginal speculum examination** should be performed to rule out cervical or vaginal sources of bleeding.
- **Laboratory findings** (Table 26.4) associated with placental abruption such as prolonged PT, prolonged PTT,

Table 26.4 Laboratory Results in Women with Abruption

Test	% Positive
D-dimer	66
Thrombocytopenia (<100,000/mm^3)	13
Prolonged prothrombin time	20
Prolonged thromboplastin time	7
Hypofibrinogenemia	7

Source: Adapted from Ref. 29.

hypofibrinogenemia, and thrombocytopenia are markers of DIC or a consumptive coagulopathy and typically not present until later in the course of disease. D-dimer, a fibrin degradation product, has a sensitivity and specificity for placental abruption of 66% and 93%, respectively, in one study (44).

General Principles

Once the diagnosis of placental abruption has been made, attention should be focused on ensuring maternal and fetal well-being. **Maternal status** should be addressed with attention paid to signs or symptoms of hemorrhage, hypovolemic shock, and DIC. The frequency of repeated evaluations is dependent primarily on the acuity and severity of the abruption. Preparations should be made in anticipation of potential maternal complications. This should include **intravenous access; two large-bore peripheral lines** will allow for rapid fluid or blood component replacement. The **availability of blood** or blood components may be life saving; therefore, close cooperation with blood banking services is essential.

Fetal status is typically assessed with **continuous electronic fetal monitoring**, at least in the acute setting. For women with a chronic abruption, once clinically stable, intermittent monitoring may be a consideration.

Timing of Delivery (Fig. 26.1)

Near-Term Abruption: ≥34 Weeks
Prompt delivery is indicated if the pregnancy is near term (45–47). Fortunately rapid labor often ensues as a result of the abruption.

Preterm Abruption: <34 Weeks
Maternal or fetal compromise necessitates delivery. In selected patients with mild (grade 1) abruption, with no evidence of maternal or fetal compromise, expectant management may allow time for glucocorticoid administration and appears to be a safe option (1,9,47). Antepartum testing should be frequent, and at least initially continuous. There does not appear to be any increased morbidity or mortality associated with tocolytic use in selected patients (9,48). In this setting, magnesium sulfate is the tocolytic agent used most frequently in the United States due to its cardiovascular side effect profile, but its effectiveness has not been sufficiently studied (48).

Mode of Delivery

Deciding on the method of delivery is dependent primarily on the condition of the mother and fetus.

Mild Abruption (Grade 1): No Evidence of Maternal or Fetal Compromise
With close monitoring of the mother and fetus, **vaginal delivery** may be accomplished. In studies of women with mild (or grade 1) abruptions, those who delivered vaginally had a

similar perinatal mortality rates compared with those with a cesarean delivery (45).

Moderate Abruption (Grade 2): Evidence of Fetal Compromise
Rapid delivery: typically **cesarean delivery** is indicated. In a recent study of placental abruption complicated by fetal bradycardia, a decision-to-delivery interval of ≤20 minutes was associated with substantially reduced neonatal morbidity and mortality (49).

Severe Abruption (Grade 3): Fetal Death, Often with DIC
Vaginal delivery is preferred in this group as a cesarean delivery may exacerbate maternal hemorrhage. If present, DIC will typically resolve with evacuation of the uterus, with possible improvement in clotting parameters even prior to delivery (50,51).

Anesthesia

No specific suggestions. Anesthesia support is particularly important with DIC, hemorrhagic shock, and massive transfusion cases.

Postpartum

Attention should be paid to hemodynamic state and possible late hemorrhage from uterine atony after abruption.

REFERENCES

1. Hurd WW, Miodovnik M, Hertzberg V, et al. Selective management of abruptio placentae: a prospective study. Obstet Gynecol 1983; 61(4):467–473. [II-2]
2. Ananth CV, Oyelese Y, Yeo L, et al. Placental abruption in the United States, 1979 through 2001: temporal trends and potential determinants. Am J Obstet Gynecol 2005; 192(1):191–198. [Epidemiological review]
3. Oyelese Y, Ananth CV. Placental abruption. Obstet Gynecol 2006; 108:1005–1016. [Review]
4. Brosens I, Pinjenborg R, Vercruysse L, et al. The "Great Obstetrical Syndromes" are associated with disorders of deep placentation. Am J Obstet Gynecol 2011; 204(3):193–201. [Review]
5. Dommisse J, Tiltman AJ. Placental bed biopsies in placental abruption. Br J Obstet Gynaecol 1992; 99(8):651–654. [II-3]
6. Signore C, Mills JL, Qian C, et al. Circulating angiogenic factors and placental abruption. Obstet Gynecol 2006; 108: 338–344. [II-2]
7. Naeye RL, Harkness WL, Utts J. Abruptio placentae and perinatal death: a prospective study. Am J Obstet Gynecol 1977; 128(7):740–746. [II-3]
8. Couvelaire A. Classic pages in obstetrics and gynecology: Alexandre Couvelaire. Am J Obstet Gynecol 1973; 116(6):875. [II-3]
9. Sholl JS. Abruptio placentae: clinical management in nonacute cases. Am J Obstet Gynecol 1987; 156(1):40–51. [II-3]
10. Toivonen S, Heinonen S, Anttila M, et al. Reproductive risk factors, Doppler findings, and outcome of affected births in placental abruption: a population-based analysis. Am J Perinatol 2002; 19(8):451–460. [II-2]
11. Rasmussen S, Irgens LM, Dalaker K. The effect on the likelihood of further pregnancy of placental abruption and the rate of its recurrence. Br J Obstet Gynaecol 1997; 104(11):1292–1295. [II-2]
12. Ananth CV, Smulian JC, Vintzileos AM. Incidence of placental abruption in relation to cigarette smoking and hypertensive disorders during pregnancy: a meta-analysis of observational studies. Obstet Gynecol 1999; 93(4):622–628. [Meta-analysis: 13 studies, *n* = 1,358,083]
13. Sibai BM, Lindheimer M, Hauth J, et al. Risk factors for preeclampsia, abruptio placentae, and adverse neonatal outcomes

among women with chronic hypertension. N Engl J Med 1998; 339(10):667–671. [II-2; secondary analysis of RCT data]

14. Higgins SD, Garite TJ. Late abruptio placenta in trauma patients: implications for monitoring. Obstet Gynecol 1984; 63(3 suppl):10S–12S. [II-2]

15. Dombrowski MP, Wolfe HM, Welch RA, et al. Cocaine abuse is associated with abruptio placentae and decreased birth weight, but not shorter labor. Obstet Gynecol 1991; 77(1):139–141[II-2]

16. Getahun D, Oyelese Y, Salihu HM, et al. Previous cesarean delivery and risks of placenta previa and placental abruption. Obstet Gynecol 2006; 107:771–778. [II-2]

17. Sheiner E, Shoham-Vardi I, Hallak M, et al. Placental abruption in term pregnancies: clinical significance and obstetric risk factors. J Matern Fetal Neonatal Med 2003; 13(1):45–49. [II-2]

18. Salihu HM, Bekan B, Aliyu MH, et al. Perinatal mortality associated with abruptio placenta in singletons and multiples. Am J Obstet Gynecol 2005; 193(1):198–203. [II-2, $n = 1.6$ million births]

19. Ananth CV, Oyelese Y, Srinivas N, et al. Preterm premature rupture of membranes, intrauterine infection, and oligohydramnios: risk factors for placental abruption. Obstet Gynecol 2004; 104(1):71–77. [II-2, $n = 11,777$]

20. Salafia CM, Lopez-Zeno JA, Sherer DM, et al. Histologic evidence of old intrauterine bleeding is more frequent in prematurity. Am J Obstet Gynecol 1995; 173(4):1065–1070. [II-2]

21. Lockwood CJ, Toti P, Arcuri F, et al. Mechanisms of abruption-induced premature rupture of the fetal membranes: thrombin-enhanced interleukin-8 expression in term decidua. Am J Pathol 2005; 167(5):1443–1449. [II-2]

22. Stout MJ, Odibo AO, Graseck AS, et al. Leiomyomas at routine second-trimester ultrasound examination and adverse obstetric outcomes. Obstet Gynecol 2010; 116:1056–1063. [II-3]

23. Norman SM, Odibo A, Macones GA, et al. Ultrasound-detected subchorionic hemorrhage and the obstetric implications. Obstet Gynecol 2010; 116:311–315. [II-2]

24. Ananth CV, Oyelese Y, Prasad V, et al. Evidence of placental abruption as a chronic process: associations with vaginal bleeding early in pregnancy and placental lesions. Eur J Obstet Gynecol Reprod Biol 2006; 128:15–21. [II-2]

25. Katz VL, Chescheir NC, Cefalo RC. Unexplained elevations of maternal serum alpha-fetoprotein. Obstet Gynecol Surv 1990; 45 (11):719–726. [II-2]

26. Chandra S, Scott H, Dodds L, et al. Unexplained elevated maternal serum alpha-fetoprotein and/or human chorionic gonadotropin and the risk of adverse outcomes. Am J Obstet Gynecol 2003; 189(3):775–781. [II-2]

27. Kupferminc MJ, Eldor A, Steinman N, et al. Increased frequency of genetic thrombophilia in women with complications of pregnancy. N Engl J Med 1999; 340(1):9–13. [II-2]

28. Alfirevic Z, Roberts D, Martlew V. How strong is the association between maternal thrombophilia and adverse pregnancy outcome? A systematic review. Eur J Obstet Gynecol Reprod Biol 2002; 101(1):6–14. [II-2]

29. Dizon-Townson D, Miller C, Sibai B, et al. The relationship of the factor V Leiden mutation and pregnancy outcomes for mother and fetus. Obstet Gynecol 2005; 106(3):517–524. [II-2]

30. Kjellberg U, van Rooijen M, Bremme K, et al. Factor V Leiden mutation and pregnancy-related complications. Am J Obstet Gynecol 2010; 203:469e.1–469e8. [II-1]

31. Silver RM, Zhao Y, Spong CY, et al.; for the Eunie Kennedy Shriver National Institute of Child Health and Human Development for Maternal-Fetal Medicine Units (NICHD MFMU) Net-

work. Prothrombin gene G20210A mutation and obstetric complications. Obstet Gynecol 2010; 115(10):14–20. [II-1]

32. Warren JE, Simonsen SE, Brance W, et al. Thromboprophylaxis and pregnancy outcomes in asymptomatic women with inherited thrombophilias. Am J Obstet Gynecol 2009; 200:281.e1–281.e5. [II-2]

33. Said JM, Higgins JR, Moses EK, et al. Inherited thrombophilia polymorphisms and pregnancy outcomes in nulliparous women. Obstet Gynecol 2010; 115(1):5–13. [II-2]

34. Kramer MS, Usher RH, Pollack R, et al. Etiologic determinants of abruptio placentae. Obstet Gynecol 1997; 89(2):221–226. [II-2]

35. Yogev Y, Melamed N, Bardin R, et al. Pregnancy outcome at extremely advanced maternal age. Am J Obstet Gynecol 2010; 203:558e.1–558e7. [II-2]

36. Chang J, Elam-Evans LD, Berg CJ, et al. Pregnancy-related mortality surveillance—United States, 1991–1999. MMWR Surveill Summ 2003; 52(2):1–8. [Epidemiological review]

37. Page EW, King EB, Merrill JA. Abruptio placentae; dangers of delay in delivery. Obstet Gynecol 1954; 3(4):385–393. [II-2]

38. Ananth CV, Wilcox AJ. Placental abruption and perinatal mortality in the United States. Am J Epidemiol 2001; 153(4):332–337. [II-2, $n = 53,371$]

39. Nath CA, Ananth CV, DeMarco C, et al.; for the New Jersey-Placenta Abruption Study Investigators. Low birthweight in relation to placental abruption and maternal thrombophilia status. Am J Obstet Gynecol 2008; 198:293e.1–293e5. [II-2]

40. Gilbert W, Jacoby BN, Xing G, et al. Adverse obstetric events are associated with significant risk of cerebral palsy. Am J Obstet Gynecol 2010; 203:328e.1–328e5. [II-2]

41. Glantz C, Purnell L. Clinical utility of sonography in the diagnosis and treatment of placental abruption. J Ultrasound Med 2002; 21(8):837–840. [II-2]

42. Nyberg DA, Cyr DR, Mack LA, et al. Sonographic spectrum of placental abruption. AJR Am J Roentgenol 1987; 148(1):161–164. [II-2]

43. Manriquez M, Srivivas G, Bollepalli S, et al. Is computed tomography a reliable diagnostic modality in detecting placental injuries in the setting of acute trauma? Am J Obstet Gynecol 2010; 202:611e.1–611e5. [II-2]

44. Nolan TE, Smith RP, Devoe LD. A rapid test for abruptio placentae: evaluation of a D-dimer latex agglutination slide test. Am J Obstet Gynecol 1993; 169(2 pt 1):265–268; discussion 8–9. [II-2]

45. Knab DR. Abruptio placentae. An assessment of the time and method of delivery. Obstet Gynecol 1978; 52(5):625–629. [II-2]

46. Combs CA, Nyberg DA, Mack LA, et al. Expectant management after sonographic diagnosis of placental abruption. Am J Perinatol 1992; 9(3):170–174. [II-2]

47. Bond AL, Edersheim TG, Curry L, et al. Expectant management of abruptio placentae before 35 weeks gestation. Am J Perinatol 1989; 6(2):121–123. [II-2]

48. Towers CV, Pircon RA, Heppard M. Is tocolysis safe in the management of third-trimester bleeding? Am J Obstet Gynecol 1999; 180(6 pt 1):1572–1578. [II-2]

49. Kayani SI, Walkinshaw SA, Preston C. Pregnancy outcome in severe placental abruption. Br J Obstet Gynaecol 2003; 110(7):679–683. [II-2]

50. Twaalfhoven FC, van Roosmalen J, Briet E, et al. Conservative management of placental abruption complicated by severe clotting disorders. Eur J Obstet Gynecol Reprod Biol 1992; 46(1):25–30. [II-2]

51. Sher G, Statland BE. Abruptio placentae with coagulopathy: a rational basis for management. Clin Obstet Gynecol 1985; 28(1):15–23. [II-2]

27

Postpartum care[a]

Alison M. Stuebe

BREASTFEEDING
Key Points
- **In normal reproductive physiology, lactation follows pregnancy.** For the infant, use of artificial breast milk substitutes is associated with increased acute and chronic disease risk. For mothers, never or curtailed (e.g., short-term) breastfeeding is associated with increased risks of malignancy and metabolic disease.
- **All major medical organizations recommend 6 months of exclusive breastfeeding**, with continued breastfeeding through 1 year, and even beyond.
- **Infant demand drives maternal milk supply.** To ensure adequate milk production, encourage **frequent, on-demand feeding in response to infant cues, continuing until the infant is satisfied.**
- **Pre- and postnatal lay and/or professional support and evidence-based physician training** improve breastfeeding duration and exclusivity.
- **Maternity care practices affect breastfeeding initiation and duration.** Implementation of the United Nations International Children's Emergency Fund (UNICEF)/World Health Organization (WHO) Baby Friendly Hospital Initiative (BHI) improves breastfeeding duration, intensity, and infant health outcomes.
- Prenatal treatment of inverted nipples does not increase breastfeeding success.
- Distribution of formula company marketing materials and samples adversely affects breastfeeding outcomes. **Formula company materials should not be distributed in health care facilities.**
- At birth, early skin-to-skin contact increases breastfeeding duration. **Healthy infants should be placed skin-to-skin on the mother's chest** and remain there, undisturbed, until the first feeding is accomplished.
- Treatment for mastitis begins with frequent removal of milk, hydration, and analgesia. **Healthy term infants can continue to feed on the affected side.** Antibiotics are used if conservative management is ineffective or the patient is acutely ill.
- There is limited evidence that galactogogues increase milk production in placebo-controlled trials. Optimal breastfeeding education can increase milk supply among women with low production.
- Most medications are compatible with breastfeeding, or a safe alternative medication exists. **The physiology of the placenta differs from the breast**, and providers should not extrapolate drug safety information from pregnancy to lactation.

- Breastfeeding is contraindicated in the setting of an infant with classic galactosemia, active maternal use of illicit drugs, maternal medications that are contraindicated in breastfeeding, or maternal infection with T-cell lymphotropic virus type I or II (e.g., HTLV). Breastfeeding is **temporarily contraindicated** during perinatal maternal varicella infection, or from a breast with an active herpetic lesion. Recommendations for breastfeeding in the setting of maternal HIV or tuberculosis vary by region.

Definition
Breastfeeding is the physiologic form of infant nutrition. Breastfeeding is defined as the infant receiving any amount of human milk. **Exclusive breastfeeding** is defined as receiving human milk alone for nutrition. **Predominant breastfeeding** is defined as receiving human milk and nonformula supplements, and **mixed feeding** is defined as receiving both human milk and infant formula.

Breastfeeding Physiology
Secretory differentiation occurs during pregnancy, as placental hormones stimulate development of mammary alveoli. After birth, secretory activation occurs, as progesterone levels fall and milk production increases from 50 mL/day to approximately 500 mL/day in the first 2 to 3 days after birth. **Positive feedback via infant stimulation** of the breast causes secretion of prolactin from the anterior pituitary and oxytocin from the posterior pituitary. **Prolactin** stimulates continuous milk synthesis, whereas **oxytocin** stimulates intermittent milk secretion, when myoepithelial cells contract to transfer milk from the alveoli to the areola. If milk is not removed regularly, negative feedback downregulates prolactin receptors and reduces production (1). Frequent, on-demand feeding is essential to establish and maintain lactation.

Health Effects of Infant Feeding
Infants who are artificially fed face higher risks of infectious morbidity and chronic disease than infants who are breastfed. An Agency for Healthcare Research and Quality (AHRQ) meta-analysis of outcomes in developed countries found that **artificially fed infants** faced a 2.0-fold risk of **otitis media**, a 3.6-fold risk of **pneumonia**, and a 2.8-fold risk of **gastrointestinal infection** compared with infants who were exclusively breastfed (2). Artificial feeding is also associated with a 1.6- (2) to 2.1-fold (3) risk of **sudden infant death syndrome** (SIDS), a 1.1- (4) to 1.3-fold (5) risk of **child obesity**, and a 1.6-fold risk of **type 2 diabetes** (2,6,7) compared with breastfeeding. Artificial or mixed feeding is also associated with higher risks of **asthma**, OR 1.4 (2), and **atopic dermatitis**, OR 1.7 (8), compared with exclusive breastfeeding. Among preterm infants, artificial feeding is associated with a 5% absolute increased

---

[a]Includes breastfeeding, contraception, postpartum endometritis, and postpartum wound infection.

risk of **necrotizing enterocolitis** compared with being fed mother's milk (2).

For mothers, artificial feeding is similarly associated with increased health risks. Compared with women who have breastfed, parous women who have never breastfed or weaned early face **higher rates of breast cancer** (9,10), **ovarian cancer** (11), **retained gestational weight gain** (12), **type 2 diabetes** (13–16), **hyperlipidemia** (17), **metabolic syndrome (18,19), hypertension (15,20), and myocardial infarction (15,21).**

Based on these data, the U.S. Preventative Health Services Task Force (USPSTF) (22) concluded that **there is convincing evidence that breastfeeding provides substantial health benefits for children and adequate evidence that breastfeeding provides moderate health benefits for women.**

Optimal Duration of Exclusive Breastfeeding

Six months of exclusive breastfeeding, compared with 3 to 4 months of exclusive breastfeeding with mixed feeding through 6 months, reduces infant risk of gastrointestinal and respiratory tract infections without any adverse effect on infant growth (23). For mothers, longer exclusive breastfeeding was associated with delayed resumption of menses and, in one study, with greater maternal weight loss (24).

Infant Feeding Recommendations

All major medical organizations (25–29) recommend exclusive breastfeeding for the first 6 months of life. The WHO recommends continued breastfeeding up to 2 years of age or beyond (29). The American Academy of Pediatrics (AAP) recommends continued breastfeeding for at least the first year of life and beyond for as long as mutually desired by mother and child (26).

Promoting Breastfeeding

Antenatal interventions can increase breastfeeding initiation and duration (Table 27.1) (30). Breastfeeding education improves initiation rates among low-income U.S. populations. In subgroup analyses, one-on-one, needs-based, informal education sessions were more effective (RR 2.40, 95% CI 1.57–3.67) than generic, formal antenatal sessions (RR 1.26, 95% CI 1.00–1.60) (31). Both lay and professional supports for mothers after birth improve breastfeeding duration and exclusivity (32). A USPSTF review similarly found that interventions to promote and support breastfeeding increase initiation, duration, and exclusivity of breastfeeding (grade B). Interventions that include both prenatal and postnatal components may be most effective (33).

Training of Providers

Breastfeeding education for health care providers is inconsistent (34,35). A meta-analysis (32) found that training breastfeeding support personnel using the WHO/UNICEF breastfeeding training course (36) increases duration of exclusive breastfeeding. In a cluster-randomized trial, implementation of a breastfeeding training curriculum for residents improved provider knowledge, practice patterns, and confidence, and increased exclusive breastfeeding rates at 6 months (OR 4.1) compared with control sites (37). **Health care providers who work with mother and infants should receive comprehensive breastfeeding training.**

The Baby Friendly Initiative

Maternity care affects breastfeeding outcomes. The Baby Friendly Initiative (BFI) is WHO-developed set of maternity

Table 27.1 Successful Breastfeeding Recommendations

Offer additional breastfeeding support to women who have had a narcotic/general anesthetic, a caesarean, or delayed contact with their baby.

Ensure breast pumps are available for women who have been separated from their babies, and give instruction on how to use them.

Encourage unrestricted breastfeeding frequency and duration.

Reassure women about breast milk supply and help them gain confidence.

Advise women that babies will stop feeding when satisfied.

Advise women of the signs that a baby is successfully feeding:
- Swallowing is audible and visible.
- There is a sustained rhythmic suck.
- The arms and hands are relaxed.
- The mouth is moist.
- Regular soaked/heavy nappies.

Reassure women that they may feel the following:
- Brief discomfort at the start of feeds in the first few days; this is not uncommon but should not persist.
- Softening of their breast during the feed.
- No compression of the nipple at the end of the feed.
- Relaxed and sleepy.

Attachment and positioning

Advise women of the following signs of good attachment and positioning:
- The baby's mouth is wide open.
- There is less areola visible underneath the chin than above the nipple.
- The baby's chin is touching the breast, the lower lip is rolled down, and the nose is free.
- There is no pain.

If the baby is not attaching effectively, advise teasing the baby's lips with the nipple to open the mouth.

Source: From Ref. 30.

Table 27.2 The Ten Steps to Successful Breastfeeding

Every facility providing maternity services and care for newborn infants should

1. Have a written breastfeeding policy that is routinely communicated to all health care staff.
2. Train all health care staff in skills necessary to implement this policy.
3. Inform all pregnant women about the benefits and management of breastfeeding.
4. Help mothers initiate breastfeeding within a half-hour of birth.
5. Show mothers how to breastfeed, and how to maintain lactation even if they should be separated from their infants.
6. Give newborn infants no food or drink other than breast milk unless medically indicated.
7. Practice rooming in—allow mothers and infants to remain together—24 hr a day.
8. Encourage breastfeeding on demand.
9. Give no artificial teats or pacifiers (also called dummies or soothers) to breastfeeding infants.
10. Foster the establishment of breastfeeding support groups and refer mothers to them on discharge from the hospital or clinic.

Source: From Ref. 38.

care recommendations designed to increase initiation and duration of breastfeeding. The BFI requires maternity centers to implement The Ten Steps to Successful Breastfeeding (Table 27.2) (38). Each country is responsible for establishing processes and procedures for maternity center designation as baby friendly (38). In a cluster-randomized trial in Belarus, BFI implementation improved breastfeeding exclusivity at 3 months (43.3% vs. 6.4%, $p < 0.001$) and 6 months (7.9% vs. 0.6%, $p = 0.01$) and increased any breastfeeding rates at 12 months (19.7% vs. 11.4%). Infants born in intervention hospitals had lower rates of gastrointestinal illness and atopic eczema in the first year of life (39). Observational studies in the United States have found a dose-response association between implementation of BFI steps and maternal achievement of breastfeeding goals (40,41).

The National Institute for Health and Clinical Excellence (NICE) postnatal care guideline recommends that all health care providers should implement a structured program that encourages breastfeeding, using the BFI as a minimum standard (30) (Table 27.1).

Breastfeeding in Clinical Care
Antenatal Breast Exam
Clinical guidelines recommend evaluation of breast anatomy as part of prenatal care (27,42). However, there are no randomized controlled trials (RCTs) regarding the effects of an antenatal breast exam on breastfeeding outcomes or maternal satisfaction (43). **There is no evidence that antenatal manipulation for inverted nipples improves breastfeeding outcomes** (44,45).

Avoiding Commercial Infant Feeding Materials
In randomized trials, provision of formula company materials and gift packs during prenatal care (46) or during the maternity hospitalization (47–49) reduces exclusive breastfeeding. **Formula company marketing materials should not be distributed in the health care setting.**

Skin-to-Skin Contact at Birth
Early skin-to-skin contact improves breastfeeding outcomes. Skin-to-skin contact is defined as placing the naked infant prone on the mother's bare chest, with the infant's back covered with a warm blanket, ideally beginning immediately after birth. In a Cochrane meta-analysis, early skin-to-skin contact increased breastfeeding at 1 to 4 months postbirth (OR 1.82), and increased duration of total breastfeeding by about 6 weeks. Based on these data, the NICE (50), AAP (26), and American College of Obstetricians and Gynecologists (ACOG) (27) recommend that **all healthy infants should be placed skin-to-skin at birth.** Infants should remain with their mothers for at least 1 hour, and providers should encourage mothers to recognize when the infant is ready to feed and offer help if needed (38). Routine procedures, such as weighing, bathing, and vitamin K and eye prophylaxis, should be avoided during the first hour, or performed on the mother's chest.

Anticipatory Guidance to Support Normal Physiology
Human milk production is driven by infant demand. Therefore, **frequent feeding, on demand in response to infant feeding cues, continuing until the infant is satisfied, is the cornerstone of breastfeeding success** (51). NICE clinical guidelines have outlined anticipatory guidance for successful breastfeeding (Table 27.1).

Management of Breastfeeding Complications
Engorgement
Breast engorgement typically occurs between 2 and 5 days postpartum. A meta-analysis found insufficient evidence to support any single treatment strategy for engorgement (52).

Cold packs and cabbage leaves may be helpful, and acupuncture was associated with some improvement in symptoms. NICE guidelines recommend **breast massage, continued breastfeeding, and analgesia** for symptom relief (30).

Mastitis
Mastitis is defined as acute inflammation of connective tissue within the breast, which may or may not be accompanied by infection (53). Interventions to prevent mastitis have not proven effective (54). A Cochrane meta-analysis ($N = 125$) concluded that there is insufficient evidence to support treatment with antibiotics. A recent RCT found that lactobacilli strains isolated from breast milk were superior to antibiotics for treatment of mastitis (55).

Clinical guidelines emphasize **effective milk removal, hydration, and analgesia** as key elements of clinical management of mastitis. Healthy term infants may continue to breastfeed on the affected breast. If symptoms do not improve with conservative management or the woman is acutely ill, antibiotics are recommended. Penicillinase-resistant penicillins are preferred (56).

Breastfeeding and Maternal Medications
Most medications are compatible with breastfeeding, or a safe alternative medication exists. The physiology of the placenta differs from that of the maternal breast and infant gut, so the provider should not assume that a drug's pregnancy safety profile applies to breastfeeding. Many drug databases utilized by commercial pharmacies do not contain accurate information on drug safety in lactation (57). The National Library of Medicine's LactMed database (http://lactmed.nlm.nih.gov/) provides a comprehensive set of monographs on medication safety in lactation.

Milk Expression
If mothers and infants are separated, milk expression is necessary to maintain supply and provide milk to the infant. Evidence suggests that **early initiation of milk expression, simultaneous pumping of both breasts, breast massage, and relaxation techniques** improve milk production among neonatal intensive care unit (NICU) mothers (58–62).

Galactogogues
There is **limited evidence to support pharmacotherapy for low milk supply** (63,64). Two small randomized, placebo-controlled, blinded studies have found that domperidone increases milk supply among mothers of preterm infants (65,66). Domperidone is not approved by the U.S. Food and Drug Administration for any indication. Routine use of metoclopramide in the early postpartum period does not improve milk production (67,68). In two studies among women with low milk supply who received education on optimal breastfeeding (69,70), metoclopramide provided no additional benefit compared with placebo.

Maternal Diet During Lactation
In two small trials, maternal dietary restrictions during lactation did not reduce the incidence of atopic eczema or the severity of existing disease (71). Maternal supplementation with long-chain polyunsaturated fatty acids (LCPUFA) during lactation does not improve infant neurodevelopmental outcomes. In two studies, LCPUFA supplementation increased infant head circumference (72). **There is insufficient evidence to recommend LCPUFA supplementation during breastfeeding.**

Contraindications

Breastfeeding is contraindicated in the setting of the following:

- Infant with classic galactosemia (galactose-1-phosphate uridyltransferase deficiency)
- Maternal medications:
  - Mothers with current, active illicit drug use, unless approved by the pediatric provider
  - Mothers requiring medications that are contraindicated in breastfeeding
- Maternal infectious disease:
  - Mothers with varicella onset within 5 days before until 48 hours after delivery, until she is no longer infectious
  - Mothers with active herpetic lesions on the breast(s). Mothers can continue to breastfeed on the unaffected breast.
  - Mothers who are human T-cell lymphotropic virus type I or II positive (e.g., HTLV)

Tuberculosis

The AAP lists active, untreated tuberculosis as a contraindication to breastfeeding. According to AAP guidelines, the infant may continue to receive expressed milk while the mother is treated, but mother and infant should be separated until the mother has three negative sputum cultures (73). The WHO recommends continued breastfeeding in the setting of maternal tuberculosis. The infant should be treated with 6 months of isoniazid preventive therapy, followed by immunization with BCG (74).

HIV

Artificial infant feeding is efficacious in preventing maternal-child transmission of HIV, but RCTs in regions of the world where access to clean water is limited demonstrate similar mortality and malnutrition among breastfed and artificially fed infants. If infants are breastfed, early exclusive breastfeeding and extended antiretroviral prophylaxis reduce the risk of HIV transmission (75).

Women with HIV in the United States are advised not to breastfeed because of the risk of maternal-infant transmission and the availability of safe artificial feeding (26).

The WHO recommends that national or subnational health authorities determine recommendations regarding infant feeding for HIV-positive mothers, balancing HIV prevention with protection from other causes of child mortality (76). In countries where breastfeeding is recommended, antiretroviral prophylaxis for mothers and infants reduces HIV transmission. Exclusive breastfeeding is recommended for the first 6 months, continuing through 1 year. When mothers decide to stop breastfeeding, they are advised to wean gradually, over 1 month, and mothers or infants receiving antiretroviral prophylaxis should continue for 1 week after breastfeeding is fully stopped.

CONTRACEPTION
Key Points

- **Postpartum educational interventions can increase contraceptive use and delay repeat pregnancy.**
- **Intrauterine device (IUD) placement <48 hours postpartum** is not associated with infectious morbidity, but expulsion rates are higher than with placement >4 weeks. Since many women do not show up at postpartum follow-up, overall **IUD use is highest when inserted in the immediate postpartum period.**
- Postpartum tubal ligation (PPTL) is highly effective. However, risk of regret is higher for PPTL than for interval TL.
- Lactation amenorrhea is an effective but not perfect method of contraception, until the infant is 6 months old, begins complementary feeding, or the mother's menses resume.
- Barrier methods are preferred during lactation compared with hormonal contraception because of theoretical effects of hormonal methods on milk supply and hormone exposure for the infant.

Background

Two-thirds of women have unmet contraceptive needs after childbirth (77). Educational interventions during the postpartum hospitalization increase contraceptive use, compared with no intervention. Home visit programs reduce repeat pregnancies among teenagers (78).

Contraceptive Guidelines

A detailed review of contraception is behind the scope of this book. The WHO has published detailed guidelines regarding timing of initiation of postpartum contraception and other relative and absolute contraindications. Postpartum recommendations for healthy women are summarized in Tables 27.3 and 27.4. The full guidelines are available online (79).

Table 27.3 WHO Guidelines for Postpartum Contraception: Hormonal Contraception

	Progestin-only methods[a]	Combined hormonal contraceptives[b]
Breastfeeding		
<6 weeks postpartum	3	4
>6 weeks to <6 months postpartum (primarily breastfeeding)	1	3
>6 months postpartum	1	2
Not breastfeeding		
<21 days postpartum	1	(i) Without other risk factors for VTE: 3
		(ii) With other risk factors for VTE: 3/4
>21 days to 42 days	1	(i) Without other risk factors for VTE: 2
		(ii) With other risk factors for VTE: 2/3
>42 days	1	1

1: A condition for which there is no restriction for the use of the contraceptive method.
2: A condition where the advantages of using the method generally outweigh the theoretical or proven risks.
3: A condition where the theoretical or proven risks usually outweigh the advantages of using the method.
4: A condition that represents an unacceptable health risk if the contraceptive method is used.
[a]Progestogen-only pills, levonorgestrel and etonogestrel implants, depot medroxyprogesterone acetate, and norethisterone enantate.
[b]Combined oral contraceptives, combined contraceptive patch, combined contraceptive vaginal ring, and combined injectable contraceptives.
Abbreviation: VTE, venous thromboembolism.

Table 27.4 WHO Guidelines for Intrauterine Devices

	Breastfeeding	Not breastfeeding
Levonorgestrel-releasing (LNG) IUD, <48 hr postpartum	3	1
Copper-bearing (Cu) IUD, <48 hr postpartum	1	1
LNG-IUD or Cu-IUD >48 hr to <4 wk	3	3
>4 wk	1	1
Puerperal sepsis	4	4

1: A condition for which there is no restriction for the use of the contraceptive method.

2: A condition where the advantages of using the method generally outweigh the theoretical or proven risks.

3: A condition where the theoretical or proven risks usually outweigh the advantages of using the method.

4: A condition that represents an unacceptable health risk if the contraceptive method is used.

Intrauterine Devices

IUDs are highly effective methods of contraception. Immediate postpartum placement allows women to access contraception during the maternity hospitalization but is associated with an increased risk of expulsion compared with delayed insertion (80). In an RCT of postplacental versus delayed insertion, women randomized to postplacental insertion were more likely to have a device inserted (98% vs. 90.2%, $p = 0.20$). There were no differences between groups in IUD use at 6 months postpartum (84.3% vs. 76.5%). However, among women who were ineligible for the study and were advised to follow-up for IUD placement as part of routine postpartum care, only 26.8% were using an IUD at 6 months postpartum (81). These results suggest that **women undergoing postplacental placement are more likely to use an IUD than those advised to follow-up for placement during routine postpartum care.**

Postpartum Sterilization

Sterilization is the most commonly used form of contraception worldwide. Postpartum partial salpingectomy has a failure rate of 7.5/1000, which compares favorably with other sterilization methods (82). In a small RCT, operative times were shorter with postpartum Filshie clip placement compared with the Pomeroy technique, but failure rates were not evaluated (83). Maternal age <30 increases risk of regret and request for tubal reversal (84). Risk of regret is higher among women undergoing PPTL compared with interval TL. Other risk factors include ligation at the time of C-section, abrupt decision to undergo PPTL, and sterilization performed for obstetrical indications (85).

In a cohort study of women planning postpartum sterilization, one-third did not receive the procedure prior to hospital discharge. Of these women, 47% were pregnant within 1 year, compared with 22% of women who had not planned a postpartum sterilization (86). Women who desire but do not undergo postpartum sterilization are at high risk for unplanned pregnancy.

Contraception During Breastfeeding

Breastfeeding reduces fertility and prolongs amenorrhea after childbirth. In the first 6 months after birth, women who are fully breastfeeding and amenorrheic are unlikely to become pregnant (87,88). To maintain effective protection against pregnancy, another method of contraception must be used as soon as menstruation resumes, the frequency or duration of breastfeeds is reduced, bottle feeds are introduced, or the baby reaches 6 months of age (79).

Barrier methods are the preferred method of contraception during breastfeeding (89). The fall in progesterone after birth triggers lactogenesis, raising theoretical concerns that progesterone-containing contraceptives may interfere with lactation, particularly in the early postpartum period. Existing RCTs of combined versus progesterone-only contraceptives during lactation are insufficient to determine effects on milk production and quality (90). WHO recommendations regarding hormonal contraception during breastfeeding are listed in Table 27.3.

Insertion of the levonorgestrel intrauterine device (LNG-IUD) in breastfeeding women is not recommended in the first 4 weeks postpartum (79). In a small RCT (91), immediate postpartum placement of an LNG-IUD decreased breastfeeding rates at 3 and 6 months postpartum compared with insertion at 6 to 8 weeks. A study comparing insertion at 6 to 8 weeks of the LNG-IUD with the Cu T380A IUD found no differences in breastfeeding outcomes, infant growth, or development (92). WHO recommendations regarding timing of IUD insertion are listed in Table 27.4.

POSTPARTUM ENDOMETRITIS
Key Points

- The **diagnosis** of postpartum endometritis is based on the presence of ≥ 2 of the following: fever >100.3°F, at least twice, ≥ 6 hours apart; fundal tenderness; tachycardia (heart rate >100 beats/min); and foul-smelling lochia. Endometrial cultures are usually not necessary.
- As postpartum endometritis is most often associated with cesarean delivery, **prevention** is effective by **administration of preoperative antibiotics** (either ampicillin or first-generation cephalosporin for just one dose), **spontaneous placental removal, nonclosure of both visceral and parietal peritoneum,** and **suture closure of the subcutaneous tissue when thickness is ≥ 2 cm.**
- **Gentamicin** and **clindamycin** intravenously, preferably **once-daily dosing,** are most effective for the **treatment** of postpartum endometritis.
- Once uncomplicated endometritis has clinically improved with intravenous therapy (usually 24–48 hours afebrile), oral therapy is not needed.

Diagnosis/Definition

The diagnosis is based on clinical criteria. Table 27.5 describes criteria for diagnosis.

Symptoms/Signs

Those described in Table 27.5, plus abdominal pain, malaise, and elevated white blood cell count.

Table 27.5 Diagnosis of Postpartum Endometritis (≥ 2 of the Following)

- Fever >100.3°F, at least twice, ≥ 6 hr apart
- Fundal tenderness
- Tachycardia (heart rate >100 beats/min)
- Foul-smelling lochia

Table 27.6 Microorganisms More Frequently Associated with Postpartum Endometritis

Facultative gram positive: 51%
Group B streptococci
Enterococci
Staphylococcus epidermidis
Lactobacillus
Diphtheroids
S. aureus
Others

Facultative gram negative: 28%
Gardnerella vaginalis
Escherichia coli
Enterobacter spp.
Proteus mirabilis
Others

Anaerobic: 49%
Bacteroides bibius
Peptococcus asaccharolyticus
Bacteroides spp.
Peptostreptococcus spp.
Bacteroides fragilis
Veillonella spp.
Others

Source: From Ref. 95.

Table 27.7 Risk Factors for Postoperative Endometritis

Cesarean delivery (directly correlated to its length)
Labor (directly correlated to its length)
Rupture of membranes (directly correlated to its length)
Socioeconomic status
Number of vaginal examinations
Internal fetal monitoring
Manual extraction of placenta
Episiotomy
Forceps delivery
Young age (younger than 17 years old) (98)
Obesity (BMI > 30) (99)
Operative time
Blood loss (96)
Bacterial vaginosis (102)
GBS colonization (100,101)
Diabetes (94)

Source: From Ref. 97.
Abbreviations: BMI, body mass index; GBS, group B streptococcus.

Epidemiology/Incidence

Endometritis complicates about 1% of vaginal and about 5% to 27% of cesarean deliveries (93). The lower incidence in certain cesarean delivery populations is due to infection precautions at delivery and antibiotic prophylaxis (see chap. 13). In specific populations such as diabetic patients the risk might be higher (94).

Etiology/Basic Pathophysiology

Endometritis is an inflammatory process that involves both the endometrium and decidual tissue, secondary to infection. Other factors different than colonization itself play a role in pathogenesis, since 94% of postpartum patients have positive cultures from endometrial samples, but only a small fraction actually develop the infection. Although the bacteria usually ascend from the vagina and colonize the innermost layer of the endometrial cavity at first, if this is not treated, infection might spread locally and through the bloodstream giving rise to complications that can be life threatening. The use of prophylactic antibiotics has impacted the appearance of such complication dramatically, but not eliminated the risk.

Microbiology

The bacteria are usually gram-positive cocci, gram-negative rods, or anaerobes that might be present in normal female genital tract and reach the endometrium ascending from the vagina (Table 27.6) (95). The infection is usually polymicrobial, as in the vast majority of cases more than one bacterium is found. The presence of these microorganisms and the colonization of the decidua generate multiple microabscesses that trigger the invasion of inflammatory cells. These cells release chemical mediators responsible for the different manifestations of endometritis. The presence of two microorganisms in the vagina as assessed by smears or cultures has been associated to the subsequent development of postpartum endometritis.

Risk Factors/Associations

"Classic" risk factors for postpartum endometriosis are shown in Table 27.7 (94,96–102). The longer is the labor, the longest is rupture of membranes, the higher is the number of vaginal exams, or the longer is cesarean delivery; the higher is the risk of infection. HIV-positive women with CD-4 count ≤500 cells/μL have similar risks of postpartum endometritis and wound infection as HIV-negative women if they receive prophylactic antibiotics (103,104).

Complications

Sepsis is a rare complication.

Management

Workup
Endometrial cultures are usually not necessary, as the antibiotic regimens used are usually so successful that whichever microorganism is identified it is usually susceptible (105). Although not a current standard of care (105), some authors recommend the use of endometrial cultures at the time of diagnosis, advocating the need for specific antibiotic coverage (106), but no trials are available to assess their efficacy. Elevation of temperature may be the only sign found in patients with endometritis. Since one single episode of temperature ≥100.4°F (38°C) is commonly present in postpartum patients, and most of them will not develop any infection, **it is recommended that two episodes of temperature elevation are identified in order to consider the diagnosis** (107). Physical exam is the cornerstone for adequate assessment (108). Although laboratory studies are not criteria for diagnosis, an increased neutrophil count, as well as elevated proportion of bands, may suggest the presence of an infectious disease (109). However, **urine analysis and culture** should be obtained, and **blood cultures** at the time of temperature spikes should be taken, particularly in immunocompromised patients or in those at increased risk for bacterial endocarditis. In selected patients, chest X rays can be taken. Differential diagnosis includes at least atelectasis, pneumonia, viral syndrome, engorgement, mastitis, pyelonephritis, and appendicitis.

Prevention
Prophylactic antibiotics (either ampicillin or first-generation cephalosporin for just one dose about 30 minutes before skin incision), spontaneous placental removal, nonclosure of

both visceral and parietal peritoneum, and suture closure of the subcutaneous tissue when thickness is ≥2 cm should routinely be performed in cesarean delivery (see chap. 13). Each of these interventions decreases the incidence of postpartum endometritis and/or fever. In particular, both ampicillin and first-generation cephalosporins have similar efficacy in reducing postoperative endometritis from about 18% to 12% (a 61% decrease), with no added benefit found in using more broad-spectrum agents (110,111). In urban, indigenous, mainly Afro-American women with incidence of postpartum endometritis over 24% despite first-generation cephalosporin prophylaxis, the addition of doxycycline 100 mg together with the cephalosporin and azithromycin 1 g orally 6 to 12 hours postoperatively can decrease the incidence of endometritis to 17%, possibly by targeting *Ureaplasma urealyticum* (112). The number of vaginal examinations, nulliparity, early gestational age, and cefazolin use were predictors of prophylaxis failure in one study (113). Cleansing of the vagina with povidone-iodine prior to cesarean delivery has been associated with a reduction in the risk of postpartum endometritis, particularly among women with ruptured membranes (114) (see chap. 13).

Therapy
Since more than one microorganism is usually involved, a combination of antibiotics is used to assure proper coverage and prevent resistance. Parenteral, broad-spectrum antibiotics should be initiated and continued until patient is afebrile. The combination of **gentamicin and clindamycin is appropriate** for the treatment of endometritis (13) Compared with other regimens, clindamycin and an aminoglycoside are associated with 44% less treatment failures (115). Regimens with **activity against penicillin-resistant anaerobic bacteria** are better than those without, as failures of those regimens with poor activity against penicillin-resistant anaerobic bacteria are 94% more likely. Compared with other regimens, either clindamycin/gentamicin or piperacillin/tazobactam, a regimen with aminoglycoside and penicillin or ampicillin is associated with about twice more treatment failures. There was no evidence of difference in incidence of allergic reactions. Cephalosporins were associated with fewer diarrheas. There is no evidence that any one regimen is associated with fewer side effects (115).

In four studies comparing once-daily with thrice-daily dosing of **gentamicin,** there were fewer failures with **once-daily dosing.** Once-daily gentamicin can be given 5 mg/kg, and once-daily clindamycin phosphate 2700 mg, both intravenously (116). Thrice-daily dosing consists of clindamycin 900 mg and gentamicin 1.5 mg/kg every 8 hours. It is recommended that levels (peak/trough) of gentamicin should be taken after the third dose, to make sure therapeutic regimens are achieved.

Once uncomplicated endometritis has clinically improved with intravenous therapy (usually 24–48 hours afebrile), oral therapy is not needed, as, compared with continued oral antibiotic therapy after intravenous therapy, **no oral therapy** is associated with similar recurrent endometritis or other outcomes in four trials (115).

Response is usually prompt. If fever persists >48 hours (<10% of women), the addition of ampicillin for refractory cases can be considered. If fever still persists, pelvic abscess, wound infection, pelvic septic thrombophlebitis, inadequate antibiotic coverage, and retained placental tissue should be ruled out. Also, the likelihood of a resistant organism, a nongenital source of infection (pyelonephritis, pneumonia, and

intravenous catheter phlebitis), or noninfectious fever are part of the entities to be ruled out (106).

Because of neonatal implications, information on the mother's condition should be provided to the neonate's health care provider (105).

Breastfeeding
Most antibiotics, including clindamycin, gentamicin, and penicillin, are considered safe in breastfeeding, although they may cause changes in infant gastrointestinal flora (117).

POSTPARTUM WOUND INFECTION
Key Points
- **Risk factors** for postcesarean wound infection are **chorioamnionitis, maternal preoperative condition or infection, preeclampsia, higher body mass index, nulliparity, increased surgical blood loss,** and **diabetes.**
- **Prophylactic antibiotics (either ampicillin or first-generation cephalosporin for just one dose)** and **suture closure or drainage of subcutaneous fat in women with ≥2 cm thickness** reduce the risk of postcesarean wound infection.
- **Penicillin** is an antibiotic often used as first line for wound infection. Wound **drainage and debridement of necrotic tissue** may be necessary.
- Compared with healing by secondary intention, **reclosure of the disrupted laparotomy wound** after the infection has resolved **is associated with success in >80% of women, faster healing times, and fewer office visits.**

Diagnosis/Definition
The Center for Disease Control defines and classifies surgical site infection (SSI) as either superficial, deep or organ/space, as shown in Table 27.8. These criteria should be addressed at the time of diagnosis (118). The vast majority of significant wound infections in obstetrics are postpartum following cesarean delivery.

Symptoms
Pain, redness, swelling or heat, and fever.

Epidemiology/Incidence
The incidence of wound infection after cesarean delivery ranges from 2.8% (119) to 3.5% (in obese patients) (99) to 9.8% (120).

Etiology/Basic Pathophysiology
The most common microorganisms identified by cultures from wound infections after cesarean delivery include *Staphylococcus epidermidis*, *Enterococcus faecalis*, *S. aureus*, *Escherichia coli*, and *Proteus mirabilis*. The pathophysiology involves seeding of bacteria either from the uterine cavity or from the skin (119).

Classification
See Table 27.8.

Risk Factors/Associations
Risk factors described are **preoperative remote infection, chorioamnionitis, maternal preoperative condition, preeclampsia, higher body mass index, nulliparity,** and

Table 27.8 Classification of Surgical Site Infection

A. **Superficial:** Occurs within 30 days after surgical procedure, involves skin and subcutaneous tissue only, and *at least one* of the following:
1. Purulent drainage from incision
2. Organism isolated from culture of fluid or tissue from SSI
3. At least one of the following: pain, redness, swelling or heat, and superficial incision is deliberately opened by the surgeon
4. Diagnosis of superficial SSI by surgeon or attending physician
B. **Deep:** Occurs within 30 days from surgical procedure and involves deep soft tissues (fascia, muscle) of the incision, and at least one of the following:
1. Purulent drainage from incision
2. Spontaneous dehiscence or deliberately opened by a surgeon when the patient presents at least one of the following: fever, pain, and tenderness.
3. An abscess involving the deep incision is found on direct examination during reoperation, or by histopathologic or radiologic examination.
4. Diagnosis of deep SSI by surgeon or attending physician
C. **Organ/Space:** Occurs within 30 days from surgical procedure and the infection appears to be related to the operation, and infection involves any part of the anatomy (organs, spaces) other than the incision, which was opened or manipulated during an operation, and at least one of the following:
1. Purulent drainage from a drain placed in the organ/space
2. Organisms isolated from a culture of fluid or tissue in the organ/space
3. An abscess involving the organ/space found on direct examination during reoperation, or by histopathologic or radiologic examination
4. Diagnosis of an organ/space SSI by surgeon or attending physician

increased surgical blood loss (99,120,121). **Diabetes** has also long been considered a classic risk factor, with five times the risk of wound infection compared with women without diabetes (122).

Management
Workup
In early-onset wound infection (<48 hours after the procedure), the microorganisms are likely to be either group A streptococcus or *Clostridium*. A **wound culture** can be taken and a Gram stain will depict either gram-positive cocci or gram-positive rods, respectively. There are no trials to confirm the efficacy of obtaining a wound culture.

Prevention
Prophylactic antibiotics (either ampicillin or first-generation cephalosporin for just one dose) are associated with a 59% decrease in the incidence of wound infection compared with no antibiotics in women undergoing cesarean delivery (111). The timing for prophylaxis should be **before cord clamp**, as while it is not associated with significant change in neonatal outcomes (123), it reduces risk of maternal infectious morbidity (124). **Suture closure of subcutaneous fat in women with ≥2 cm thickness** is associated with a significant decrease in wound disruptions, including infections (32,125) (see also chap. 13).

Therapy
The onset of the infection defines the need for **antibiotics.** For infection arising <48 hours after cesarean, **penicillin** is the drug of choice, but this is based more on expert opinion than on level 1 evidence. Empiric therapy for cellulitis is reasonable with dicloxacillin, cephalexin, or clindamycin (126). Wound **drainage and debridement of necrotic tissue** may be necessary.

In late-onset wound infection (4–8 days postoperatively), the management consists purely of drainage. Antibiotics are not considered indicated in this setting, unless extensive cellulitis is present, or if the patient does not improve after drainage (necrotizing fasciitis should be considered.) (106).

Disrupted (Open) Laparotomy Wound, After Infection Has Resolved
There are different ways to manage the open wound (127).

Compared with healing by secondary intention, **reclosure of the disrupted laparotomy wound is associated with success in >80% of women, faster healing times** (16–23 vs. 61–72 days), **and fewer office visits** (128). No serious morbidity or mortality is associated with either method. There is insufficient evidence to assess optimal timing (probably 4–6 days after disruption if noninfected) and technique (superficial vertical mattress or "en bloc" reclosure of entire wound thickness with absorbable sutures, or adhesive tape) of reclosure, as well as utility of antibiotics. After the wound is free of infection and is granulating properly, local anesthesia can be applied at bedside, and polypropylene mattress stitches can be used to close the skin.

Compared with reclosure using sutures, reclosure using permeable, adhesive tape (Cover-Roll; Biersdorf Inc., Norwalk, Connecticut, U.S.) was a faster procedure with lower pain scores and similar healing times in a small trial (129). However, a subsequent study found shorter healing times (16.1 vs. 23.0 days) with suture closure compared with surgical tape (130).

Secondary intention with negative pressure wound therapy (NPWT), also called vacuum-assisted closure, has not been studied in any trials after cesarean section (131). A recent meta-analysis in non-pregnant adults found some evidence of improved healing with NPWT but concluded that existing data are insufficient to establish clinical benefit (132).

OTHER POSTPARTUM ISSUES
There is insufficient evidence for general postpartum advice on common issues such as lifting, climbing stairs, driving, exercise, vaginal intercourse, and return to work. Suggestions based on this limited evidence and mostly expert opinion are shown in Table 27.9 (134,135). For other postpartum issues, see also chapter 1, chapter 9 (third stage of labor and its complications—includes repair of vaginal lacerations, etc.), chapter 13 (cesarean delivery—especially for prevention of postpartum endometritis and postpartum wound infection), and chapters pertinent to specific

Table 27.9 Postpartum (Including Postcesarean) Advice Regarding Common Daily Life Activities

Advice	Evidence	Suggested recommendations
Lifting	Lifting increases intra-abdominal pressure much less than Valsalva, forceful coughing, or rising from supine to erect position (134).	(1) Patients should continue lifting patterns as before prepregnancy. (2) Patients need an adequate postoperative analgesic regimen as necessary.
Climbing stairs	Climbing stairs increases intra-abdominal pressure much less than Valsalva, forceful coughing, or rising from supine to erect position (134).	(1) Patients should continue climbing stairs as before pregnancy. (2) Patients need an adequate postoperative analgesic regimen as necessary.
Driving	No retrospective or prospective evidence	(1) Patients need an appropriate postoperative analgesic regimen that does not cause a clouded sensorium when driving. (2) Patients may resume driving when comfortable with hand and foot movements required for driving.
Exercise	Limited retrospective and prospective evidence. Forceful coughing increases intra-abdominal pressure as much as jumping jacks (134).	(1) Patients need an appropriate postoperative analgesic regimen as necessary. (2) Patients may resume prepregnancy exercise level. (3) Exercise program may need to be tailored for postpartum women. (4) Preprocedure and postprocedure recommendations should be consistent.
Vaginal intercourse	No consistent retrospective evidence; no prospective evidence	(1) Women and their partners should make the decision to resume intercourse mutually. (2) Women should use appropriate contraception after childbirth. (3) There is insufficient evidence as to when to resume vaginal intercourse.
Returning to work	No consistent prospective or retrospective evidence	(1) Women should be encouraged to return to work relatively soon postpregnancy; the usual times in the United States are 6 wk after vaginal and 8 wk after cesarean delivery, but these are not based on level 1 evidence. (2) Consider graded return to work, as tolerated.

Source: Adapted from Ref. 133.

conditions in both this book and its companion *Maternal-Fetal Evidence Based Guidelines*.

REFERENCES

1. Pang WW, Hartmann PE. Initiation of human lactation: secretory differentiation and secretory activation. J Mammary Gland Biol Neoplasia 2007; 12(4):211–221. [Review]
2. Ip S, Chung M, Raman G, et al. Breastfeeding and maternal and infant health outcomes in developed countries. Evid Rep Technol Asses (Full Rep) 2007; 153:1–186. [II-2]
3. McVea KL, Turner PD, Peppler DK. The role of breastfeeding in sudden infant death syndrome. J Hum Lact 2000; 16(1):13–20. [II-2]
4. Owen CG, Martin RM, Whincup PH, et al. Effect of infant feeding on the risk of obesity across the life course: a quantitative review of published evidence. Pediatrics 2005; 115(5):1367–1377. [II-2]
5. Arenz S, Ruckerl R, Koletzko B, et al. Breast-feeding and childhood obesity—a systematic review. Int J Obes Relat Metab Disord 2004; 28(10):1247–1256. [II-2]
6. Horta BL, Bahl R, Martines JC, et al. Evidence on the Long-term Effects of Breastfeeding: Systematic Review and Meta-analyses. Geneva: World Health Organization, 2007. [Review]
7. Owen CG, Martin RM, Whincup PH, et al. Does breastfeeding influence risk of type 2 diabetes in later life? A quantitative analysis of published evidence. Am J Clin Nutr 2006; 84(5):1043–1054. [II-2]
8. Gdalevich M, Mimouni D, David M, et al. Breast-feeding and the onset of atopic dermatitis in childhood: a systematic review and meta-analysis of prospective studies. J Am Acad Dermatol 2001; 45(4):520–527. [II-2]
9. Collaborative Group on Hormonal Factors in Breast Cancer. Breast cancer and breastfeeding: collaborative reanalysis of individual data from 47 epidemiological studies in 30 countries, including 50302 women with breast cancer and 96973 women without the disease. Lancet 2002; 360(9328):187–195. [II-2]
10. Stuebe AM, Willett WC, Xue F, et al. Lactation and incidence of premenopausal breast cancer: a longitudinal study. Arch Intern Med 2009; 169(15):1364–1371. [II-2]
11. Danforth KN, Tworoger SS, Hecht JL, et al. Breastfeeding and risk of ovarian cancer in two prospective cohorts. Cancer Causes Control 2007; 18(5):517–523. [II-2]
12. Dewey KG, Heinig MJ, Nommsen LA. Maternal weight-loss patterns during prolonged lactation. Am J Clin Nutr 1993; 58 (2):162–166. [II-3]
13. Stuebe AM, Rich-Edwards JW, Willett WC, et al. Duration of lactation and incidence of type 2 diabetes. JAMA 2005; 294 (20):2601–2610. [II-2]
14. Villegas R, Gao YT, Yang G, et al. Duration of breast-feeding and the incidence of type 2 diabetes mellitus in the Shanghai Women's Health Study. Diabetologia 2008; 51(2):258–266. [II-2]
15. Schwarz EB, Ray RM, Stuebe AM, et al. Duration of lactation and risk factors for maternal cardiovascular disease. Obstet Gynecol 2009; 113(5):974–982. [II-2]
16. Schwarz EB, Brown JS, Creasman JM, et al. Lactation and maternal risk of type 2 diabetes: a population-based study. Am J Med 2010; 123(9):863.e861–863.e866. [II-2]
17. Gunderson EP, Lewis CE, Wei GS, et al. Lactation and changes in maternal metabolic risk factors. Obstet Gynecol 2007; 109 (3):729–738. [II-2]
18. Ram KT, Bobby P, Hailpern SM, et al. Duration of lactation is associated with lower prevalence of the metabolic syndrome in

midlife-SWAN, the study of women's health across the nation. Am J Obstet Gynecol 2008; 198(3):268.e261–268.e266. [II-1]

19. Gunderson EP, Jacobs DR Jr., Chiang V, et al. Duration of lactation and incidence of the metabolic syndrome in women of reproductive age according to gestational diabetes mellitus status: A 20-year prospective study in CARDIA—the coronary artery risk development in young adults study. Diabetes 2010; 59(2):495–504. [II-2]

20. Lee SY, Kim MT, Jee SH, et al. Does long-term lactation protect premenopausal women against hypertension risk? A Korean women's cohort study. Prev Med 2005; 41(2):433–438. [II-2]

21. Stuebe AM, Michels KB, Willett WC, et al. Duration of lactation and incidence of myocardial infarction in middle to late adulthood. Am J Obstet Gynecol 2009; 200(2):138.e131–138.e138. [II-2]

22. Chung M, Raman G, Trikalinos T, et al. Interventions in primary care to promote breastfeeding: an evidence review for the U.S. Preventive Services Task Force. Ann Intern Med 2008; 149 (8):565–582. [Meta-analysis: 38 RCTs, n > 2000]

23. Kramer MS, Kakuma R. Optimal duration of exclusive breastfeeding. Cochrane Database Syst Rev 2009; (1):CD003517. [Meta-analysis: 2 RCTs, 11 observational studies]

24. Dewey KG, Cohen RJ, Brown KH, et al. Effects of exclusive breastfeeding for four versus six months on maternal nutritional status and infant motor development: results of two randomized trials in Honduras. J Nutr 2001; 131(2):262–267. [2 RCTs, n = 260]

25. American Academy of Family Physicians. Breastfeeding (Position Paper), 2001. Available at: http://www.aafp.org/online/en/home/policy/policies/b/breastfeedingpositionpaper.html. Accessed June 10, 2009. [Guideline]

26. American Academy of Pediatrics. Breastfeeding and the use of human milk. Pediatrics 2005; 115(2):496–506. [Guideline]

27. American College of Obstetricians and Gynecologists. Special report from ACOG. Breastfeeding: maternal and infant aspects. ACOG Clinical Review. 2007; 12(1 suppl):1S–16S. [Guideline]

28. Department of Health. Infant feeding recommendation, 2003. Available at: http://www.dh.gov.uk/en/Publicationsandstatistics/Publications/PublicationsPolicyAndGuidance/DH_4097197. Accessed December 16, 2010. [Guideline]

29. World Health Organization. Global Strategy for Infant and Young Child Feeding. Geneva: World Health Organization, 2003. [Guideline]

30. National Institute for Health and Clinical Excellence. Quick Reference Guide. NICE Clinical Guideline No. 37: Routine postnatal care of women and their babies, 2006. [Guideline]

31. Dyson L, McCormick F, Renfrew MJ. Interventions for promoting the initiation of breastfeeding. Cochrane Database Syst Rev 2005; (2):CD001688. [Meta-analysis: 11 RCTs, n = 1553]

32. Britton C, McCormick F, Renfrew M, et al. Support for breastfeeding mothers. Cochrane Database Syst Rev 2007; (1): CD001141. [Meta-analysis]

33. U.S. Preventative Services Task Force. Primary Care Interventions to Promote Breastfeeding: U.S. Preventive Services Task Force Recommendation Statement. Ann Intern Med 2008; 149 (8):560–564. [Guideline]

34. Freed GL, Clark SJ, Sorenson J, et al. National assessment of physicians' breast-feeding knowledge, attitudes, training, and experience. JAMA 1995; 273(6):472–476. [II-2]

35. Walton DM, Edwards MC. Nationwide survey of pediatric residency training in newborn medicine: preparation for primary care practice. Pediatrics 2002; 110(6):1081–1087. [II-2]

36. World Health Organization, UNICEF. BFHI Section 3: Breastfeeding Promotion and Support in a Baby-Friendly Hospital, a 20-Hour Course for Maternity Staff. Geneva: World Health Organization, 2009. [Guideline]

37. Feldman-Winter L, Barone L, Milcarek B, et al. Residency curriculum improves breastfeeding care. Pediatrics 2010; 126 (2):289–297; [Epub July 5, 2010]. [Cluster-randomized trial, n = 417 residents, 6 interventions, and 7 control sites]

38. World Health Organization, UNICEF. Baby Friendly Hospital Initiative: Revised, Updated and Expanded for Integrated Care. Geneva: World Health Organization, 2009. [Guideline]

39. Kramer MS, Chalmers B, Hodnett ED, et al. Promotion of Breastfeeding Intervention Trial (PROBIT): a randomized trial in the Republic of Belarus. JAMA 2001; 285(4):413–420. [RCT, n = 17,046]

40. Declercq E, Labbok MH, Sakala C, et al. Hospital practices and women's likelihood of fulfilling their intention to exclusively breastfeed. Am J Pub Health 2009; 99(5):929–935. [II-2]

41. DiGirolamo AM, Grummer-Strawn LM, Fein SB. Effect of maternity-care practices on breastfeeding. Pediatrics 2008; 122(suppl 2):S43–S49. [II-2]

42. Academy of Breastfeeding Medicine Protocol Committee. Clinical Protocol No. 19: Breastfeeding promotion in the prenatal setting. Breastfeed Med 2009; 4(1):43–45. [Guideline]

43. Lee Sue J, Thomas J. Antenatal breast examination for promoting breastfeeding. Cochrane Database Syst Rev 2008; (3): CD006064. [Meta-analysis, no RCTs identified]

44. The MAIN Trial Collaborative Group. Preparing for breast feeding: treatment of inverted and non-protractile nipples in pregnancy. Midwifery 1994; 10(4):200–214. [RCT, n = 463]

45. Alexander JM, Grant AM, Campbell MJ. Randomised controlled trial of breast shells and Hoffman's exercises for inverted and non-protractile nipples. BMJ Clin Res 1992; 304(6833):1030–1032. [RCT, n = 96]

46. Howard CR, Howard FM, Lawrence RA, et al. Office prenatal formula advertising and its effect on breast-feeding patterns. Obstet Gynecol 2000; 95(2):296–303. [RCT, n = 547]

47. Bergevin Y, Dougherty C, Kramer MS. Do infant formula samples shorten the duration of breast-feeding? Lancet 1983; 1 (8334):1148–1151. [RCT, n = 448]

48. Frank DA, Wirtz SJ, Sorenson JR, et al. Commercial discharge packs and breast-feeding counseling: effects on infant-feeding practices in a randomized trial. Pediatrics 1987; 80(6):845–854. [RCT, n = 343]

49. Dungy CI, Christensen-Szalanski J, Losch M, et al. Effect of discharge samples on duration of breast-feeding [see comment]. Pediatrics 1992; 90(2 pt 1):233–237. [RCT, n = 146]

50. National Institute for Health and Clinical Excellence. NICE Clinical Guideline No. 55: Intrapartum care: care of healthy women and babies during childbirth 2007. [Guideline]

51. De Carvalho M, Robertson S, Friedman A, et al. Effect of frequent breast-feeding on early milk production and infant weight gain. Pediatrics 1983; 72(3):307–311. [II-3]

52. Mangesi L, Dowswell T. Treatments for breast engorgement during lactation. Cochrane Database Syst Rev 2010; (9): CD006946. [Meta-analysis: 8 RCTs, n = 744]

53. Barbosa-Cesnik C, Schwartz K, Foxman B. Lactation mastitis. JAMA 2003; 289(13):1609–1612. [Review]

54. Crepinsek Maree A, Crowe L, Michener K, et al. Interventions for preventing mastitis after childbirth. Cochrane Database Syst Rev 2010; (8):CD007239. [Meta-analysis: 5 trials, n = 960]

55. Arroyo R, Martin V, Maldonado A, Jimenez E, Fernandez L, Rodriguez JM. Treatment of infectious mastitis during lactation: antibiotics versus oral administration of lactobacilli isolated from breast milk. Clin Infect Dis 2010; 50(12):1551–1558. [RCT, n = 352]

56. Academy of Breastfeeding Medicine. Clinical protocol #4: mastitis. Breastfeed Med 2008; 3(3):177–180. [Guideline]

57. Akus M, Bartick M. Lactation safety recommendations and reliability compared in 10 medication resources. Ann Pharmacother 2007; 41(9):1352–1360. [III]

58. Furman LM, Minich N, Hack M. Correlates of lactation in mother of VLBW infants. Pediatrics 2002; 109(4):e57. [II-3]

59. Becker Genevieve E, McCormick Felicia M, Renfrew Mary J. Methods of milk expression for lactating women. Cochrane Database Syst Rev 2008; (4):CD006170. [Meta-analysis, 6 RCTs, n = 397]

60. Jones E, Dimmock PW, Spencer SA. A randomised controlled trial to compare methods of milk expression after preterm delivery. Arch Dis Childhood Fetal Neonatal Ed 2001; 85(2): F91–F95. [RCT, n = 36]

61. Morton J, Hall JY, Wong RJ, et al. Combining hand techniques with electric pumping increases milk production in mothers of preterm infants. J Perinatol 2009; 29(11):757–764. [II-3]

62. Feher SDK, Berger LR, Johnson JD, et al. Increasing breast milk production for premature infants with a relaxation/imagery audiotape. Pediatrics 1989; 83(1):57–60. [RCT, $n = 71$]

63. Anderson PO, Valdes V. A critical review of pharmaceutical galactogogues. Breastfeed Med 2007; 2(4):229–242. [Review]

64. Academy of Breastfeeding Medicine. Clinical protocol #9: Use of galactogogues in initiating or augmenting the rate of maternal milk secretion. Breastfeed Med 2011; 6(1). [Guideline]

65. Wan EW, Davey K, Page-Sharp M, et al. Dose-effect study of domperidone as a galactagogue in preterm mothers with insufficient milk supply, and its transfer into milk. Br J Clin Pharmacol 2008; 66(2):283–289. [Crossover RCT, $n = 6$]

66. Campbell-Yeo ML, Allen AC, Joseph KS, et al. Effect of domperidone on the composition of preterm human breast milk. Pediatrics 2010; 125(1):e107–e114. [RCT, $n = 46$]

67. Lewis PJ, Devenish C, Kahn C. Controlled trial of metoclopramide in the initiation of breast feeding. Br J Clin Pharmacol 1980; 9(2):217–219. [RCT, $n = 20$]

68. Hansen WF, McAndrew S, Harris K, et al. Metoclopramide effect on breastfeeding the preterm infant: a randomized trial. Obstet Gynecol 2005; 105(2):383–389. [RCT, $n = 69$]

69. Seema, Patwari AK, Satyanarayana L. Relactation: an effective intervention to promote exclusive breastfeeding. J Trop Pediatr 1997; 43(4):213–216. [RCT, $n = 50$]

70. Sakha K, Behbahan AG. Training for perfect breastfeeding or metoclopramide: which one can promote lactation in nursing mothers? Breastfeed Med 2008; 3(2):120–123. [RCT, $n = 20$]

71. Kramer MS, Kakuma R. Maternal dietary antigen avoidance during pregnancy or lactation, or both, for preventing or treating atopic disease in the child. Cochrane Database Syst Rev 2006; (3):CD000133. [Meta-analysis: 4 RCTs, $n = 334$]

72. Delgado-Noguera Mario F, Calvache Jose A, Bonfill Cosp X. Supplementation with long chain polyunsaturated fatty acids (LCPUFA) to breastfeeding mothers for improving child growth and development. Cochrane Database Syst Rev 2010; (12): CD007901. [Meta-analysis: 6 RCTs, 1280 women]

73. American Academy of Pediatrics. Committee on Infectious Diseases. Report of the Committee on Infectious Diseases. Elk Grove Village, IL: American Academy of Pediatrics, 2010. [Guideline]

74. World Health Organization. Treatment of Tuberculosis: Guidelines. 4th ed. Geneva: World Health Organization, 2010. [Guidelines]

75. Horvath T, Madi Banyana C, Iuppa Irene M, et al. Interventions for preventing late postnatal mother-to-child transmission of HIV. Cochrane Database Syst Rev 2009; (1):CD006734. [Meta-analysis: 6 RCTs, 1 cohort intervention study]

76. World Health Organization. Guidelines on HIV and Infant feeding: Principles and Recommendations for Infant Feeding in the Context of HIV and a Summary of the Evidence. Geneva: World Health Organization, 2010. [Guideline]

77. Ross JA, Winfrey WL. Contraceptive use, intention to use and unmet need during the extended postpartum period. Int Family Planning Persp 2001; 27(1):20–27. [II-3]

78. Lopez LM, Hiller JE, Grimes DA. Education for contraceptive use by women after childbirth. Cochrane Database Syst Rev 2010; (1):CD001863. [Meta-analysis]

79. World Health Organization. Medical Eligibility Criteria for Contraceptive Use. 4th ed. Geneva: World Health Organization, 2010. Accessed December 23, 2010. [Review]

80. Grimes DA, Lopez LM, Schulz KF, et al. Immediate post-partum insertion of intrauterine devices. Cochrane Database Syst Rev 2010(5):CD003036. [Meta-analysis, 9 RCTs]

81. Chen BA, Reeves MF, Hayes JL, et al. Postplacental or delayed insertion of the levonorgestrel intrauterine device after vaginal delivery: a randomized controlled trial. Obstet Gynecol 2010; 116(5):1079–1087. [RCT, $n = 102$]

82. Peterson HB, Xia Z, Hughes JM, et al. The risk of pregnancy after tubal sterilization: findings from the U.S. Collaborative Review of Sterilization. Am J Obstet Gynecol 1996; 174(4):1161–1168; discussion 1168–1170. [II-2]

83. Kohaut BA, Musselman BL, Sanchez-Ramos L, et al. Randomized trial to compare perioperative outcomes of Filshie clip vs. Pomeroy technique for postpartum and intraoperative cesarean tubal sterilization: a pilot study. Contraception 2004; 69(4):267–270. [RCT]

84. Curtis KM, Mohllajee AP, Peterson HB. Regret following female sterilization at a young age: a systematic review. Contraception 2006; 73(2):205–210. [Review]

85. Chi IC, Jones DB. Incidence, risk factors, and prevention of poststerilization regret in women: an updated international review from an epidemiological perspective. Obstet Gynecol Surv 1994; 49(10):722–732. [Review]

86. Thurman AR, Janecek T. One-year follow-up of women with unfulfilled postpartum sterilization requests. Obstet Gynecol 2010; 116(5):1071–1077. [II-3]

87. Van der Wijden C, Brown J, Kleijnen J. Lactational amenorrhea for family planning. Cochrane Database Syst Rev 2003; (4): CD001329. [Meta-analysis of observational studies, II-2]

88. Kennedy KI, Visness CM. Contraceptive efficacy of lactational amenorrhoea. Lancet 1992; 339(8787):227–230. [II-2]

89. Academy of Breastfeeding Medicine. ABM Clinical Protocol #13: contraception during breastfeeding. Breastfeed Med 2006; 1 (1):43–51. [Guideline]

90. Truitt Sarah T, Fraser Anna B, Gallo Maria F, et al. Combined hormonal versus nonhormonal versus progestin-only contraception in lactation. Cochrane Database Syst Rev 2003; (2): CD003988. [Meta-analysis: 5 trials, poor quality]

91. Chen BA, Reeves MF, Creinin MD, et al. Postplacental or delayed levonorgestrel intrauterine device insertion and breast-feeding duration. Contraception 2011; 84:499–504. [RCT, $n = 96$]

92. Shaamash AH, Sayed GH, Hussien MM, et al. A comparative study of the levonorgestrel-releasing intrauterine system Mirena versus the Copper T380A intrauterine device during lactation: breast-feeding performance, infant growth and infant development. Contraception 2005; 72(5):346–351. [II-1]

93. Brown CE, Stettler RW, Twickler D, et al. Puerperal septic pelvic thrombophlebitis: incidence and response to heparin therapy. Am J Obstet Gynecol 1999; 181(1):143–148. [II-2]

94. Diamond MP, Entman SS, Salyer SL, et al. Increased risk of endometritis and wound infection after cesarean section in insulin-dependent diabetic women. Am J Obstet Gynecol 1986; 155(2):297–300. [II-2]

95. Rosene K, Eschenbach DA, Tompkins LS, et al. Polymicrobial early postpartum endometritis with facultative and anaerobic bacteria, genital mycoplasmas, and Chlamydia trachomatis: treatment with piperacillin or cefoxitin. J Infect Dis 1986; 153 (6):1028–1037. [RCT]

96. Wolfe HM, Gross TL, Sokol RJ, et al. Determinants of morbidity in obese women delivered by cesarean. Obstet Gynecol 1988; 71 (5):691–696. [II-3]

97. Gibbs RS. Clinical risk factors for puerperal infection. Obstet Gynecol 1980; 55(5 suppl):178S–184S. [II-2]

98. Magee KP, Blanco JD, Graham JM, et al. Endometritis after cesarean: the effect of age. Am J Perinatol 1994; 11(1):24–26. [II-2]

99. Myles TD, Gooch J, Santolaya J. Obesity as an independent risk factor for infectious morbidity in patients who undergo cesarean delivery. Obstet Gynecol 2002; 100(5 Pt 1):959–964. [II-2]

100. Krohn MA, Hillier SL, Baker CJ. Maternal peripartum complications associated with vaginal group B streptococci colonization. J Infect Dis 1999; 179(6):1410–1415. [II-2]

101. Minkoff HL, Sierra MF, Pringle GF, et al. Vaginal colonization with group B beta-hemolytic streptococcus as a risk factor for post-cesarean section febrile morbidity. Am J Obstet Gynecol 1982; 142(8):992–995. [II-2]

102. Watts DH, Krohn MA, Hillier SL, et al. Bacterial vaginosis as a risk factor for post-cesarean endometritis. Obstet Gynecol 1990; 75(1):52–58. [II-2]

103. Ferrero S, Bentivoglio G. Post-operative complications after caesarean section in HIV-infected women. Arch Gynecol Obstet 2003; 268(4):268–273. [II-2]

104. Watts DH, Lambert JS, Stiehm ER, et al. Complications according to mode of delivery among human immunodeficiency virus-infected women with CD4 lymphocyte counts of < or = 500/microL. Am J Obstet Gynecol 2000; 183(1):100–107. [II-3]

105. American College of Obstetrians and Gynecologists, American Academy of Pediatrics. Guidelines for Perinatal Care. 6th ed. Washington, D.C.: ACOG, 2007. [Review]

106. Sweet, RL, Gibbs RS. Infectious Diseases of the Female Genital Tract. Philadelphia, PA: Wolters Kluwer Health/Lippincott Williams & Wilkins, 2009. [Review]

107. Monif GR, Baker DA. Infectious Diseases in Obstetrics and Gynecology. 5th ed. New York, NY: Parthenon Publishing, 2004. [Review]

108. Gabbe SG, Niebyl JR, Simpson JL, eds. Obstetrics: Normal and Problem Pregnancies. Philadelphia, PA: Churchill Livingstone/Elsevier, 2007. [Review]

109. Chen K. Postpartum endometritis. UpToDate. 2010. Accessed December 23, 2010. [Review]

110. Hopkins L, Smaill FM. Antibiotic prophylaxis regimens and drugs for cesarean section. Cochrane Database Syst Rev 1999; (2). Available at: http://www.mrw.interscience.wiley.com/cochrane/clsysrev/articles/CD001136/frame.html. [Meta-analysis]

111. Hofmeyr GJ, Smaill FM. Antibiotic prophylaxis for cesarean section. Cochrane Database Syst Rev 2010; (1):CD000933. Available at: http://www.mrw.interscience.wiley.com/cochrane/clsysrev/articles/CD000933/frame.html. [Meta-analysis]

112. Andrews WW, Hauth JC, Cliver SP, et al. Randomized clinical trial of extended spectrum antibiotic prophylaxis with coverage for Ureaplasma urealyticum to reduce post-cesarean delivery endometritis. Obstet Gynecol 2003; 101(6):1183–1189. [RCT, n = 597]

113. Chang PL, Newton ER. Predictors of antibiotic prophylactic failure in post-cesarean endometritis. Obstet Gynecol 1992; 80 (1):117–122. [II-2]

114. Haas David M, Morgan Al Darei S, Contreras K. Vaginal preparation with antiseptic solution before cesarean section for preventing postoperative infections. Cochrane Database Syst Rev 2010; (3):CD007892. [Meta-analysis: 4 RCTs, n = 1198]

115. French L, Smaill FM. Antibiotic regimens for endometritis after delivery. Cochrane Database Syst Rev 2004; (4):CD001067. Available at: http://www.mrw.interscience.wiley.com/cochrane/clsysrev/articles/CD001067/frame.html. [Meta-analysis]

116. Livingston JC, Llata E, Rinehart E, et al. Gentamicin and clindamycin therapy in postpartum endometritis: the efficacy of daily dosing versus dosing every 8 hours. Am J Obstet Gynecol 2003; 188(1):149–152. [RCT, n = 110]

117. National Library of Medicine. LactMed. Available at: http://toxnet.nlm.nih.gov/cgi-bin/sis/htmlgen?LACT. Accessed December 22, 2010. [Review]

118. Mangram AJ, Horan TC, Pearson ML, et al. Guideline for prevention of surgical site infection, 1999. Hospital Infection Control Practices Advisory Committee. Infect Control Hosp Epidemiol 1999; 20(4):250–278; quiz 279–280. [Guideline]

119. Martens MG, Kolrud BL, Faro S, et al. Development of wound infection or separation after cesarean delivery. Prospective evaluation of 2,431 cases. J Reprod Med 1995; 40(3):171–175. [II-1]

120. Tran TS, Jamulitrat S, Chongsuvivatwong V, et al. Risk factors for postcesarean surgical site infection. Obstet Gynecol 2000; 95 (3):367–371. [II-2]

121. Vermillion ST, Lamoutte C, Soper DE, et al. Wound infection after cesarean: effect of subcutaneous tissue thickness. Obstet Gynecol 2000; 95(6 pt 1):923–926. [II-2]

122. Cruse PJ, Foord R. A five-year prospective study of 23,649 surgical wounds. Arch Surg 1973; 107(2):206–210. [II-1]

123. Wax JR, Hersey K, Philput C, et al. Single dose cefazolin prophylaxis for postcesarean infections: before vs. after cord clamping. J Matern Fetal Med 1997; 6(1):61–65. [RCT, n = 90]

124. Sullivan SA, Smith T, Chang E, et al. Administration of cefazolin prior to skin incision is superior to cefazolin at cord clamping in preventing postcesarean infectious morbidity: a randomized, controlled trial. Am J Obstet Gynecol 2007; 196(5):455e.451–455e.455. [RCT, n = 357]

125. Anderson Elizabeth R, Gates S. Techniques and materials for closure of the abdominal wall in caesarean section. Cochrane Database Syst Rev 2004; (4):CD004663. Available at: http://www.mrw.interscience.wiley.com/cochrane/clsysrev/articles/CD004663/frame.html. [Meta-analysis]

126. Baddour L. Cellulitis and erysipelas. UpToDate. 2010. Accessed 12/23/2010. [Review]

127. Sarsam SE, Elliott JP, Lam GK. Management of wound complications from cesarean delivery. Obstet Gynecol Surv 2005; 60 (7):462–473. [Review]

128. Wechter ME, Pearlman MD, Hartmann KE. Reclosure of the disrupted laparotomy wound: a systematic review. Obstet Gynecol 2005; 106(2):376–383. [Review]

129. Harris RL, Magann EF, Sullivan DL, et al. Wound dehiscence: secondary closure with suture versus noninvasive adhesive bandage. Female Pelvic Med Reconst Surg 1995; 1(1):88–91. [RCT, n = 27]

130. Zaid TM, Herring WP, Meeks GR. A randomized trial of secondary closure of superficial wound dehiscence by surgical tape or suture. Female Pelvic Med Reconst Surg 2010; 16(4):246–248. [RCT, n = 30]

131. Eginton MT, Brown KR, Seabrook GR, et al. A prospective randomized evaluation of negative-pressure wound dressings for diabetic foot wounds. Ann Vasc Surg 2003; 17(6):645–649. [RCT, n = 10]

132. Gregor S, Maegele M, Sauerland S, et al. Negative pressure wound therapy: a vacuum of evidence? Arch Surg 2008; 143 (2):189–196. [Meta-analysis, n = 602]

133. Minig L, Trimble EL, Sarsotti C, et al. Building the evidence base for postoperative and postpartum advice. Obstet Gynecol 2009; 114:892–900. [Review]

134. Wier LF, Nygaard IE, Wilken J, et al. Postoperative activity restrictions: any evidence? Obstet Gynecol 2006; 107:305–309. [Review]

28

The neonate

Gary A. Emmett and Melissa Skibo

KEY POINTS

- **Necessary equipment** for neonatal stabilization must be available at every delivery.
- **Personnel trained in neonatal resuscitation** should be present at every delivery.
- An infant who is 38+ weeks of gestation, is crying or breathing, and has good muscle tone does not require resuscitation. Dry the baby, place the baby skin-to-skin with the mother, and cover the baby with dry linen to maintain temperature.
- Provide routine care, provide warmth, assure open airway, dry, and continuously evaluate color, activity and breathing.
- Neonatal resuscitation begins if child does not proceed through successful transition. Stimulate the baby and open the airway. Routine suctioning is no longer suggested. If further resuscitation is needed, it is frequently due to poor respiratory transition and can usually be resolved with bag-and-mask **support of airway and breathing**.
- A difficult transition may be anticipated by infants at risk and may be due to hypothermia, hypoglycemia, or congenital anomalies.
- **Low-risk infants** are 36 weeks of gestation or older and have birth weight between 2500 and 4200 g, Apgar scores of 7 or above at 5 minutes, normal vital signs, and no signs of congenital anomalies or respiratory distress.
- **The preterm infant** (especially 35 weeks of gestation or less) is at **greater risk** for complications in the delivery room and in the well nursery. With high-risk infants, there must be immediate access to means of establishing **intravenous (IV) access and airway pressure**.
- Every nursery should have preexisting protocols to institute best stabilization practices and should have clear statements of what conditions and degree of illness require transfer.
- Initial bag-and-mask resuscitation should be with room air.
- **The majority of cases of cerebral palsy do *not* result from isolated intrapartum hypoxia with resultant asphyxia and organ damage.**

DELIVERY ROOM MANAGEMENT

The perinatal period is the riskiest time in a child's life (1–3). Every newborn has the right to a resuscitation performed at a high level of competence. A competent resuscitation means that the proper equipment and well-trained personnel must be at every delivery. **Necessary equipment** is shown in Table 28.1.

Initiation of Resuscitation

Due to the complex physiologic changes that occur at birth, many newborns will experience apnea or bradycardia that will require opening the airway, stimulation, and ventilation. The need for medication is rare.

The first steps include the following:

1. **Thermal management:** Placing the infant under a pre-heated radiant warmer, drying and stimulating the newborn, and frequently replacing wet blankets with dry ones.
2. **Opening the airway:** Because of evidence that suctioning of the nasopharynx can lead to bradycardia during resuscitation, the first step is simply opening the airway. Clearing the airway should be reserved for babies with obvious obstruction of the airway or who require positive pressure ventilation. Most historic methods of removing meconium from the airway (suctioning of the oral pharynx before delivery of the shoulders and elective endotracheal intubation and direct suctioning of the trachea) have not been shown to improve outcomes. There is insufficient evidence to recommend a change in the current practice of endotracheal suctioning of non-vigorous babies with meconium stained amniotic fluid, but if this cannot be done easily and quickly, start bag-mask ventilation, especially if child is bradycardic.
3. **Tactile stimulation:** Rubbing the baby's back may occasionally be necessary to stimulate the baby to normal breathing and heart rate. Drying the baby is not sufficient stimulation, and suctioning the airway is no longer recommended.

On rare occasions, medications are necessary and should be available (refer to Table 28.2 for the full list.). The most commonly used are as follows:

1. Epinephrine 1:10,000; 0.1–0.3 mL/kg IV or via endotracheal tube (ETT) given rapidly
2. Volume expanders: normal saline, 5% albumin, Ringer's lactate, or whole blood. Dose is 10 mL/kg IV over 5 minutes.
3. Sodium bicarbonate 0.5 mEq/mL: 2 mEq/kg IV given over at least 2 minutes
4. Naloxone hydrochloride 0.4 mg/mL: 0.1 mg/kg ETT or IV given rapidly

Delivery Room Resuscitation

The Apgar score assesses the need to treat the newborn (refer to Table 28.3 for specifics.). The algorithm in Figure 28.1 can be used as a guideline for the resuscitation of a term or near-term infant.

The Difficult Transition

Successful transition to extrauterine life generally occurs over the first hours after birth. Delay in transition can occur for many reasons. Common causes of delayed transition are listed in Table 28.4.

Table 28.1 Necessary Equipment for Neonatal Resuscitation in the Delivery Room

1. Suction equipment:
   a. Bulb syringe
   b. Mechanical suction and tubing
   c. Suction catheters of various sizes (recommended: 5, 8, 10, and 12 or 14 Fr)
   d. Feeding tubes (8 Fr with 20-mL syringe)
   e. Meconium aspirator
2. Bag mask equipment
   a. Device for delivering PPV such as neonatal resuscitation bag with manometer or T-piece resuscitator
   b. Face masks in newborn and premature sizes
   c. Oxygen source and tubing (blender preferable due to varying oxygen requirements)
   d. Oxygen flow meter
3. Intubation equipment
   a. Laryngoscope with 0 and 1 blades (for preterm and term infants)
   b. Endotracheal tubes (ETT) (2.5–4.0 mm)
   c. Stylet
   d. CO_2 detector
4. Other equipment
   a. Alcohol
   b. Stethoscope
   c. Gloves
   d. Scissors
   e. Tape (for securing ETT and lines)
   f. Stopcocks
   g. Syringes (1–20 mL)
   h. Umbilical artery and vein tray with catheters (3.5 and 5 Fr)
   i. Warmer
   j. Needles (25, 21, and 18 gauge)
   k. Pulse oximeter
   l. Transporter

Abbreviations: PPV, positive pressure ventilation; CO_2, carbon dioxide.

Table 28.2 Medications Required for Resuscitation

1. Epinephrine 1:10,000 (0.1 mg/mL)
2. Crystalloid fluids (Normal saline or Ringer's lactate)
3. Sodium bicarbonate 4.2% (5 mEq/10 mL)
4. Dextrose 10%
5. Normal saline flushes

In infants with signs of poor transition (tachypnea, cyanosis, mottled skin or pallor, tremors, and/or jitteriness), additional measurements of the child's vital signs should be considered. These include temperature, blood glucose, and arterial blood saturation (by pulse oximetry or blood gas). Some of the more common reasons for delayed transition are discussed below.

Hypoglycemia
Low blood glucose in the newborn is a common problem often associated with a diabetic mother or with abnormal in utero growth–either too small or too large. A less common cause is congenital abnormalities of the pancreas. The exact definition of hypoglycemia is not agreed upon but all *symptomatic* infants should be treated. Treatment should be initiated immediately. Specific guidelines vary with the institution.

According to the 2011 report by the Committee of Fetus and Newborn of the American Academy of Pediatrics (AAP), treatment should proceed as in Table 28.5. Screening should be limited to term babies who are symptomatic (see Table 28.5), or ones that are at high-risk which include babies that are less than 36 weeks gestation, SGA, LGA, and/or IDM. Routine screening of blood glucose is not needed in healthy, term newborns after uneventful pregnancy and delivery, except if they are symptomatic. No studies have demonstrated harm from asymptomatic hypoglycemia in the first 12 hours of life. Screening in late preterm infants and SGA infants should continue up to at least 24 hours. After 24 hours, any infant with glucose that is persistently <45 mg/dL should continue to be screened until stable. If glucose is not stable at 24 hours of age, or symptoms continue in spite of treatment, transfer to a higher level of care is necessary.

Meconium
Meconium is the thick, green bowel movement of a newborn infant. All newborns should have a bowel movement within 24 hours of birth. Intrauterine stress or stress during delivery may cause the meconium to pass early. Meconium-stained fluid may be present in 8% to 20% of deliveries and is almost exclusively found in term or postterm infants. The fluid may be lightly stained and thin or very dark and thick, but all meconium-stained fluid presents a risk to the baby. The treatment is based on the condition of the infant at birth. If the baby is vigorous and cries immediately, resuscitation should proceed normally. If the infant is limp or lethargic, he or she should be delivered immediately and placed on the warmer. Meconuim suctioning, by intubating the baby and directly suctioning the trachea with a meconuim aspirator attached to the ETT, may be helpful if it can be done quickly and easily. If not, simply bag the baby with room air. Current recommendation is to not suction the baby before delivery of the shoulders and to apply mask-and-bag resuscitation with room air as soon as possible to a baby who is not vigorous.

Respiratory Distress
Respiratory distress and/or tachypnea may occur and can be the manifestation of underlying illnesses. Etiologies include abnormalities of the lung (respiratory distress or aspiration syndromes, infections, pneumothorax, and congenital lung abnormalities), structural airway problems (choanal atresia, tracheal-esophageal fistula, and micrognathia), abnormalities of the cardiovascular system (primarily congenital heart disease—cyanotic or not, congestive heart failure, and pulmonary hypertension), abnormalities of the neurologic system [central nervous system (CNS) infections, hypoxic injury, and hydrocephalus], blood dyscrasia (anemia or polycythemia), infections, metabolic problems, or exposure to maternal drugs. Specific treatment should be aimed at the underlying etiology. Screening laboratory tests and imaging studies such as

Table 28.3 Apgar Score

	0	1	2
Color	Blue/Pale	Acrocyanosis	Pink
Heart rate	Absent	<100/min	>100/min
Reflex/Irritability	No response	Grimace	Cry/Active withdrawal
Tone	Limp	Some flexion	Active motion
Respirations	Absent	Weak cry/Hypoventilation	Good/Crying

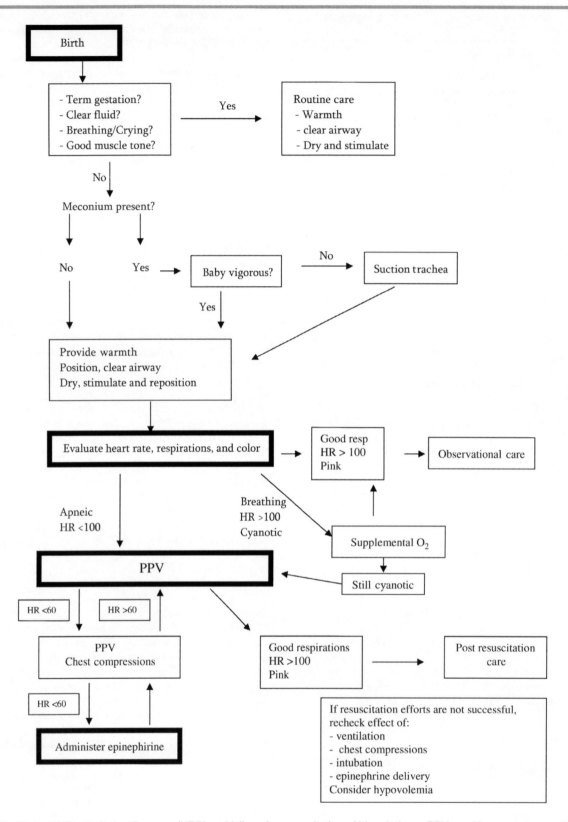

Figure 28.1   Neonatal Resuscitation Program (NRP); guidelines for resuscitation. *Abbreviations*: PPV, positive pressure ventilation; HR, heart rate.

complete blood count (CBC), C-reactive protein (CRP), blood gas, and chest X ray should be initiated if gudicated.

Clear evidence exists that either insufficient or excessive oxygen can be harmful to the newborn infant. Hypoxia/ Ischemia can result in injury to the brain and other organs, but even brief exposure to excessive oxygen can result in vision or other neurological problems. Newborn babies do not have high levels of blood oxygen until at least 10 minutes after birth, so pulse oximetry below 90 is completely normal just after birth. Also, because of circulation changes at birth,

Table 28.4 Factors Associated with Delayed Transition

Infant
Hypothermia
Hypoglycemia
Retained pulmonary fluid
Preterm birth (<37 wk)
Multiple births
Small or large for gestational age (<2500 g or >4200 g)
Postterm birth (≥42 wk gestation)
Meconium
Low Apgar scores (i.e., <7 at 5 minutes)
Congenital problems (i.e., chromosomal abnormalities and
    structural problems)
Infection
Mother
Diabetes
Tocolysis
Licit or illicit drugs

cyanosis does not always mean lack of oxygen and a pink color of the skin does not always mean presence of oxygen in the newborn. When using pulse oximetry on the newborn in the first hour of life, it should be applied preductally (the right, upper extremity).

Resuscitation in newborns 34 weeks and older should always begin with room air. Goals for children not going successfully through transition are presented in Table 28.6 and range from 65% blood oxygenation/pulse oximetry in the first minute of life to 85% or higher after 10 minutes. This major change in the use of oxygen during the initial resuscitation of the newborn will seem dramatic to delivery room personnel and a well-organized educational program where clear posting of the new protocol in every venue where neonates are resuscitated is of the utmost importance.

Transient Tachypnea of the Newborn
In the newborn, tachypnea without respiratory distress may be a benign condition called transient tachypnea of the newborn (TTN). These infants are usually term or near term and will develop tachypnea following birth. They may have respiratory rates up to 120 breaths/min, nasal flaring, grunting, and retractions, but upon physical examination, they do not appear to be in serious distress. Risk factors include cesarean delivery, precipitous delivery, fetal polycythemia, and delivery to a diabetic mother. There is no clear etiology to this disorder, but it is thought to be due to a combination of delayed resorption of fetal lung fluid from the lymph system, pulmonary immaturity, and a mild surfactant deficiency. Unfortunately, TTN is not easily distinguishable from other

causes of tachypnea, such as pneumonia or sepsis. If the condition does not quickly resolve, these infants should have screening laboratory tests, including a CBC, CRP, and blood culture, along with a chest X ray and a pediatric or neonatal consult. In TTN, the lab work will be normal and the chest X

Table 28.6 Disorders Recommended by the American College of Medical Genetics Task Force for Inclusion in Newborn Screening[a]

Disorders of organic acid metabolism
Isovaleric acidemia
Glutaric aciduria type 1
3-hydroxy-3-methylglutaric aciduria
Multiple carboxylase deficiency
Methylmalonic acidemia, mutase deficiency form
3-methylcrotonyl-CoA carboxylase deficiency
Methylmalonic acidemia, Cb1 A and Cb1 B forms
Propionic acidemia
Beta-ketothiolase deficiency

Disorders of fatty acid metabolism
Medium-chain acyl-CoA dehydrogenase deficiency
Very long chain acyl-CoA dehydrogenase deficiency
Long-chain L-3-hydroxy acyl-CoA dehydrogenase deficiency
Trifunctional protein deficiency
Carnitine uptake defect

Disorders of amino acid metabolism
Phenylketonuria
Maple syrup urine disease
Homocystinuria
Citrullinemia
Argininosuccinic acidemia
Tyrosinemia type 1

Hemoglobinopathies
Sickle cell anemia
Hemoglobin S-β-thalassemia
Hemoglobin SC disease

Other disorders
Congenital hypothyroidism
Biotinidase deficiency
Congenital adrenal hyperplasia
Galactosemia
Hearing deficiency
Cystic fibrosis

[a]The American College of Medical Genetics task force also recommended reporting an additional 25 disorders ("secondary targets") that can be detected through screening but that do not meet the criteria for primary disorders (6). At this time, there is a state-to-state variation in newborn screening; a list of the disorders that are screened for by each state is available at http://genes-r-us.uthscsa.edu.
Abbreviations: CoA, coenzyme A; Cb1 A, cobalamin A; Cb1 B, cobalamin B.
Source: Adapted from Refs. 4,5.

Table 28.5 Hypoglycemia Management in the Child After 34 Weeks of Gestation At Risk (34–36 Weeks' Gestation, Small for Gestation Age, Infants of Diabetic Mothers, and/or Large for Gestational Age)

Symptomatic* with serum glucose < 40 mg/dL	Asymptomatic (Birth to 4 hr of age)		Asymptomatic (4–24 hr of age)	
Use IV glucose	Initial feed within 1 hr		Continue feeds every 2–3 hr	
	Screen glucose 30 min after first feed		Screen glucose prior to each feed	
	If initial screen is <25 mg/dL, feed and recheck in 1 hr		If screen <35 mg/dL, feed and recheck in 1 hr	
	If repeat glucose is still <25 mg/dL, start IV glucose	If 25–40 mg/dL, re-feed and use IV glucose as needed	If repeat glucose is still <35 mg/dL, start IV glucose	If repeat glucose is 35–45 mg/dL, re-feed and use IV glucose as needed

*Symptomatic hypoglycemia: irritability, tremors, jitteriness, exaggerated reflexes, high-pitched cry, seizures, lethargy, floppiness, cyanosis, apnea, and poor feeding.
TARGET GLUCOSE > 45 mg/dL PRIOR TO ROUTINE FEEDINGS. IV infusion, if needed, at 5–8 mg/kg/min (80–100 mL/kg/24 hr).

ray will have increased pulmonary vascular markings and fluid in the fissures. More seriously affected infants may be treated with broad-spectrum antibiotics until infection can be excluded. In addition, those infants with respiratory rates above 60 breaths/min should not be fed by mouth, and some will require either nasogastric (NG) tube feeds or IV fluids if the tachypnea lasts more than 12 hours.

Common Malformations Affecting Transition
Some congenital abnormalities of the newborn can present as problems in the delivery room. Below is a list of common malformations and best stabilization practices before transfer to a tertiary care nursery.

1. Choanal atresia (blockage of the nasal passageway): Secure an oral airway.
2. Pierre–Robin sequence (small mandible with relatively large tongue): Secure an oral airway, but consider intubation if inadequate.
3. Congenital diaphragmatic hernia: At birth, immediate insertion of an NG tube to decompress the stomach and intubation of the airway are required.
4. Abdominal wall defects (omphalocele and gastroschisis): Cover the defect with a silo as soon as possible after birth. Gastroschisis may require prompt surgical correction; therefore, surgery should be called as soon as the baby is born.
5. Neural tube defects: Best emergent management is controversial, but the goal is to keep the area moist and free of contamination. The area may be covered with sterile plastic wrap, or the baby may be placed in a sterile plastic bag to just above the lesion.

TYPE OF NURSERY: LOW- VS. ELEVATED-RISK NEONATES

Minimal intervention is needed for the infant with no risks and a normal delivery. Therefore, it is important to distinguish which infants are at low risk and can go to the well baby nursery, and which infants are at high risk and require further evaluation.

Low Risk

These infants can be admitted without pediatric specialist consultation. Low-risk infants are 36 weeks of gestation or older and have birth weight between 2200 and 4200 g, Apgar scores of 7 or above at 5 minutes, normal vital signs, and no signs of congenital anomalies or respiratory distress.

Elevated Risk

Elevated-risk infants require pediatric specialist consultation prior to admission to the well baby nursery. Criteria include infants at risk for neonatal abstinence syndrome, sepsis, rupture of membranes greater than 16 hours, exposure to group B streptococcus (GBS) that was inadequately treated, maternal temperature of greater than 100.4°F (38°C) within 24 hours of delivery, infants of diabetic mothers, infants born outside of the hospital, infants of uncertain gestation, infants 35 weeks' gestation or less, infants less than 2200 g, and infants greater than 4200 g.

CARE OF THE 'WELL' NEWBORN AFTER L&D CARE

All infants must be observed until they complete transition. A skilled staff member must assess the vital signs every 30 minutes for at least 2 hours and observe that the newborn is completely stable on its own. Completion of transition includes thermostability, respiratory rate less than 60 breaths/min, heart rate greater than 100 beats/min, and good muscle tone and sucking reflex.

NEWBORN SCREENING

Neonatal screening has arisen from the politics of medicine and of government, and has not been subject to consistent cost-benefit analysis or evidence-based medicine (4,5). The required tests vary from state to state, but each state requires screening after 24 hours of life. Both the American College of Medical Genetics and Centers for Disease Control (CDC) have made model screening lists, but there is no single list of tests universally required in 2012. The tests suggested are referenced in Table 28.6.

CIRCUMCISION

The American Academy of Pediatrics (AAP) recommends that circumcision should be **parental choice** and only agreed to after a discussion with a health care provider about the risks and benefits (7). The World Health Organization has recommended universal circumcision as a method to reduce the risk of acquiring HIV infection in populations at high risk for HIV. Circumcision is often a social decision rather than a medical decision. The pediatric practitioner should delay or prevent circumcision in the following cases:

- Suspected sepsis or bacteremia
- Family history of bleeding problems (until the child is fully assessed by hematologist)
- Genital abnormalities, including ambiguous genitalia, micropenis (<2.5 cm from pubic bone to penile tip), hypospadias, epispadias, or chordae.

Performing a Circumcision

Prior to circumcision, infants should have completed transition, voided at least once, and been fasting for 1 hour prior to the procedure. Pain control should be utilized and can include a dorsal penile nerve block, topical analgesic, or subcutaneous ring block. Sucrose water or sweet wine also provides some pain control. Techniques for circumcision include the Plastibell™ and Gomco™. After the procedure, breast- or bottle-feeding is an excellent pain control method. If needed, the dose of acetaminophen is 12–15 mg/kg/dose. A gauze wrap is no longer recommended after the procedure. The area should be kept clean with plain water and covered with lubricant for up to 1 week until completely healed. The parents should be told to expect a white yellow discharge for 5 to 7 days.

CARE OF THE PRETERM INFANT

The delivery of a preterm infant follows many of the guidelines generated for the term infant (1–3). These infants born at 36 weeks' gestation or less are at high risk for problems immediately following birth and in the subsequent newborn period. If a preterm delivery is anticipated, the delivery should be attended by a team of neonatal intensive care unit (NICU) personnel (physician, nurse, and respiratory therapist). Management of the infant includes accentuated attention to drying and maintaining thermal stability and close observation of blood glucose, fluid requirements, and respiratory function. In high-risk infants, the prophylactic placement of an umbilical venous line should be considered.

Also, early institution of positive airway pressure may be necessary to prevent respiratory failure. Preparation for and anticipation of the delivery with the availability of the proper equipment and personnel for stabilization and transport will optimize survival (8).

NEONATAL ENCEPHALOPATHY AND CEREBRAL PALSY
Neonatal Encephalopathy

Neonatal encephalopathy is a clinically defined syndrome of disturbed neurologic function in the earliest days of life in the term infant, manifested by difficulty initiating and maintaining respiration, depression of tone and reflexes, subnormal level of consciousness, and, often, seizures. It can result from a myriad of conditions and may or may not result in permanent neurologic impairment (9).

Hypoxic-Ischemic Encephalopathy

Hypoxic-ischemic encephalopathy (HIE) is a subset of neonatal encephalopathy for which the etiology is considered to be a limitation of oxygen and blood flow near the time of birth. The usual progression of events is as follows:

Intrapartum hypoxic-ischemic injury
↓
Neonatal encephalopathy
↓
Cerebral palsy

Cerebral Palsy

Cerebral palsy is a chronic static neuromuscular disability characterized by aberrant control of movement or posture, appearing early in life and not the result of recognized progressive disease. Spastic quadriplegia is the only type of cerebral palsy associated with birth asphyxia. Cerebral palsy affects 2 to 3/1000 live births.

Prevention is elusive. **The majority of cases of cerebral palsy do *not* result from isolated intrapartum hypoxia with resultant asphyxia and organ damage** (9).

Known factors associated with cerebral palsy are as follows:

- Prematurity
- Developmental malformations
- Metabolic defects
- Autoimmune and coagulation disorders
- Infections
- Hypoxia

Historically, four nonspecific clinical signs were often assumed to be adequate evidence of birth asphyxia and hypoxic-ischemic neonatal encephalopathy in the absence of objective criteria:

- Meconium staining
- Nonreassuring fetal heart rate (FHR) pattern
- Low Apgar score
- Neonatal encephalopathy

In fact, **abnormal FHR patterns thought to predict subsequent cerebral palsy actually have a 98% false-positive rate**. Less than one-quarter of infants with neonatal encephalopathy have evidence of hypoxia or ischemia at birth. Intrapartum hypoxia is uncommonly the sole cause of neonatal encephalopathy or cerebral palsy.

Timing of Neonatal Encephalopathy

Estimating the time when neonatal encephalopathy occurred is extremely difficult. Some (9) have reported risk factors related to this condition:

- 69% Only antepartum risk factors
- 25% Both antepartum risk factors and evidence for intrapartum hypoxia
- 4% Intrapartum hypoxia without antepartum risk factors
- 2% No recognized risk factors

Therefore, the incidence of neonatal encephalopathy attributed to intrapartum hypoxia in absence of other preconception or antepartum abnormalities is about 1.6/10,000 infants (9).

Apgar Scores and Cerebral Palsy

0–3 at 5 min:	0.3–1.0% of babies with cerebral palsy
0–3 at 10 min:	10% of babies with cerebral palsy (but rates drop to 5% if scores improve at 15 and 20 min)
<3 at 15 min:	53% mortality, 36% of survivors with cerebral palsy
<3 at 20 min:	60% mortality, 57% of survivors with cerebral palsy

Seventy-five percent of children with **cerebral palsy** had **normal Apgar scores** at birth.

Criticism of the management of labor should not be confused with cerebral palsy causation because the two often may not be linked.

Criteria to Define an Acute Intrapartum Event Sufficient to Cause Cerebral Palsy

Essential criteria (must meet all four):

- Metabolic acidosis in fetal umbilical artery: pH <7.0 and base deficit >12 mmol/L
- Early onset of neonatal encephalopathy born at or >34 weeks' gestation
- Cerebral palsy of the spastic quadriplegic or dyskinetic type
- Exclusion of other identifiable etiologies

Criteria That Collectively Suggest Intrapartum Timing but Nonspecific to Asphyxial Insults

- Sentinel (signal) hypoxic event immediately before or during labor
- Sudden and sustained fetal bradycardia or absence of FHR variability with persistent late or variable decelerations, when pattern was previously normal
- Apgar score 0 to 3 beyond 5 minutes
- Onset of multisystem organ involvement within 72 hours
- Early neuroimaging with evidence of acute nonfocal cerebral abnormality

REFERENCES

1. Gomella TL, Cunningham MD, Eyal FG, et al., eds. Neonatology: Management, Procedures, On-Call Problems, Diseases, and Drugs. 6th ed. New York: McGraw-Hill, 2009. [Review]
2. Kattwinkel J, ed. Textbook of Neonatal Resuscitation. 5th ed. Elk Grove Village, IL: American Academy of Pediatrics, 2006. [Review]
3. American Heart Association, American Academy of Pediatrics. 2005 American Heart Association guidelines for cardiopulmonary resuscitation (CPR) and emergency cardiovascular care

(ECC) of pediatric and neonatal patients: neonatal resuscitation guidelines. Pediatrics 2006; 117(5):e1029–e1038. [Review]

4. Natowicz M. Newborn screening—setting evidence-based policy for protection. N Engl J Med 2005; 353:867–870. [Review]

5. Watson MS, Mann MY, Lloyd-Puryear MA, et al.; American College of Medical Genetics Newborn Screening Expert Group. Newborn Screening: Toward a Uniform Screening Panel and System. Rockville, MD: Maternal and Child Health Bureau, 2005. [Review]

6. http://www.acmg.net/resources/policies/NBS/NBS-sections. htm. Accessed September 30, 2011. [Review]

7. American Academy of Pediatrics, Task Force on Circumcision. Circumcision policy statement. Pediatrics 1999; 103(3):686–693. [Review; reaffirmed September 1, 2005]

8. Larson JE, Desai SA, McNett W. Perinatal care and long-term implications. In: Berghella V, ed. Preterm Birth: Prevention and Management. Oxford, UK: Wiley-Blackwell, 2010. [Review]

9. Hankins GD, Speer M. Defining the pathogenesis and pathophysiology of neonatal encephalopathy and cerebral palsy. Obstet Gynecol 2003; 102:628–636. [Review]

29

Management of early pregnancy failure

Aileen M. Gariepy and Beatrice A. Chen

KEY POINTS

- The diagnosis of early (e.g., first trimester) pregnancy failure (aka loss) may be suspected on symptoms, but is usually made by **transvaginal ultrasound**, and/or symptoms and serial beta human chorionic gonadotrophin (BHCG) levels.
- **Early pregnancy failure (EPF)** is an inclusive term that comprises the following: incomplete, complete, or inevitable spontaneous abortion (SAB); anembryonic gestation (blighted ovum); and embryonic demise (missed abortion).
- There are **three options** for management of EPF: **expectant, medical, and surgical management**. Choice of management for EPF **does not affect future fertility**.
- **Patient preference should guide treatment choice**.
  - **Successful management** of EPF consists of complete evacuation of the uterus. The success of each of these approaches depends on several factors, for example, the type of loss (e.g., with or without symptoms).
- **Medical management**
  - **Medical management** is a **safe and effective** alternative to expectant management or surgical curettage for EPF.
  - Medical management of EPF is more effective than expectant management. **Misoprostol 800 µg vaginally, with a repeated dose on day 3 if complete evacuation is not confirmed**, has a success rate of **93% with incomplete or inevitable abortion, 88% with embryonic or fetal death, and 81% with anembryonic gestation** in women at <**13 weeks** of gestation.
  - Misoprostol 800 µg per vagina is the most studied regimen for medical management of EPF. Success of medical management of EPF increases with **multiple-dose** regimens. Whether there is added benefit from adding **mifepristone** to misoprostol is still uncertain.
  - Women choosing medical management of EPF report an **average of 12 days of bleeding**. Hemorrhage after medical management of EPF is rare.
  - **Follow-up:** Transvaginal ultrasound after medical management of EPF can be used to confirm successful expulsion of the gestational sac. Measurement of endometrial thickness is not predictive of success.
  - **Advantages of medical management** of EPF: Avoidance of surgery and anesthesia, perception of more natural treatment, increased privacy, and increased control.
- **Surgical management**
  - Surgical management has a high (>97%) success rate.
  - Endometritis or hemorrhage rates are ≤1%.
  - Maternal safety is highest with vacuum aspiration, when regional or general anesthesia can be avoided.

DEFINITIONS

Pregnancy loss (PL) (or pregnancy failure, PF): Spontaneous loss of pregnancy from conception to <20 weeks. The term SAB is often used as an equivalent but should be avoided since women may associate negative feelings with this term. This guideline does not discuss voluntary (elective) termination (induced abortion).

    Miscarriage: Lay term signifying pregnancy loss.

    Early pregnancy failure: Inclusive medical term describing inevitable abortion, incomplete abortion, anembryonic pregnancy, and embryonic/fetal demise at <**14 weeks** (1). It can also be called "first-trimester" PF. Early first-trimester PF is a loss of pregnancy between conception and 9 6/7 weeks. Late first-trimester PF is a loss of pregnancy between 10 and 13 6/7 weeks.

- **Spontaneous abortion** (aka loss)
  - **Complete:** Clinical definition describing an EPF that is characterized by a history of a positive pregnancy test, vaginal bleeding with passage of tissue, and a closed cervical os at the time of diagnosis. Transvaginal ultrasound exam shows a thin endometrial stripe.
  - **Incomplete:** Clinical definition describing a history of positive pregnancy test, vaginal bleeding, and a cervical os that may be open or closed. Transvaginal ultrasound exam shows heterogeneous tissue distorting the endometrial canal with or without a gestation sac. There is no agreement on a measurement of endometrial thickness that can distinguish incomplete from complete abortion (2).
  - **Inevitable:** Clinical definition describing an EPF that is characterized by a history of a positive pregnancy test, vaginal bleeding without passage of tissue, and an open cervical os.
- **Anembryonic pregnancy:** Previously described as "blighted ovum." It occurs when the embryonic disk has failed to develop or has already been resorbed (1). Anembryonic pregnancy is defined by **absence of a visible yolk sac with a mean sac diameter (MSD) of ≥13 mm, absence of an embryonic pole with MSD of ≥20 mm, or the presence of an empty amnion** (2,3).
- **Embryonic/Fetal demise:** Previously described as "missed abortion." It is defined by the failure of an embryo, previously identified, to grow and/or retain cardiac activity over time, or **by the absence of cardiac motion in embryos measuring 5 mm or more** (4) (see also chap. 15).

    Expectant management: No intervention and awaiting natural passage of tissue.

    Medical management: The use of medications to expel uterine tissue.

    Surgical management: The mechanical removal of tissue from the uterus.

DIAGNOSIS OF EPF
Transvaginal Ultrasound

- **Anembryonic pregnancy:** Absence of a visible yolk sac with an MSD of ≥13 mm, absence of an embryonic pole with MSD of ≥20 mm, or the presence of an empty amnion (2,3).
- **Embryonic/Fetal demise:** Defined by the failure of an embryo to grow over time or by the absence of cardiac motion in embryos measuring 5 mm or more (4).

Beta human chorionic gonadotrophin

- Abnormal pregnancies (EPF and ectopic pregnancies) usually have <15% increase in BHCG over ≥48 hours. If the BHCG is >1500 to 2000, a gestational sac should be visualized by transvaginal ultrasound; if the gestational sac is not seen in the uterus, suspect ectopic pregnancy.

SYMPTOMS OF EPF

Vaginal bleeding, lower abdominal cramping, and dilation of cervix. Women with EPF may also be asymptomatic.

EPIDEMIOLOGY/INCIDENCE OF EPF

Fifteen to twenty percent of clinically recognized pregnancies end in EPF (5). It is estimated that up to 60% of conceptions end up in early losses, most not clinically recognized (e.g., "late cycle") (see chap. 15).

ETIOLOGY OF EPF

Chromosomal abnormalities are responsible for >50% of all spontaneous EPF, most commonly translocations and aneuploidy. Many spontaneous losses may be secondary to other genetic defects that are impossible to discern by simple karyotype. Many other factors are also associated with spontaneous losses (see also chap. 15).

MANAGEMENT OF EPF
General Principles

- There are **three main options** for the woman with EPF (unless the spontaneous loss is complete): **expectant, medical,** and **surgical management**.
- Successful management of EPF entails complete evacuation of the uterus. The success of each of these approaches depends on several factors, for example, the type of loss (e.g., with or without symptoms).
- Failure of expectant or medical management results in the need for surgical evacuation.
- There are **several types of medical management approaches and several surgical approaches**.

Principles of Surgical Management

- **Procedure:** Surgical management of EPF can be accomplished via **vacuum aspiration or sharp curettage**.
- In comparisons of vacuum aspiration versus sharp curettage, **vacuum aspiration is preferred**, as it is associated with:
  - less blood loss [mean difference (MD) −17.10 mL, 95% CI −24.05 to −10.15 mL]
  - less pain during the procedure (RR 0.74, 95% CI 0.61–0.90)

- shorter duration of the procedure (MD −1.20 minutes, 95% CI −1.53 to −0.87 minutes)
- The small sample sizes of the trials were too small to evaluate rare complications such as uterine perforation and other morbidity (6).
- Vacuum aspiration can be accomplished with **electric vacuum aspiration (EVA) or manual vacuum aspiration (MVA)**. Both EVA and MVA can be types of dilation and curettage (D&C).
- **Location:** Vacuum aspiration can be accomplished in the operating room or in the office.
- **MVA is a safe alternative** for gestations 6 to 12 weeks with EPF, and can be performed in the **office under local anesthesia**.
- **There is no significant difference in the success or complication rates for MVA versus EVA** (7).

Principles of Medical Management
- **Medications used:**
  - **Misoprostol** is a prostaglandin E1 analogue. It is a uterotonic that results in cervical softening and contractions that expel the products of conception. Its route of administration may be vaginal, oral, buccal, or sublingual. Side effects vary based on route of administration (8).
  - **Mifepristone** is an antiprogestin that results in weakening of the uterine attachment of a pregnancy. This results in capillary breakdown and synthesis of prostaglandins.
  - **Methotrexate** (IM or oral) antagonizes folic acid, a cofactor needed for synthesis of nucleic acids. It is toxic to the rapidly dividing cells of the trophoblast. There is no role for methotrexate in the treatment of EPF (9).
- **Success** of medical management should be determined by expulsion of the gestational sac and not by endometrial thickness on transvaginal ultrasound. Studies that use an endometrial thickness of >15 mm to define failure of medical management may underestimate success rates of expectant and medical management (1).
- **Success** of medical management is **higher in patients with symptoms**, such as cramping and bleeding (10).
- **Contraindications:** The contraindications listed in Table 29.1 apply to medical management but can also apply to expectant management (7,11,12).
- **Complications:**
  - Complications are rare.
  - The incidence of gynecologic infection after surgical, expectant, or medical management of EPF is low (2–3%). There is no evidence to show a differential risk of infection by management choice (13).

Table 29.1 Contraindications to Medical (or Expectant) Management

- Hemodynamically or medically unstable patients
- Signs of pelvic infection and/or sepsis
- Suspected molar or ectopic pregnancy
- Caution should be used in women with hemoglobin ≤9.5 g/dL
- History of coagulopathy or current use of anticoagulants
- Allergy to prostaglandins[a]

[a]Specific to medical management.
Source: Modified from Refs. 7,12.

- In the largest randomized controlled trial (RCT) ($n = 652$) comparing medical with surgical management, there was no difference in the following complications (7):
  - Hemorrhage requiring hospitalization with or without blood transfusion (1%)
  - Hospitalization for endometritis (<1%)
  - Fever (3–4%)
  - Emergency visit to hospital within 24 hours of treatment (2–3%)
  - Unscheduled hospital visits (17–23%)
  - Decrease in hemoglobin ≥ 2 g/dL (4–9%)
  - Decrease in hemoglobin ≥ 3 g/dL (1–5%)

Principles of Expectant Management

- Expectant management of EPF is an option for women who would like to avoid surgical or medical treatment of EPF; however, time until resolution of EPF is unpredictable and may take as long as 6 weeks.
- Success of expectant management can range from 25% to 83%, depending on length of time of follow-up, definition of "failed" expectant management, and inclusion criteria (14–16).

Medical Vs. Surgical Management

- **Misoprostol versus surgical management:**
  - **Cochrane review**
    - Nine RCTs, $n = 1766$ with incomplete abortion before 13 weeks; misoprostol route: four oral, four vaginal, one vaginal and oral (17)
    - No significant difference in complete miscarriage (RR 0.96, 95% CI 0.92–1.00)
    - Not surprisingly, women using misoprostol have fewer surgical procedures (RR 0.07, 95% CI 0.03–0.18)
    - Risk of unplanned procedure is higher with misoprostol (RR 6.32, 95% CI 2.90–13.77)
    - Deaths and "serious complications" with either management are too rare to compare
  - **Largest multicenter RCT**
    - $n = 652$; 491 treated with **800 µg vaginal misoprostol** versus 161 by vacuum aspiration (7)
    - Participants
      - 94% anembryonic gestation, embryonic/fetal demise
      - 6% incomplete/inevitable abortion
    - **Medical regimen: 800 µg vaginal misoprostol, repeated on day 3 if incomplete expulsion (diagnosed by persistence of gestational sac or endometrial lining greater than 30 mm on transvaginal ultrasound), vacuum aspiration on day 8 if still incomplete**
    - **Success**
      - 97% success with vacuum aspiration
      - **84% success with misoprostol overall**
    - **71% success with one dose misoprostol**
      - Success increases to 84% with second dose of 800 µg vaginal misoprostol if gestational sac still present on ultrasound on day 3
    - **Success by type of EPF**
      - 93% for incomplete/inevitable abortion
      - 88% embryonic/fetal demise
      - 81% anembryonic pregnancy
    - Success did not vary by gestational age
    - Increased rates of nausea, vomiting, and diarrhea and abdominal pain in misoprostol group

- No difference in hemorrhage or endometritis between groups (<1%)
- Success of medical management associated with cramping, vaginal bleeding, and nulliparity (10)
- **Conclusion: Medical management with misoprostol is an acceptable alternative to surgical evacuation. Patient preference** should guide decision-making (17)

Medical Vs. Expectant Management

- Medical management involved mostly vaginal misoprostol (9)
- 24 RCTs, $n = 1888$, of embryonic/fetal demise or anembryonic pregnancy
- **Vaginal misoprostol** compared with expectant management:
  - Shortens the time to achieve complete uterine evacuation:
    - At less than 24 hours after treatment (RR 4.73, 95% CI 2.70–8.28)
    - At less than 48 hours after treatment (RR 5.74, 95% CI 2.70–12.19)
  - Results in less need for uterine curettage
  - Does not show a significant difference in need for blood transfusion (RR 0.2, 95% CI 0.01–4.0)
  - Does not have a significant increase in nausea (RR 1.38, 95% CI 0.43–4.40) or diarrhea (RR 2.21, 95% CI 0.35–14.06)
  - **Dosage** of vaginal misoprostol: When compared with lower dosages, **800 µg** vaginal misoprostol is more effective at completing uterine emptying (RR 0.85, 95% CI 0.72–1.00) with similar incidence of nausea
  - No advantage of "wet" versus "dry" preparation of vaginal misoprostol or of adding methotrexate
- Oral misoprostol is less effective than vaginal misoprostol in emptying the uterus (RR 0.90, 95% CI 0.82–0.99)
- Sublingual misoprostol is equivalent to vaginal misoprostol in inducing complete uterine emptying but was associated with more frequent diarrhea
- **Mifepristone:** Two trials of mifepristone added to misoprostol show conflicting results
- **Conclusion: Medical management with 800 µg of vaginal misoprostol is significantly more effective than expectant management** (9,17)

Expectant Vs. Surgical Management

- Cochrane review of five RCTs, $n = 689$ (18)
  - Expectant management has a higher incidence of the following:
    - Incomplete miscarriage (RR 5.3, 95% CI 2.57–11.22)
      - Of note, time interval to diagnose incomplete miscarriage differed among studies
    - Need for unplanned or additional surgical emptying of the uterus (RR 4.78, 95% CI 1.99–11.48)
    - Bleeding
      - More days of bleeding [weighted mean difference (WMD) 1.59, 95% CI 0.74–2.45]
      - Greater amount of bleeding (WMD 1.00, 95%CI 0.60–1.40)
  - Expectant management has a lower incidence of infection (RR 0.29, 95% CI 0.09–0.87)
  - Although differences were found between expectant versus surgical management, none of these differences were clinically serious
  - **Patient preference** should guide decision-making (18)

Misoprostol: Route, Dose, and Safety

- There is published literature on a wide range of therapeutic regimens (1,12,19).
- Optimal dose and route of administration of misoprostol have not been determined by randomized trials.
- **Misoprostol 800 µg per vagina** is the most studied regimen for medical management of EPF.
- Success of medical management of EPF increases with **multiple-dose regimens** (7).
- WHO recommends a single oral dose of 600 µg misoprostol for medical management of incomplete abortion (11).
- WHO recommends a single vaginal dose of 800 µg misoprostol for medical management of anembryonic pregnancy and embryonic/fetal demise (20). Misoprostol 600 µg sublingual is an alternative regimen (20).
- Overall, misoprostol is safe and well tolerated (8).
- Side effects of prostaglandins include diarrhea, nausea, and vomiting. These are increased when misoprostol is given orally.
- Patients receiving misoprostol vaginally have decreased gastrointestinal side effects and prolonged duration of action when compared with oral administration (8).

Antibiotics

There is no sufficient evidence to recommend or to abandon prophylactic antibiotics for surgical evacuation in women with an incomplete abortion. Clinical judgment is recommended (12,21).

Follow-Up

- There are no RCTs to assess optimal management of follow-up after PL in the first trimester. A clinical history and bimanual exam during a follow-up visit at 7 to 14 days after medication use is suggested (11).
- Endometrial thickness after medical or expectant management is not predictive of retained products of conception (POCs) and/or need for surgical evacuation (22).
- If chorionic villi or a gestational sac is obtained at D&C, there is usually no need for BHCG follow-up.
- After expectant or medical management of a known intrauterine pregnancy, BHCG, in general, do not need to be followed. Ultrasound can be used to confirm expulsion of the gestational sac.

FUTURE FERTILITY

- Choice of management for EPF does not affect future fertility.
- In long-term follow-up of women participating in an RCT of expectant, medical, or surgical management of EPF, there was no significant difference in the live birth rate 5 years after the index miscarriage (23).
  - Expectant management: 177/224 (79%, 95% CI 73–84%)
  - Medical management: 181/230 (79%, 95% CI 73–84%)
  - Surgical management: 192/235 (82%, 95% CI 76–86%)

PATIENT COUNSELING

- Patients choosing medical management of EPF should have appropriate counseling regarding expected symptoms.
- Bleeding
  - Bleeding with medical management is heavier and longer in duration than with surgical management (24).

- Women experienced approximately 12 days of bleeding after medical management of EPF (24).
- Bleeding will most likely be heavy for about 3 to 4 days, followed by light bleeding or spotting for several weeks (11).
- Bleeding associated with medical management of EPF rarely requires intervention (24).
- Patients should be counseled to contact their physician if they experience heavy vaginal bleeding (soaking through more than two extra large sanitary pads per hour for 2 consecutive hours) or signs of infection (11).
- Fever and/or chills
  - Some women experience fever and/or chills during the first 24 hours after misoprostol use.
  - Patients should call their doctor and be evaluated for infection if fever and/or chills persist beyond 24 hours after using misoprostol (11).
- Nausea and vomiting
  - May occur with use of misoprostol and will usually resolve 2 to 6 hours after taking misoprostol (11).

PATIENT ACCEPTABILITY

- In one study, the majority of women would prefer medical management of EPF with misoprostol to surgical management if its efficacy is >65% (25).
- In a large RCT comparing medical versus surgical management of EPF, women receiving medical management had significantly higher reports of treatment-related symptoms (cramping and bleeding), but overall quality of life and treatment acceptability were similar (26).
- In a large RCT comparing medical versus surgical management of EPF, 83% of women with EPF randomized to medical management with misoprostol would recommend medical management to others and 78% would probably/absolutely use medical management again (7).

PATIENT PREFERENCE

- Most women have strong preferences regarding management of EPF (27).
- Preferences are diverse and different women place different values on the advantages and disadvantages of avoiding the OR or of miscarrying at home, for example (27).
- Patient preference will depend on individual circumstances, expectations, and awareness of the advantages and disadvantages of each management option (27).
- Women have greater satisfaction when treated according to their preferences (27).
- Due to the comparable safety and efficacy of all current treatment options for EPF, patient preference should be the guiding force deciding management of EPF.

REFERENCES

1. Chen BA, Creinin MD. Medical management of early pregnancy failure: efficacy. Semin Reprod Med 2008; 26(5):411–422; [Epub September 29, 2008]. [Review]
2. Perriera L, Reeves MF. Ultrasound criteria for diagnosis of early pregnancy failure and ectopic pregnancy. Semin Reprod Med 2008; 26(5):373–382; [Epub September 29, 2008]. Erratum in: Semin Reprod Med 2009; 27(1):103. [Review]
3. McKenna KM, Feldstein VA, Goldstein RB, et al. The empty amnion: a sign of early pregnancy failure. J Ultrasound Med 1995; 14:117–121. [II-2]

4. Brown DL, Emerson DS, Felker RE, et al. Diagnosis of early embryonic demise by endovaginal sonography. J Ultrasound Med 1990; 9:631–636. [II-3]

5. Hemminki E. Treatment of miscarriage: current practice and rationale. Obstet Gynecol 1998; 91:247–253. [Review]

6. Tunçalp O, Gülmezoglu AM, Souza JP. Surgical procedures for evacuating incomplete miscarriage. Cochrane Database Syst Rev 2010; (9):CD001993.[Meta-analysis: 2 RCTs, *n* = 550]

7. Zhang J, Gilles JM, Barnhart K, et al.; National Institute of Child Health Human Development (NICHD) Management of Early Pregnancy Failure Trial. A comparison of medical management with misoprostol and surgical management for early pregnancy failure. N Engl J Med 2005; 353(8):761–769. [RCT, *n* = 652]

8. Tang OS, Gemzell-Danielsson K, Ho PC. Misoprostol: pharmacokinetic profiles, effects on the uterus and side-effects. Int J Gynaecol Obstet 2007; 99(suppl 2):S160–S167; [Epub October 26, 2007]. [Review]

9. Neilson JP, Hickey M, Vazquez J. Medical treatment for early fetal death (less than 24 weeks). Cochrane Database Syst Rev 2006; 3:CD002253.[Review]

10. Creinin MD, Huang X, Westhoff C, et al.; National Institute of Child Health and Human Development Management of Early Pregnancy Failure Trial. Factors related to successful misoprostol treatment for early pregnancy failure. Obstet Gynecol 2006; 107(4):901–907. [II-2]

11. Blum J, Winikoff B, Gemzell-Danielsson K, et al. Treatment of incomplete abortion and miscarriage with misoprostol. Int J Gynaecol Obstet 2007; 99(suppl 2):S186–S189; [Epub October 24, 2007]. [Review]

12. Royal College of Obstetricians and Gynaecologists (RCOG). Green-Top Guideline No. 25: The management of early pregnancy loss. London, UK: RCOG, 2006.[Guideline; 75 references]

13. Trinder J, Brocklehurst P, Porter R, et al. Management of miscarriage: expectant, medical, or surgical? Results of randomised controlled trial (miscarriage treatment (MIST) trial). BMJ 2006; 332(7552):1235–1240; [Epub May 17, 2006]. [RCT]

14. Blohm F, Friden B, Platz-Christensen J-J, et al. Expectant management of first trimester miscarriage in clinical practice. Acta Obstet Gynecol Scand 2003; 82:654–658. [II-2]

15. Jurkovic D, Ross JA, Nicolaides KH. Expectant management of missed miscarriage. Br J Obstet Gynaecol 1998; 105:670–671. [II-2]

16. Luise C, Jermy K, May C, et al. Outcome of expectant management of spontaneous first trimester miscarriage: observational study. BMJ 2002; 324:873–875. [II-2]

17. Neilson JP, Gyte GML, Hickey M, et al. Medical treatments for incomplete miscarriage (less than 24 weeks). Cochrane Database Syst Rev 2010; (1):CD007223.[Meta-analysis: 15 RCTs, *n* = 2750]

18. Nanda K, Peloggia A, Grimes DA, et al. Expectant care versus surgical treatment for miscarriage. Cochrane Database Syst Rev 2006; (2):CD003518.[Meta-analysis: 5 trials, *n* = 689]

19. Dempsey A, Davis A. Medical management of early pregnancy failure: how to treat and what to expect. Semin Reprod Med 2008; 26(5):401–410; [Epub September 29, 2008]. [Review]

20. Gemzell-Danielsson K, Ho PC, Gómez Ponce de León R, et al. Misoprostol to treat missed abortion in the first trimester. Int J Gynaecol Obstet 2007; 99(suppl 2):S182–S185; [Epub October 24, 2007]. [II-2]

21. May W, Gülmezoglu AM, Ba-Thike K. Antibiotics for incomplete abortion. Cochrane Database Syst Rev 2007; (4):CD001779. [Review]

22. Reeves MF, Lohr PA, Harwood BJ, et al. Ultrasonographic endometrial thickness after medical and surgical management of early pregnancy failure. Obstet Gynecol 2008; 111(1):106–112. [II-3]

23. Smith LF, Ewings PD, Quinlan C. Incidence of pregnancy after expectant, medical, or surgical management of spontaneous first trimester miscarriage: long term follow-up of miscarriage treatment (MIST) randomised controlled trial. BMJ 2009; 339:b3827. [II-1]

24. Davis AR, Hendlish SK, Westhoff C, et al. Bleeding patterns after misoprostol vs surgical treatment of early pregnancy failure: results from a randomized trial. Am J Obstet Gynecol 2007; 196:31.e1–31.e7. [RCT]

25. Graziosi GC, Bruinse HW, Reuwer PJ, et al. Women's preferences for misoprostol in case of early pregnancy failure. Eur J Obstet Gynecol Reprod Biol 2006; 124:184–186. [II-3]

26. Harwood B, Nansel T for the National Institute of Child Health and Human Development Management of Early Pregnancy Failure Trial. Quality of life and acceptability of medical versus surgical management of early pregnancy failure. Br J Obstet Gynecol 2008; 115:501–508. [II-2]

27. Wallace RR, Goodman S, Freedman LR, et al. Counseling women with early pregnancy failure: utilizing evidence, preserving preference. Patient Educ Couns 2010; 81(3):454–461; [Epub November 18, 2010]. [II-3]

30

The adnexal mass

George Patounakis and Norman G. Rosenblum

KEY POINTS

- There are **no trials** on any intervention for adnexal mass in pregnancy.
- **Ultrasound,** with transvaginal and Doppler capabilities, **is the mainstay of diagnosis and prognosis.**
- Complications related to the **persistent adnexal mass** in gravid patients may include **severe pain** (5–26%), **ovarian torsion** (7–12%), **cyst rupture** (9%), **pelvic impaction and obstruction of labor** (17%), and **ovarian cancer** (<5%).
- Management in the **first trimester** is almost uniformly **expectant** when the clinical presentation is not acute.
- For **persistent adnexal mass in pregnancy**, early preoperative **consultation with gynecologic oncologist, anesthesiologist, and neonatologist** is recommended.
- **Surgery** in pregnancy can be reserved for adnexal masses that persist in the second trimester, and are either **complex, with papillations and/or bilateral and >5 cm, or increase by >30% in size, or simple but >10 cm.**
- When necessary and feasible, **surgery should be scheduled in the early second trimester** when organogenesis is complete, most spontaneous abortions have occurred, and the risk for premature delivery is low.
- Intervention in the **third trimester** is typically **deferred until delivery or the postpartum period**.
- **Intervention** should be considered **at any point** in gestation **if a mass is complex or suspicious for malignancy and increases in size**.
- If a suspicious **adnexal mass** is **identified incidentally at the time of cesarean section**, it should be **removed** and not simply aspirated.
- **If** a **malignant neoplasm of the ovary** is found at the time of exploration, the surgeon's first obligation is to properly **stage the disease**.
- For more advanced ovarian cancer, the degree of cytoreductive surgery and the timing of initiation of chemotherapy will depend on fetal viability and maternal choice.

DEFINITION/DIAGNOSIS

An adnexal mass is any mass in the ovary or tube or attached to them (adnexa). The vast majority (>90%) of adnexal masses in pregnancy are ovarian. Table 30.1 outlines the differential diagnosis of an adnexal mass during pregnancy (1). The diagnosis is most accurately made **by ultrasound**, even if it is possible to diagnose an adnexal mass by bimanual physical exam. A persistent adnexal mass is one that does not resolve by the second trimester.

EPIDEMIOLOGY/INCIDENCE

In earlier studies, approximately 1% to 4% of women were diagnosed with an adnexal mass in pregnancy with persistence of only 1 in 200 to 1 in 600 into the second trimester (2). A more recent study of adnexal masses that performed ultrasound of asymptomatic women during nuchal translucency evaluation (11–14 weeks) found an **incidence of almost 25%, with 85% of those resolving during the pregnancy without intervention** (3). This dramatic increase in incidence is likely secondary to the early prevalence of functional cysts that spontaneously resolve during the pregnancy. The majority of the adnexal masses are simple cysts such as corpus luteum or other functional cysts. **Most of them** (up to 90%) **when identified during pregnancy will spontaneously regress prior to the second trimester.** The likelihood of regression is inversely related to size. Only 6% of cysts <6 cm compared with 39% of cysts >6 cm persist into the second trimester of pregnancy (4–6). Two adnexal conditions are specifically associated with pregnancy and spontaneously regress in the postpartum period requiring no further treatment—luteomas of pregnancy and theca lutein cysts. Only **1% to 5% of adnexal masses are malignant ovarian tumors** (4,7). The incidence of ovarian cancer in pregnancy is rare, 1 in 18,000 to 1 in 47,000 deliveries (8,9).

CLASSIFICATION

Among persistent adnexal masses diagnosed during pregnancy (age group 18–35 years), **mature teratomas are the most common** followed by benign serous or mucinous cystadenomas (Table 30.2). Most of the literature on ovarian cancer in pregnancy is based on case reports and series. In the largest case series, the most common ovarian cancers found in pregnancy are serous and mucinous tumors of low malignant potential (1).

RISK FACTORS/ASSOCIATIONS

Maternal age is a risk factor for malignancy, but ovarian malignancies can occur at any reproductive age. A recent study assessing the accuracy of combining patient demographics, serum CA-125, and ultrasonographic features in predicting the risk of malignancy of an ultrasonographically confirmed adnexal mass in nonpregnant women found age, menopausal status, weight, tumor morphology, presence of ascites, tumor laterality, tumor diameter, and CA-125 level to be associated with risk of malignancy (11). Specifically, **age ≤55, premenopausal weight >200 lb, cystic morphology, negative ascites, unilaterality, diameter <10 cm, and CA-125 <35 were associated with benign masses.** None of the cystic tumors in that study were malignant. Furthermore, a large study in postmenopausal women with unilocular cystic masses <10 cm found none to have malignancy (12). **Assisted reproductive technologies** increase the incidence of enlarged ovaries, cysts, and therefore adnexal masses.

Table 30.1 Differential diagnosis of most common adnexal masses in pregnancy

Benign	Malignant
Corpus luteum	Germ cell tumor
Simple cyst	Cystadenocarcinoma
Hemorrhagic cyst	Borderline tumors
Dermoid	Sex-cord stromal tumor
Endometrioma	Metastatic cancer to ovary
Myoma	
Luteoma	
Hyperstimulated ovary	
Hydrosalpinx	
Theca lutein cyst	
Ectopic/Heterotopic pregnancy	
Cystadenoma	
Peritoneal cyst	
Paraovarian/Paratubal cyst	

Source: From Ref. 1.

Table 30.2 Relative Frequency of Adnexal Masses Diagnosed in Pregnancy

Diagnosis	Percent
Mature teratoma	43.0
Serous or mucinous cystadenoma	18.6
Corpus luteum	12.0
Follicular cyst	9.0
Endometrioma	7.1
Fibroids	6.3
Malignancy	2.4
Other	1.6

Source: From Ref. 10.

COMPLICATIONS

Complications related to the persistent adnexal mass in gravid patients include **severe pain** (26%), **ovarian torsion** (12%), **cyst rupture** (9%), and **pelvic impaction and obstruction of labor** (17%) (13). Ovarian torsion, the most common significant complication in pregnancy, occurs usually in less than 15% of the cases and is most common in adnexal masses with sizes between 6 and 8 cm (14). Approximately 60% of torsion happens between 10 and 17 weeks' gestation and less than 6% happens after 20 weeks' gestation (14). The risk of **ovarian cancer** is usually <5% (15). Most malignancies are either germ cell, stromal, or epithelial tumors of low malignant potential (16).

MANAGEMENT
Principles

There are **no trials** available to assess any intervention in the management of adnexal masses in pregnancy. **As about 90% of these masses resolve and the risk of malignancy is <5%, in general, expectant management with serial ultrasounds is usually appropriate in the vast majority of, but not all, clinical situations.** If malignancy is suspected, the best gestational age for surgery is about 16 to 18 weeks, as the risk of loss is lowest.

Workup
Ultrasound

Highly skilled ultrasonographers may be able to accurately diagnose complications of adnexal masses in pregnancy (e.g., cancer and torsion) without surgical intervention. Suspicious characteristics of an adnexal mass include **complex** masses consisting of both **solid and cystic components** with nodular-

ity, thick septations, irregular borders, solid masses containing irregular echoes, and papillary projections (17). While cancer can be present in a cyst of any size, adnexal masses of ≤5 cm have an incidence of malignancy less than 1% (15). Even unilocular cysts <10 cm in postmenopausal women can be safely followed by serial ultrasounds until they resolve or develop solid and/or wall abnormalities prompting surgical intervention secondary to a high suspicion of malignancy (12). In addition to routine ultrasonography, color **Doppler** studies may be used to distinguish between malignant and benign adnexal masses (18). Low pulsatility index of <1.0 and low impedance are associated with ovarian neoplasms. **Transvaginal** ultrasound may also help to better visualize the adnexal mass. The overall sensitivity of high-resolution ultrasound in distinguishing malignant from benign adnexal masses is 96.6%, specificity of 77%, and negative predictive value of 99% (18). After 20 weeks, adnexal masses are more difficult to see by ultrasound given the larger uterine size. However, definitive diagnosis requires pathologic confirmation.

Magnetic Resonance Imaging

Magnetic resonance imaging (MRI) has been used in addition to ultrasound to characterize adnexal masses. There are insufficient data to assess the effect of MRI on management of adnexal masses in pregnancy, but a review of the topic with respect to each type of adnexal mass and the usefulness of MRI has been recently published (19). The conclusions are that MRI can assist ultrasound in distinguishing an exophytic leiomyoma, the red degeneration of a leiomyoma, an endometrioma, a dermoid cyst, and a decidualized endometrioma, from other masses. Furthermore, it supports the value in MRI of detecting massive ovarian edema and distant findings such as widespread ascites, peritoneal implants, and lymphadenopathy that can help distinguish benign from malignant masses.

Laboratory

Most tumor markers may be elevated in normal pregnancy and are generally **not helpful** in distinguishing between a benign or malignant ovarian mass in pregnancy. For example, up to 16% of pregnant patients may have an elevated **CA-125** (20). Levels of CA-125 peak in the first trimester (range, 7–251 units/mL), and decrease consistently thereafter. Low-level elevations in pregnancy are typically not associated with malignancy (16).

Therapy

Treatment planning is dependent upon the timeliness of detection of an adnexal mass in pregnancy. When an adnexal mass is diagnosed in the first trimester, the likelihood of a functional etiology is high, as is the probability of spontaneous resolution. In pregnant women, most simple cysts <6 cm have been shown to spontaneously resolve (21–24). Given the high obstetrical risk during this period, **the management in the first trimester is almost uniformly expectant when the clinical presentation is not acute** (15). Similarly, **intervention in the third trimester is typically deferred until delivery or the postpartum period as the risk of delaying therapy rarely outweighs the risk of surgery to the mother and the fetus.** When necessary and feasible, **surgery should be scheduled in the early second trimester** after most functional cysts have resolved, organogenesis is complete, most spontaneous losses have occurred, and the risk for premature delivery is low. **Intervention should be considered at any point in gestation if a mass is complex or highly suspicious for malignancy and increases in size** (Fig. 30.1). In addition to suspected

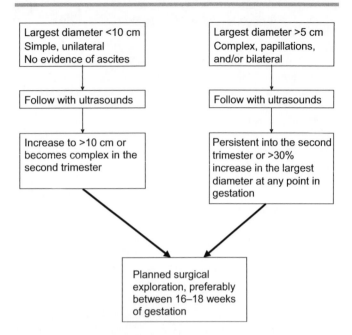

Figure 30.1   Management of the ovarian mass in pregnancy.

Table 30.3   Preoperative, Intraoperative, and Postoperative Considerations

Preoperative management	Preoperative hydration—to reduce risk of hypotension, uteroplacental insufficiency, and resultant fetal hypoxemia
Placement	15% left lateral tilt if the uterus is >20 wk to shift the uterus off the inferior vena cava/wedge placement under the right hip
Monitoring	All viable fetuses (≥24 wk) may be continuously monitored
Anesthesia	Preoxygenation with 100% oxygen administered by face mask for 3–5 min
	Halothane, isoflurane, and enflurane decrease uterine tone and may inhibit labor during the operative procedure
	Cocaine hydrochloride is a vasoconstrictor and contraindicated during pregnancy

Source: From Refs. 26–28.

malignancy, **surgical intervention may be indicated if torsion, rupture, or hemorrhage is identified.**

For persistent adnexal masses in pregnancy, **early preoperative consultation with a gynecologic oncologist, anesthesiologist, and neonatologist is recommended** (25). Consultation at <15 weeks is recommended for better operative planning.

Surgery
When exploration is necessary, all efforts should be made to **avoid unnecessary manipulation of the uterus** to minimize premature uterine contractions. Other intraoperative and postoperative considerations should be kept in mind when operating on a pregnant patient (Table 30.3) (26–28). While traditionally a laparotomy was the standard recommendation used to explore the abdomen of a pregnant patient with an adnexal mass, **laparoscopy** is currently not only an acceptable alternative (in experienced hands) but also is

Table 30.4   FIGO Staging for Ovarian Cancer

Stage I—Growth limited to the ovaries
    Stage Ia—Growth limited to one ovary, no ascites, no tumor on external surface, and capsule intact
    Stage Ib—Growth limited to both ovaries, no ascites, no tumor on external surface, and capsule intact
    Stage Ic—Tumor either stage Ia or Ib but with tumor on surface of one or both ovaries, ruptured capsule, ascites with malignant cells, or positive peritoneal washings
Stage II—Growth involving one or both ovaries, with pelvic extension
    Stage IIa—Extension and/or metastases to the uterus or tubes
    Stage IIb—Extension to other pelvic tissues
    Stage IIc—Stage IIa or IIb but with tumor on surface of one or both ovaries, ruptured capsule, ascites with malignant cells, or positive peritoneal washings
Stage III—Tumor involving one or both ovaries, with peritoneal implants outside the pelvis and/or positive retroperitoneal or inguinal nodes; superficial liver metastases
    Stage IIIa—Tumor grossly limited to pelvis, negative lymph nodes but histological proof of microscopic disease on abdominal peritoneal surfaces
    Stage IIIb—Confirmed implants of abdominal peritoneal surfaces; no implant exceeds 2 cm in diameter and lymph nodes are negative.
    Stage IIIc—Abdominal implants >2 cm in diameter and/or positive lymph nodes
Stage IV—Distant metastases; pleural effusion must have a positive cytology to be classified as stage IV; parenchymal liver metastases

Abbreviation: FIGO, Fédération Internationale de Gynécologie et d'Obstétrique (International Federation of Gynecology and Obstetrics).

preferred in cases with low suspicion of malignancy, as it offers the benefit of a more expeditious recovery (29–31). Laparoscopic surgery can be safely performed for ovarian torsion during pregnancy (32,33). Abdominal surgery during pregnancy, in particular laparotomy, has been associated with higher rates of miscarriage and preterm birth compared with no surgery (15).

If a suspicious adnexal mass is identified incidentally **at the time of cesarean section**, it should be removed and not simply aspirated (2). With aspiration and cytologic evaluation, malignancy could be missed (34).

If a malignant neoplasm of the ovary is found at the time of exploration, the surgeon's first obligation is to properly stage the disease (Table 30.4). Since most present as stage I disease, a unilateral salpingo-oophorectomy, omentectomy, and limited pelvic and paraaortic lymph node dissection is the procedure of choice. If the disease appears to be confined to the pelvis, comprehensive surgical staging is indicated. The staging procedure includes peritoneal cytology, multiple peritoneal biopsies, omentectomy, and pelvic and paraaortic lymph node sampling. Rarely is a hysterectomy indicated. **For more advanced disease, the degree of cytoreductive surgery and the timing of initiation of chemotherapy will depend on fetal viability and maternal choice, and should be managed by a gynecologic oncologist.**

REFERENCES

1. Schwartz N, Timor-Tritsch I, Wang E. Adnexal masses in pregnancy. Clin Obstet Gynecol 2009; 52:570–585. [Review]
2. Koonings PP, Platt LD, Wallace R. Incidental adnexal neoplasms at cesarean section. Obstet Gynecol 1988; 72:767–769. [II-3]

3. Yazbek J, Salim R, Woelfer B, et al. The value of ultrasound visualization of the ovaries during the routine 11-14 weeks nuchal translucency scan. Eur J Obstet Gynecol Reprod Biol 2007; 132:154–158. [II-3, *n* = 2925]

4. Hess LW, Peaceman A, O'Brien WF, et al. Adnexal mass occurring with intrauterine pregnancy: report of fifty-four patients requiring laparotomy for definitive management. Am J Obstet Gynecol 1988; 158:1029–1034. [II-3]

5. Whitecar MP, Turner S, Higby MK. Adnexal masses in pregnancy: a review of 130 cases undergoing surgical management. Am J Obstet Gynecol 1999; 181:19–24. [II-3]

6. Beischer NA, Buttery BW, Fortune DW, et al. Growth and malignancy of ovarian tumours in pregnancy. Aust NZ J Obstet Gynaecol 1971; 11:208–220. [II-3]

7. El Yahia AR, Rahman J, Rahman MS, et al. Ovarian tumors in pregnancy. Aust NZ J Obstet Gynecol 1991; 31:327–330. [II-3]

8. Munnell EW. Primary ovarian cancer associated with pregnancy. Clin Obstet Gynecol 1963; 6:983–993. [III]

9. Dgani R, Shoham Z, Atar E, et al. Ovarian carcinoma during pregnancy: a study of 23 cases in Israel between the years of 1963 and 1984. Gynecol Oncol 1989; 33:326–331. [II-3]

10. Liu JR, Lilja JF, Johnston C. Adnexal masses in pregnancy. In: Trimble EL, Trimble CL, eds. Cancer Obstetrics and Gynecology. Philadelphia, PA: Lippincott Williams & Wilkins, 1999:239–248. [III]

11. McDonald JM, Doran S, DeSimone CP, et al. Predicting risk of malignancy in adnexal masses. Obstet Gynecol 2010; 115:687–694. [II-2, *n* = 395]

12. Modesitt SC, Pavlik EJ, Ueland FR, et al. Risk of malignancy in unilocular ovarian cystic tumors less than 10 centimeters in diameter. Obstet Gynecol 2003; 102:594–599. [II-2, *n* = 3259]

13. Struyk AP, Treffers PE. Ovarian tumors in pregnancy. Acta Obstet Gynecol Scand 1984; 63:421–424. [II-3]

14. Yen C, Lin S, Murk W, et al. Risk analysis of torsion and malignancy for adnexal masses during pregnancy. Fertil Steril 2009; 91:1895–1902. [II-3, *n* = 174]

15. Schmeler KM, Mayo-Smith WW, Peipert JF, et al. Adnexal masses in pregnancy: surgery compared with observation. Obstet Gynecol 2005; 105:1098–1103. [II-3]

16. American College of obstetricians and Gynecologists. ACOG Practice Bulletin No. 83: Management of adnexal masses. Obstet Gynecol 2007; 110:201–214. [Review]

17. Bromley B, Benacerraf B. Adnexal masses during pregnancy: accuracy of sonographic diagnosis and outcome. J Ultrasound Med 1997; 16:447–454. [II-3]

18. Wheeler TC, Fleischer AC. Complex adnexal mass in pregnancy: predictive value of color Doppler ultrasonography. J Ultrasound Med 1997; 16:425–428. [II-2, *n* = 34]

19. Telischak NA, Yeh BM, Joe BN, et al. MRI of adnexal masses in pregnancy. Am J Roentgenol 2008; 191:364–370. [Review]

20. Niloff JM, Knapp RC, Schaetzi E, et al. CA125 antigen levels in obstetric and gynecology patients. Obstet Gynecol 1984; 64:703–707. [II-3]

21. Hogston P, Lilford RJ. Ultrasound study of ovarian cysts in pregnancy: prevalence and significance. Br J Obstet Gynaecol 1986; 93:625–628. [II-3]

22. Thornton JG, Wells M. Ovarian cysts in pregnancy: does ultrasound make traditional management inappropriate? Obstet Gynecol 1987; 69:717–721. [II-3]

23. Bernhard LM, Klebba PK, Gray DL, et al. Predictors of persistence of adnexal masses in pregnancy. Obstet Gynecol 1999; 93:585–589. [II-3]

24. Zanetta G, Mariani E, Lissoni A, et al. A prospective study of the role of ultrasound in the management of adnexal masses in pregnancy. Br J Obstet Gynecol 2003; 110:578–583. [II-2, *n* = 79]

25. American College of obstetricians and Gynecologists. ACOG Committee Opinion No. 284: Nonobstetric surgery in pregnancy. Obstet Gynecol 2003; 102:431. [Review]

26. Caspi B, Appelman Z, Rabinerson D, et al. Pathognomonic echo patterns of benign cystic teratomas of the ovary: classification, incidence and accuracy rate of sonographic diagnosis. Ultrasound Obstet Gynecol 1996; 7:275–279. [II-2, *n* = 115]

27. Granberg S, Wikland M, Jansson I. Macroscopic characterization of ovarian tumors and the relation to the histological diagnosis: criteria to be used for ultrasound evaluation. Gynecol Oncol 1989; 35:139–144. [II-3]

28. Hata K, Hata T. Intratumoral blood flow analysis in ovarian cancer: what does it mean? J Ultrasound Med 1996; 15:571–575. [II-3]

29. Soriano D, Yefet Y, Seidman DS, et al. Laparoscopy versus laparotomy in the management of adnexal masses during pregnancy. Fertil Steril 1999; 71:955–960. [II-2, *n* = 88]

30. Yuen PM, Ng PS, Leung PL, Rogers MS. Outcome in laparoscopic management of persistent adnexal mass during the second trimester of pregnancy. Surg Endosc 2004; 18(9):354–357. [II-3]

31. Mathevet P, Nessah K, Dargent D, et al. Laparoscopic management of adnexal masses in pregnancy: a case series. Eur J Obstet Gynecol Reprod Biol 2003; 108(2):217–222. [II-3]

32. Shalev E, Peleg D. Laparoscopic treatment of adnexal torsion. Surg Gynecol Obstet 1993; 176:448–450. [II-3]

33. Cohen SB, Oelsner G, Seidman DS, et al. Laparoscopic detorsion allows sparing of the twisted ischemic adnexa. J Am Assoc Gynecol Laparosc 1999; 6:139–143. [II-3]

34. Rodin A, Coltart TM, Chapman MG. Needle aspiration of simple ovarian cysts in pregnancy. Case reports. Br J Obstet Gynaecol 1989; 96:994–946. [II-3]

31

Cervical cancer screening

Cheung K. Kim

KEY POINTS

- Cervical cancer screening guidelines for nonpregnant women can be followed in pregnant women. These suggest **initiating Pap smear screening at age 21, regardless of onset of sexual activity. Routine screening intervals have also been extended to every 2 years for women in their 20s and every 3 years in women over 30 who have had three consecutive normal Pap smears.**
- **The only cervical diagnosis** that is considered **to alter management in pregnancy** is **invasive cancer.**
- New guidelines recommend a more **conservative approach to managing cervical intraepithelial neoplasia (CIN).**
- Due to risks of bleeding and premature rupture of membranes, **endocervical curettage (ECC)** is **generally precluded in pregnancy.**
- **Diagnostic conization** during pregnancy should **only be considered when** either the biopsy or cytology is **suggestive of invasive cancer** and the diagnosis of invasion would result in a modification of treatment recommendations, timing, or mode of delivery.
- **If** the histologic diagnosis of **invasive cervical cancer (ICC)** is made and a **grossly visible** lesion is detected, **cesarean delivery** is indicated and results in better survival outcomes as well as a decreased risk of obstetrical bleeding in the intrapartum and postpartum periods.
- **If a microinvasive** (stage IA1) **or a nonvisible invasive lesion** (stage IA2) is identified, **either the abdominal or vaginal route of delivery is acceptable,** depending upon obstetrical and gynecologic circumstances.
- Once the diagnosis of cervical cancer is established, individualized recommendations for the **management of the malignancy** as well as the **pregnancy** are formulated **with consideration for the stage of disease, gestational age at the time of diagnosis, and maternal desires regarding the continuation of her pregnancy.**
- Fertility-sparing surgery and neoadjuvant chemotherapy for earlier stage cervical cancer found in pregnancy may be considered without worsening survival.

HISTORIC NOTES

The cytologic evaluation of the cervix, known as the Pap smear, was developed in the 1940s by George Papanicolaou. The Bethesda System standardized terminology for reporting Pap smears in 1988 (1), and was subsequently revised in 2001 (2).

DIAGNOSIS/DEFINITION

Microinvasive cervical cancer (MCC) is defined as cancer spread to no more than 5 mm into the tissues of the cervix. Invasive cervical cancer (ICC) is defined as cancer spread from the surface of the cervix to tissue deeper in the cervix, possible spread to part of the vagina, to the lymph nodes, to other tissues surrounding the cervix, within the pelvis, or beyond the pelvic areas into nearby organs.

EPIDEMIOLOGY/INCIDENCE

The overall rate of an abnormal Pap smear [atypical squamous cells–undetermined significance (ASC-US) or higher] in the United States from 1995 to 2001 was 6% (3,4). The peak age incidence of cervical cancer is in the mid-40s. Cervical cancer is the second most common cancer among women worldwide, the third most common cause of cancer-related death, and the most common cause of mortality from gynecologic malignancy worldwide. Although in the majority of developing countries cervical cancer remains the number-one cause of cancer-related deaths among women, Pap smear screening in developed countries became a preventive medicine issue by accurately detecting preinvasive and early-invasive cervical disease. In the United States, the incidence of cervical cancer ranges from 1.5 to 12 cases in 100,000 pregnancies (5). About 1% of the women who have cervical cancer are pregnant at the time of diagnosis. However, the likelihood that a pregnant woman with ASC pathology has a detectable high-risk human papillomavirus (HR HPV) is 84% (6).

CLASSIFICATION

The Pap smear report consists of the following (2):

Specimen Type

For example, conventional Pap smear or liquid-based cytology.

Specimen Adequacy

Satisfactory for Evaluation

- Defined as a minimum of 5000 well-visualized squamous cells on a liquid-based preparation or 8000 to 12,000 well-visualized squamous cells on a conventional smear.
- The presence of endocervical cells indicates that the area at risk for neoplasia, the transformation zone, has been adequately sampled.
- In contrast, absence of endocervical cells may reflect inadequate sampling of the transformation zone. If recent Pap smears have been normal, then repeat Pap in 12 months is acceptable. Otherwise, repeating the Pap smear in 6 months is recommended. Pregnant patients with a normal Pap lacking endocervical cells may repeat the Pap smear postpartum (7).

Unsatisfactory for Evaluation

- Defined as more than 75% of the cells being uninterpretable or unlabeled specimen.
- Since women with this result are more likely to have intraepithelial lesions or cancer on follow-up than women with satisfactory Pap smears (8), test should always be repeated in 2 to 4 months (9). If Pap smear is repeatedly unsatisfactory, evaluation with colposcopy and/or biopsies is appropriate (9).

Interpretation/Result

Squamous Epithelial Cell Abnormalities

- ASC of either of the following:
  - Undetermined significance (ASC-US) or
  - Suspicious for high-grade squamous intraepithelial lesions (HSIL) (ASC-H).
- Low-grade squamous intraepithelial lesions (LSIL)
  - Changes consistent with HPV, mild dysplasia, or grade 1 cervical intraepithelial neoplasia (CIN I).
- HSIL
  - HSIL includes moderate or severe dysplasia, CIN II, CIN III, carcinoma in situ (CIS) and should indicate if there are features suspicious for invasive disease. When glandular cell abnormalities are present, it should be noted whether there are changes favoring neoplasia.
- Carcinoma

Glandular Cell Abnormalities

- Atypical glandular cells (AGC) may be of endocervical, endometrial, or other glandular origin
- Endocervical adenocarcinoma in situ (AIS)
- Adenocarcinoma

Any Ancillary Testing Done

For example, HPV testing—important in management of ASC-US Pap smear.

- HPV infection is the leading etiologic agent in the development of premalignant and malignant lower genital tract disease (10).
- The most well-studied HPV test is the Hybrid Capture 2 HPV DNA Assay (Digene Corporation, Beltsville, Maryland, U.S.), which uses a probe mix for high-risk (HR) HPV types 16, 18, 31, 33, 35, 39, 45, 51, 52, 56, 58, 59, and 68. A newer assay for detecting HR HPV was approved for FDA use in 2009. Cervista^{TM} HR HPV (Hologic Corporation, Waltham, Massachusetts, U.S.) includes the 13 HPV types above and adds type 66 (7). The use of HPV testing was validated in 2001 by a consensus group of the American Society for Colposcopy and Cervical Pathology (see below) (11).
- Cervista HPV 16/18 is another diagnostic test that specifies type 16 and 18. These two represent the most common types found in cervical squamous cell carcinomas and adenocarcinomas, respectively. Subsequently, 2009 guidelines incorporating testing for HPV 16/18 were added in the specific instance of women over 30 who were cytology normal but HPV positive, to determine if colposcopy was indicated by the presence of these two high-risk types (7).
- Ongoing research looks promising in improving specificity and positive predictive value of screening for CIN2+ by looking at mRNA instead of DNA for HR HPV (12).

MANAGEMENT
Pregnancy Considerations

Pregnancy-induced changes in the cervix include hyperemia, eversion of columnar epithelium, more prominent glands, and increased production and volume of mucus. The decidual changes may exaggerate the colposcopic appearance of CIN. A biopsy during pregnancy may cause substantial bleeding (9). In pregnancy, the general philosophy for the treatment of intraepithelial neoplasia of the cervix has become expectant management after careful diagnosis.

Screening

The Pap smear is used to screen for cellular abnormalities that are associated with an increased risk for the development of cervical cancer. It selects those women who should have further evaluation, such as HPV DNA testing, colposcopy, and/or biopsy, which then are used for treatment decisions. The National Comprehensive Cancer Network (NCCN) panel has adopted recommendation set forth by the American Cancer Society on initiation and frequency of Pap smear. New recommendations for 2009 include **initiating Pap smear screening at age 21, regardless of onset of sexual activity. Routine screening intervals have also been extended to every 2 years for women in their 20s and every 3 years in women over 30 who have had three consecutive normal Pap smears.** The rationale is that ICC is rare in women under 21. The evidence for increasing the interval is based on studies which suggested no statistical difference between annual surveillance and 2- to 3-year intervals. More frequent surveillance is recommended for patients with known immunosuppression from HIV or organ transplantation, women exposed to diethylstilbestrol in utero, or those who have been previously treated for CIN 2, CIN 3, or cervical cancer. Pap smears are often obtained at the first prenatal visit by many providers, but the **guidelines for nonpregnant women can be followed in pregnant women** (7). There is no difference in unsatisfactory rates, cytology classifications, and accuracy between conventional and liquid-based cervical cytology (13).

Consultations Required

Consultation with gynecologic oncologists is recommended in cases of cervical cancer (14). Consultation should occur as early as possible after the diagnosis of cervical cancer for better therapeutic planning.

Natural History/Prenatal Care/Pregnancy Course

As in nonpregnant women, **women with abnormal Pap smears during pregnancy should undergo colposcopy with directed biopsies** of suspicious areas to rule out invasive disease. While necessary colposcopically directed cervical biopsies can be safely performed at any time during pregnancy, many defer biopsy until the second trimester when the risk of incidental pregnancy loss is minimal. Due to risks of bleeding and premature rupture of membranes, ECC is generally not recommended in pregnancy.

Termination Issues

Once the diagnosis of cervical cancer is established, individualized recommendations for the management of the malignancy as well as the pregnancy are formulated with consideration for the stage of disease, gestational age at the time of diagnosis, and maternal desires regarding the continuation of her pregnancy (see chap. 41 in *Maternal-Fetal Evidence Based Guidelines*).

Therapy

There are **no randomized trials** assessing any aspect of management of abnormal Pap smear in pregnancy. Most of the recommendations are based on expert opinion and anecdotal experience (15,16). **The only diagnosis that is considered to alter management in pregnancy is invasive cancer.** Management of abnormal Pap smears in pregnancy should follow the recommendations delineated in Figure 31.1.

Recommendations for **colposcopy** in pregnant patients are similar to those in the nongravid state, with certain

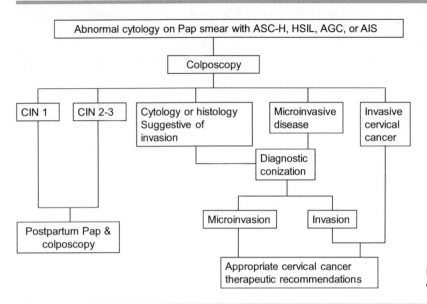

Figure 31.1 Algorithm for the workup of abnormal cytology in pregnancy. See text for abbreviations.

Table 31.1 Cervical Screening Considerations During Pregnancy

- Endocervical brush cytology is safe.
- Cervical biopsy is safe.
- Endocervical curettage (ECC) should be avoided.
- For ASC and LSIL, colposcopy is preferred but can be done postpartum.
- For CIN 2 or CIN 3, Pap and colposcopy can be repeated postpartum if cancer is not suspected.
- Delay treatment of any level of CIN until postpartum period.
- Cervical conization is recommended if invasion is suspected.

See text for abbreviations.

Table 31.2 Indications for Conization in Pregnancy

- Histologic presence of microinvasive or invasive disease
- Persistent cytologic impression of invasive cancer (in absence of histologic confirmation)
- Histologic presence of adenocarcinoma in situ

exceptions as listed in Table 31.1. Newer guidelines for colposcopy in pregnancy state that colposcopy is preferred for ASC-US associated with positive HR HPV type or LSIL Pap smears, but also that colposcopy can be deferred by the clinician until after pregnancy for these two categories. Colposcopy during pregnancy has as its **primary goal to assess for invasive cancer**. It is reasonable to follow expectantly cytology results that are not associated with cancer, such as ASC and LSIL, normal Pap but absence of endocervical cells, or colposcopic impression of CIN I (12) during pregnancy, with just postpartum follow-up. Biopsy proven or colposcopic impressions of CIN 2 or CIN 3 can be followed by repeat Pap and colposcopy at 6 weeks postpartum. Repeat Pap and colposcopy are acceptable if invasive cancer is suspected but not yet proven.

Endocervical sampling is **not performed** in pregnancy.

Cervical biopsy(ies) may be omitted with ASC and LSIL, with colposcopic evaluation either during pregnancy or 6 to 12 weeks postpartum (12,17). Biopsies should be performed for women with colposcopic impression of **CIN 3, AIS, or cancer**, with the purpose to exclude invasive cancer.

Cervical conization in pregnancy is primarily utilized as a diagnostic measure with **limited indications** (Table 31.2). Unlike standard recommendations for cervical conization in nonobstetrical patients with inadequate colposcopies or discordance between Pap smears and colposcopic biopsies, pregnant women with these findings can defer further examination until after pregnancy if invasive cancer has been ruled out.

In general, diagnostic conization during pregnancy should only be considered **when either the biopsy or cytology is suggestive of invasive cancer** and the diagnosis of invasion would result in a modification of treatment recommendations, timing, or mode of delivery.

For staging and management please refer to Table 31.3 and chapter 41 in *Maternal-Fetal Evidence Based Guidelines* (18). If a microinvasive (stage IA1) or a nonvisible invasive lesion (stage IA2) is identified, either the abdominal or vaginal route of delivery is acceptable, dependent upon obstetrical and gynecologic circumstances. If the histologic diagnosis of ICC is made and a grossly visible lesion is detected, cesarean delivery with radical hysterectomy is indicated and results in better survival outcomes as well as a decreased risk of obstetrical bleeding in the intrapartum and postpartum periods. More studies involving fertility-sparing cancer surgery (radical trachelectomy vs. hysterectomy) with neoadjuvant chemotherapy have shown promising results regarding improved fetal outcomes with maternal benefits (19).

Recurrence and Follow-Up Treatment

Seventy-five percent of patients with CIN diagnosed during pregnancy have persistent or progressive disease at postpartum evaluation (20). A regression rate of only 12% is found in pregnant women with CIN III, emphasizing the importance of **reevaluation 6 weeks postpartum** (12,21).

Routine surveillance can be resumed if there is no recurrence after the first year.

This is established by two Pap smears at 6-month intervals or HPV testing at 1-year intervals. Postpregnancy surveillance intervals are modified if the Pap smear or colposcopic biopsies reveal CIN 2, CIN 3, or CIS, and are the same as the nonpregnant guidelines (12).

Table 31.3 Staging and Management of Cervical Cancer in Pregnancy

Stage 0	Carcinoma in situ		**Preinvasive** disease—not treated in pregnancy
Stage I	The tumor is confined to the cervix.		
	IA	Microinvasive disease, with the lesion not grossly visible: no deeper than 5 mm and no wider than 7 mm	**Microinvasive cervical cancer** (MCC)—not treated during pregnancy
		IA1 invasion <3 mm and no wider than 7 mm	
		IA2 invasion >3 mm but <5 mm and no wider than 7 mm	
	IB	Larger tumor than in IA or grossly visible, confined to cervix	Histologically confirmed, **invasive cervical cancer (ICC)** is the only indication to treat during pregnancy.
		IB1 Clinical lesion <4 cm	
		IB2 Clinical lesion >4 cm	
Stage II	Extends beyond the cervix but does not involve the pelvic side wall or lowest third of the vagina		
	IIA	Involvement of the upper two-third of vagina, without lateral extension into the parametrium	
	IIB	Lateral extension into parametrial tissue	
Stage III	Involves the lowest third of the vagina or pelvic side wall, or causes hydronephrosis		
	IIIA	Involvement of the lowest third of the vagina	
	IIIB	Involvement of pelvic side wall or hydronephrosis	
Stage IV	Extensive local infiltration or has spread to a distant site		
	IVA	Involvement of bladder or rectal mucosa	
	IVB	Distant metastases	

Prevention

HPV-16 vaccine reduces the incidence of both HPV-16 infection and HPV-16-related CIN (22). The quadrivalent vaccine is currently most recommended (23) (see chap. 38 in *Maternal-Fetal Evidence Based Guidelines*).

REFERENCES

1. National Cancer Institute Workshop. The 1988 Bethesda System for reporting cervical/vaginal cytological diagnoses. JAMA 1989; 262:931. [Review, guideline]
2. Solomon D, Davey D, Kurman R, et al. The 2001 Bethesda system: terminology for reporting results of cervical cytology. JAMA 2002; 287:2114. [Review, guideline]
3. Benard VB, Eheman CR, Lawson HW, et al. Cervical screening in the National Breast and Cervical Cancer Early Detection Program, 1995-2001. Obstet Gynecol 2004; 103:564. [II-3]
4. Insinga RP, Glass AG, Rush BB. Diagnosis and outcomes in cervical cancer screening: a population-based study. Am J Obstet Gynecol 2004; 191:105–113. [II-3]
5. Hunter MI, Krishnansu T, Bradley JM. Cervical neoplasia in pregnancy. Part 2: current treatment of invasive disease. Am J Obstet Gynecol 2008; 199:10–18. [Review]
6. Lu DW, Pirog EC, Zhu X, et al. Prevalence and typing of HPV DNA in atypical squamous cells in pregnant women. Acta Cytol 2003; 47(6):1008–1016. [II-3]
7. ACOG Committee on Practice Bulletins—Gynecology. ACOG Practice Bulletin No. 109: Cervical cytology screening. Obstet Gynecol 2009; 114(6):1409–1420. [Review]
8. Ransdell JS, Davey DD, Zaleski S. Clinicopathologic correlation of the unsatisfactory Papanicolaou smear. Cancer 1997; 81:139. [II-3]
9. Davey DD, Austin RM, Birdsong G, et al. ASCCP patient management guidelines: Pap test specimen adequacy and quality indicators. J Lower Genital Tract Dis 2002; 6:195. [Guideline]
10. Bosch FX, Manos MM, Munoz N, et al. Prevalence of human papillomavirus in cervical cancer: a worldwide perspective. International Biological Study on Cervical Cancer (IBSCC) Study group. J Natl Cancer Inst 1995; 87:796. [II-3]
11. American College of Obstetricians and Gynecologists. ACOG Practice Bulletin No. 99: Management of abnormal cervical cytology and histology. Obstet Gynecol 2008; 112(6):1419–1444. [Review]
12. Burger EA, Kornør H, Klemp M, et al. HPV nRMA tests for the detection of cervical intraepithelial neoplasia: a systematic review. Gynecol Oncol 2011; 120(3):430–438; [Epub December 4, 2010]. [Review]
13. Davey E, Barratt A, Irwig L, et al. Effect of study design and quality on unsatisfactory rates, cytology classifications, and accuracy in liquid-based versus conventional cervical cytology: a systematic review. Lancet 2006; 367:122–132. [Meta-analysis]
14. ACOG Committee on Obstetric Practice. ACOG Committee Opinion No. 284, August, 2003: nonobstetric surgery in pregnancy. Obstet Gynecol 2003; 102(2):431. [Review]
15. Hunter MI, Krishnansu T, Bradley JM. Cervical neoplasia in pregnancy. Part 1: screening and management of preinvasive disease. Am J Obstet Gynecol 2008; 199:3–9. [Review]
16. Massad SL, Wright TC, Cox TJ, et al. Managing abnormal cytology results in pregnancy. J Lower Genital Tract Dis 2005; 9(3):146–148. [III]
17. Wright JD, Pinto AB, Powell MA, et al. Atypical squamous cells of undetermined significance in girls and women. Obstet Gynecol 2004; 103:632. [II-3]
18. Wright TC Jr., Massad LS, Dunton CJ, et al. 2006 consensus guidelines for the management of women with abnormal cervical cancer screening tests. 2006 American Society for Colposcopy and Cervical Pathology–sponsored Consensus Conference. Am J Obstet Gynecol 2007; 197:346–355. [Level III]
19. Gien LT, Covens A. Fertility-sparing options for early stage cervical cancer. Gynecol Oncol 2010; 117(2):350–357; [Epub February 16, 2010]. [Review]
20. Palle C, Bangsball S, Andreasson B. Cervical intraepithelial neoplasia in pregnancy. Acta Obstet Gynecol Scand 2000; 79:306–310. [II-3]
21. Coppola A, Sorosky J, Casper R, et al. The clinical course of cervical carcinoma in situ diagnosed during pregnancy. Acta Obstet Gynecol Scand 1997; 67:162–165. [II-3]
22. Koutsky LA, Ault KA, Wheeler CM, et al. A controlled trial of a human papillomavirus type 16 vaccine. N Engl J Med 2002; 347:1645–1651. [RCT, $n = 2392$]
23. Markowitz LE, Dunne EF, Saraiya M, et al.; Centers for Disease Control and Prevention; Advisory Committee on Immunization Practices (ACIP). Quadrivalent Human Papillomavirus Vaccine. Recommendations of the Advisory Committee on Immunization Practices (ACIP). MMWR Recomm Rep 2007; 56(RR-2):1–32. [Guideline]

Index

Page numbers followed by *f* and *t* indicate figure and table respectively.